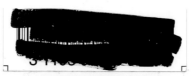

Promoting the Oral Health of Children

2ª edition

Promoting the Oral Health of Children

2ª edition

Aubrey Sheiham

Samuel Moysés

Richard G Watt

Marcelo Bönecker

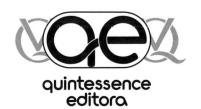

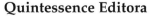

Quintessence Editora

Sao Paulo, Berlin, Chicago, Tokyo, Barcelon, Bucharest, Istanbul, London, Milan, Moscow, Now Delhi, Paris, Beijing, Prague, Riyadh, Seoul, Singapore, Warsaw e Zagreb

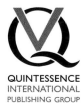

QUINTESSENCE
INTERNATIONAL
PUBLISHING GROUP

Title:	Promoting the Oral Health of Children
Authors:	Aubrey Sheiham
	Samuel Moysés
	Richard G Watt
	Marcelo Bönecker
Translation:	Nicola Jean Shellard
Diagramming:	Luiz Felipe May dos Santos
	Vannier Soares Carvalho
Design and Cover:	Gilberto R. Salomão

© 2014 Quintessence Editora Ltda
Quintessenz Verlags-GmbH, Berlin
Quintessence Publishing Co, Inc

1ª edition, 2006
2ª edition, 2014

Dados Internacionais de Catalogação na Publicação (CIP)
(Câmara Brasileira do Livro, SP, Brasil)

Promoting the oral health of children / Aubrey Sheiham...[et al.] ; [traduzido por Nicola Jean Shellard]. -- 2. ed. -- São Paulo : Quintessence Editora, 2014.

Outros autores: Samuel Moysés, Richard G. Waltt, Marcelo Bönecker
Título original: Promoting the oral health of children.
Bibliografia
ISBN 978-85-7889-037-7

1. Materiais dentários 2. Odontologia 3. Odontologia - Aspectos estéticos 4. Odontologia - Congressos 5. Prótese dentária - Periódicos 6. Tecnologia odontológica - Periódicos I. Sheiham, Aubrey. II. Moysés, Samuel. III. Watt, Richard G.. IV. Bönecker, Marcelo.

14-08996

CDD-617.6
NLM-WU 100

Índices para catálogo sistemático:
1. Odontologia : Ciências médicas 617.6

Quintessence Publishing Co Inc
4350 Chandler Drive
Hanover Park, IL 60133
www.quintpub.com

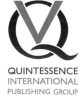

QUINTESSENCE
INTERNATIONAL
PUBLISHING GROUP

Authors

Claides Abegg

- Associate Professor. Department of Community Dentistry, Federal University of Rio Grande do Sul (UFRGS), Brazil.

Jun Aida

- Associate professor. Department of International and Community Oral Health, Tohoku University Graduate School of Dentistry, Miyagi, Japan.

Saeed Alzahrani

- Assistant Professor. Department of Public Health, College of Medicine, Imam University, Saudi Arabia.

Thiago Machado Ardenghi

- Associate Professor. Department of Stomatology, Federal University of Santa Maria (Santa Maria-RS, Brazil.

Vibeke Baelum

- Professor. Section for Oral Epidemiology & Public Health, Department of Dentistry, Health, Aarhus University, Denmark.

Marcelo Bönecker

- Professor in Paediatric Dentistry. Department of Orthodontics and Paediatric Dentistry, University of Sao Paulo (USP), Brazil.

Maria Ilma Cortes

- Associate Professor. Department of Restorative Dentistry, School of Dentistry, Federal University of Minas Gerais. Associate Professor of Department of Dentistry, Pontifical Catholic University of Minas Gerais, Brazil.

Jaime Aparecido Cury

- Professor. Piracicaba Dental School, UNICAMP, Brazil

Ruth Freeman

- Professor. Dental Health Services Research Unit, Dundee Dental School, University of Dundee, Scotland.

Maria do Carmo Matias Freire

- Associate Professor. Department of Dental Public Health. Federal University of Goias (UFG), Brazil.

Sabrina Susan Fuller

- Head of Health Improvement, NHS England, Manchester, England. Specialist in Dental Public Health. Honorary Lecturer in Oral Health Promotion, University of Manchester, England

Lisa Gibbs

- Associate Director, Jack Brockhoff Child Health and Wellbeing Program, University of Melbourne, Australia.

Paulo Goes

- Associate Professor Department of Preventive Dentistry, Federal University Pernambuco (UFPE), Brazil.

Wagner Marcenes

- Professor of Oral Epidemiology Institute of Dentistry, Barts and The London School of Medicine & Dentistry, University of London. England.

Valeria Coelho Catão Marinho

- Senior Lecturer. Institute of Dentistry, Queen Mary University of London, UK.
- Editor of the Cochrane Oral Health Group.

Bella Elizabeth Monse

- Director of the Regional Fit for School Program (Philippines, Cambodia, Indonesia and Lao PDR). Deutsche Geselschaft fur Internationale Zusammenarbeit (GIZ) Gmbh (German Development Cooperation), Manila Office, Philippines.

Samuel Jorge Moysés

- Professor. Department of Epidemiology and Public Health - School of Health and Bioscience, Pontifical Catholic University of Paraná. Professor. Department of Epidemiology and Public Health, Federal University Parana (UFPR) Brazil.

Simone Tetu Moysés

- Professor. Department of Epidemiology and Public Health, School of Health and Bioscience, Pontifical Catholic University of Paraná, Brazil. Member of the Board of the Technical Group of Health Promotion and Integrated and Sustainable Local Development, Brazilian Association of Collective Health, ABRASCO.

Jonathon Timothy Newton

- Professor of Psychology as Applied to Dentistry, Unit of Social and Behavioural Sciences, Dental Institute, King's College London.

Richard Niederman

- Professor and Chair, Department of Epidemiology and Health Promotion
- Director Center for Evidence-Based Dentistry College of Dentistry, New York University. USA.

Saul Martins Paiva

- Professor. Department of Paediatric Dentistry and Orthodontics, School of Dentistry, Federal University of Minas Gerais (UFMG), Brazil.

Marco Aurélio Peres

- Professor of Population Oral Health, School of Dentistry. Director of the Australian Research Centre for Population Oral Health, School of Dentistry, The University of Adelaide, Adelaide, Australia.

Isabela Almeida Pordeus

- Professor. Department of Paediatric Dentistry and Orthodontics Dental School. Federal University of Minas Gerais, Brazil.

Cecile Soriano Rodrigues

- Associate Professor. Department of Community Dentistry. University of Pernambuco (UPE), Brazil.

John Rogers

- Principal Population Oral Health Advisor. Manager Oral Health Promotion.
- Department of Health, Victoria, Australia

Julie Satur

- Associate Professor. Melbourne Dental School, University of Melbourne, Melbourne, Australia.

Andrea De Silva-Sanigorski

- Associate Professor. Population Oral Health Research Unit, Dental Health Services Victoria, Australia. Melbourne School of Population and Global Health, University of Melbourne, Australia.

Aubrey Sheiham

- Emeritus Professor of Dental Public Health. Department of Epidemiology and Public Health, University College London, London.

John Spencer

- Emeritus Professor, Australian Research Centre for Population Oral Health. The University of Adelaide

Livia Maria Andaló Tenuta

- Associate Professor of Biochemistry and Cariology. Piracicaba Dental School, UNI-CAMP, Brazil

William Murray Thomson

- Professor of Dental Epidemiology and Public Health. Sir John Walsh Research Institute, School of Dentistry, The University of Otago, Dunedin, New Zealand.

Georgios Tsakos

- Senior Lecturer in Dental Public Health. Department of Epidemiology and Public Health, University College London, England.

Jefferson Traebert

- Professor of Epidemiology and Vice-Chair of the Post-Graduation Programme in Health Sciences. School of Medicine and Post-Graduation Programme in Health Sciences, University of Southern Santa Catarina, Brazil.

Mario Vianna Vettore

- Lecturer in Dental Public Health. Unit of Dental Public Health, School of Clinical Dentistry, University of Sheffield, England.

Elizabeth Waters

- Jack Brockhoff Professor of Child Public Health. Jack Brockhoff Child Health & Wellbeing Program. The Melbourne School of Population & Global Health. The University of Melbourne. Australia.

Richard G. Watt

- Professor of Dental Public Health and Head of Department. Research Department of Epidemiology and Public Health, University College London, London.

Preface

In many economically rich countries child oral health dramatically improved across the first four decades following WW2, but then improvements stalled, or have even marginally reversed. It is as though the application of existing knowledge about the use of fluorides at a population-level and oral hygiene measures and clinical preventive dentistry at an individual-level have largely been exhausted. At the same time countries with developing economies have generally seen deteriorating child oral health as the growth in the availability of refined carbohydrates has outpaced growth in dental resources and efforts to implement approaches that initially served developed countries well. This situation calls for a serious examination of what is new and different that can be brought to bear once again to improving child oral health across the World.

Improvements in child oral health are required for two straightforward reasons. First, oral diseases in children, predominantly dental caries, cause infection, discomfort, pain and suffering for the child, and impacts on the family through occasionally distressing symptoms and the burden of costly and sometimes difficult treatment. Dental caries remains one of the most common reasons for children's hospitalization in economically rich countries, creating a risk of complications and a substantial healthcare cost. In countries with developing economies where dental services are severely rationed, dental caries can progress to advanced stages with infection of deeper tissues and possible severe adverse sequela. Second, experience of poor oral health early in life is the strongest predictor of further oral disease and the mutilation of the adult dentition when the technical resources of the dental profession are scarce or largely beyond the reach of people.

As a result, it is timely to examine a broad array of approaches, their detail and implications for intervening to improve child oral health. Two strands are relevant. There is an opportunity to improve the provision of individual-level prevention, ranging from what is practised in the home to what services are provided in dental practices. These domains need to be driven more by evidence than enthusiasm. There needs to be a clear understanding of what works and why, then a considered implementation. Too many common practices are without supportive evidence and too many efficacious practices are not widely practised.

However there is also a growing understanding of the wider determinants of child oral health, operating in a linked and interdependent way across individual-, family-, school- and community-levels. These determinants are actively shaping child oral health at each stage of development. Oral health has borrowed from the wider health field a number of concepts that are helpful in building the intellectual foundations for this expanded understanding of child oral health: a life-course approach; social determinants; common risk factors; health promotion; evidence-based practices; integrated primary care.

In this book each of these concepts has been described and then considered in their applicability to child oral health. The concepts provide the grounding for changes in how child oral health is viewed and how existing interventions might be better shaped and delivered and new interventions developed and pursued. There is an emphasis on improving the effectiveness of downstream clinical preventive services and self-care. However, more importantly there is the addition of many upstream contextual factors and mid-stream psychological or behavioural factors at the community-, family and child-level, that are positioned in the chain of 'causes of the causes' that offer great scope for new activities.

The identification of the numerous factors and the relation between them at an individual-, family-, school- and community-level poses both difficulties and opportunities for activities to improve child oral health and reduce social inequalities in child oral health. The critical understanding and skills needed to implement and evaluate the activities that might be pursued are the focus of this book. The understanding required is new to many in dentistry who were educated in a biological model of oral disease and in clinical interventions that are implemented at the individual-level and best evaluated in randomized clinical trials. Instead, social models of oral health and disease with points of intervention at multiple levels are presented which would be usually evaluated in non-randomized community-level research. This shift in focus is a large step for many in dentistry, but one which this book makes quite possible.

The contributors to this book are a mix of the leading international academics in the field of 'population oral health' and numerous academics out of Brazil, an emerging powerhouse of population oral health research. They provide informative, interesting and useful perspectives on the determinants of child oral health and how to improve child oral health. The book, and especially individual chapters, will be useful to academics, graduate students and critical thinking dental practitioners who want to explore the 'new public health'.

There is something in this book for every reader. The opportunity exists for some selectivity in the concepts explored and activities pursued. The existence of a number of factors at a single level actually creates a smorgasbord from which to choose. At present there is insufficient experience to know what works best beyond the population activity of fluoridation (water, salt or milk). Therefore, activities need to be developed and evaluated to help build the evidence-base to inform all involved. Such evaluation needs to be conducted under a set of criteria on the quality of the largely non-randomized, population-level research involved.

There is a compelling argument to give early priority to activities to improve child oral health that seem more universal, i.e., reach large numbers of children, are more passive, i.e., require little individual effort to change behaviours, and are more proportionate, i.e., benefit most those with the greatest burden of oral disease. Certainly these characteristics need to be purposefully examined when developing activities and evaluating their outcomes. It is applying the understanding of what shapes child oral health detailed in this book that will help dentistry move from preaching to informing about what is effective, efficient and equitable in further improving child oral health to all involved.

John Spencer
Emeritus Professor
Australian Research Centre for Population Oral Health
The University of Adelaide.

Contents

Introduction

Aubrey Sheiham
Samuel Moysés
Richard G Watt
Marcelo Bönecker

Oral health is an essential component of good health, and good oral health is a fundamental human right. The provision of high quality evidence-based treatment and care is the primary function of the dental profession. In addition, dentists and their team members have an important role to play in the prevention of oral diseases and the promotion of oral health and general health. Traditionally, the approach to oral health has overwhelmingly focused on treatment more than on disease prevention and oral health promotion. The prevention of oral diseases and promotion of oral health has received relatively little attention, in terms of resources, research and teaching. The education and dental payment systems in most countries focus on treatment of dental problems. This approach however has limitations. It is becoming increasingly recognised that treatment services alone will never successfully tackle oral health problems of the population. Even in very rich countries with highly developed dental services and large numbers of dental personnel, oral health problems are frequent and there are marked inequalities in oral health. Dental treatment does not cure oral diseases. No dentist or dental care system can treat away oral diseases. Moreover, it is apparent that despite the fact that there are effective methods of preventing dental caries and periodontal disease, very few of the methods are effectively implemented. There is an unacceptable gap between what is known about prevention and what is carried out by dentists.[1] A treatment dominated approach not viable in most countries and particularly in developing countries where more than 90% of dental caries remains untreated. Yet, most developing countries have adopted the relatively ineffective methods used in developed countries to improve oral health for their communities. In low income countries the cost to restore one tooth per the child in low-income nations would cost between $US1618 and $US3513 per 1000 children of mixed ages from 6 to 18 years. That exceeds the available resources for the provision of an essential public health care package for the children of many low-income countries.[2]

The time is now right for developing a new model for oral health care, which considers oral health as an integral part of general health and addresses the needs and demands of populations. Greater recognition is therefore now being placed on effectively promoting oral health. Preventive interventions, as with modern treatments, need to be developed based upon current sound scientific knowledge. There is growing evidence worldwide of the benefits and effectiveness of investing in health promotion programs, through an integrated approach. Integrated health promotion programs deliver benefits for the community through promoting positive wellbeing, strengthening community capacity and minimizing the burden of serious diseases, such as diabetes and cardiovascular disease. A health promotion approach moves health from an individual lifestyle/choice model to a broad community issue. Health is created where people live, love, work and play. Therefore a public health promotion strategy starts from settings of everyday life within which health is promoted, rather with disease categories, and with strengthening the health potential of the respective settings. Because, to change behaviours one needs to change the environment that predisposed people to health compromising behaviours. That is why the Ottawa Charter[3,4] suggests that concern for social and physical environments supportive of health is pivotal to improving health. A re-orientation from prescription to health promotion, should redress the balance of influence and make healthier choices easier, facilitate decision-making skills rather than be prescriptive. It includes combatting the influences of those interests which produce and profit from ill health. That involves controls on industry sponsored educational materials in schools, advertising, and campaigns to reduce barriers and enable and empower people.

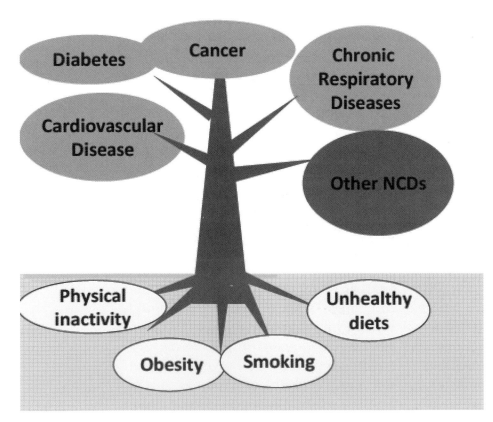

Fig. 1 – Common risk factors for Non-communicable disease.[5]

There is a growing realization that oral health is an integral part of overall health, and shares many common risk factors with leading chronic diseases, commonly referred to as non-communicable disease (NCDs) because there are associations between oral disease and major NCDs (Fig. 1).[5] This realization led the WHO to re-orient its Global Oral Health Programme to foster its integration with chronic disease prevention and general health promotion.[6] The World Health Assembly's resolution on "Oral health: action plan for promotion and integrated disease prevention"[6] urged Member States to adopt measures "to ensure that oral health is incorporated as appropriate into policies for the integrated prevention and treatment of chronic non-communicable disease and communicable disease, and into maternal and child health policies".[6] That reorientation lead to a High-level Meeting of the General Assembly of the United Nations on the Prevention and Control of Non-communicable Diseases, whose final statement recognizes that: "Renal, oral and eye diseases pose a major health burden for many countries and that these diseases have common risk factors and can benefit from common responses to non-communicable diseases".[7] The High-level Meeting on Prevention and Control of Noncommunicable Disease concluded with a political declaration that commits governments of theworld to significant and sustained action to address the rising burden of noncommunicable diseases (NCDs) such as diabetes, cancer, cardiovascular and respiratory diseases, with oral diseases as an integral part. The Declaration calls for integrated and cross-sectoral approaches to tackle noncommunicable diseases – an approach highly appropriate for most oral diseases. It is appropriate because the risk factors for oral diseases are common to other major chronic diseases. Therefore using the Common Risk Factor Approach (CRFA)[8,9] will become mainstream for all health sectors.

This introduction to this book on a public health approach to prevention of oral diseases and promotion of oral health of children will highlight the limitations of traditional approaches to prevention and outline the principles of oral health promotion as health promotion is a more effective means of promoting oral health and reducing inequalities for child populations everywhere.

The traditional preventive approach

In dentistry, preventive activities have followed a very clinical dental practice based model. In this approach clinical preventive agents such as topical fluorides and fissure sealants are used in conjunction with chair side educational counselling. This approach, often referred to as the "medical model" relies on the expertise, skill and philosophy of the dentist. The patient is required to comply with the dentists' instructions. Regular dental attendance is considered an essential requirement to secure good oral health. The educational component focuses primarily on developing the patients' oral health knowledge based on the belief that this will lead to changes in the their oral hygiene and dietary behaviours. That erroneous educational approach, known as the KAB approach where Knowledge (K) is considered to lead to Attitude (A) change and that is considered to lead to Behaviour (B) change, does not change behaviours in the long term. Such an educational approach to prevention has been applied to both individual chair side and school based programmes and has been the dominant style of preventive action in dentistry. As chapters in this book will demonstrate, such approaches have been relatively unsuccessful in preventing oral diseases and promoting oral health. The measrues are relatively ineffective because the conditions, the determinants, which promoted the health compromising behaviours are not changed. The question that needs addressing is 'What good does it do to treat people's illnesses without changing the conditions that made them ill? (Fig. 2).

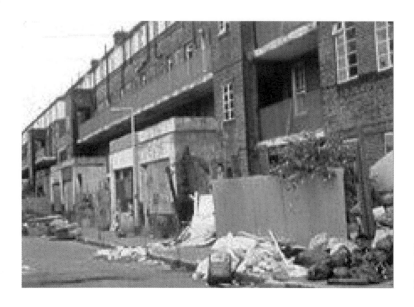

Fig. 2 – What good does it do to treat people's illnesses without changing the conditions that made them ill?

A critique of oral health approaches to prevention

The limitations of most current approaches to improve oral health and reduce inequities in oral health is cogently summed up by Kwan and Petersen[10] of the WHO. They concluded that "Measures that focus on downstream factors only, such as lifestyle and behavioural influences, may have limited success in reducing oral health inequities. ... Such approaches may be counterproductive; they are often ineffective and costly and fail to address the wider social determinants that cause people to get ill in the first place. ... Approaches that take into account the principles of the common risk factor approach, which promotes coordinated work across a range of disciplines, and the Ottawa Charter for Health Promotion, may be promising."

The principal shortcomings of current approaches to prevention and to reducing inequalities in oral health is the failure of dental practitioners and policy-makers to collaborate with groups involved in implementing policies on the determinants of health that are common to most noncommunicable diseases. Policies should therefore be based on the Common Risk Factor Approach to preventing noncommunicable diseases (NCDs). These common risk factors can be altered as they relate to dietary habits, use of tobacco and excessive consumption of alcohol, and standards of hygiene. Moreover, dentists continue to use dental education approaches that have been shown to be ineffective. Their failure to recognize that what they are doing is ineffective, would be considered unethical practice if the information on ineffectiveness was applied to a clinical intervention. Another shortcoming is the gap between what is known and not implemented by dental policy makers. That has been repeatedly emphasized by chief dental officers such as Professor Petersen, I lead of the Global Oral Health Programme at the World Health Organization. Petersen said "The major challenges of the future will be to translate knowledge and experiences of disease prevention and health promotion into action programmes." "Global health urgently needs to apply the body of evidence based policies, strategies and approaches of health promotion developed over the past twenty years."[11] Why is good evidence not being implemented by dentists in a systematic manner? This book therefore sets out to provide dentists and dental educators with a philosophy and the body of evidence on disease prevention and health promotion to promote oral health in patients and child populations.

Not only are there serious limitations associated with individual level risk factor intervention approaches to prevention commonly used by dentists but such approaches "... divert limited resources away from upstream healthy public policies; blame the victim; produce a lifestyle approach to health policy, instead of a social policy approach to healthy lifestyles; decontextualize risk behaviors and overlook the ways in which such behaviors are culturally generated and structurally maintained; seldom assess the relative contribution of non-modifiable genetic factors and modifiable social and behavioral factors; can actually be harmful to the health of the targeted populations".[12] "Most interventions (both at the individual and community levels) remain focused on "downstream" tertiary treatments or one-on-one interventions. These efforts have their origins in the biomedical paradigm and risk factor epidemiology and the behavioral science research methods that serve as their handmaidens."[12] That prevailing paradigm is currently being challenged because it does not work and is costly. We need to move beyond these "downstream" efforts towards a more appropriate whole population public health approach to health policy.[13]

There are three levels of public health interventions to improve health of the population; "Downstream efforts comprise treatments, rehabilitation counseling and patient education for those already experiencing some disease and disability. This is the level which, while consuming most of the available resources, encompasses a very small segment of the general population; Mid-stream prevention efforts to improve a population's health should involve two main areas A) secondary prevention efforts which attempt to modify the risk levels of those individuals and groups who are very likely to experience some untoward outcome; B) primary prevention actions to encourage people not to commence risky behaviors that may unnecessarily increase their changes of experiencing a negative health event; Even further upstream are healthy public policy interventions which include governmental, institutional, and organizational actions directed at entire populations which require adequate support through tax structures, legal constraints and reimbursement mechanisms for health promotion and primary prevention."[12]

So, instead of the individualized high-risk strategies, that are widely used by dentists, a rigorous exploration of the upstream determinants of the major decline in caries and periodontal disease would provide much information that can be applied to promoting oral health. It will also point to the greater importance of health and oral health promotion; a subject with a low priority in the education of dentists in dental schools and in dental policies.

The way forward is that policy makers and deans of dental schools need to address the imbalance of resources allocated to oral health promotion directed at the social determinants of risk factors common to a number of diseases, the Common Risk Factor Approach (CRFA), and to behavioural and political factors.[8,9] The WHO Commission on Social Determinants of Health[14] defines social determinants of health (SDH) as 'the structural determinants and conditions of daily life responsible for a major part of health inequities between and within countries'. Health determinants include 1. social and physical environment, individual behaviours, genetics and, 2. the health care system. Social Determinants of Health Inequalities (SDHI) combines the two concepts in order to emphasize the role of social and economic conditions in people's different rates of health and illness. "This link between social conditions and health is not a footnote to the 'real' concerns with health – health care and unhealthy behaviours – it should become the main focus."[15] The concept of 'social determinants of health' (SDH) has a dual meaning.[16,17] SDH refers both to the "social factors promoting and undermining the health of individuals and populations and to the social processes underlying the unequal distribution of these factors between groups occupying unequal positions in society. The central concept of 'social determinants' thus remains ambiguous, referring simultaneously to the determinants of health and to the determinants of inequalities in health." "But the evidence points to marked socioeconomic differences in access to material resources, health-promoting resources, and in exposure to risk factors. Furthermore, policies associated with positive trends in health determinants (e.g. a rise in living standards and a decline in smoking) have also been associated with persistent socioeconomic disparities in the distribution of these determinants (marked socioeconomic differences in living standards and smoking rates)".[16,17] The determinants of health and health inequalities - the "causes of the causes, are socially patterned and this patterning may pass from generation to generation.

Little attention is given to the causes of behaviours, the underlying social and environmental conditions that influence behaviours. Environmental conditions deserves much more attention. They should become the main focus.[15] When behaviours are addressed by dentists they are mainly in terms of problems of compliance; how to attract high-risk individuals to dental surgeries because the preventive measures dentists use demand regular reinforcement and lifelong attention and monitoring by professionals.

The gap between what is known and not implemented by dental policy makers

The gap between what is practiced by dentists worldwide and what is being widely discussed and implemented by other health disciplines to promote general health needs to be addressed as a matter of urgency. Petersen[11] has pointed out that the objectives of the WHO Global Oral Health Programme, is to place greater emphasis on developing global policies based on common risk factors approaches and which are coordinated more effectively with other programmes in public health because a core group of modifiable proximal and distal causes of oral disease are common to the major chronic diseases[8,9] Although evidence-based clinical care can reduce dental diseases and dental discomfort and retain a natural dentition for longer periods, the aggregate impact of these interventions is limited by lack of use of evidence –based approaches and to access to dental health care resources.

Most dental policies are dominated by concerns about access to dental services. They ignore the findings from the WHO/USPHS International Collaborative Study of Dental Manpower Systems in a range of countries with differing systems of dental care. The study found that availability and accessibility of the best dental care system did not reduce the incidence of disease or lead to a satisfactory level of oral health.[18] Yet, despite these findings from many diverse countries with differing systems of dental care, few policies were changed. There is something intrinsically wrong with an approach, such as the dominant one used by dentistry, that calls for regular annual treatment and re-education from infancy to old age. Not only does such a dental approach lead to unjustified policies to concentrate on improving access to services to improve oral health and reduce inequalities at considerable cost, but the ineffective approach is adopted

by developing countries, where its high cost makes even treatment to alleviate oral pain unavailable to the majority of people.

There has been dramatic reductions in the major oral disease, caries in the past four decades, and a sustained decrease in the second most important disease, periodontal disease, and a remarkable increase in the percentages of adults retaining their natural teeth for their lifetime. No other chronic disease has decreased in severity as dramatically as caries has in such a short time span. This improvement has come about as a result of changes in behaviours in populations together with an alteration in food manufacturing practices and the addition of fluoride to toothpaste. The common dental view, that modern dentistry can take much of the credit by having identified the causes and methods of prevention, is far from the truth. Yet, dental services explained only 3% of the variation in changes in 12-yearold caries levels in the 1970s and early 1980s whereas broad socioeconomic factors explained 65%.[19] The implication of these findings is that major improvements in the prevention of disease tend to follow social changes - alterations in dietary patterns and breastfeeding, smoking, oral cleanliness, contraception and in the availability of key preventive productssuch as fluoridated toothpaste. There is no reason why a similar approach, if applied more widely, should not prove equally successful in the future. The improvements in oral health demonstrate that the means for effectively controlling caries are known and widely used by populations. Declines in periodontal disease are most probably due to declines in smoking and availability of anti--calculus toothpastes.[20,21]

Public health approaches to disease prevention

What does a public health approach mean? Most health professionals work at an individual level providing clinical treatment and care to their patients. A minority of doctors, dentists and other health professionals operate at a community and population level. All health professionals however need to understand the relevance of a public health perspective in disease prevention. Table 1 lists a set of core public health principles relevant to prevention.

Oral diseases are important public health problems (Table 2). Although oral health improvements have taken place in recent years, oral diseases are prevalent and their impact on both society and the individual are significant. Pain, discomfort, sleepless nights and time off school are common problems for many children. The costs of treatment are high, although the causes of the diseases are known and are largely preventable. Indeed many middle class children now enjoy good oral health. Nevertheless, addressing social inequalities in oral health is a key challenge facing the dental profession.

Applying the criteria for a condition being a public health problem to oral health, it is apparent that oral diseases are a major public health problem (Table 3).

Table 1 – A public health agenda in prevention.

- Focuses action on public health problems using population rather than high-risk approaches
- Addresses the underlying 'causes of the causes' of disease in populations
- Aims to reduce health inequalities and promote equity
- Works in partnership with a range of agencies and sectors
- Utilises an evidence based approach to the design and evaluation of interventions
- Facilitates self care and autonomy amongst the population

Table 2 – Criteria for public health problem.

- High prevalence of condition. If not prevalent, then severe (eg. oral cancer)
- Impact of condition on individual is great (mortality, morbidity, impact on quality of life)
- Impact of condition on wider society (costs of treatment, time off school, lost productivity)
- The causes are known
- The condition is preventable.

Table 3 – Public health importance of Oral Diseases.

- Oral diseases are highly prevalent
- Impact on individuals and society is great. Dental pain and discomfort are common as are functional limitation and handicap. They affect the quality of life. The financial cost to individuals and the community is considerable. Dental diseases are more expensive to treat
- Causes are known – diet, dirt (plaque), smoking – the risk factors common to other non-communicable diseases.
- Preventable. There are simple and cheap public health methods available to prevent and control oral Diseases.

Limitations of conventional dental health education

In line with the evidence-based movement in medicine, the effectiveness of preventive interventions has been scrutinised to determine what interventions are effective and identify those that produce minimal benefit. The key features of current preventive approach is that it is:

- individualistic, 'top down',
- paternalistic and prescriptive,
- focuses on knowledge to change "lifestyle",
- uses threats and fear arousal,
- ignores broader context and it is theoretically flawed,
- it is ineffective in reducing inequalities,
- conventional dental health education fails to tackle causes of the causes,
- it is costly as needs high professional input,
- nonsustainable,
- duplicates effort,
- engenders public apathy and resistance (see Chapter 16).

A range of areas of prevention, including cessation of smoking, alcohol, injury, improving diet and nutrition and oral health have been subjected to effectiveness reviews. How effective have oral health interventions been in improving oral health? Since 1994 a series of reviews have attempted to answer this question. These effectiveness reviews will be discussed in Chapter 16. Overall, consistent results were identified by the reviewers (Table 4).

Publication of these reviews caused a good deal of debate and discussion within the international dental public health community. Some people concluded that the disappointing results indicated that oral health interventions were ineffective and a waste of resources. Others took a more constructive approach and identified that the majority of the interventions reviewed were in fact educational in nature and that other types of approaches needed to be implemented and fully evaluated.

The findings and conclusions of the oral health effectiveness reviews are consistent with the results of reviews in other areas of prevention. Clinical prevention and health education approaches alone have been found to be unsuccessful in achieving sustainable improvements in health. A conceptual movement away from the traditional biomedical downstream' and victim blaming approaches, to one addressing the 'upstream' underlying social determinants of oral health is necessary.

Table 4 – Common findings of effectiveness reviews.

- Many oral health education studies were poorly designed and lacked detailed evaluation
- Improving individuals' knowledge of oral health can be achieved in the short term but the effects on behaviour and clinical outcomes are very limited
- Provision of health information alone does not produce long term behaviour changes
- Interventions at an individual level are effective at reducing plaque levels only in the short term
- School based toothbrushing campaigns aimed at improving oral hygiene are largely ineffective
- Mass media campaigns are ineffective at promoting either knowledge or behaviour change
- Very few studies have assessed the effects of interventions on sugars consumption at an individual or population level

Thus, there is a need for more supportive rather than judgemental approaches to oral health behaviour change.[22] An important body of international evidence demonstrates the need for a radically different approach to disease prevention. Educational approaches alone have limited effects and may increase inequalities (see Chapter 16). The World Health Organisation and a range of government expert reports have identified a new way forward to promote health and well being. It is essential that those working in dentistry are not left behind but become actively involved in a range of exciting and innovative developments.

Because many policy analysts have recognized that health education is not the solution to the problem of how to promote oral health and improve the quality of lives of people, there has been a major shift in emphasis to health promotion.

Health Promotion – concepts and principles

The modern health promotion movement emerged out of the need for a fundamental change in strategy to improve health and reduce inequalities. Recognition and frustration with the limited improvements in health education interventions could achieve in isolation, led to a rediscovery of a public health approach to prevention. Health promotion focuses on the underlying determinants of health, on the upsteream social causes of ill health rather than a victim-blaming approach. Thereby acknowledging the limited real choices available to individuals. The strategy should incorporate general health strategies and tackle causes common to a number of chronic diseases.

The upstream-downstream allegory illustrates the present dominant approach point very clearly. A person was standing by the side of a river and heard a cry of a drowning person (Fig. 3). He jumped in to rescue him, pulled him to the bank and applied artificial respiration. Just as the rescued man was recovering there were more cries from other drowning people. The rescuer jumped in again and again and brought some back and resuscitated them. The rescuer could not cope on his own so he got some helpers and life support machines. Still he could not cope. So they worked faster in teams - four-handed and six-handed dentistry - with more complex equipment. The numbers of drowning people become so numerous that some could not be rescued before permanent damage to their bodies occurred. How could he stop them from drowning? The traditional approach is to teach people to swim. These rescuing and training activities kept the man so busy that at no time did he stop to consider why people who could not swim were in the river. Who was pushing them in upstream?[23,24] The dentist's concentration on 'downstream' victim-blaming distracts attention from the 'upstream' activities of the confectionery, food and drink and tobacco companies who are 'pushing people into the water'. Health workers usually intervene only after the damage has been done. Instead of concentrating so much effort on downstream and midstream activities, more efforts should be directed at making the river shallower sothat people do not have to learn to swim - making healthier choices the easier choices[25-27] - and controlling the activities of those pushing people into the water - a direct attack on the determinants of health.

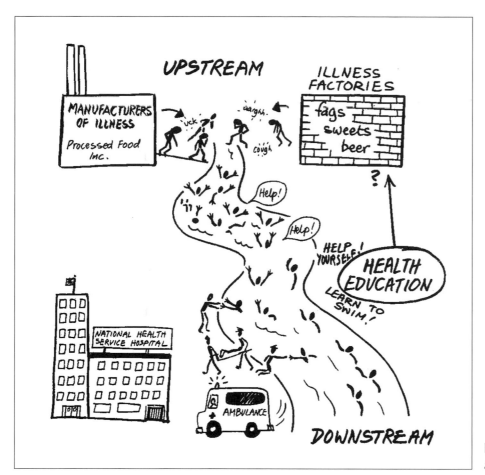

Fig. 3 – Upstream-downstream approaches to improving health.

The dental profession have largely concentrated their efforts on 'downstream' action when the damage has already been done. Some motivated members of the profession have tackled the midstream factors and have focused their efforts on developing educational action to promote better oral health. As mentioned above, these educational approaches are relatively ineffective in changing sustained health promoting behaviours. The effects if any, were short term. If they were more effective, why do they need to be repeated? If it did work, why is it necessary to repeat the instructions on how to brush so frequently? The answer is that chairside downstream or midstream dental health education is not very effective. What about 'upstream' action? Instead of concentrating so much time and effort on 'downstream and midstream' activities, more effort should be directed at making the "river shallower" – making the healthier choices the easier choices. Structural and environmental interventions are likely to affect the population more evenly than educational programs aimed at individual behaviour change and thereby have a greater potential to reduce health inequalities.[28] So it is more effective to change the environment than to try and change the individual behaviour by health education. Change the social determinants of health and there will be improvements in health behaviours, in health and in health equity.

The modern health promotion movement is a fundamental change in strategy to achieve and maintain health. It recognizes that health is more than a matter of personal choice. The decisions people make about health or are health related are shaped by the environment in which they are raised as children and live their adult lives. The movement is based on a public health philosophy that encompasses the prevention of disease at a primary care level, and secondly the promotion of health using public health approaches.[25] These concepts, when applied to developing environments which promote healthier choices for people in their everyday lives, needs to be adopted in a manner that encourages the health promoting choices to be the easiest choices.

In 1978, the 1978 WHO-UNICEF Alma-Ata Declaration set the visionary goal of "Health for All" (HFA).[29] The Alma-Ata declaration emerged as a major milestone of the 20th century in the field of public health, emphasizing the need for broad intersectoral collaboration between governments to protect and promote the health of all people of the world. During that conference, health was defined as a state of complete physical, mental and social wellbeing, and not merely the absence of disease or infirmity, and was prominently affirmed as a fundamental human right. It was also pointed out that primary health care (PHC) was the way to attain the goal of HFA, namely to maintain a level of health to permit people to lead socially and economically productive lives. The spirit of the Alma-Ata Declaration was carried forward in 1986 during the first international conference on health promotion, widely known as the Ottawa Charter for health promotion. The Ottawa Charter states that improvement

in health requires a secure foundation in basic conditions and resources, including peace, shelter, education, food, income, stable ecosystem, sustainable resources, social justice and equity. The Ottawa Charter for health promotion has three basic prerequisites:

- To advocate health as a resource for development. WHO defined advocacy for health as the "combination of individual and social actions designed to gain political commitment, policy support, social acceptance and systems support for a particular health goal or programme".[30]
- To enable health equity so as individuals become able to reach the highest attainable quality of life.
- To mediate that the success of health promotion is dependent upon the collaboration between the health sector and other governmental sectors and independent organizations, such as the media and industry.

Delegates at Ottawa declared that policies by all sectors, such as finance, education, industry, agriculture should consider health when developing all their policies. Five priority policies are needed to improve public health of individuals and societies;

- Build healthy public policy.
- Create supportive environments,
- Strengthen community action,
- Develop personal skills, and
- Reorient health services.

The declaration of Ottawa Charter on health promotion has been significantly expanded during future conferences. The first update occurred in 1988 with the Adelaide conference on public health policies.[31] The Adelaide declaration was followed by the Sundsvall conference on supportive environments for health in 1991,[31] the Jakarta declaration on leading health promotion into the 21st century, held in 1997,[31] and the Bangkok 2005 Charter for health promotion in a globalised world.[31] Overall, these conferences emphasized that health promotion must be placed among WHO's main commitments because it represents one of the most viable processes to ensure equitable health development.

By definition, health promotion is the process of enabling individuals to increase control over their health and improve it. Health promotion focuses on achieving equity in health. Its actions aim at reducing differences in current health status and ensuring equal opportunities for all people to achieve their highest health potential.[32] The advocacy for health through health promotion should not be just the responsibility of the health sector, but should go beyond healthy lifestyles to achieve good health and well-being for everyone through coordinated actions conducted by governments, social and economic sectors, voluntary organizations, local authorities, industry and media.[33]

Definitions of health promotion

"Health promotion goes beyond health care. It puts health on the agenda of policy makers in all sectors and at all levels, directing them to be aware of the health consequences of their decisions and to accept their responsibilities for health. Health promotion policy combines diverse but complementary approaches including legislation, fiscal measures, taxation and organizational change. It is coordinated action that leads to health, income and social policies that foster greater equity. Joint action contributes to ensuring safer and healthier goods and services, healthier public services and cleaner, more enjoyable environments. Health promotion policy requires the identification of obstacles to the adoption of healthy public policies in non-health sectors and ways of removing them. The aim must be to make the healthier choice the easier choice for policy makers as well."[4]

There are many definitions of health promotion. Health promotion can be considered `as the combination of educational and environmental supports for actions and conditions of living conducive to health'.[34] Strategies to change the range of options available to people and to make health-promoting choices easier and/or to diminish health damaging options by making them more difficult to choose.[26-28] Health promotion is described by the World Health Organization as "the science and art of helping people change their lifestyle to move toward a state of optimal health." Health promotion is the process of enabling people to increase control over, and to improve, their health. It is a positive concept emphasising personal, social, political and institutional resources, as well as physical capacities.[35] Health promotion is any combination of health, education, economic, political, spiritual or organisational initiative designed to bring about positive attitudinal, behavioural, social or environmental changes conducive to improving the health of populations. It is directed towards action on the determinants or causes of health. Therefore it requires a close co-operation of sectors beyond health services, reflecting the diversity of conditions which influence health.

The following World Health Organisation definition has been widely adopted.

"Health promotion is the process of enabling individuals and communities to increase control over the determinants of health and thereby improve their health. Health promotion represents a mediating strategy between people and their environment, combining personal choice and social responsibility for health to create a healthier future."[35]

The Bangkok Charter for Health Promotion in a Globalized World added the following to that definition. "It is a core function of public health and contributes to the work of tackling communicable and noncommunicable diseases and other threats to health."

Health promotion was considered to:
- involve the population as a whole in the context of everyday lives,
- be directed towards action on the determinants of health, the causes of the casuses,
- combine diverse but complementary methods or approaches,
- aim for effective and concrete public participation,
- involve health professionals, mainly as advocates.

Some of the critical factors that now influence health include: increasing inequalities within and between countries, new patterns of consumption and communication, the nutrition transition, commercialization and the market society, global environmental change, and increasing rates of urbanization. Other factors that influence health include rapid and often adverse social, economic and demographic changes that affect working conditions, learning environments, family patterns, and the culture and social fabric of communities. Women and men are affected differently. The vulnerability of children and exclusion of marginalized, disabled and indigenous peoples have increased.[36]

The Ottawa Charter for Health Promotion[4] and subsequent charters have emphasized the importance of policy for health, healthy environments, healthy

lifestyles and the need for orientation of health services towards health promotion and disease prevention.

"In tackling the determinants of health, health promotion will include both actions directed towards changing determinants within more immediate control of individuals, including individual health behaviours, and those factors largely outside the control of individual, including social, economic, and environmental conditions. Thus, actions which support healthy lifestyles and create supportive environments for health are valued outcomes to health promotion." **"Health promotion policy combines diverse but complimentary approaches including legislation, fiscal measures, taxation and organizational change. It is coordinated action that leads to health, income and social policy that foster greater equity. Joint action contributes to ensuring safer and healthier goods and services, healthier public services, and cleaner, more enjoyable environments."[4]

The 6th Global Conference on Health Promotion, Bangkok, Thailand, 2005 and The Bangkok Charter recognized that the global context for health promotion has changed markedly since the development of the Ottawa Charter. The Bangkok Charter for Health Promotion spelt out four new commitments in a Globalized World:
- to make the promotion of health central to the global development agenda,
- a core responsibility for all of government,
- a key focus of communities and civil society,
- a requirement for good corporate practices.

In addition to advocacy for health based on health rights and solidarity, the Bangkok Charter urges all sectors and settings to:

- invest in sustainable policies, actions and infrastructure;
- to build capacity to promote health;
- to regulate, including through legislation, for a high level of protection against harm; and
- to build alliances with public and other sectors.

The Bangkok Charter also calls for more conscientious effort to sustain the effectiveness of health promotion by developing benchmarks for monitoring and plans for implementation of a worldwide partnership to fulfill its four commitments.[37]

Why consider policy as a health promotion strategy?

As a strategy for health promotion, a policy should serve one of the following purposes:

- make healthy choices easier;
- make unhealthy choices more difficult; and/or
- provide equitable access to the key determinants of health, such as income, education, housing, employment, clean air, nutritious food and a safe water supply.

Health promotion has shifted the focus from behavioural change at the individual level to health-oriented behaviour and other determinants such as a healthy diet, physical activity, personal hygiene, education for women and social connectedness, through the use of combinations of the five Ottawa Charter Action Areas and being directed to the underlying determinants as well as the immediate causes of health. If implemented well, policies addressing a health issue can have a profound impact on the health status of individuals and communities. For example, a 10% increase in the prices of cigarettes through taxation policies decreased consumption by 4% among adults and up to 14% among youth. A significant aspect of policy is that it is long lasting. This can be very important since people in positions of influence may change, but a policy is harder and slower to change. Similarly, educational programs may be short lived if funding for these initiatives is withdrawn. Accordingly, it is very important to consider policy as a way of sustaining change over time.

Principles of health promotion

The six key principles of health promotion outlined by WHO are:

- Health promotion involves the population as a whole in the context of their everyday life, rather than focusing on people at risk from specific diseases.
- Government at both local and national levels has a unique responsibility to act appropriately and in a timely way to ensure that the 'total' environment, which is beyond the control of individuals and groups, is conducive to health.
- Health promotion is directed towards action on the determinants or cause of health. This requires a close co-operation between sectors beyond health care reflecting the diversity of conditions which influence health.
- Health promotion combines diverse, but complementary methods or approaches including communication, education, legislation, fiscal measures, organisational change, community change, community development and spontaneous local activities against health hazards.

- Health promotion aims particularly at effective and concrete public participation. This requires the further development of problem-defining and decision-making life skills, both individually and collectively, and the promotion of effective participation mechanisms.
- Health promotion is primarily a societal and political venture and not medical service, although health professionals have an important role in advocating and enabling health promotion.

The Strategies and Practices of Health Promotion

There are a number of approaches used in the promotion of health. These approaches are necessary to enhance the health of communities. The main strategies and practices of health promotion include:

- Awareness raising – Increasing the public and individual's knowledge of the issue, usually through media campaigns and publications e.g. speed awareness.
- Regulation and policies – Passing laws and developing policies to prevent health endangering practices, for example, pesticides in food), and to promote good health (for example, seat belt legislation, smoke free areas).
- Education – Equipping people of all ages with the knowledge and skills necessary to look after their own health and the health of others e.g. learning about disease transmission; skills in food purchase and preparation; skills in stress management; learning to drive a car safely.
- Advocacy – Enabling individuals and groups to lobby for changes which prevent ill health and promote opportunities for health to be advanced, for example lobbying for non-smoking work environments, vehicle safety.
- Mediation – Facilitating the balance between groups with differing interests in the pursuit of health, e.g. between the proponents of processed food and unprocessed food.
- Resources and services – The development of appropriate resources and services which enable people to access information and facilities which will enhance their health, for example, electronic and print material to support drug management, telephone advisory services.

When it comes to devising health promotion and health education programmes, dentists should take into account all of the processes involved. Planning, implementation and evaluation are all essential components of health promotion programmes (Fig. 4). The planning and implementation stages of any health-related programme are vital for ensuring successful outcomes. Effective planning and implementation allows dentists to look ahead towards the most appropriate evaluation activity.

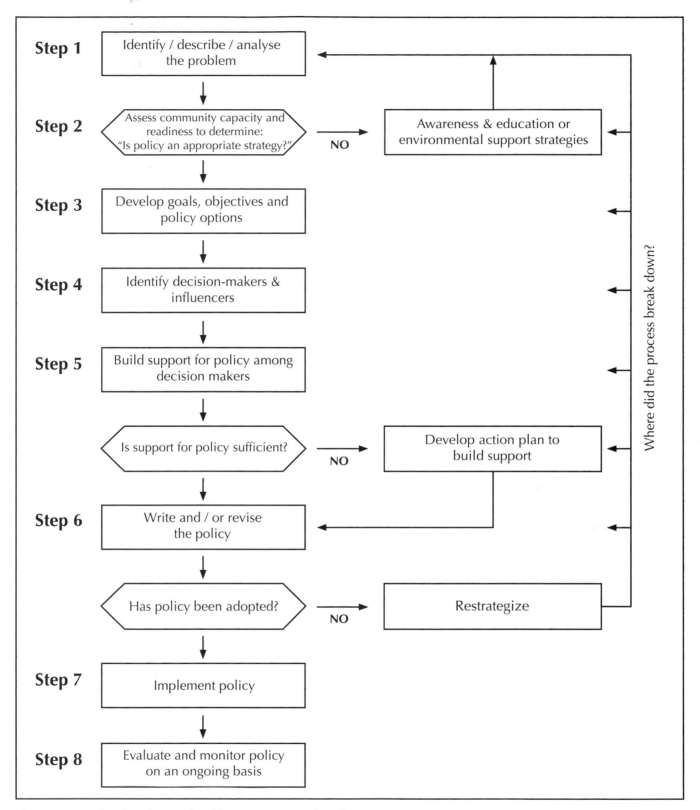

Fig. 4 – Steps for developing health promotion policy.[38]

What is evaluation as applied to health promotion practice?

The health promotion community have been able to identify a number of common elements about what constitutes evidence. They have also identified what is meant by effectiveness. Nutbeam[39] argued that "effective health promotion leads to changes in the determinants of health". There are many determinants of health. Some are within an individual's capacity to change, e.g. behaviour, use of facilities. Many, such as creating improved environmental, economic and social conditions, are outside individual control. Addressing these involves collective actions. Different groups and individuals place different levels of importance on what should be measured. They also often have different interpretations as to what the evidence means. Nutbeam[39] developed a framework to assist funders, policy makers, practitioners, researchers and target populations to better understand the variety of outcomes from a health promotion activity. Many different evaluation methods and approaches are needed to assess the effectiveness of health promotion activities (see Chapter 20). Health and Social Outcomes are the end point of the actions. Intermediate Health Outcomes are the actual determinants of the Health and Social Outcomes which are amenable to modification. Health Promotion Outcomes 'represent those personal, social and structural factors that can be modified in order to change the determinants of health'. Health Promotion Actions are the activities occurring in health promotion which are designed to produce certain health promotion outcomes, which modify the determinants of health to produce the required health and social outcomes.

Successful health promotion interventions are based on a thorough interrogation of the evidence from epidemiological, behavioural and social research are theoretically based according to the type of intervention create the conditions for successful implementation of the program; need to be of an appropriate size, of reasonable duration (3+years) and complexity to be able to have a chance of success and to be amenable to evaluation.[39-41]

Health promotion evaluation is a planned and continuous process that is carried out with regard to stated health criteria that may involve measurement. Tones and Tilford[42,43] state that it is a process that is primarily concerned with assessing health related activity against values and goals in such a way that the results contribute to future decision-making. Health promotion evaluation is viewed as a research approach in its own right that involves assessing the capacity and/or performance of an intended action for health improvement, in terms of its effectiveness and efficiency.[44,45] It is conducted for three overarching reasons: accountability, future programme development and knowledge-building.

Downie et al.[46] suggest that there are essentially two main types of evaluation in health promotion. First, there is evaluation that involves assessing an activity in terms of specific aims or objectives (outcome assessment/evaluation). Essentially, this refers to the measurement of 'what has been achieved' and necessitates that the researcher refers back to the original programme objectives. The second evaluation approach is concerned with measuring an activity against a standard that may or may not be related to the specific objectives of the activity (process assessment/evaluation). This approach focuses more on 'how the intervention has been achieved'. Process assessment therefore may not necessarily consider only the success rates of health promotion programmes, but also the processes of how this is achieved, how it is measured and at what cost. It is primarily directed at resources and procedures. When process and outcome evaluation are combined, the evaluation focuses on monitoring the process of change that occurs as the result of a health intervention as well as the factors that facilitate or prevent desired changes.[45,47]

What are the causes of the causes of dental diseases?

Traditionally dental health education interventions have sought to alter behaviours and lifestyles that are seen to be the cause of dental problems. Programmes therefore focus on oral hygiene skills, changing inappropriate dietary patterns and encouraging frequent dental attendance. However this narrow and very often 'victim blaming' approach fails to recognise the mounting evidence highlighting the importance of, what is termed the social determinants of health. The causes of the causes. Social conditions and structure are the true aetiological agents in most chronic diseases. Therefore health promotion is directed at the underlying determinants, the causes of the causes.

Health status and behaviours are determined above all by social conditions.

People's behaviour and health bears the imprints of what positions they occupied and currently occupy in the social hierarchy. Poor early social conditions "cast long shadows" over health in later adult life.[48] Children living in low SES conditions may "produce a negative behavioural and psychosocial health dividend to be reaped in the future."[49] Adverse social conditions and negative life events become literally biologically embodied. Health related behaviours are an expression of the circumstances that condition and constrain people's behaviours. People respond to psychological stress and adverse social circumstances by smoking, excessive alcohol consumption, comfort eating and risk taking.[50]

The effects of the social environment on health behaviours are related to how individuals of different socioeconomic statuses with varying personal propensities, vulnerabilities and capabilities interact with each other and with others, and their social and economic environments. The resultant patterns of health related behaviours are related to personal vulnerabilities and capabilities, and control over resources and access to information. The clustering of behaviours can therefore be viewed as the way in which social groups "translate their objective situation into patterns of behaviour".[51] Indeed the propensity for risk behaviours to cluster in certain groups, indicates that behaviours are determined by social environments and conditions in which people live (see Chapters 3 and 8).[52] Clustering of social conditions are important in shaping individual health behaviours encompassed in the CRFA because resources shape access to health relevant circumstances.[53]

An Integrated Common Risk Factor Approach

One of the major criticisms of traditional dental health education has been the narrow, isolated and compartmentalised approach, essentially separating the mouth from the rest of the body. All too often programmes have been developed in isolation from other health promoting activities. This non-integrated approach can lead to a duplication of effort but often results in conflicting and contradictory messages being delivered to the public. The common risk factor approach recognises that the chronic conditions which are the major public health problems across the globe such as heart disease, stroke, cancers, diabetes, mental illness and oral diseases share a set of common risks (Fig. 6). An inadequate diet, smoking, poor hygiene, stress and trauma are factors linked to the development of several chronic conditions including oral diseases.[9] The key concept of the integrated common risk approach is that by directing action on these common risks and their underlying social determinants, improvements in a range of chronic conditions will be achieved more efficiently and with greater effectiveness. The common risk factor approach provides a rationale for integrated working, a key principle of health promotion practice. Namely, making alliances and partnerships and integrating evidence based approaches.

The Common Risk Factor Approach (CRFA) is the core concept that will be used throughout this book because it is so fundamental to effective oral health promotion. The key concept underlying the integrated common risk approach is that promoting general and oral health by controlling a small number of important risk factors, may have a major impact on a large number of diseases at a lower cost, greater efficiency and effectiveness than disease specific approaches.[8,9] Governments and important decision-makers and individuals will be more readily influenced by measures directed at preventing heart diseases, obesity, stroke, cancers, diabetes than they will by disease-specific measures to, for example, only prevent dental caries or periodontal disease than are made alone. Using a CRFA will not only reduce heart disease and obesity and all the chronic non-communicable diseases, but should also lead to a reduction in most oral diseases.

The common risk factor approach has influenced the integration of oral health into general health improvement strategies. Unfortunately, dental policy makers and oral health promoters have interpreted the CRFA too narrowly. They focused mainly on the common behavioural risks, rather than on the broader shared social determinants of chronic diseases. As mentioned earlier in this chapter, a behavioural preventive approach alone will have minimal impact in promoting sustained improvements in health and tackling oral health inequalities. Based upon recent WHO policy recommendations, the CRFA has been updated in accordance with the social determinants agenda (see Chapter 7).[9]

A Lifecourse approach to health promotion

Epidemiologists have concluded that social factors have profound influences on health and behaviour. The economic and social conditions - the social determinants of health - under which individuals live their lives have a cumulative effect upon the probability of developing any number of diseases. Children are particularly sensitive to social determinants. For much of the 20th century, adult chronic diseases such as heart disease, obesity, diabetes and cancer were regarded mainly as products of adult behaviour and lifestyles. Consequently, most health promotion strategies are mainly based on modifying health related behaviours of adults. However, an extensive body of evidence now links adult chronic disease to processes and experiences occurring in childhood. Social environmental influences early in life continue to exert effects on health into mid-life and beyond. So behavioural factors are influenced by social and material conditions experienced by children at sensitive periods of their development. Adverse early social exposures become programmed into biological systems, setting off chains of risk that can result in chronic illness in mid-life and beyond (see Chapter 1). When exposures occur during sensitive periods of development, their effects can become permanently incorporated into regulatory physiological processes. Based on the abovementioned concepts positive health promoting influences in children can set in motion a positive and health-affirming cycle, leading to more optimal health trajectories. Health trajectories apply to dental diseases such as caries as well as a number of chronic conditions and indicate that social conditions in childhood are embodied in the person and affect caries rates in later life. The phenomenon is known as 'tracking' because an individual or group with a particular level of caries follow a 'track' allowing their caries level at a later age to be predicted from their earlier level. Groups with a particular severity level of caries at 6 years of age would follow a 'channel' or track representing their dental caries increment. The groups with the higher severity level at 6 years of age would follow a higher 'channel' or track representing the higher dental caries increment.[54] This tracking feature of caries highlights the importance of implementing oral health promotion directed at children at sensitive developmental periods using life course concepts. Adopting a life-course perspective directs attention to how social determinants of health operate at every level of development — early childhood, childhood, adolescence, and adulthood — to both immediately influence health as well as provide the basis for health or illness during later stages of the life course.

Partnership working

Many dentists may feel very uncertain and anxious how they can become involved in health promotion practice which seems so far removed from clinical dentistry. How can dentists change the living conditions of the most vulnerable children in society? How can clinicians take on the power of multi-national companies? The answer to these questions is quite simply that dentists alone cannot expect to achieve meaningful results in promoting oral health. However when effective partnerships are formed with a range of relevant and influential groups then results can indeed be achieved. The challenge is to place oral health issues onto the broader agenda. A collection of different partners have a direct influence on oral health (Table 5).

Table 5 – Potential partners in oral health promotion.

Other health professionals: doctors, pharmacists, nurses, community health workers
Education services: head teachers, education planners, teachers, support staff
Local government services: planning departments, social workers, catering services, local politicians
Voluntary sector: community groups, religious groups
Industry and commerce: food retailers, advertisers, water industry, drug companies.
National government: education department, agriculture, trade.

Traditionally dentists have been trained in isolation from other health professionals. The knowledge and skills required to work in a collaborative manner are not covered in most under graduate dental curriculae. How can this style of working be facilitated? Partnership working needs to satisfy three basic points:

• Demonstrating relevance and importance
• Acknowledging common agendas for change and shared goals
• Offering unique expertise, contacts and skills

Oral diseases are rarely fatal conditions and to many may seem rather unimportant and peripheral. Socio-dental research has however highlighted the wide range of impacts oral conditions can have on both individual quality of life and at a societal level. For example, pain, discomfort, sleepless nights and time off school are all effects of oral diseases on children's quality of life. Lost productivity due to time off work attending dental services and economic costs to the health services of providing dental services are examples of society wide impacts. Many groups in society can be persuaded of the importance of oral health when meaningful and relevant impacts are demonstrated.

As outlined above, the common risk factor approach provides a rational agenda for setting shared goals with other sectors and agencies. For example, diets high in sugar are not only linked to the development of dental caries but also have an effect on obesity and nutrient depletion. The World Health Organisation has recommended that sugars should be reduced to a maximum of 10% of energy intake or 60 g/day/person.[55] Essentially oral health should be considered an integral part of general health and action focused on common risks and conditions.

What expertise and skills can dentists offer other groups? This clearly depends on many diverse factors but often public health dentists may already have established good working relationships with sectors such as the local education service. Oral health epidemiological data on children is often more readily available than other health data. As a consequence oral health population based data can be used as an indicator of general health status and as a marker for health inequalities. Another potential unique feature is the fact that unlike most other health services, young people often attend dental services on a regular basis. This provides an opportunity of working with young people directly and assessing more clearly their needs and concerns.

From prescription to participation

Rather than adopting the conventional 'top down' approach in which professionals control decisions and dictate action to the community, effective health promotion requires professionals to work with members of the community in a participative manner. A 'bottom up' approach aims to share control and facilitate joint decision-making. This approach respects the expertise and knowledge nonprofessionals have and aims to harness collective skills for the benefit of promoting better health and achieving sustainable improvements.

Working with the community takes time, resources and appropriate skills. In addition identifying relevant and appropriate community representatives requires knowledge of the local community groups and organisations. In parts of Brasil community representation and involvement in social and health policy has developed much further than in many other parts of the world. This provides a valuable resource in health promotion action.

Complementary actions to improve oral health

A key finding from the oral health promotion effectiveness reviews was recognition of the limitations of health education as the sole means of promoting oral health and reducing inequalities. Increasing individual's knowledge is one element of improving oral health. However a change in knowledge does not lead automatically to any sustained alteration in behaviour. Indeed improved oral health knowledge may be of limited value for those who live in an environment where positive oral health choices are not available. In these circumstances other strategies will be required. A shift in emphasis is needed away from a sole reliance on educational actions to one in which a range of complementary strategies can be implemented appropriate to the needs and circumstances of the target population.

It is important to consider the set of guiding principles for effective action outlined at the first international health promotion conference in Ottawa. The Ottawa Charter provides a radical agenda for change and is frequently used as a framework to guide good practice. In many countries dental professionals are using these principles to inform the development of oral health strategies. As mentioned earlier, the Ottawa Charter outlines five key areas of health promotion action. As they are so important they are repeated here.

- Promoting health through public policy: by focusing attention on health of public policies from all sectors, and not just the health sector
- Creating supportive environments: by assessing the impact of the environment and clarifying opportunities to make changes conducive to health
- Developing personal skills: by moving beyond the transmission of information, to promote understanding, and to support the development of personal, social and political skills which enable individuals to take action to promote their health
- Strengthening community action: by supporting concrete and effective community action in defining priorities, making decisions, planning strategies and implementing them to achieve better health.
- Reorienting health services: by refocusing attention away from the responsibility to provide curative and clinical services towards the goal of achieving health gain

Role of dental profession in oral health promotion

An important question to consider is what is the role of the dental profession in oral health promotion? For the majority of clinical dentists their active role may be limited. Their major function is the provision of high quality clinical care and reinforcing the health promoting messages based on sound scientific evidence. However, every clinician has an ethical and professional responsibility to focus on the preventive needs of their patients. To undertake this role effectively requires an understanding of the principles of health promotion. In particular, recognition of the over-riding influence of the social determinants on individual behaviours is critical. Clinicians need to adopt an understanding and supportive manner with their patients who are attempting to change their oral health behaviours.

Public health dentists in contrast, have a key role to play in health promotion as advocates of oral health gain. The significant role as health advocates involves educating and influencing decision makers, including senior government officers, national and international agencies, community leaders, and the public. A wealth of opportunities exist within the field of health promotion for those public health dentists willing to engage in a different style of working. Rather than being the professional expert in a hierarchical organisation, health promotion work will often involve being a partner in a team. Public health dentists can become advocates for public health policy development to create a more enabling supportive social environment for oral health. These actions often start at a very local level working within antenatal clinics, nurseries, schools, colleges and community centres. In addition, lobbying and putting pressure on decision makers and politicians for change at local, regional and a national level is an essential role of advocates for health.

Roles of advocates for health

- The role of advocacy should be the cornerstone of dentists activities in the framework of NCDs and the social determinants of health.
- Advocacy involves implementing well planned interventions outside the health sector and considering ways to create and enhance links between different sectors.
- Advocacy also involves informing and educating government and community leaders and decision makers about specific issues that will have an impact on the oral health and well being. This includes influencing the food industry and to changing tobacco control policies.

Dental academics within universities also have an important role to play in oral health promotion. As previously highlighted, there is a need to implement, evaluate and then publish the findings of different types of oral health promotion interventions. They should t ensure that all that is taught is based on sound scientific evidence Researchers may be able to support practitioners in the appropriate design and evaluation of interventions. Publication of different approaches in oral health promotion is essential to guide good practice and innovation.

Conclusions

To improve the oral health of children and reduce inequalities requires a public health approach. Conventional dental health education and preventive activities will have a minimal effect and may increase inequalities across society. A health promotion agenda which seeks to tackle the underlying causes of poor oral health amongst children using a range of complementary actions provides the best way forward. The success of this approach depends upon establishing good working partnerships with the relevant agencies and sectors across society. A central pillar of any oral health promotion policy policy is to address risk factors and their social determinants integrated with approaches directed at all chronic non-communicable diseases (NCDs) thereby preventing and controlling many chronic health conditions, including oral diseases. In addition it is essential that the population are involved in all stages of action.

The causes of inequalities in health and oral health are due to the structural determinants and conditions of daily life and poor social policies and programs which emanate from the failure to address these social determinants of health. If widespread improvements in the health of societies are to be achieved then all sectors of society must become engaged, and not just the health sector. This principle has fundamental implications for the promotion of oral health and reduction in oral health inequalities. It points to the need to ensure that oral health promotion and disease prevention are incorporated more widely into the policies of ministries beyond those which carry the health portfolio.

The chapters in this book will provide detailed insights into the issues raised in this introductory chapter. Public health approaches to the prevention and measurement of dental caries, periodontal diseases and trauma, will be outlined. Using the Ottawa Charter as a framework, oral health initiatives in creating supportive environments, developing personal skills, building healthy public policies, strengthening community action and re-orientating health services will be presented.

Case Study 2 – Upstream-downstream approaches

A woman was standing by the side of a river enjoying the fine view when she heard a cry of a drowning person. Immediately she jumped in to rescue him, pulled him to the bank and applied artificial respiration. Just as the rescued man was recovering there were more cries from other drowning people in the river. In jumped the rescuer, brought more back and resuscitated them one by one. Exhausted by the numerous cries for help, she then enlisted the help of some helpers and resuscitation equipment. Still she could not cope with the increasing numbers of people in need. The teams worked faster and brought more advanced equipment. However the numbers of drowning people became so numerous that some could not be saved. How could she stop them drowning? Someone suggested swimming lessons were the solution. Midstream swimming lessons were then organised for those in the water. Different educational techniques were used but still more and more people kept flowing down the river crying for help. These rescuing and training activities kept everyone so busy that at no time did anyone stop to consider why people who could not swim were in the river in the first place. Who or what was pushing them in upstream?

Discussion point:
(i) What factors 'upstream' create poor oral health?
(ii) Outline actions that could be implemented 'upstream' to promote and maintain oral health?

Case Study 2 – An example of oral health promotion practice.

Case study 2

Dr Isabela Da Silva has worked for 20 years as a public health dentist. Her main area of interest has been focusing on the oral health needs of pre-school children in her local area. She spends two days providing clinical care and the rest of her time is devoted to oral health promotion activities.

Ten years ago a group of local nurses, doctors, pharmacists and dentists formed a community health action group. Isabela has been an active member of this group and has become involved in the development of food policies in nurseries and schools across her city. Through this work the nutritional status of children has improved greatly. Another initiative has been her involvement in a citywide injury prevention programme. This has involved working with the local government and planning authorities to improve the design and safety of public areas, including playgrounds and leisure facilities.

Three years ago Isabela was invited onto the local parents community group to represent oral health issues. This group was formed by anxious parents concerned about their children's poor education and health status. The group have successfully lobbied the education authority for improvements in the resources directed towards pre-school groups. Isabela has also been involved in advocating a shift to prescribing and selling sugar free medicines within local pharmacists and clinics. She worked with some interested hospital paediatricians on developing a policy on sugar free medicines in the main teaching hospital in her city.

Discussion points:

(i) What types of skills would Isabela require to be effective in the above activities?

(ii) In what ways could she evaluate her work?

Appendix

Glossary of Terms used in Health Promotion

Because it is important to be precise about what terms one uses when describing health promotion activities the WHO developed a glossary of terms. These are quoted verbatim here;
(See: Health Promotion Glossary.[35]
http://www.who.int/healthpromotion/about/HPR%20Glossary%201998.pdf)

Health promotion – Health promotion is the process of enabling people to increase control over, and to improve their health. Ottawa Charter for Health Promotion. (WHO, Geneva, 1986). Health promotion represents a comprehensive social and political process, it not only embraces actions directed at strengthening the skills and capabilities of individuals, but also action directed towards changing social, environmental and economic conditions so as to alleviate their impact on public and individual health. Health promotion is the process of enabling people to increase control over the determinants of health and thereby improve their health. Participation is essential to sustain health promotion action.

The Ottawa Charter identifies three basic strategies for health promotion. These are advocacy for health to create the essential conditions for health indicated above; enabling all people to achieve their full health potential; and mediating between the different interests in society in the pursuit of health. These strategies are supported by five priority action areas as outlined in the Ottawa Charter for health promotion:

- Build healthy public policy
- Create supportive environments for health
- Strengthen community action for health
- Develop personal skills, and
- Re-orient health services

The Jakarta Declaration on Leading Health Promotion into the 21st Century from July 1997 confirmed that these strategies and action areas are relevant for all countries. Furthermore, there is clear evidence that:

Comprehensive approaches to health development are the most effective. Those that use combinations of the five strategies are more effective than single-track approaches; Settings for health offer practical opportunities for the implementation of comprehensive strategies; Participation is essential to sustain efforts. People have to be at the centre of health promotion action and decision-making processes for them to be effective; Health literacy/ health learning fosters participation. Access to education and information is essential to achieving effective participation and the empowerment of people and communities. For health promotion in the 21st century the Jakarta Declaration identifies five priorities:

- Promote social responsibility for health
- Increase investments for health development
- Expand partnerships for health promotion
- Increase community capacity and empower the individual
- Secure an infrastructure for health promotion

Health for All – The attainment by all the people of the world of a level of health that will permit them to lead a socially and economically productive life. Health for All has served as an important focal point for health strategy for WHO and its Member States for almost twenty years. Although it has been interpreted differently by each country in the light of its social and economic characteristics, the health status and morbidity patterns of its population, and the state of development of its health system, it has provided an aspirational goal, based on the concept of equity in health. The Health for All strategy is currently being redeveloped to ensure its continued relevance into the next century. A new policy is being developed, to be adopted by the World Health Assembly in 1998.

Public health – The science and art of promoting health, preventing disease, and prolonging life through the organized efforts of society. Public health is a social and political concept aimed at the improving health, prolonging life and improving the quality of life among whole populations through health promotion, disease prevention and other forms of health intervention. A distinction has been made in the health promotion literature between public health and a new public health for the purposes of emphasizing significantly different approaches to the description and analysis of the determinants of health, and the methods of solving public health problems. This new public health is distinguished by its basis in a comprehensive understanding of the ways in which lifestyles and living conditions determine health status, and a recognition of the need to mobilize resources and make sound investments in policies, programmes and services which create, maintain and protect health by supporting healthy lifestyles and creating supportive environments for health. Such a distinction between the "old" and the "new" may not be necessary in the future as the mainstream concept of public health develops and expands.

Primary health care – As defined above will do much to address many of the pre-requisites for health indicated earlier. In addition, at a very practical level, there is great scope for both planned and opportunistic health promotion through the day to day contact between primary health care personnel and individuals in their community. Through health education with clients, and advocacy on behalf of their community, PHC personnel are well placed both to support individual needs and to influence the policies and programmes that affect the health of the community.

Disease prevention – Disease prevention covers measures not only to prevent the occurrence of disease, such as risk factor reduction, but also to arrest its progress and reduce its consequences once established. Primary prevention is directed towards preventing the initial occurrence of a disorder. Secondary and tertiary prevention seeks to arrest or retard existing disease and its effects through early detection and appropriate treatment; or to reduce the occurrence of relapses and the establishment of chronic conditions through, for example, effective rehabilitation. Disease prevention is sometimes used as a complementary term alongside health promotion. Although there is frequent overlap between the content and strategies, disease prevention is defined separately. Disease prevention in this context is considered to be action which usually emanates from the health sector, dealing with individuals and populations identified as exhibiting identifiable risk factors, often associated with different risk behaviours.

Health education – Health education comprises consciously constructed opportunities for learning involving some form of communication designed to improve health literacy, including improving knowledge, and developing life skills which are conducive to individual and community health. Health education is not only concerned with the communication of information, but also with fostering the motivation, skills and confidence (self-efficacy) necessary to take action to improve health. Health education includes the communication of information concerning the underlying social, economic and environmental conditions impacting on health, as well as individual risk factors and risk behaviours, and use of the health care system. Thus, health education may involve the communication of information, and development of skills which demonstrates the political feasibility and organizational possibilities of various forms of action to address social, economic and environmental determinants of health. In the past, health education was used as a term to encompass a wider range of actions including social mobilization and advocacy. These methods are now encompassed in the term health promotion, and a more narrow definition of health education is proposed here to emphasize the distinction.

Advocacy for health – A combination of individual and social actions designed to gain political commitment, policy support, social acceptance and systems support for a particular health goal or programme. Such action may be taken by and/or on behalf of individuals and groups to create living conditions which are conducive to health and the achievement of healthy lifestyles. Advocacy is one of the three major strategies for health promotion and can take many forms including the use of the mass media and multi-media, direct political lobbying, and community mobilization through, for example, coalitions of interest around defined issues. Health professionals have a major responsibility to act as advocates for health at all levels in society.

Alliance – An alliance for health promotion is a partnership between two or more parties that pursue a set of agreed upon goals in health promotion. Alliance building will often involve some form of mediation between the different partners in the definition of goals and ethical ground rules, joint action areas, and agreement on the form of cooperation which is reflected in the alliance.

Community action for health – Community action for health refers to collective efforts by communities which are directed towards increasing community control over the determinants of health, and thereby improving health. The Ottawa Charter emphasises the importance of concrete and effective community action in setting priorities for health, making decisions, planning strategies and implementing them to achieve better health. The concept of community empowerment is closely related to the Ottawa Charter definition of community action for health. In this concept an empowered community is one in which individuals and

organizations apply their skills and resources in collective efforts to address health priorities and meet their respective health needs. Through such participation, individuals and organizations within an empowered community provide social support for health, address conflicts within the community, and gain increased influence and control over the determinants of health in their community.

Determinants of health – The range of personal, social, economic and environmental factors which determine the health status of individuals or populations. The factors which influence health are multiple and interactive. Health promotion is fundamentally concerned with action and advocacy to address the full range of potentially modifiable determinants of health – not only those which are related to the actions of individuals, such as health behaviours and lifestyles, but also factors such as income and social status, education, employment and working conditions, access to appropriate health services, and the physical environments. These, in combination, create different living conditions which impact on health. Achieving change in these lifestyles and living conditions, which determine health status, are considered to be intermediate health outcomes.

Empowerment for health – In health promotion, empowerment is a process through which people gain greater control over decisions and actions affecting their health. Empowerment may be a social, cultural, psychological or political process through which individuals and social groups are able to express their needs, present their concerns, devise strategies for involvement in decision-making, and achieve political, social and cultural action to meet those needs. Through such a process people see a closer correspondence between their goals in life and a sense of how to achieve them, and a relationship between their efforts and life outcomes. Health promotion not only encompasses actions directed at strengthening the basic life skills and capacities of individuals, but also at influencing underlying social and economic conditions and physical environments which impact upon health. In this sense health promotion is directed at creating the conditions which offer a better chance of there being a relationship between the efforts of individuals and groups, and subsequent health outcomes in the way described above. A distinction is made between individual and community empowerment. Individual empowerment refers primarily to the individuals' ability to make decisions and have control over their personal life. Community empowerment involves individuals acting collectively to gain greater influence and control over the determinants of health and the quality of life in their community, and is an important goal in community action for health.

Enabling – In health promotion, enabling means taking action in partnership with individuals or groups to empower them, through the mobilization of human and material resources, to promote and protect their health. The emphasis in this definition on empowerment through partnership, and on the mobilization of resources draws attention to the important role of health workers and other health activists acting as a catalyst for health promotion action, for example by providing access to information on health, by facilitating skills

development, and supporting access to the political processes which shape public policies affecting health.

Equity in health – Equity means fairness. Equity in health means that people's needs guide the distribution of opportunities for well-being. The WHO global strategy of achieving Health for All is fundamentally directed towards achieving greater equity in health between and within populations, and between countries. This implies that all people have an equal opportunity to develop and maintain their health, through fair and just access to resources for health. Equity in health is not the same as equality in health status. Inequalities in health status between individuals and populations are inevitable consequences of genetic differences, of different social and economic conditions, or a result of personal lifestyle choices. Inequities occur as a consequence of differences in opportunity which result, for example in unequal access to health services, to nutritious food, adequate housing and so on. In such cases, inequalities in health status arise as a consequence of inequities in opportunities in life.

Health behaviour – Any activity undertaken by an individual, regardless of actual or perceived health status, for the purpose of promoting, protecting or maintaining health, whether or not such behaviour is objectively effective towards that end. It is possible to argue that almost every behaviour or activity by an individual has an impact on health status. In this context it is useful to distinguish between behaviours which are purposefully adopted to promote or protect health (as in the definition above), and those which may be adopted regardless of consequences to health. Health behaviours are distinguished from risk behaviours which are defined separately as behaviours associated with increased susceptibility to a specific cause of ill-health. Health behaviours and risk behaviours are often related in clusters in a more complex pattern of behaviours referred to as lifestyles.

***Health communication* –** Health communication is a key strategy to inform the public about health concerns and to maintain important health issues on the public agenda. The use of the mass and multi media and other technological innovations to disseminate useful health information to the public, increases awareness of specific aspects of individual and collective health as well as importance of health in development. Health communication is directed towards improving the health status of individuals and populations. Much of modern culture is transmitted by the mass and multi media which has both positive and negative implications for health. Research shows that theory-driven mediated health promotion programming can put health on the public agenda, reinforce health messages, stimulate people to seek further information, and in some instances, bring about sustained healthy lifestyles. Health communication encompasses several areas including edutainment or enter-education, health journalism, interpersonal communication, media advocacy, organizational communication, risk communication, social communication and social marketing. It can take many forms from mass and multi media communications to traditional and culture-specific communication such as story telling, puppet shows and songs. It may take the form of discreet health messages or be incorporated into existing media for communication such as soap operas. Advances in communication media, es-

pecially in the multi media and new information technology continue to improve access to health information. In this respect, health communication becomes an increasingly important element to achieving greater empowerment of individuals and communities.

***Health literacy* –** Health literacy represents the cognitive and social skills which determine the motivation and ability of individuals to gain access to, understand and use information in ways which promote and maintain good health. Health literacy implies the achievement of a level of knowledge, personal skills and confidence to take action to improve personal and community health by changing personal lifestyles and living conditions. Thus, health literacy means more than being able to read pamphlets and make appointments. By improving people's access to health information, and their capacity to use it effectively, health literacy is critical to empowerment. Health literacy is itself dependent upon more general levels of literacy. Poor literacy can affect people's health directly by limiting their personal, social and cultural development, as well as hindering the development of health literacy.

***Health promotion evaluation* –** Health promotion evaluation is an assessment of the extent to which health promotion actions achieve a "valued" outcome. The extent to which health promotion actions enable individuals or communities to exert control over their health represents a central element of health promotion evaluation. In many cases it is difficult to trace the pathway which links particular health promotion activities to health outcomes. This may be for a number of reasons, for example, because of the technical difficulties of isolating cause and effect in complex, "real-life" situations. Therefore, most recent outcome models in health promotion distinguish between different types of outcomes and suggest a hierarchy among them. Health promotion outcomes represent the first point of assessment and reflect modifications to those personal, social and environmental factors which are a means to improve people's control over their health. Changes in the determinants of health are defined as intermediate health outcomes. Changes in health status represent health outcomes. In most cases, there is also "value" placed on the process by which different outcomes are achieved. In terms of valued processes, evaluations of health promotion activities may be participatory, involving all those with a vested interest in the initiative; interdisciplinary, by involving a variety of disciplinary perspectives; integrated into all stages of the development and implementation of a health promotion initiative; and help build the capacity of individuals, communities, organizations and governments to address important health problems.

References

1. Sheiham A, Alexander D, Cohen L, Marinho V, Moysés S, Petersen PE, *et al.* (2011). IADR global oral health inequalities: implementation and delivery of oral health research and strategies. *Adv Dent Res.* 2011; 23(2):259-267.

2. Yee R, Sheiham A. The burden of restorative dental treatment for children in Third World Countries. International Dental J. 2002; 52:7-10.

3. WHO. World Health Organization. The Ottawa Charter for Health Promotion. Geneva: WHO; 1986 [Acessado em 12/09/2006]; Available from: Available at: https://www.who.int/healthpromotion/conferences/previous/ottawa/en/.

4. WHO. World Health Organization. Ottawa Charter for Health Promotion. Health Promotion. 1987; 1(4):iii-v.

5. Bovet P. Chronic diseases: structural prevention and health promotion. Swiss Public Health Conference. August 2011.

6. WHO. Sixtieth World Health Assembly. Oral health: action plan for promotion and integrated disease prevention. 2007. http://apps.who.int/gb/ebwha/pdf_files/WHA60/A60_16-en.pdf

7. UN. United Nations General Assembly. Political declaration of the High-level Meeting of the General Assembly on the Prevention and Control of Non-communicable Diseases. Resolution A/66/L1. 2011. http://www.un.org/en/ga/ncdmeeting2011/

8. Sheiham A, Watt R. The common risk factor approach - a rational basis for promoting oral health. Community Dent Oral Epidemiol. 2000; 28:399-406

9. Watt RG, Sheiham A. Integrating the common risk factor approach into a social determinants framework. Community Dent Oral Epidemiol. 2012; 40:289-296.

10. Kwan S, Petersen PE. Oral health: equity and social determinants. In: Equity, social determinants and public health programmes. Edited by Erik Blas and Anand Sivasankara Kurup. World Helath Organization. Geneva. pp.159-176. *2010.*

11. Petersen PE. Global policy for improvement of oral health in the 21st century – implications to oral health research of World Health Assembly 2007, World Health Organization. Community Dent Oral Epidemiol. 2009; 37:1-8.

12. McKinlay JB. Paradigmatic obstacles to improving the health of populations: implications for health policy. *Salud publica Mex.* 1998; 40:369-379

13. Rose's Strategy of Preventive Medicine. Geoffrey Rose, Commentary by Kay-Tee Khaw, Michael Marmot . Oxford University Press, Oxford. 2008.

14. World Health Organization. Closing the gap in a generation. Health equity

through action on social determinants of health. Commission on Social Determinants of Health Final Report. WHO, Geneva. 2008. http://www.who.int/social_determinants/thecommission/final-report/en/index.html

15. Marmot M. Fair Society, Healthy Lives The Marmot Review Strategic review of health inequalities in England post-2010 Published by The Marmot Review. February 2010. http://www.ucl.ac.uk/gheg/marmotreview/FairSocietyHealthyLives and www.ucl.ac.uk/gheg/marmotreview/Documents.

16. Graham H. Social determinants and their unequal distribution: clarifying policy understandings. Milbank Quarterly. 2004; 82:101-124.

17. Graham H. Health inequalities, social determinants and public health policy. Policy & Politics. 2009; 37:463-79.

18. Cohen LK. Dental care delivery in seven countries: the international collaborative study of dental manpower systems in relation to oral health status. Ingle JE and Blair P. Editors. International dental care delivery systems: issues in dental health policies. Cambridge (Mass), Ballinger; 1978. pp.201-214. 1978.

19. Nadanovsky P, Sheiham A. The relative contribution of dental services to the changes in caries levels of 12 year-old children in 18 industrialized countries in the 1970s and early 1980s. Community Dent Oral Epidemiol. 1995; 23:231-239.

20. Netuveli GS. Public Health aspects of dental calculus. An analysis of trends and future scenarios. PhD University of London Mimeo. 2002.

21. Netuveli GA, Sheiham A. A systematic review of the effectiveness of anticalculus dentifrices. Oral Health Prev Dent. 2004; 2:49-58.

22. Yevlahova D, Satur J. Models for individual oral health promotion and their effectiveness: a systematic review. Australian Dental Journal. 2009; 54:190-197.

23. McKinlay JB. 'A case for refocusing upstream – the political economy of illness', In: A.J. Enelow and J.B. Henderson (eds) *Applying behavioural science to cardio-*

24. Cowell CR, Sheiham A. The promotion of dental health. King Edward's Hospital Fund.1981.

25. Milio N. Promoting health through public policy. Philadelphia: F.A. Davis Company; 1983.

26. Milio N. Making healthy public policy; developing the science of art: an ecological framework for policy studies. *Health Promotion*. 1988; 2(3):236-274.

27. Milio N. Glossary: healthy public policy. *Journal of Epidemiology and Community Health*. 2001; 55:622-623.

28. Woodward A, Kawachi I. Why reduce health inequalities? J Epidemiol Community Health 2000;54: 923-929.

29. WHO. Declaration of Alma-Ata: international conference on primary health care, Alma-Ata, USSR, September 6–12, 1978. http://www.who.int/hpr/NPH/docs/declaration_almaata.pdf.

30. WHO. *Advocacy Strategies for Health and Development: Development Communication in Action*. World Health Organization. Geneva. 1995.

31. Milestones in Health Promotion Statements from Global Conferences. WHO/NMH/CHP/09.01. World Health Organization; 2009. http://www.who.int/healthpromotion/conferences/en/ and http://www.who.int/healthpromotion/Milestones_Health_Promotion_05022010.pdf.

32. Mechanic D. Issues in promoting health. Social Science & Medicine. 1999; 48:711-718.

33. WHO. The World Health Report 1995. Bridging the Gap. Geneva; *1999*. http://www.who.int/whr/1995/en/whr95_en.pdf

34. Green LW, Kreuter MW. Health promotion planning: An education and environmental approach (2nd ed.). Mountain View, California: Mayfield; 1991.

35. WHO. Health Promotion Glossary WHO, Geneva. 1998. http://www.who.int/healthpromotion/about/HPR%20Glossary%201998.pdf

36. WHO. World Health Organization. Bangkok charter for health promotion in the a globalized world. Geneve: WHO;

2005 [Acessado em 13/03/2007]; Available at: https://www.who.int/healthpromotion/conferences/en/.

37. Tang KC, Beaglehole R, O'Byrne D. Policy and partnership for health promotion - addressing the determinants of health. Bull World Health Organ. 2005; 83:884-5.

38. Policy in health promotion. The Health Communications Unit, Centre for Health Promotion, University of Toronto Developing Health Promotion Policies Version 1.0 March 31, 2004. http://www.thcu.ca

39. Nutbeam D The challenge to provide 'evidence' in health promotion. Health Promot. Int. 1999;14(2): 99-101.

40. Nutbeam D, Harris E. Health Promotion and Health Education in Schools – Trends, Effectiveness and Possibilities June 2006. Royal Automobile Club of Victoria. 1998.

41. Nutbeam D, Harris E. Theory in a nutshell: A practitioners guide to commonly used theories and models in health promotion. Sydney: National Centre for Health Promotion. 1998.

42. Tones K, Tilford S. Health Education: Effectiveness, Efficiency & Equity, 2nd edn. Chapman & Hall, London; 1994.

43. Tones K. Evaluating health promotion: a tale of three errors. Patient Education and Counseling. 2000; 39:227-236.

44. Wimbush E, Watson J An Evaluation Framework for Health Promotion: Theory, Quality and Effectiveness. Evaluation. 2000; 6(3):301-321.

45. Health Education Board for Scotland (HEBS), Evaluation of Health Promoting Health Service Framework: Final Report Health Scotland. http://www.healthscotland.com/documents/browse/443/0.aspx http://www.healthscotland.com/uploads/documents/RE-004Final-031104.pdf

46. Downie RS, Tannahill C, Tannahill A. Health Promotion: Models and Values. Oxford University Press. 1996.

47. Whitehead D. Evaluating health promotion: a model for nursing practice Journal of Advanced Nursing. 2003; 41(5):490-498.

48. Davey Smith G, Chaturvedi N, Harding S, Nazroo J, Williams R. Ethnic inequalities in health: a review of UK epidemiological evidence. Crit Public Health. 2000; 10:375-408.

49. Lynch JW, Kaplan GA, Salonen JT. Why do poor people behave poorly? Variation in adult health behaviours and psychosocial characteristics by stages of the socioeconomic lifecourse. Soc Sci Med. 1997; 44:809-19.

50. Dean K. Methodological issues in the study of health-related behaviour. In: Anderson R, Davies JK, Kickbusch I, McQueen DV, Turner J. Health behavior research and health promotion. Oxford: Oxford University Press. pp.83-99. 1988

51. Ma J, Betts NM, Hampl JS. Clustering of lifestyle behaviours. Am J Health Promot. 2000; 15:107-17.

52. Link BG, Phelan JC. Social conditions as fundamental causes of disease. J Health Soc Behav. 1995; 35:80-94.

53. Link BG, Northridge ME, Phelan JC, Ganz ML. Social epidemiology and the fundamental cause concept: on the structuring of effective cancer screens by socioeconomic status. Millbank Quart. 1998; 76:375-402.

54. Sheiham A, Sabbah W. Using Universal Patterns of Caries for Planning and Evaluating Dental Care. (A. Sheiham W. Sabbah) Caries Res. 2010; 44:141-150.

55. WHO. Diet, Nutrition and the Prevention of Chronic Diseases. WHO Technical Report Series 916. WHO. Geneva. 2003.

Chapter 1

The Life Course Approach: Healthy Children as a Sound Basis for a Healthy Society, with Particular Reference to Oral Health

William Murray Thomson
Saul Martins Paiva
Thiago Machado Ardenghi

This chapter considers the life course approach and its usefulness in helping us to think about the oral health of children and their families. After first defining the approach, we examine the ways in which life course research can be conducted, and then we consider its applicability to the main oral conditions affecting children. We then examine some recent life course oral research findings, together with their relevance for promoting the oral health among children and their families.

Defining the life course approach

The life course approach is a way of looking at chronic disease occurrence by considering the longer-term effects of exposures occurring through life. The life course can be thought of as our journey from gestation through childhood, adolescence, early and middle adulthood, and finally to old age and eventual death. Life course epidemiology seeks to understand the links between exposures and chronic conditions while considering as-

pects of the former, such as their timing, duration and intensity.[1] Its relevance for child oral health promotion is that it can assist us to understand the scale of the challenges which face us.

Four main models have been described,[2] and all four emphasise the incremental, developmental nature of health and chronic disease occurrence (Table 1.1). The four models can be summarised as: (1) the critical period model, in which exposure during a key period early in life produces a condition much later in life; (2) the critical period with effect modifier model, in which key early-life exposures interact with later-life exposures to increase or ameliorate the risk of a condition later in life; (3) the accumulation risk model, in which detrimental and beneficial exposures accumulate through life to affect health; and (4) the chain of risk model, in which one detrimental or beneficial exposure leads in a fairly linear way to another, and so on, to influence health. All of these have direct relevance for oral health, and how they apply is discussed later in this chapter.

Table 1.1 – Overview of life course models, with dental examples.

Model	Dental example	Mode of action
Critical period Exposure during a key developmental period leads to the condition later in life	Demarcated opacity defects of enamel	Interruption of enamel maturation by infection of carious deciduous predecessor[10]
Critical period with effect modifier Key early-life exposures interact with later ones in the occurrence of the condition later in life	Periodontitis	Low household SES and poor maternal nutrition, along with smoking later in adolescence and early adulthood[16]
Accumulation risk Detrimental and beneficial exposures accumulate through life to affect health	Dental caries	Prolonged inadequate removal of plaque and associated lower exposure to topical fluoride in dentifrices[15]
Chain of risk One detrimental or beneficial exposure leads in a fairly linear way to another (and so on) to influence health	Orofacial trauma	Growing up in deprived neighbourhood leading to greater exposure to family violence, leading to aggressive behaviour, leading to trauma[20]

Doing life course research

It is worthwhile to consider the various scientific methods which inform the lifecourse perspective. The prospective cohort study is the one which fits it most readily. In such a study, a sample (ideally, a representative one) is followed over time, with periodic measurement of the exposures and outcomes which are of interest. It is a very powerful design for determining the incidence and natural history of conditions. Its prospective measurement of exposure to putative determinants and potential confounders means that it is ideally suited to the life course approach.[2] This is particularly so for chronic, progressive, noncommunicable conditions (such as dental caries) which usually develop slowly over time

and for which the accumulation model is most relevant. Of course, the major disadvantage of the prospective cohort study design is that such studies take a long time, especially if the research aims to elucidate the life course aspects of a condition's occurrence rather than to merely determine whether a specific exposure is likely to be causally related to that condition. They are also prone to attrition: participants may move, die, decide that they no longer wish to take part, and so on. If it is substantial, that loss to follow-up can compromise the inferences which can be drawn from the study. The nature of the condition(s) under study is also an important consideration. A condition with a long latency period between exposure and disease presentation would require that a cohort be followed for many decades. A condition such as dental caries—which manifests at a relatively constant rate throughout life—might also demand decades of follow-up, but for reasons more to do with elucidating its natural history (and whether the various risk factors maintain their relative importance).

Other designs also have their merits, particularly in settings which lack the resources, expertise or political support to initiate and sustain a cohort study of sufficient duration and assessment periodicity. Retrospective cohort studies involve identifying a cohort which has been assembled in the past (usually in connection with another line of enquiry), and then using the measurements which have been made previously. With this method, the researcher has no meaningful control over the nature of the sample or the assessments which have been undertaken. Descriptive studies (surveys) can also contribute to understanding of a condition from the life course perspective, in that they can pinpoint important associations with exposures which have been measured retrospectively (such as maternal self-reported smoking through pregnancy in a survey of dental caries experience among five-year-old children). Such information would be prey to the usual recall biases, of course, but it is better than having none at all, and it can be useful (indeed, necessary but not sufficient) in building a life-course-informed understanding of a condition's aetiology.

While these other study designs can make important contributions to our understanding of a condition, the prospective cohort study is by far the most useful one. So, does having such a study necessarily mean that life course research is being undertaken? To an-swer this question satisfactorily, it is necessary to remind ourselves that the nature of life course enquiry involves investigating the accumulation of risk through the life course.[2] In essence, the longer a prospective study's duration, the greater the contribution it can make to understanding. Thus, one would be hard-pressed to describe a study which followed a birth cohort of infants from birth to five years of age as a life course study, but continued follow-up of the same cohort (especially if it is sizable) through the various important developmental epochs of mid-to-late childhood and adolescence would indeed take the study into the realm of life course enquiry. Further follow-up through adulthood and into old age with minimal attrition would, of course, make it an excellent life course study. One consideration with such a study would be that the researchers who initiated it would no longer be there at its conclusion (underlining the need for those involved in such studies to develop and mentor younger researchers who can continue the work).

In using the life course approach to consider the common chronic diseases which afflict humans, Darnton-Hill and co-workers outlined the issues which are specific to particular life stages.[3] They also made the point that distinctions among those developmental epochs are somewhat arbitrary. The stages and associated concerns are summarised in Table 1.2. Not only do they merge more or less seamlessly and imperceptibly into one another as we age, the relative effects of the various influences which are operative during those stages vary in their impact through the life course.

Table 1.2 – Developmental stages and issues which are specific to them.

Developmental stage	Specific issues for chronic diseases
Foetal life	Intrauterine growth retardation Premature birth (with normal growth for gestational age) Overnutrition in utero Intergenerational influences
Infancy and childhood	Breastfeeding Postnatal growth in weight and height Other factors (such as growing up in socio-economic disadvantage)
Adolescence	Development of risk factors Tracking of risk factors from earlier in life Development of healthy or unhealthy habits which tend to persist through life
Adulthood	The extent to which risk factors continue to be important in chronic disease development The extent to which modifying those risk factors will make a difference Role of risk factor modification in secondary prevention/treatment among those with disease
Old age	Most chronic conditions will have manifested themselves by now Benefits can still be gained from addressing risk factors The need to maximise health and quality of life by avoiding/delaying preventable disability

Oral health and the life course

The common oral conditions — dental caries and periodontitis — are eminently suited to the lifecourse perspective.[1] Both are chronic conditions which are largely irreversible and cumulative in nature. Their chronicity means that, once theyhave developed, their detection during an assessment is far more likely than an acute condition, which might have developed and then resolved between assessments, thus going unrecorded (a cold sore is an example of this type of condition). Cumulative conditions allow individuals to be distinguished by their extent and severity of disease development. They should be able to be validly and reliably measured, which requires that the evidence of disease experience (and therefore the diagnosis) be incontrovertible. They are reasonably common, so that the number of individuals required in the cohort is not too large (and therefore expensive). The common oral conditions also have public health importance, meaning that studies of them are ethically justifiable and (often) able to attract the necessary funding.

It is appropriate here to focus on the chronic oral conditions of childhood. Dental caries is by far the most common. It rightly deserves the majority of our attention, being responsible for a great deal of suffering and effects on the day-to-day lives of children and their families.[4-6] However, developmental defects of enamel are interesting conditions to consider with the life course perspective, and the contrast with dental caries — which may be considered to be an acquired defect of enamel — emphasises the different ways in which the life course approach can be used to inform understanding of oral diseases in children and how best to deal with them.[7] Developmental defects of enamel have been defined as a disturbances arising in hard tissue matrices and in their mineralisation during odontogenesis. Because of the non-remodelled nature of teeth, such defects can provide a window into the "metabolic memory" of the developmental process through the relevant stage of the life course.[8]

For the purposes of this discussion, it is useful to divide enamel defects into either opacities or hypoplastic defects. The former can be further subdivided into demarcated opacities and diffuse opacities (Table 1.3). The different types of enamel defect have different aetiologies, although our understanding is not complete, and some may merely be idiopathic. Demarcated opacities and hypoplastic defects of enamel tend to be isolated and sporadic in their distribution; thus, a local cause is most likely. For example, it was reported from a population-based prospective cohort study that children who had had chicken pox before age 3 were more likely by age 9 to have a hypoplastic defect in a permanent tooth (indicating that a febrile illness may disrupt the secretion of enamel by ameloblasts).[9] They also found that a history of trauma to a deciduous tooth was a risk factor for enamel hypoplasia in the permanent dentition. From more recent work using generalised estimating equation model analyses with the same cohort (these allow individual matching of deciduous teeth with their permanent successors, something that the statistical packages available at the time of the earlier analyses did not allow), Broadbent and coworkers reported that, if a deciduous incisor tooth was carious by age 5, its permanent successor was twice as likely to have a demarcated opacity when the child was next examined, at 9 years of age.[10]

Table 1.3 – Taxonomy and characteristics of enamel defects.

Defect type	Characteristic features
Hypoplasia	A defect involving the surface of the enamel and a localised reduction in its thickness. It can occur as pits, grooves or the partial or complete absence of enamel over a considerable area of dentine.
Demarcated opacities	In enamel of normal thickness and with an intact surface, there is a discrete area of different enamel translucency. It is demarcated from the adjacent enamel and has a clear, distinct boundary. It can be white, cream, yellow or brown in colour.
Diffuse opacities	In enamel of normal thickness and with an intact surface, there is a difference in translucency, with no clear boundary between it and the adjacent normal enamel. The opacity can be linear or patchy, or it can have a confluent distribution.

[a]World Health Organization. Oral health surveys. Basic methods. 4th Edition. (1997)

In contrast, diffuse opacities more frequently affect multiple teeth which have undergone enamel secretion and maturation during the same period, meaning that a systemic cause (such as consumption of fluoridated water) is more likely. A Brazilian study showed an association between life course events (such as malnutrition and pre- and postnatal infections) and the occurrence of any enamel defects in a cohort of socioeconomically underprivileged children.[7]

What is particularly fascinating is that, despite those differing aetiologies, the occurrence of developmental defectsof enamel is best understood through the critical period life course model: for a given tooth, enamel secretion and maturation occurs during a specific period.[11] Only a perturbation which occurs during that period can result in a developmental defect. Whether that defect is hypoplastic or a diffuse or demarcated opacity depends upon the nature and timing of the disturbance. For example, an apical infection to a deciduous central incisor may result in a hypoplastic defect if it occurs while the permanent successor is undergoing enamel secretion, but the same infection occurring during the enamel maturation phase after secretion is complete may result in a demarcated opacity in that successor tooth. For enamel hypoplasia in particular, such defects are routinely used as stress indicators in studies of past and contemporary populations.[12]

By contrast, dental caries can be considered to be an "acquired" defect of enamel, in that it develops after eruption (other examples of acquired enamel defects are erosion, attrition, traumatic enamel loss and, of course, the loss of enamel through surgical removal with a bur). Where dental caries is concerned, there is a steadily accumulating body of evidence that its occurrence is consistent with the accumulation risk model. Data from cohort studies have been invaluable in confirming this. For example, the longstanding Dunedin Multidisciplinary Health and Development Study has shown that the caries increment in the permanent dentition is remarkably constant, at an average 0.8 surfaces per year up to age 32 across the entire cohort, and that it is also constant within each of three identified trajectories of caries experience.[13] Preliminary data from the age-38 assessments in that study (underway at the time of writing) confirm the continuation of that pattern. Earlier data from the same study demonstrated a strong association between caries experience in the deciduous dentition at age 5 and the permanent dentition two decades later,[14] further underlining the continuity of caries experience throughout life.

The Dunedin study finding which really underlines the applicability of the accumulation risk model to dental caries occurrence was reported recently.[15] Using records of dental plaque accumulation at 5, 9, 15, 18, 26 and 32 years of age, they were able to identify three distinct plaque life course trajectories (Fig. 1.1). After controlling for confounders, those in the High plaque trajectory (who thus had the consistently "dirtiest" teeth through life from childhood to age 32) were almost 5 times as likely to have lost 1 or more teeth due to caries, and their DMFT score by age 32 was (on average) 40% higher than those in the Low trajectory. Those following the Medium plaque trajectory had better oral health than those in the High group, but their age-32 caries experience was still significantly worse than that of the Low group. Together with the constancy of

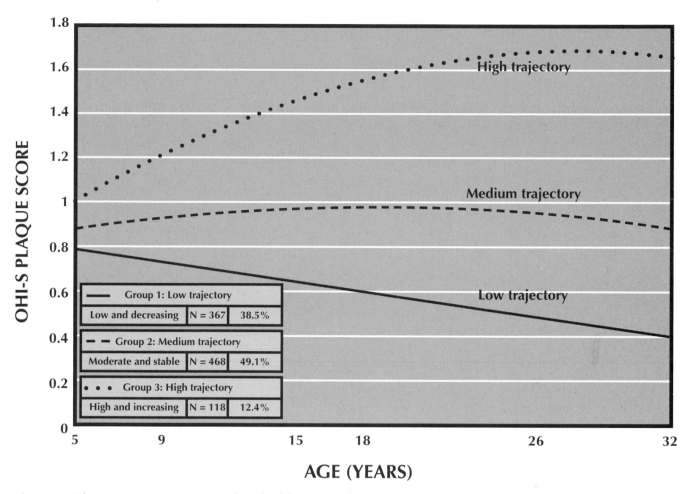

Fig. 1.1 – Plaque trajectory groups identified from Simplified Oral Hygiene Index (OHI-S) scores in the Dunedin Multidisciplinary Health and Development Study (Reprinted by permission from: Broadbent JM, Thomson WM and colleagues. Dental plaque and oral health during the first 32 years of life. JADA 2011;142(4):415-426. Copyright ©2011 American Dental Association. All rights reserved).

the caries increment through life, these gradients strongly support an accumulation risk model for dental caries and its sequelae. Even further support for this comes from the striking finding in the Dunedin Study that there is intergenerational continuity in oral health, with maternal self-rated oral health when the child was aged 5 years being strongly associated with that "child's" caries and tooth-loss experience by age 32, more than a quarter century later.[16]

Other life course studies provide support for these findings, and particularly for the observation that deleteri-

ous social conditions in early life predispose individuals to poor oral health later in the life course. For example, the 1982 Pelotas Birth Cohort study in Brazil collected data on family income trajectories and the number of episodes of poverty.This information was then examined against the number of unsound teeth among participants at 15 and 24 years of age. Poverty at birth and subsequent chronic exposure to poverty during the life course was positively associated with the number of unsound teeth by 24 years of age.[17] Other research using the same birth cohort study estimated the association between possible risk factors and the use of (and need for) dental prostheses. The findings supported the hypothesis that life-course socioeconomic, behavioural, and clinical determinants influenced the need for dental prostheses.[18] Other work by the same authors in Brazil investigated oral health impacts among 12-year-old adolescents and their association with life course socioeconomic characteristics. The findings highlighted the importance for adolescents' quality of life of early-life factors such as the social environment, maternal education level and occupational status, along with their dental status in early and later childhood.[19]

Another Brazilian example of the use of the life course perspective in oral health research is the work by Nicolau and coworkers,[20-23] who investigated life course circumstances and oral health in adolescents in Cianorte-PR. Despite the cross-sectional nature of the project, its findings provide interesting life course hypotheses which could be further examined in longitudinal research. The project comprised two phases. In the first phase, all 13-year-old adolescents who attended private or public schools in the town were invited to participate. For the second phase, 330 families were randomly selected for an in-depth interview on the adolescents' birth and early infancy circumstances, as well as information on several indicators of socio-economic status at two life stages (birth and 13 years of age). Adolescents who were low birth weight babies had high levels of dental caries by 13 years of age.[20] There was also an association between height and caries experience in adolescence, with taller adolescents having lower caries scores.[21] In that study, height was used as a surrogate marker of early development

and social and physical environment exposures in early life. The potential impact of the psychosocial environment in infancy and childhood on oral health later in life was also assessed, with the best predictors of gingival bleeding among 13-year-old adolescents being family socio-economic status (SES) at birth and 13 years of age, family structure, failing a school year(s) and plaque levels.[22] Similar observations were made in respect of traumatic dental injury, with higher rates observed among adolescents from a nonnuclear family, in lower school grades, or who reported high levels of paternal punishment.[23]

These examples of findings from life course studies of oral health underline the importance of not only the early years but also the path (or trajectory) which is followed through life.[24] Life course research in oral health is attracting more and more attention is the utility and importance of the findings is becoming clear, and it is likely that more such studies will be initiated in years to come. After all, cohort study findings are bounded by time and place; what applies in one setting or period may not necessarily hold in another, and the replication and extension of cohort study findings is a necessary feature of the life course research approach.[25]

Implications for promoting the oral health of children and their families

The life course approach for understanding oral health determinants has received growing attention in recent years. The findings from such studies could be useful in planning public health policies and promoting oral health through a multidisciplinary framework integrated into a common risk factor approach.[26]

They also offer a chance to conceptualise how the underlying social determinants of oral health can influence the development of dental diseases at different life course stages, as mediated through proximal, specific biological processes.[27] Life course epidemiological findings clearly show the importance of early life for the oral health of children and adolescents, in that those who get a compromised start to life are much more likely to follow a trajectory which will lead to poor oral health in adult hood and later life. The findings also show that getting a good start is necessary but not sufficient; the relative constancy of the caries increment through life means that efforts to maintain the integrity of the dentition must be ongoing. Promoting oral health must be a rational, sustained and evidence--based undertaking which is integrated with wider efforts to improve health.[26]

For conditions (such as enamel defects) which arise out of exposures and stressors occurring during a critical period, the avoidance of pre-, peri- and postnatal stressors is the key. Those for which the accumulation model applies (such as dental caries) require the commencement of a supportive environment as early as possible, especially in the light of the strong intergenerational influences which are operative. The establishment and maintenance of salutogenic environments and self-care practices cannot come too early.

There are formidable challenges to achieving this. For example, the poor health behaviour of low-SES groups has recently been shown by Nettle to be an adaptive response to the stressful conditions they are faced with in their day-to-day lives and environment.[28] Rogers and coworkers highlighted some years ago the tendency of health professionals to neglect the social context of poor health behaviours, and that this is not a feature of the lay view, which emphasises instead the connected ness of day-to-day life, health experience and behaviour.[29] The social context of health-affecting behaviours is a complex nexus of family/household, peers, social status, neighbourhood deprivation, ethnicity, societal structure and so on. Such social inequalities could affect oral health at different times in the life course, operating at both the individual and population levels, and by the psychosocial or material deprivation causal pathways. Therefore, improving the oral health of children requires sustained, multifaceted efforts directed at many of those aspects,[26] and a long-term political and societal consensus on how that should be done.

References

1. Nicolau B, Thomson WM, Steele JG, Allison PJ. Life-course epidemiology: concepts and theoretical models with particular reference to oral chronic conditions. Community Dent Oral Epidemiol. 2007; 35: 241-249.

2. Kuh D, Ben-Shlomo Y. A life course approach to chronic disease epidemiology (Second edition). Oxford: Oxford Medical Publications. 2004.

3. Darnton-Hill I, Nishida C, James WPT. A life course approach to diet, nutrition and the prevention of chronic diseases. Public Health Nutr. 2004; 7(1A): 101-121.

4. Locker D, Jokovic A, Stephens M, Kenny D, Thomson B, Guyatt G. Family impact

of child oral and oro-facial conditions. Community Dent Oral Epidemiol. 2002; 30: 438-448.

5. Thomson WM, Malden PE. Assessing change in the family impact of caries in young children after treatment under general anaesthesia. Acta Odont Scand. 2011; 69: 257-262.

6. Malden PE, Thomson WM, Jokovic A, Locker D. Changes in parent-assessed oral health-related quality of life among young children following dental treatment under general anaesthetic.Community Dent Oral Epidemiol. 2008; 36: 108-117.

7. Chaves AM, Rosenblatt A, Oliveira OF. Enamel defects and its relation to life course events in primary dentition of Brazilian children: a longitudinal study. Community Dent Health. 2007; 24: 31-36.

8. Berbesque JC, Doran GH. Brief communication: physiological stress in the-Florida Archaic-enamel hypoplasia and patterns of developmental insult in earlyNorth American hunter-gatherers. Am J Phys Anthropol. 2008;136:351-356.

9. Suckling GW, Herbison GP, Brown RH. Etiological factors influencing the prevalence of developmental defects of dental enamel in nine-year-old New Zealand children participating in a health and development study. J Dent Res. 1987; 66: 1466-1469.

10. Broadbent JM, Thomson WM, Williams SM. Does caries in primary teeth predict enamel defects in permanent teeth? A longitudinal study. J Dent Res. 2005; 84: 260-264.

11. Evans RW, Darvell BW. Refining the estimate of the critical period for enamel fluorosis in human maxillary incisors. J Public Health Dent. 1995; 55: 238-249.

12. Newell EA, Guatelli-Steinberg D, Field M, Cooke C, Feeney RN. Life history,enamel formation, and linear enamel hypoplasia in the Ceboidea. Am J Phys Anthropol. 2006; 131:252-60

13. Broadbent JM, Thomson WM, Poulton R. Trajectory patterns of dental caries experience in the permanent dentition to the fourth decade of life. J Dent Res. 2008; 87: 69-72.

14. Thomson WM, Poulton R, Milne BJ, Caspi A, Broughton JR, Ayers KMS. Socio-economic inequalities in oral health in childhood and adulthood in a birth cohort. Community Dent Oral Epidemiol. 2004; 32: 345-353.

15. Broadbent JM, Thomson WM, Boyens JV, Poulton R. Dental plaque and oral health during the first 30 years of life. JADA. 2011; 142: 415-426.

16. Shearer DM, Thomson WM, Broadbent JM, Poulton R. Maternal oral health predicts their children's caries experience in adulthood. J Dent Res. 2011; 90: 672-677.

17. Peres MA, Peres KG, Thomson WM, Broadbent JM, Gigante DP, Horta BL. The influence of family income trajectories from birth to adulthood on adult oral health: findings from the 1982 Pelotas birth cohort. Am J Public Health. 2011; 101: 730-736.

18. Correa MB, Peres MA, Peres KG, Horta BL, Gigante DP, Demarco FF. Life-course determinants of need for dental prostheses at age 24. J Dent Res. 2010; 89:733-738.

19. Peres KG, Peres MA, Araujo CL, Menezes AM, Hallal PC. Social and dental status along the life course and oral health impacts in adolescents: a population-based birth cohort.Health Qual Life Outcomes. 2009; 7:95.

20. Nicolau B, Marcenes W, Bartley M, Sheiham A. A life course approach to assessing causes of dental caries experience: the relationship between biological, behavioural, socio-economic and psychological conditions and caries in adolescents. Caries Res. 2003; 37:319-26.

21. Nicolau B, Marcenes W, Allison P, Sheiham A. The life course approach:explaining the association between height and dental caries in Brazilian adolescents. Community Dent Oral Epidemiol. 2005; 33:93-8.

22. Nicolau B, Marcenes W, Bartley M, Sheiham A. Associations between socio-economic circumstances at two stages of life and adolescents' oral health status. J Public Health Dent. 2005; 65:14-20.

23. Nicolau B, Marcenes W, Sheiham A. The relationship between traumatic dental

injuries and adolescents' development along the life course. Community Dent Oral Epidemiol. 2003; 31:306-13.

24. Sheiham A, Sabbah W. Using universal patterns of caries for planning and evaluating dental care. Caries Res. 2010; 44:41-150.

25. Peres MA, Thomson WM, Peres KG, Gigante DP, Horta BL, Broadbent JM, Poulton R. Challenges in comparing the methods and findings of cohort studies of oral health: the Dunedin (New Zealand) and Pelotas (Brazil) studies. Aust NZ J Public Health. 2011; 35: 549-556.

26. Sheiham A, Watt RG. The Common Risk Factor Approach: a rational basis for promoting oral health. Community Dent Oral Epidemiol. 2000; 28: 399-406.

27. Lynch J, Smith GD. A life course approach to chronic disease epidemiology. Annu Rev Public Health 2005;26:1-35.

28. Nettle D. Why are there social gradients in preventative health behavior? A perspective from behavioral ecology. PLoS One. 2010; 5:e13371

29. Rogers A, Popay J, Williams G, Latham M. Inequalities in health and health promotion: insights from the qualitative research literature. London: Health Education Authority. 1997.

Chapter 2

Epidemiology of Oral Health Problems in Children and Adolescents

Marcelo Bönecker
Isabela Almeida Pordeus
Jun Aida
Marco Aurelio Peres

Epidemiology and health promotion are closely associated when it comes to the health of the population. The study of the determinants and the distribution of a disease in specific populations provides relevant information for control of the health problem by strategies that include health education, change of public policies, changes in environments and community action.[1]

This chapter focuses on epidemiological perspectives, yet it is geared more towards the global distribution of oral diseases and problems that most frequently affect children and adolescents. The determinants of these diseases are discussed in depth in the other chapters of this book.

Oral disorders that most frequently affect children and adolescents are dental caries, periodontal disease, dental trauma, dental erosion and malocclusion. In order to better to organize the epidemiological data on the main oral health problems affecting children and adolescents in the world, data will be presented for four age groups; under[5] years; 5-6 years; 12 years and 15 years or over, and data on prevalence, severity and trends will be presented. Among the numerous epidemiological studies we preferentially selected national studiesor those that presented well-defined methodological criteria and more recent representative samples.

Dental caries

Summarized information is presented here that allows us to establish the global epidemiological picture of dental caries in early childhood. The use of nationwide studies was prioritized.

Children under 5 years of age

Prevalence and extent

Few national baseline studies are available for under 5 year olds.[2-11] Prevalences rangefrom about 30% in the United Kingdom and Australia to close on 70% in Brazil and the Middle East (Fig. 2.1).

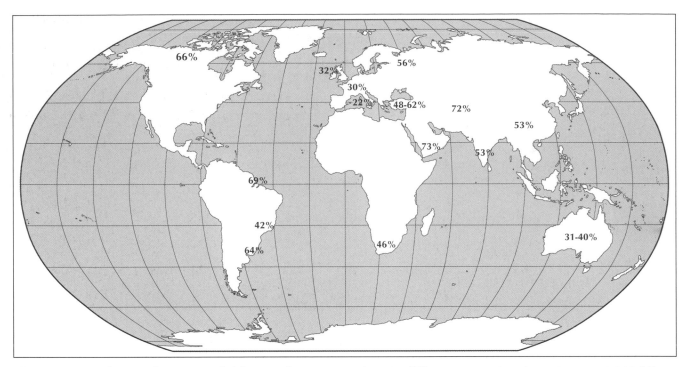

Fig. 2.1 – Prevalence of caries in children under 5 years of agein different countries, from 2005 to 2010.[2-11]

Trends

Few countries have data on trends in dental caries in children under 5 years of age. For 3-year-old children (Fig. 2.2) the data are only available in England,[12] Japan,[13] South Africa,[14] USA[15] and Brazil.[16-18]

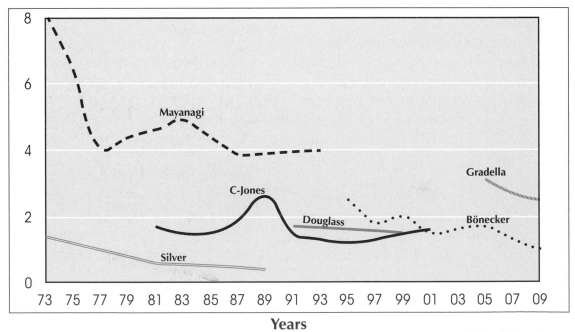

Fig. 2.2 – Trend in the prevalence of dental caries (dmf-t decayed, missing and filled deciduous teeth) in 3-year-old children, according to the study years.[12-18]

For 4-year-old children epidemiological caries trend studies are available fromJapan,[13] South Africa,[14] Brazil[16-18] and Sweden[19] (Fig. 2.3).

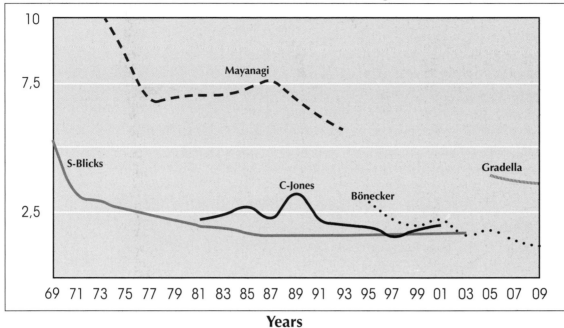

Years

Fig. 2.3 – Trend in the prevalence of dental caries (dmf-t) in 4-year-old children, according to the study years.[13-19]

5-6 year-old children

Prevalence and extent

There is a variation of methods and age composition in the studies (Table 2.1). The lowest prevalence was in Thailand (12.6%) and the highest in Denmark (75%),while the mean dental caries experience indices (mean dmf-t) ranged from 0.1 in Singapore to 5.97 in Thailand.

Table 2.1 – Prevalence (% dmf-t>0) and mean dmf-t index for 5 and 6 year olds by country and study year.

Country	Study year	Prevalence (% dmf-t>0)	mean dmf-t
Australia	2003-4	43.5	1.83
Barbados	2001	64.0	1.25
Brazil	2010	53.4	2.43
Singapore	2002	-	0.10
Denmark	2005	75.0	0.80
England and Wales	2006	61.2	1.50
New Zealand	2005	52.0	2.20
United Kingdom	2006	60.6	1.57
Czech Rep.	2001	31.3	3.32
Thailand	2001	12.6	5.97

Source:[20-22]

Trend

Only Australia, the United Kingdom and Brazil have data on epidemiological indicators of dental caries in 5-6 yearold children. In the United Kingdom, the prevalence of caries at 5 years of age decreased from 44% in 1995-6 to 39% in 2005-6 and the mean dmf-tindex decreased from 1.84 in 1995-96 to 1.1 in 2007-8.[23-28] In Australia the mean dmf-tindex ranged from 2.15 in 1989 to 1.83 in 2003-4. In recent years there has been relative stabilization and a slight increase in the index.[22] In Brazil the prevalence of caries and mean dmf-t index in 2002-3 at 6 years of age was 59% and 2.80 respectively, while in 2010 at 5 years of age it was 53% and 2.4 respectively, a slight decline.[21,29]

12 year-old children

Prevalence and extent

Prevalences ranged from 15% in Japan and 37% in Hong Kong to approximately 50% in Australia, Israel, Nigeria and New Zealand, and reach more than 85% in Croatia, Brazil and the Philippines (Fig. 2.4). The mean DMFT(decayed, missing and filled permanent teeth) index at 12 years exhibited considerable variation. Considering only national baseline studies conducted in the 2000s, Croatia has the highest DMF[6.7] and Denmark (0.7), the lowest.[30]

Trend

A limited number of low and mediumincome countries have national baseline studies over time that allow them to

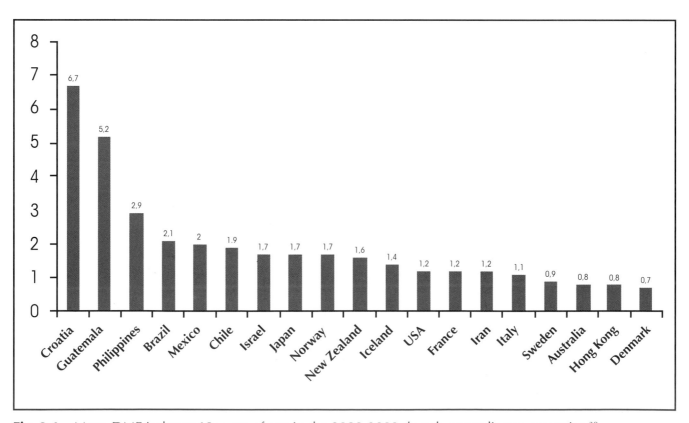

Fig. 2.4 – Mean DMF index at 12 years of age in the 2000-2009 decade according to countries.[30]

establish the dental caries extent trend. In the group of countries with available data (Fig. 2.5). Almost all presented a decline in the extent of dental caries with the exception of Nigeria.[31,32]

In high income countries there was a markeddecline in caries between 1985 and 2009 with an uptrend in recent years in some countries such as Australia and Norway (Fig. 2.6).[33-40]

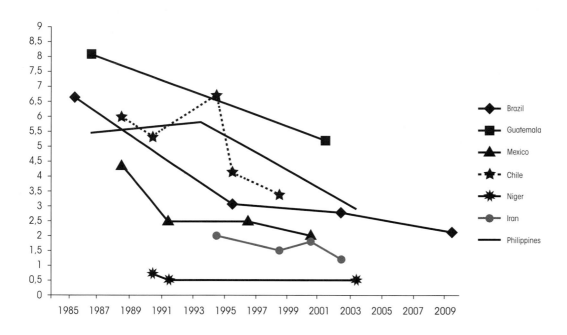

Fig. 2.5 – Trends in caries in the permanent dentition of 12-year-old children in medium and low income countries in the period of 1985-2010.[21,31,32]

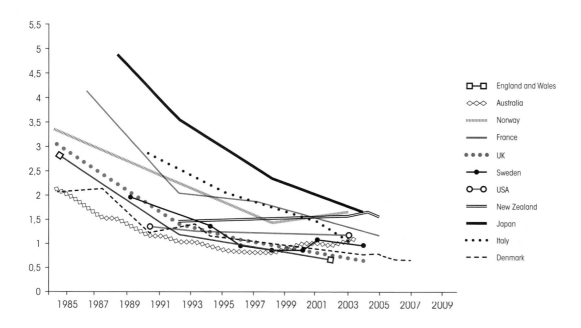

Fig. 2.6 – Trend in caries in the permanent dentition of 12-year-old children in high income countries in the period of 1985-2010.[33-40]

Periodontal disease

Various measures of periodontal disease have been developed[41,42] that makes comparison difficult. In addition, there have been few studies on periodontal disease in young children.[43,44] Therefore, no comprehensive international prevalence of periodontal disease is shown for o 6 years or younger children.

Children under 5 years of age

Prevalence

A survey on 3-5 years children which represented a selected health district was conducted in Brazil in 1999.[45] The Periodontal Screening and Recording (PSR) index was used.[46,47] Table 2.2 shows the prevalence of PSR code according to age.

Table 2.2 – Percentage distribution of PSR code according to age (Brazil).[5]

PSR code	3 years	4 years	5 years
0 (Healthy gingiva)	27.5	10.7	11
1 (Bleeding)	1.3	0.6	0.6
2 (Calculus and/or defective margine)	71.1	88.8	88.5

Source:[45]

5-6 year-old children

Prevalence

The prevalence of gingival inflammation was reported in the 2003 Children's Dental Health Survey, a series of decennial national children's dental health surveys in United Kingdom.[48] In 2003, 32% of 5 years children and 63% of the 8 years children had gingival inflammation.[48]

12 year-old children

Prevalence

WHO conducted oral health surveys in selected countries[49] using the Community Periodontal Index of Treatment Needs (CPITN).[50,51] The results were shown in table 2.3.

Table 2.3 – Percentage distribution of periodontal statuson 12-13 years children.

Site	Healthy	Bleeding	Calculus
Erfurt,Germany	54	37	9
Yamanashi,Japan	23	10	67
New Zealand	73	5	21
Lodz, Poland	60	22	18
Baltimore,USA	20	35	45
HIS Navajo, USA	4	26	70
HIS Lakota, USA	21	59	20

Source:[49]

Distribution

School children aged 5-12 years attending a hospital in Australia were investigated the prevalence of alveolar bone loss around the first permanent molars, and first and second deciduous molars.[52] The overall prevalence of bone loss was 26%. Second deciduous molars were the most affected teeth with almost 75% lesions being distal. Among the young children, second deciduous molars showed highest prevalence of periodontal disease.

Adolescents older than 15 years of age

Prevalence

The Community Periodontal Index of Treatment Needs (CPITN) in various countries among the children older than 15 years were available from the WHO Oral Health Country/Area Profile Programme database.[53] Figure 2.7 shows the 20 countries with the highest percentage of the child with healthy periodontal status (CPTIN=0). Figure 2.8 shows the 20 countries with the lowest percentage of children with healthy periodontal status (CPTIN=0).

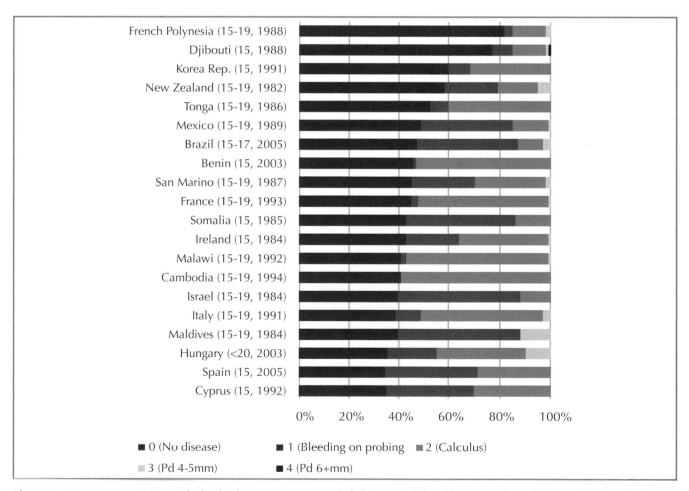

Fig. 2.7 – Twenty countries with the highest percentage of children with healthy periodontal status (CPTIN=0) (county, years of child, survey year).[53]

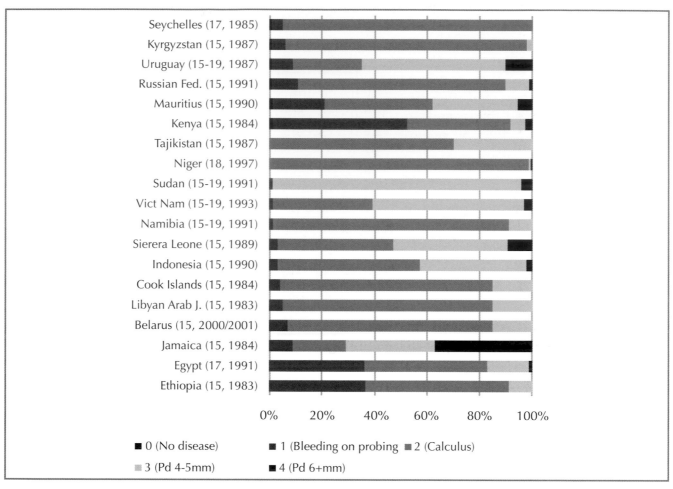

Fig. 2.8 – Twenty countries with the lowest percentage of children with healthy periodontal status (CPTIN=0) (county, years of child, survey year).

There were relatively large differences on periodontal status between countries among the children older than 15 years[53] compared to the results among 12 year olds.[49] The WHO Oral Health Country/Area Profile Programme databasehave data from various surveys. Dentists were not calibrated between the surveys in different settings. That partially explained the large variation of periodontal status on the WHO Oral Health Country/Area Profile Programme database.

Distributions

From the data in UK, periodontal disease among children and adolescent seems to increasing. A longitudinal study in Norway described the distribution of those with 2 mm or more attachment loss.[54] Among the 16-24 year olds, the first molars and first premolars had the highest prevalence of attachment loss.

Trends in periodontal diseases among children and adolescents

Among children, data from the Children's Dental Health Survey in United Kingdom are shown in figure 2.9.[48] Among adults, a review showed a reduction of periodontitis in recent years.[55]

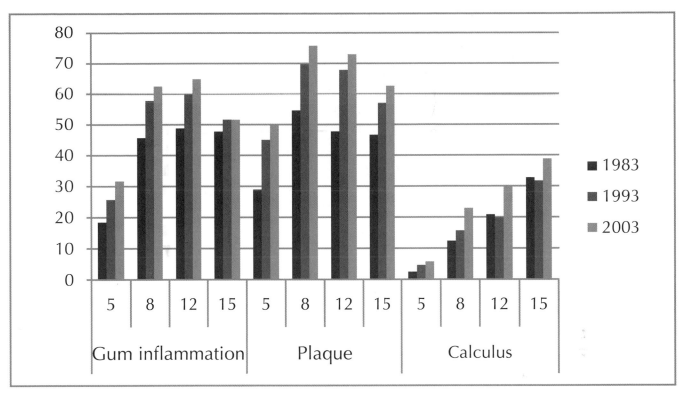

Fig. 2.9 – Prevalence of gum inflammation, plaque and calculus among children in 1983, 1993 and 2003 in the United Kingdom.[48]

Traumatic Dental Injuries (TDI)

The prevalence of traumatic dental injuries in children and adolescentsis high all over the world. The high prevalence of traumatic dental injuries can be more frequently observed in several studies using a cross-sectional epidemiological design of representativeness. However, it is known that this type of design tends to underestimate prevalenceas it is unable to assess all the types of dental trauma.

The differences in prevalence found in epidemiological studies conducted in the same country or even between countries can be attributed to methodological concerns and differences of socioeconomic conditions between the regions where the data were collected.

Most traumatic dental injuries involve upper anterior teeth regard-less of the age group studied. In very young children the most prevalent traumatic dental injuries in deciduous teeth are related to displacements and avulsions while in permanent the most common severe events are fractures involving the different dental tissues and roots.

There are few studies reporting trends in traumatic dental injuries. The only study on trends in traumatic dental injuries in children under 5 years of age available in international dental literature was carried out in Brazil.[56] It clearly indicates an uptrend in the prevalence of traumatic dental injuries in recent years (Fig. 2.10). A sequence of national baseline studies conducted in the United Kingdom indicates that dental trauma in 15-year-old adolescents between the years 1973 and 2003 decreased from 22% to 13%.[57,58]

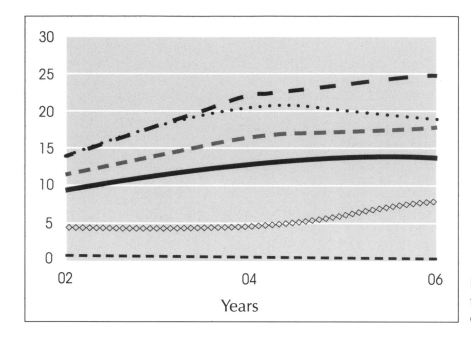

Fig. 2.10 – Trends in traumatic dental injuries in children under 5 years of age, Brazil.

Children under 5 years of age

Prevalence

The data from Table 2.4 indicate that prevalence ranged between 6.2% and 41.6%. Note that there is considerable variation in the prevalence of traumatic dental injuries within, between and among countries.

Trends

Table 2.4 – Prevalence of traumatic dental injuries in children under 5 years of age.

YEAR	AUTHORS	COUNTRY	AGE GROUP (YEARS)	n	PREVALENCE (%)
2008	Feldens et al.	Brazil	1-1.5	376	15
2009	Jorge et al.	Brazil	1-3	519	41,6
2009	Avsar et al.	Turkey	0-3	563	17,4
2009	Robson et al.	Brazil	0-5	419	39,1
2009	Ferreira et al.	Brazil	0-5	3489	14,9
2009	Vasconcelos et al.	Brazil	0-5	1265	13,9
2010	Feldens et al.	Brazil	3-5	888	36,4
2010	Wendt et al.	Brazil	1-5	571	36,6
2010	Granville-Garcia et al.	Brazil	1-5	820	20,1
2010	Goettems et al.	Brazil	2-5	608	29,4
2011	Piovesan et al.	Brazil	1-5	455	31,5
2011	Shekhar et al.	India	3-5	1126	6,2
2011	Assunção et al.	Brazil	0-5	1703	24
2011	Tümen et al.	Turkey	2-5	727	8

Source:[56,59-71]

5-6 year-old children

Prevalence

There are few studies concerning the prevalence of traumatic dental injuries in 5-and 6-year-old children in the world (Table 2.5). Between the years 2008 and 2012 only 2 studies were selected and the prevalence are very different.

Table 2.5 – Prevalence of traumatic dental injuries in 5- and 6-year-old children.

YEAR	AUTHORS	COUNTRY	AGE GROUP (YEARS)	n	PREVALENCE (%)
2009	Noori et al.	Iraq	6-7	1325	3,9
2010	Viegas et al.	Brazil	5-6	388	62,1

Source:[72,73]

12 year-old children

Prevalence

The prevalence of traumatic dental injuries in studies that include 12-year-old children (Table 2.6) appears lower than inchildren under 5 years of age, and ranged between 6% and 22.5%.

Table 2.6 – Prevalence of traumatic dental injuries in 12 year-old children.

YEAR	AUTHORS	COUNTRY	AGE GROUP (YEARS)	n	PREVALENCE (%)
2008	Fakhruddin et al.	Canada	12-14	2422	11.4
2008	Gopinath et al.	Malaysia	12	250	11.2
2009	Naidoo et al.	South Africa	11-13	1665	6.4
2009	AdekoyaSofowora et al.	Nigeria	12	415	12.8
2009	Noori et al.	Iraq	12-13	288	11.5
2009	David et al.	India	12	838	6
2010	Piovesan et al.	Brazil	12	792	9.7
2010	Bendo et al.	Brazil	11-14	1612	17.1
2010	Livny et al.	Israel	11-12	804	17.7
2010	Traebert et al.	Brazil	12	405	22,5
2010	Castro et al.	Brazil	11-12	571	9.4
2011	Ravishankar et al.	India	12	1020	15.1
2011	Taiwo et al.	Nigeria	12	719	15.2

Source:[74-86]

Adolescents older than 15 years of age

Prevalence

The prevalence of TDI in adolescents over than 15 years of age (Table 2.7) ranged between 8.9% and 19.9%.

Table 2.7 – Prevalence of traumatic dental injuries in adolescents older than 15 years of age.

YEAR	AUTHORS	COUNTRY	AGE GROUP (YEARS)	n	PREVALENCE (%)
2008	Gopinath et al.	Malaysia	16	238	13.4
2009	Huang et al.	Taiwan	15-18	6312	19.9
2010	Thelen et al.	Albania	16-18	2789	8.9 (16)/ 10.5 (18)

Source:[87-89]

Dental erosion

Dental erosion is an oral health problem that particularly affects populations of children and adolescents. The prevalence data vary considerably between countries and the reasons for these divergences are the use of different diagnositic criteria, socioeconomic, cultural and demographic differences among the different countries studied and lack of standardization of which teeth considered.

There is novalidated and universally accepted index for the evaluation of erosive lesions, although several indices have already been proposed.[90-92]Accordingly, the prevalence data presented by age groupvary considerably, as different indices and methodologies were used.

There was a workshop on Dental Erosion in Switzerland in 2007, when the Basic Erosive Wear Examination (BEWE) index was proposed.[93]This is currently the most widely accepted index for the clinical assessment oferosive lesions.

Children under 5 years of age

Prevalence

There are few studies on the prevalence of erosion among children under 5 years of age (Table 2.8). Prevalence ranged from 5.7% (China) to 51.6% (Brazil).

Table 2.8 – Prevalence of dental erosion in children under 5 years of age.

YEAR	AUTHORS	COUNTRY	AGE GROUP (YEARS)	n	PREVALENCE (%)
1994	Hinds & Gregory	England	4-5	178	50
1995	Huang et al.	United Kingdom	1.5-4.5	1,522	19
1995	Jones & Nunn	United Kingdom	3	135	29
2001	Al-Malik et al.	Saudi Arabia	2-5	987	31
2005	Luo et al.	China	3-5	1,949	5.7
2011	Murakami et al.	Brazil	3-4	967	51,6

Source:[94-99]

5-6 year-old children

Prevalence

There arelimited data on prevalence in 5- and 6-year-old children (Table 2.9). The prevalence ranged between 10.9% (China) and 95% (Saudi Arabia).

Table 2.9 – Prevalence of dental erosion in 5-6 year-old children.

YEAR	AUTHORS	COUNTRY	AGE GROUP (YEARS)	n	PREVALENCE (%)
1994	O'Brien	United Kingdom	5-6	17,061	52
2002	Al-Majed et al.	Saudi Arabia	5	202	47
2003	Harding et al.	Ireland	3	135	29
2004	Deshpande&Hughar	India	5-6	100	30.7
2009	Chen et al.	China	5	1,219	10.9

Source:[92,100-103]

12 year-old children

As there are few reports in literature concerning the prevalence of dental erosion in 12-year-old children, the data will be presented in two tables (Tables 2.10 and 2.11), one showing the results of studies conducted with children who were 12 years old, and the other that included children close to 12 years of age.

Prevalence

Table 2.10 – Prevalence of dental erosion in 12 year-old children.

YEAR	AUTHORS	COUNTRY	AGE GROUP (YEARS)	n	PREVALENCE (%)
2004	Dugmore et al.	England	12	1,753	59.7
2005	Truin et al.	Netherlands	12	832	24
2005	Peres et al.	Brazil	12	391	13
2008	El-Aidi et al.	Netherlands	12	622	42.8
2009	Chen et al.	China	12	786	22.1
2009	Hou et al.	China	12	844	61.8
2010	Arnadóttir et al.	Iceland	12	2,251	15.7

Source:[103-109]

Table 2.11 – Prevalence of dental erosion in children approximately 12 years of age.

YEAR	AUTHORS	COUNTRY	AGE GROUP (YEARS)	n	PREVALENCE (%)
2000	Deery et al.	England	11-13	125	37
2000	Deery et al.	USA	11-13	129	41
2002	Al-Majed et al.	Saudi Arabia	12-14	862	95
2007	El-Karim et al.	Sudan	12-14	157	66.9
2010	Wang et al.	China	12-13	1,499	27.3

Source:[100-112]

Adolescents older than 15 years of age

Prevalence

The data on prevalence of dental erosion for adolescents older than 15 years of age (Table 2.12) indicatethat there is apparently no variation between Iceland[115] and the Netherlands[109] despite the difference of year in which the studies were carried out.

Table 2.12 – Prevalence of dental erosion in adolescents older than 15 years of age.

YEAR	AUTHORS	COUNTRY	AGE GROUP (YEARS)	n	PREVALENCE (%)
2002	Van Rijkom et al.	Netherlands	15-16	400	30
2003	Arnadóttir et al.	Iceland	15	278	21.6
2004	Jensdottir et al.	Iceland	19-22	80	39
2010	Arnadóttir et al.	Iceland	15	2,251	30.7

Source:[109,113-115]

Malocclusion

Malocclusion is defined by different clinical signs, dental and aesthetic parameters and functional and skeletal considerations. The high prevalence of malocclusion is related to genetic and environmental factors.[116] In 1997, WHO adopted the Dental Aesthetic Index - DAI as a reference for the performance of epidemiological surveys. This index is recommended for use in complete permanent dentition (generally at 12 years) and has been replaced the old index proposed by WHO in 1987 for this dentition. This is the index currently recommended by WHO.[117]

There is a high prevalence of malocclusion in several countries. The significant variation in malocclusion prevalence data is related to the different methods used, particularly differences of diagnostic criteria and the use of different malocclusion classifications. Ethnic and population variations act as determinants of this variation. The facial pattern of several populations tends to vary, since blacks, whites, Hispanics, indigenous peoples and other groups havedifferent levels of malocclusion prevalence, as a consequence of the distinct ethnic characteristics.[118]

Data in this section are organized

differently from the other topics inthis chapter.

It is important to emphasize that there are not yet any reportson malocclusion prevalence and severity trends. Thus we present data from the latest studies on the prevalence of malocclusion in children and adolescents in Brazil and in other countries.

In Brazil, there are several regional epidemiological studies and the malocclusion prevalence data are highly different, ranging from 24% to 74% (Table 2.13). The broader investigation of oral health problems existing in the Brazil reports that the prevalence of malocclusion was 36% at age 5, 58% at age 12 and 53% in the 15-19 age group.[29]

As is the case of Brazil, malocclusion is a dental condition with high prevalence in several countries. However, the prevalence varies considerably depending on population/ethnic groups and methodologies of each study. We selected some of the most up-to-date world studies to illustrate the prevalence of malocclusion in various countries (Table 2.13). These data show variability of 17% to 92% in prevalence of malocclusion.

Table 2.13 – Prevalence of malocclusion in children and adolescents.

Prevalence of malocclusion in children and adolescents - Brazil			
Author/Year	**Place**	**Age**	**Prevalence (%)**
Peres et al., 2002	Brazil	14 to 18 years	71
Frazão et al., 2002	Brazil	5 to 12 years	49 (Deciduous. D.) 71 (Deciduous. D.)
MS, 2003	Brazil	5 years 12 years 15 to 19 years	38 58 53
Katz et al., 2004	Brazil	3 years	49
Marques et al., 2005	Brazil	10 to 14 years	62
Silva Filho et al., 2007	Brazil	3 to 6 years	73
Leite-Cavalcanti et al., 2007	Brazil	3 to 5 years	87
Dhar et al., 2007	India	5 to 14 years	36
Grabowski et al., 2007	Germany	Average Age4.5 Average Age8.3 74 (Deciduous Dent.)	92 (Mixed Dent.)
Oliveira et al., 2008*	Brazil	3 to 18 years	74
Mtaya et al., 2009	Tanzania	12 to 14 years	63
Murshid et al., 2010	Saudi Arabia	13 to 15 years	91
Abanto et al., 2011	Brazil	2 to 5 years	24
Carvalho et al., 2011	Brazil	5 years	46
Aliaga-Del Castillo et al., 2011	Peru	2 to 18 years	85
Mountain et al., 2011	England	3 to 6 years	17
Bhardwaj et al., 2011	India	16 and 17 years	20

*Individuals with Downs syndrome

Source:[29,119-134]

Final considerations

According to WHO[135] epidemiological studies provide basic information about the oral health situation and/or dental treatment needs of a population, at a given time and place. The main goals of these studies are to discover the magnitude of dental problems and to monitor changes in the levels and in the patterns of diseases over time. These were also the objectives of this chapter, namely, to provide an objective and direct account of the prevalence and trends of the principal health problems that affect children and adolescents in the world to serve as a basis for discussion of these oral health issues in the following chapters of this book.

References

1. WHO: Ottawa Charter for Health Promotion. Health Promotion. 1987; 1 (44).
2. Leake J, Jozzy S, Uswak G. Severe dental caries, impacts and determinants among children 2-6 years of age in Inuvik Region, Northwest Territories, Canada. J Can Dent Assoc. 2008; 74(6):519.
3. Ardenghi TM, Sheiham A, Marcenes W, Oliveira LB, Bönecker M.Maxillary anterior caries as a predictor of posterior caries in the primary dentition in preschool Brazilian children.J Dent Child (Chic). 2008; 75(3):215-21.
4. Gradella CM, Bernabé E, Bönecker M, Oliveira LB.Caries prevalence and severity, and quality of life in Brazilian 2- to 4-year-old children.Community Dent Oral Epidemiol. 2011; 39(6):498-504.
5. Traebert J, GuimarãesLdo A, Durante EZ, Serratine AC. Low maternal schooling and severity of dental caries in Brazilian preschool children. Oral Health Prev Dent. 2009; 7(1):39-45.
6. Cleaton-Jones P, Williams S, Green C, Fatti P. Dental caries rates in primary teeth in 2002, and caries surveillance trends 1981-2002, in a South African city.Community Dent Health. 2008; 25(2):79-83
7. Slade GD, Sanders AE, Bill CJ, Do LG. Risk factors for dental caries in the five-year-old South Australian population. Aust Dent J. 2006; 51(2):130-9.
8. Simratvir M, Moghe GA, Thomas AM, Singh N, Chopra S. Evaluation of caries experience in 3-6-year-old children, and dental attitudes amongst the caregivers in the Ludhiana city. J Indian SocPedodPrev Dent. 2009; 27(3):164-9.
9. Campus G, Solinas G, Strohmenger L, Cagetti MG, Senna A, Minelli L, Majori S, Montagna MT, Reali D, Castiglia P; Collaborating Study Group. National pathfinder survey on children's oral health in Italy: pattern and severity of caries disease in 4-year-olds.Caries Res. 2009;43(2):155-62. Epub. 2009 Apr 8.
10. Pitts NB, Boyles J, Nugent ZJ, Thomas N, Pine CM. The dental caries experience of 5-year-old children in Great Britain (2005/6). Surveys co-ordinated by the British Association for the study of community dentistry.Community Dent Health. 2007; 24(1):59-63.
11. Shang XH, Li DL, Huang Y, Chen H, Sun RP. Prevalence of dental caries among preschool children in Shanghe County of Shandong Province and relevant prevention and treatment strategies. Chin Med J (Engl). 2008 20; 121(22):2246-9.
12. Silver DH. A comparison of 3-year-olds' caries experience in 1973, 1981 and 1989 in a Hertfordshire town, related to family behaviour and social class.Br Dent J. 1992;7;172(5):191-7.
13. Mayanagi H, Saito T, Kamiyama K. Cross-sectional comparisons of caries time trends in nursery school children in Sendai, Japan. Community Dent Oral Epidemiol. 1995; 23(6):344-9.

14. Cleaton-Jones P, Williams S, Fatti P. Surveillance of primary dentition caries in Germiston, South Africa, 1981-97.Community Dent Oral Epidemiol. 2000;28(4):267-73.

15. Douglass JM, Montero MJ, Thibodeau EA, Mathieu GM. Dental caries experience in a Connecticut Head Start program in 1991 and 1999. Pediatr Dent. 2002; 24(4):309-14.

16. Bönecker M, Ardenghi TM, Oliveira LB, Sheiham A, MarcenesW .Trends in dental caries in 1- to 4-year-old children in a Brazilian city between 1997 and 2008. Int J Paediatr Dent. 2010; 20(2):125-31.

17. Bönecker M, Marcenes W, Sheiham A. Caries reductions between 1995, 1997 and 1999 in preschool children in Diadema, Brazil. Int J Paediatr Dent. 2002; 12(3):183-8.

18. Gradella CM, Bernabé E, Bönecker M, Oliveira LB. Caries prevalence and severity, and quality of life in Brazilian 2- to 4-year-old children. Community Dent Oral Epidemiol. 2011; 39(6):498-504

19. Stecksén-Blicks C, Sunnegårdh K, Borssén E..Caries experience and background factors in 4-year-old children: time trends 1967-2002. Caries Res. 2004; 38(2):149-55.

20. Scottish Public Health Observatory (www.sotphp.org.uk);

21. Brasil. Ministério da Saúde. Secretaria de Vigilância em Saúde. Secretaria de Atenção à Saúde. Departamento de Atenção Básica. Coordenação Nacional de Saúde Bucal. SB Brasil 2010. Pesquisa Nacional de Saúde Bucal. Resultados Principais. Brasília: MS, 2011.

22. Australian Institute of Health and Welfare. Dental Statistics and Research series n. 52. Dental Health of Australians´ teenagers and pre-ten children.The Child Dental Survey, Australia 2003-4.Camberra: Australian Institute of Health and Welfare, 2009.

23. Pitts NB, Evans DJ.The dental caries experience of 5-year-old children in the United Kingdom. Surveys coordinated by the Britsh Association for the Study of Community Dentistry in 1995-96. Community Dent Health. 1997; 14: 47-52.

24. Pitts NB, Evans DJ, Nugent ZJ.The dental caries experience of 5-year-old children in the United Kingdom. Surveys co-ordinated by the British Association for the Study of Community Dentistry in 1997/98. Community Dent Health 1999; 16: 50-56.

25. Pitts NB, Evans DJ, Nugent ZJ. The dental caries experience of 5-year-old children in Great Britain. Surveys co-ordinated by the British Association for the study of Community Dentisrty in 1999/2000. Community Dent Health. 2001; 18: 49-55.

26. Pitts NB, Boyles J, Nugent ZJ, Thomas N, Pine CM.The dental caries experience of 5-year-old children in England and Wales. Surveys co-ordinated by the British Association for the Study of Community Dentistry in 2001/2002. Community Dent Health. 2003; 20:45-54.

27. Pitts NB, Boyles J, Nugent ZJ, Thomas N, Pine CM.The dental caries experience of 5-year-old children in England and Wales (2003/4) and in Scotland (2002/3). Surveys co-ordinated by the British Association for the Study of Community Dentistry. Community Dent Health. 2005; 22:46-56.

28. Pitts NB, Boyles J, Nugent ZJ, Thomas N, Pine CM.The dental caries experience of 5-year-old children in Great Britain (2005/6). Surveys co-ordinated by the British Association for the study of community dentistry. CommunityDent Health. 2007; 24:59-63.

29. Brasil. Ministério da Saúde. Secretaria de Atenção à Saúde. Departamento de Atenção Básica. Coordenação Nacional de Saúde Bucal. Projeto SB Brasil 2003. Condições de saúde bucal da população brasileira 2002-2003. Resultados Principais. Brasília: MS, 2004.

30. FDI http://www.fdiworldental.org/.

31. Organização Mundial da Saúde(http://www.mah.se/CAPP/Country-Oral-Health-Profiles);

32. Narvai PC, Frazão P, Roncalli AG, Antunes JLF. Cárie dentária no Brasil: declínio, polarização, iniquidade e exclusão social. Pan Am J Public Health. 2006; 19(6):385–93.

33. Downer MC. The Improving Dental Health of United Kingdom Adults and Prospects for the Future. Br Dent J 1991; 170 (4): 154-158.

34. Marthaler TM, O'Mullane DM, Vrbic V. The Prevalence of Dental Caries in Europe 1990-95. Symposium Report. Caries Res, 1996; 30: 237-255.

35. Pitts NB, Evans DJ, Nugent ZJ. The dental caries experience of 12-year-old children in the United Kingdom. Surveys coordinated by the British Association for the Study of Community Dentistry in 1996-97. Comm Dent Health, 1998; 15: 49-54.

36. Pitts NB, Evans DJ, Nugent ZJ, Pine CM. The dental caries experience of 12-year-old children in England and Wales. Surveys coordinated by the British Association for the study of Community Dentistry in 2000-01. BASCD Survey report. Comm Dent Health, 2002; 19: 46-53.

37. Bourgeois DM, Roland E, Desfontaine J. Caries prevalence 1987-1998 in 12-year-olds in France. International Dental Journal 2004; 54(4):193-200.

38. Ola H, Magne BJ. Ecological time-trend analysis of caries experience at 12 years of age and caries incidence from age 12 to 18 years: Norway 1985-2004. Acta Odontologica Scandinavica. 2006; 64(6):368-375.

39. Armfield JM, Spencer AJ. Quarter of a century of change: caries experience in Australian children, 1977-2002. Australian Dental Journal. 2008; 53(2): 151-159.

40. Australian Research Centre for Population Oral Health (ARCPOH). Dental caries trends in Australian school children. Australian Dental Journal. 2011; 56:227-230.

41. Dhingra K, Vandana KL. Indices for measuring periodontitis: a literature review. Int Dent J. 2011; 61: 76-84.

42. Savage A, Eaton KA, Moles DR, Needleman I. A systematic review of definitions of periodontitis and methods that have been used to identify this disease. J Clin Periodontol. 2009; 36: 458-67

43. Oh TJ, Eber R, Wang HL. Periodontal diseases in the child and adolescent. J Clin Periodontol. 2002; 29: 400-10.

44. Jenkins WM, Papapanou PN. Epidemiology of periodontal disease in children and adolescents. Periodontol 2000. 2001; 26: 16-32.

45. Andrade IT, Rapp GE. Prevalence assessment of periodontal disease in 3-5 year old children through PSR--population study. J Int Acad Periodontol. 2002; 4:126-31.

46. Landry RG, Jean M. Periodontal Screening and Recording (PSR) Index: precursors, utility and limitations in a clinical setting. Int Dent J. 2002; 52:35-40.

47. Salkin LM, Cuder R, Rush R. A look at the PSR impact on one dental practice. J Am Dent Assoc. 1993; 124:230-1.

48. White DA, Chadwick BL, Nuttall NM, Chestnutt IG, Steele JG. Oral health habits amongst children in the United Kingdom in 2003. Br Dent J. 2006; 200:487-91.

49. Chen M, Barmes DE, Andersen RM, Leclerq M-H. Dentition and periodontal status. In: Chen M, Andersen RM, Barmes DE, Leclerq M-H, Lyttle SC, editors. Comparing Oral Health Systems A Second International Collaborative Study. Geneva: World Health Organization. 1997; p.115-33.

50. Miyazaki H, Pilot T, Leclercq MH, Barmes DE. Profiles of periodontal conditions in adolescents measured by CPITN. Int Dent J. 1991; 41:67-73.

51. World Health Organization. Oral health survey- basic methods. 3rd ed. 3rd ed. Geneva: World Health Organization; 1987.

52. Darby IB, Lu J, Calache H. Radiographic study of the prevalence of periodontal bone loss in Australian school-aged children attending the Royal Dental Hospital of Melbourne. J Clin Periodontol. 2005; 32:959-65.

53. Periodontal Country Profiles. An overview of CPITN data in the WHO Global Oral Data Bank. [cited 2011 08/24]; Available from: http://www.dent.niigata-u.ac.jp/prevent/perio/contents.html.

54. Heitz-Mayfield LJ, Schatzle M, Loe H, Burgin W, Anerud A, Boysen H, et al. Clinical course of chronic periodontitis. II. Incidence, characteristics and

54. time of occurrence of the initial periodontal lesion. J Clin Periodontol. 2003; 30:902-8.

55. Hugoson A, Norderyd O. Has the prevalence of periodontitis changed during the last 30 years? J Clin Periodontol. 2008; 35:338-45.

56. de Vasconcelos Cunha Bonini GA, Marcenes W, Oliveira LB, Sheiham A, Bönecker M. Trends in the prevalence of traumatic dental injuries in Brazilian preschool children.Dent Traumatol. 2009 Dec; 25(6):594-8

57. Todd JE. Children's dental health in England and Wales 1973. London: Social Survey Division and Her Majesty's Stationery Office, 1975.

58. Pitts N. Children's dental health in the United Kingdom 2003. London: Her Majesty's Stationery Office.

59. Feldens CA, Kramer PF, Vidal SG, Faraco Junior IM, Vítolo MR. Traumatic dentalinjuries in the first year of life and associated factors in Brazilian infants.J Dent Child (Chic). 2008 Jan-Apr; 75(1):7-13.

60. Jorge KO, Moysés SJ, Ferreira e Ferreira E, Ramos-Jorge ML, de Araújo Zarzar PM. Prevalence and factors associated to dentaltrauma in infants 1-3 years of age. Dent Traumatol. 2009; 25(2):185-9.

61. Avsar A, Akba⊠ S, Ataibi⊠ T. Traumatic dentalinjuries in children with attention deficit/hyperactivity disorder. Dent Traumatol. 2009; 25(5):484-9.

62. Robson F, Ramos-Jorge ML, Bendo CB, Vale MP, Paiva SM, Pordeus IA. Prevalence and determining factors of traumatic injuries to primary teeth in preschool children. Dent Traumatol. 2009F; 25(1):118-22.

63. Ferreira JM, Fernandes de Andrade EM, Katz CR, Rosenblatt A. Prevalence of dentaltrauma in deciduous teeth of Brazilian children.DentTraumatol. 2009; 25(2):219-23.

64. Feldens CA, Kramer PF, Ferreira SH, Spiguel MH, Marquezan M. Exploring factors associated with traumatic dentalinjuries in preschool children: a Poisson regression analysis. Dent Traumatol. 2010; 26(2):143-8.

65. Wendt FP, Torriani DD, Assunção MC, Romano AR, Bonow ML, da Costa CT, Goettems ML, Hallal PC. Traumatic dentalinjuries in primary dentition: epidemiological study among preschool children in South Brazil. Dent Traumatol. 2010; 26(2):168-73.

66. Granville-Garcia AF, Vieira IT, Siqueira MJ, de Menezes VA, Cavalcanti AL. Traumatic dentalinjuries and associated factors among Brazilian preschool children aged 1-5 years. Acta OdontolLatinoam. 2010; 23(1):47-52.

67. Goettems ML, Ardenghi TM, Romano AR, Demarco FF, Torriani DD. Influence of maternal dental anxiety on oral health-related quality of life of preschool children. Qual Life Res. 2011; 20(6):951-9.

68. Piovesan C, Abella C, Ardenghi TM. Child oral health-related quality of life and socioeconomic factors associated with traumatic dentalinjuries in school children. Oral Health Prev Dent. 2011; 9(4):405-11.

69. Shekhar MG, Mohan R. Traumatic dentalinjuries to primary incisors and the terminal or occlusal plane relationship in Indian preschool children. Community Dent Health. 2011; 28(1):104-6.

70. Assunção LR, Ferelle A, Iwakura ML, do Nascimento LS, Cunha RF. Luxation injuries in primary teeth: a retrospective study in children assisted in an emergency service. Braz Oral res. 2011; 25(2):150-6.

71. Tümen EC, Adigüzel O, Kaya S, Uysal E, Yavuz I, Ozdemir E, Atakul F. Incisor trauma in a Turkish preschool population: prevalence and socio-economic risk factors. Community Dent Health. 2011; 28(4):308-12.

72. Noori AJ, Al-Obaidi WA. Traumatic dentalinjuries among primary school children in Sulaimani city, Iraq. Dent Traumatol. 2009; 25(4):442-6.

73. Viegas CM, Scarpelli AC, Carvalho AC, Ferreira FM, Pordeus IA, Paiva SM. Predisposing factors for traumatic dentalinjuries in Brazilian preschool children. Eur J Paediatr Dent. 2010; 11(2):59-65.

74. Fakhruddin KS, Lawrence HP, Kenny DJ, Locker D. Etiology and environment of

dentalinjuries in 12- to 14-year-old Ontario school children. Dent Traumatol. 2008; 24(3):305-8.

75. Gopinath VK, Ling KT, Haziani KN, Ismail NM. Predisposing factors and prevalence of fractured anterior teeth among 12 and 16 years old school Malaysian children. J Clin Pediatr Dent. 2008; 33(1):39-42.

76. Naidoo S, Sheiham A, Tsakos G. Traumatic dentalinjuries of permanent incisors in 11- to 13-year-old South African school children. Dent Traumatol. 2009; 25(2):224-8.

77. Adekoya-Sofowora CA, Adesina OA, Nasir WO, Oginni AO, Ugboko VI. Prevalence and causes of fractured permanent incisors in 12-year-old suburban Nigerian school children. Dent Traumatol. 2009; 25(3):314-7.

78. Noori AJ, Al-Obaidi WA. Traumatic dentalinjuries among primary school children in Sulaimani city, Iraq. Dent Traumatol. 2009; 25(4):442-6.

79. David J, Astrøm AN, Wang NJ.Factors associated with traumatic dentalinjuries among 12-year-old schoolchildren in South India. Dent Traumatol. 2009; 25(5):500-5. Epub 2009 Jul 9.

80. Piovesan C, Antunes JL, Guedes RS, Ardenghi TM. Impact of socioeconomic and clinical factors on child oral health-related quality of life (COHRQoL). Qual Life Res. 2010; 19(9):1359-66.

81. Bendo CB, Paiva SM, Oliveira AC, Goursand D, Torres CS, Pordeus IA, Vale MP. Prevalence and associated factors of traumatic dental injuries in Brazilian school children. J Public Health Dent. 2010; 70(4):313-8.

82. Livny A, Sgan-Cohen HD, Junadi S, Marcenes W. Traumatic dentalinjuries and related factors among sixth grade school children in four Palestinian towns.Dent Traumatol. 2010; 26(5):422-6.

83. Traebert J, Marcon KB, Lacerda JT. Prevalence of traumatic dentalinjuries and associated factors in schoolchildren of Palhoça, Santa Catarina State. Cien Saude Colet. 2010; 15Suppl 1:1849-55. Abstract in English

84. Castro RD, Portela MC, Leão AT, de Vasconcelos MT. Oral health-related qulity

of life of 11- and 12-years-old public school children in Rio de Janeiro. Community Dent Oral Epidemiol. 2011; 39(4):336-44.

85. Ravishankar TL, Kumar MA, Ramesh N, Chaitra TR. Prevalence of traumatic dentalinjuries to permanent incisors among 12-year-old school children in Davangere, South India.Chin J Dent Res. 2010; 13(1):57-60.

86. Taiwo OO, Jalo HP. Dentalinjuries in 12-year old Nigerian students. Dent Traumatol. 2011; 27(3):230-4.

87. Gopinath VK, Ling KT, Haziani KN, Ismail NM. Predisposing factors and prevalence of fractured anterior teeth among 12 and 16 years old school Malaysian children. J Clin Pediatr Dent. 2008; 33(1):39-42.

88. Huang B, Marcenes W, Croucher R, Hector M. Activities related to the occurrence of traumatic dentalinjuries in 15- to 18-year-olds. Dent Traumatol. 2009; 25(1):64-8.

89. Thelen DS, Bårdsen A. Traumatic dentalinjuries in an urban adolescent population in Tirana, Albania. Dent Traumatol. 2010; 26(5):376-82.

90. EcclesJD. Dental erosion of nonindustrial origin. A clinical survey and classification. J Prosthet Dent. 1979; 42(6):649-653.

91. Smith BG, Knight JK.A comparison of patterns of tooth wear with aetiological factors. Br Dent J. 1984 Jul 7; 157(1):16-19.

92. O'Brien M. Children´s dental health in the United Kingdom, 1993. London: OPCS. Her Majesty´s Stationery Office 1994; 74-76, 113.

93. Bartlett D, Ganss C, Lussi A. Basic Erosive Wear Examination (BEWE): a new scoring system for scientific and clinical needs. Clin Oral Investig. 2008; 12Suppl 1:S65-68.

94. Millward A, Shaw L, Smith AJ, Rippin JW, Harrington E. The distribution and severity of tooth wear and the relationship between erosion and dietary constituents in a group of children. Int J Paediatr Dent. 1994; 4(3):151-157.

95. Hinds K, Gregory J. National Diet and Nutrition Survey: children aged 1½ to

4½ years. Office of population censuses and surveys. London:HMSO, 1995.

96. Jones SG, Nunn JH. The dental health of 3-year-old children in east Cumbria 1993. Community Dent Health. 1995; 12(3):161-6.

97. Al-Malik MI, Holt RD, Bedi R. The relationship between erosion, caries and rampant caries and dietary habits in preschool children in Saudi Arabia. Int J Paediatr Dent. 2001; 11(6):430-9.

98. Luo Y, Zeng XJ, Du MQ, Bedi R. The prevalence of dental erosion in preschool children in China. J Dent. 2005; 33(2):115-121.

99. Murakami C, Oliveira LB, Sheiham A, Nahás Pires Corrêa MS, Haddad AE, Bönecker M. Risk indicators for erosive tooth wear in brazilian preschool children. Caries Res. 2011; 45(2):121-129

100. Al-Majed I, Maguire A, Murray JJ. Risk factors for dental erosion in 5-6 year old and 12-14 year old boys in Saudi Arabia. Community Dent Oral Epidemiol. 2002; 30(1):38-46

101. Harding MA, Whelton H, O'Mullane DM, Cronin M. Dental erosion in 5-year-old Irish school children and associated factors: a pilot study. Community Dent Health. 2003; 20(3):165-70.

102. Deshpande SD, Hugar SM. Dental erosion in children : an increasing clinical problem. J Indian SocPedodPrev Dent. 2004; 22(3):118-27.

103. Chen YG, Li X, Hu DY, Shen H, Li KZ, Zhao Y, Peng LL. [Prevalence of tooth erosion of 5-year-old and 12-year-old children in Xuzhou city].Hua Xi Kou Qiang Yi XueZaZhi. 2009 Oct; 27(5):565-7. Abstract in English

104. Dugmore CR, Rock WP. The prevalence of tooth erosion in 12-year-old children. Br Dent J. 2004 13; 196(5):279-82; Discussion 273.

105. Truin GJ, Frencken JE, Mulder J, Kootwijk AJ, Jong E. Prevalence of caries and dental erosion among school children in The Hague from 1996-2005. Ned Tijdschr Tandheelkd. 2007; 114(8):335-42. Abstract in English

106. Peres KG, Armênio MF, Peres MA, Traebert J, De Lacerda JT. Dental erosion in 12-year-old schoolchildren: a cross-sectional study in Southern Brazil. Int J Paediatr Dent. 2005; 15(4):249-255.

107. El Aidi H, Bronkhorst EM, Truin GJ. A longitudinal study of tooth erosion in adolescents. J Dent Res. 2008; 87(8):731-5.

108. Hou XM, Zhang Q, Chen XC, Wang JD. Prevalence of dental erosion and associated drinks in 12-year-old population of Beijing. Zhonghua Kou Qiang Yi XueZaZhi. 2009; 44(4):208-211

109. Arnadottir IB, Holbrook WP, Eggertsson H, Gudmundsdottir H, Jonsson SH, Gudlaugsson JO, Saemundsson SR, Eliasson ST, Agustsdottir H. Prevalence of dental erosion in children: a national survey. Community Dent Oral Epidemiol. 2010; 38(6):521-6

110. Deery C, Wagner ML, Longbottom C, Simon R, Nugent ZJ. The prevalence of dental erosion in a United States and a United Kingdom sample of adolescents. Pediatr Dent. 2000; 22(6):505-10.

111. El Karim IA, Sanhouri NM, Hashim NT, Ziada HM.Dental erosion among 12-14 year old school children in Khartoum: a pilot study. Community Dent Health. 2007; 24(3):176-80.

112. Wang X, Lussi A. Assessment and management of dental erosion. Dent Clin North Am. 2010; 54(3):565-78.

113. van Rijkom HM, Truin GJ, Frencken JE, König KG, van 't Hof MA, Bronkhorst EM, Roeters FJ. Prevalence, distribution and background variables of smooth-bordered tooth wear in teenagers in the hague, the Netherlands. Caries Res. 2002; 36(2):147-154.

114. Arnadóttir IB, Saemundsson SR, Holbrook WP. Dental erosion in Icelandic teenagers in relation to dietary and lifestyle factors. Acta Odontol Scand. 2003; 61(1):25-8.

115. Jensdottir T, Arnadottir IB, Thorsdottir I, Bardow A, Gudmundsson K, Theodors A, Holbrook WP. Relationship between dental erosion, soft drink consumption, and gastroesophageal reflux among Icelanders. Clin Oral Investig. 2004; 8(2):91-6.

116. Zhang M, McGrath C, Hägg U. The impact of malocclusion and its treatment

on quality of life: a literature review. Int J Paediatr Dent. 2006; 16:3

117. World Health Organization. Oral Health Surveys: Basic Methods. 3rd ed. Geneva: WHO 1987.

118. Johe RS, Steinhart T, Sado N, Greenberg B, Jing S. Intermaxillary tooth-size discrepancies in different sexes, malocclusion groups, and ethnicities. Am J Orthod Dentofacial Orthop 2010; 138:599-607.

119. Peres KG, Barros AJ, Peres MA, Victora CG.Effects of breastfeeding and sucking habits on malocclusion in a birth cohort study. Rev Saude Publica. 2007; 4:343-350.

120. Frazão P, Narvai PC, Latorre MRDO, Castellanos RA. Prevalência de oclusopatia na dentição decídua e permanente de crianças na cidade de São Paulo, Brasil, 1996. Cad. Saúde Pública 2002; 18:1197-1205.

121. Katz CR, Rosenblatt A, Gondim PP. Nonnutritive sucking habits in Brazilian children: effects on deciduous dentition and relationship with facial morphology.Am J Orthod Dentofacial Orthop. 2004; 126:53-57.

122. Marques LS, Barbosa CC, Ramos-Jorge ML, Pordeus IA, Paiva SM. Prevalência da maloclusão e necessidade de tratamento ortodôntico em escolares de 10 a 14 anos de idade em Belo Horizonte, Minas Gerais, Brasil: enfoque psicossocial. Cad. Saude Publica. 2005; 21:1099-1106.

123. Silva Filho OG, Santamaria Jr M, Capelozza Filho L. Epidemiologyof posterior crossbite in theprimarydentition. J. Clin Pediatr Dent. 2007; 32:73-78.

124. Leite-Cavalcanti A, Medeiros-Bezerra PK, Moura C. Breast-feeding, bottle-feeding, sucking habits and malocclusion in Brazilian preschool children. Rev Salud Publica. 2007; 9:194-204

125. Dhar V, Jain A, Van Dyke TE, Kohli A. Prevalence of gingival diseases, malocclusion and fluorosis in school-going children of rural areas in Udaipur district. J Indian Soc Pedod Prev Dent. 2007; 25:103-105.

126. Grabowski R, Stahl F, Gaebel M, Kundt G. Relationship between occlusal findings and orofacialmyofunctional status in primary and mixed dentition. Part I: Prevalence of malocclusions. J Orofac Orthop. 2007; 68:26-37.

127. Oliveira AC, Paiva SM, Campos MR, Czeresnia D. Factors associated with malocclusions in children and adolescents with Down syndrome. Am J Orthod Dentofacial Orthop. 2008; 133:489.e1-8.

128. Mtaya M, Brudvik P, Astrom AN. Prevalence of malocclusion and its relationship with socio-demographic factors, dental caries, and oral hygiene in 12- to 14-year-old Tanzanian school children. Eur J Orthod. 2009; 31:467-476.

129. Murshid ZA, Amin HE, Al-Nowaiser AM. Distribution of certain types of occlusal anomalies among Saudi Arabian adolescents in Jeddah city. Community Dent Health 2010; 27:238-241.

130. Abanto J, Carvalho TS, Mendes FM, Wanderley MT, Bönecker M, Raggio DP.Impact of oral diseases and disorders on oral health-related quality of life of preschool children.Community Dent Oral Epidemiol. 2011; 39:105-114.

131. Carvalho AC, Paiva SM, Scarpelli AC, Viegas CM, Ferreira FM, Pordeus IA. Prevalence of malocclusion in primary dentition in a population-based sample of Brazilian preschool children.Eur J Paediatric Dent. 2011; 12:107-111.

132. Aliaga-Del Castillho A, Mattos-Vela Ma, Aliaga-Del Castillo R, Del Castillo-Mendoza C. Malocclusions in children and adolescents from villages and native communities in the Ucayali Amazon region in Peru. Rev Peru Med ExpSalud Publica 2011; 28:87-91.

133. Mountain G, Wood D, Toumba J. Bite force measurement in children with primary dentition. Int J Paediatric Dent. 2011; 21:112-118.

134. Bhardwaj VK, Veeresha KL, Sharma KR. Prevalence of malocclusion and orthodontic treatment needs among 16 and 17 year-old school-going children in Shimla city, Himachal Pradesh. Indian J Dent Res. 2011; 22:556-60.

135. World Health Organization. Oral Health Surveys. Basic Methods. 4th ed. Geneva: WHO, 1997.

Chapter 3

A Social Determinants Approach to Reduce Inequalities and Promote General and Oral Health - Tackling the "Causes of the Causes"

Samuel Moysés
Aubrey Sheiham

Introduction

Most dental strategies to prevent oral diseases are directed at changing behaviours. Many of the models of behavioural change are based on the assumption of cognitively determined behaviour and psychological predispositions. Their basic premise is that preventive behaviour is a function of knowledge and perceptions of threat and other predominantly psychological models of behaviour change. Unsurprisingly, although widely used, such approaches to change behaviours have had limited positive impacts on changing behaviours and reducing chronic diseases.[1]

Policy makers should therefore recognize that people live in social, political, and economic systems that shape behaviours and access to resources they need to maintain good health.[2-5] Some behaviour change interventions can be effective in low-income groups[6] and a few well-conducted theory-based behaviour change techniques that focus on

manipulating "environmental contingencies" and enhancing self-efficacy are effective.[1,6,7] However, the individual behavioural change approach in dental settings has been relatively ineffective in changing long term behaviours[3, 8-10]. (See also Chapters 4, 5 and 16).

Whilst such behaviour change approaches need to be considered, it is very important to have a better understanding of the causes of the behaviours; "the causes of the causes".[11,12] Why do people behave in the ways they do? There is interplay between intrapersonal, behavioural and environmental determinants. The behaviours are linked to the conditions in which people are born, grow, live, work and age. While individuals make choices about how to behave, those choices are situated within economic, historical, family, cultural and political contexts. Individual behaviours, commonly referred to as proximal factors, such as smoking cigarettes, dietary patterns, drinking alcoholic beverages, drug taking and being physically inactive or leading a sedentary lifestyle, oral hygiene practices, attendance for medical and dental screening and care are largely influenced by the social environments and conditions in which people live and their status. Although those proximal behaviours are often cited as the major determinants of preventable morbidity, they account for a relatively small proportion of the variance in differences in health by socioeconomic position.[13-16]

This chapter will outline why it is essential to put the Common Risk Factor Approach (CRFA) into a broader social determinants and environmental perspective. That broader perspective requires a theoretical expansion relating to the CRFA as there is a need to refocus health promotion approaches to change behaviours by incorporating concurrent interventions at multiple levels, individual, family, community, and society.[17]

A social determinants of health (SDH) approach to improving oral health and reducing inequalities in health

To change individual behaviours, the conditions within which individuals live and work, the environments and social structures need to be changed. By changing the structure, behavioural change is allowed to occur.[18] Therefore there is a need to better understand the ways environments influence behaviours and health. Although socioeconomic differentials in mortality are due to a wider array of factors than behaviours, differentials in health outcomes persist even with improved health behaviours.[6,7] Most importantly, interventions are likely to be more effective if they target causal determinants of behaviour and behaviour change.[6] And as Watt[2, p. 716] has said "future improvements in oral health and a reduction in inequalities in oral health are dependant upon the implementation of public health strategies focusing on the underlying determinants of oral diseases".

Health is not merely a result of individual biological, psychological, and behavioural factors; it is the sum of collective social conditions created when people interact with the environment[19]. Health status is directly related to socioeconomic position across the socioeconomic gradient in all populations. Even in high-income countries where absolute poverty is uncommon, there is a fine and graduated pattern of inequality in health status across the full socioeconomic social spectrum.[20-24] There is a social gradient in health and oral health – the lower a person's social position, the worse their health.

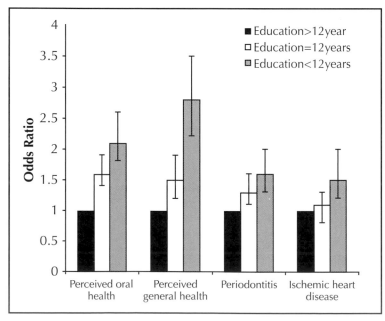

Fig. 3.1 – Social gradients in oral and general health.[25]

Rates of morbidity and mortality are successively lower at successively higher rungs on the social ladder; each unit increase in socioeconomic resource is linked to a corresponding improvement in health status. The WHO[26, p.5] recognized that "interventions which only tackle adverse health behaviours will have little success: they offer micro environmental solutions to a macro environmental problem". The behavioural decisions made by individuals are rooted in their social and economic circumstances. Childhood deprivation, the stress of poverty, overcrowding, living in a run-down area, feeling powerless at work and being unemployed do not give people the control over their lives that fosters good health and enables them to succeed in making difficult changes in behaviour.

Health is the outcome of a web of social influences.[27] It is determined by social determinants, the conditions in which people are born, grow, live, work, and age - that influence the occurrence of health problems and their risk factors in the population, such as type of housing, income, lifestyle, the economic policy of the country in which they live.[28,29] The web can be seen to constitute the social determinants of health.[30,31] The WHO Commission on Social Determinants of Health[32] defines social determinants of health (SDH) as the structural determinants and conditions of daily life responsible for a major part of health inequities between and within countries. Health determinants include: 1) social and physical environment, individual behaviours, genetics; and, 2) the health care system.

Concerns about determinants of health lead to the setting up of the WHO Commission on Social Determinants of Health – CSDH.[32] CSDH analyses the causes of ill health and the "causes of the causes" (See Box 3.1). The CSDH provides very convincing evidence that the structural factors and conditions of daily life are the major determinants of health and inequalities in health. Moreover, CSDH goes some way beyond medical care and individual responsibility as solutions to inequality in health. The social processes that produce differences in levels of health are the causes, rather than biological differences. So if we change the social determinants of health there will be dramatic improvements in health and health equity. The major conclusions of the CSDH are a wake-up call to all health professionals, policy makers and politicians. They herald a large shift in thinking about policies on promoting health and reducing inequalities. The CSDH is an optimistic report as it considers that if the actions recommended are adopted the health gap can be closed in a generation.

Box 3.1 – Smoking, obesity and heavy drinking are causes of ill-health, but what are the causes of these behaviours?

- The WHO Commission took a much broader approach to the determinants of health than the CRFA embodied.
- The Marmot Review drew attention not only to the causes of ill-health but to the causes of the causes.
- There is interplay between intrapersonal, behavioural and environmental determinants. The behaviours are linked to the conditions in which people are born, grow, live, work and age.
- That led social science and public health researchers to realize the underlying importance of psychosocial, economic, political and environmental factors to health and disease.

Social determinants are "societal risk conditions" rather than "individual risk factors" that either increase or decrease the risk for a disease in a population. Social determinants of health also determine the extent to which a person possesses the physical, social, and personal resources to identify and achieve personal aspirations, satisfy needs, and cope with the environment. Such an approach suggests a broader definition of health than the one used by dentists.[33] The primary factors that shape people's health are not medical and dental treatments or lifestyle choices. Rather, they are the conditions of life they experience. Health is also determined by the health and social services, and people's ability to obtain quality education, food and housing, among other factors. This relationship between social conditions and health is not a footnote to the "real" concerns with health – health care and unhealthy behaviours.[28] Thus, health promotion requires intense action in the broad social determinants of health, ranging from interrelationships between society's socioeconomic, cultural, and environmental policies, the educational programs and public health interventions to change personal habits.

McMichael[34, p. 634] puts risk factor epidemiology in perspective when he suggests that "modern epidemiology is thus oriented to explaining and quantifying the bobbing of corks on the surface waters, while largely disregarding the stronger undercurrents that determine where, on average, the cluster of corks ends up along the shoreline of risk." The focus on individual risks is associated with high risk strategies that have been seriously criticized and found wanting.[35-37] The limitations associated with individual level risk factor intervention approaches are that they divert limited resources away from healthy public policies; they blame the victim and produce a lifestyle approach to health policy, instead of a social policy approach to healthy lifestyles. Moreover, such intervention approaches decontextualize risk behaviours and overlook the ways in which such behaviours are culturally generated and structurally maintained. They seldom assess the relative contribution of non-modifiable genetic factors and modifiable social and behavioural factors that are harmful to the health of the targeted populations.[38-41]

The role of health-related behaviours in determining oral health

As stated above, determinants of health inequalities are different from determinants of health.[42] The fundamental differences are that determinants of health inequalities are about the "causes of the causes", the economic, social and physical environmental; that is, the fundamental structures of social hierarchy and the socially determined conditions in which people grow, live, work, and age,[12,32] whereas determinants of health are more related to proximal causes such as, in oral health, compromising behaviours: sugars consumption, smoking, poor hygiene and risk taking behaviours. Macro environmental factors, the national socioeconomic factors and the physical and social environment, are the principal determinants of inequalities in health. These factors influence living and working conditions of the individual, although their effect is moderated by local social and community conditions.

Ultimately, all these factors influence health behaviours which individuals adopt, particularly those behaviours which adversely affect health, namely, smoking, poor diet, lack of physical activity, excessive alcohol consumption and irresponsible sexual behaviour.

Many countries have goals to reduce inequalities in health, and recognize that interventions to achieve this must tackle the macro environmental factors and the physical and social environment, as well as adverse health behaviours and access to health care. The fundamental differences between micro and macro determinants of inequalities in health are highlighted by findings that individual behaviours are estimated to account for about 25% of health inequalities.[43-45] So, changing behaviours do have a role to play in improving health.[6]

Even so, if there were effective methods to alter the behaviours of the current adult population, rescuing them "downstream from the river"[11] will do little to change the socioeconomic conditions of the next generation and those conditions will generate the same behavioural and psychosocial characteristics in their children unless the conditions are changed. More people will be 'pushed in upstream' because the conditions generating the behaviours are largely unchanged. These upstream factors were referred to as the "social determinants of health" (Fig. 3.2).

The WHO report on the social determinants of health noted:[32 (p.42)] "For policy, however important an ethical imperative, values alone are insufficient. There needs to be evidence on what can be done and what is likely to work in practice to improve health and reduce health inequities". This is challenging, because understanding how to reduce health inequities between the poorest and better-off members of society may require a greater use of subgroup analysis to explore the differential effects of public health interventions.[46] While high quality evidence based health care is essential to reduce health inequalities, the effects of health care are undermined by social determinants which affect peoples' health and opportunity for good health.[47,48] This is particularly important in relation to inequalities of oral health, because effective treatments for caries and periodontal disease, for example, rely heavily on health promoting behaviours and adherence to recommended regimens.

The current position on social determinants of oral health is summed up by Sanders:[49 (p.vii)]

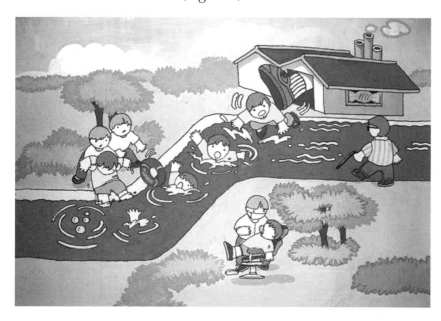

Fig. 3.2 – The upstream and downstream metaphor; a drawing by Thai children from the original by McKinlay.[11] Source: Aubrey Sheiham.

"The potency of social determinants to differentially affect population health status is influenced by the organisation of society and the ways in which society allocates resources through social service infrastructures including its health care system. Resource allocation is itself determined by the degree to which society views health as a collective public good, active responses to social policy, the balance with which it reconciles the dual objectives of maximising overall population welfare and reducing inequalities in health between social groups, and the economic philosophy it embraces in the belief in state responsibility for social expenditure versus promotion of the free market, competition and individual choice. Intriguingly, despite the wealth of evidence for the primacy of social determinants of health, public policy does not generally take action on them. Somewhere between recognition of their role and the setting of public policy, attention to the social determinants is lost. Frequently the determinants of health are reduced to behavioural risk factors such as smoking and alcohol consumption, physical inactivity and poor nutrition. Yet behaviours are not the primary determinants of health."

In spite of that, the fact that behaviours are not the primary determinants of health, social inequalities in general and oral health have been associated with social differences in lifestyle or behaviours, including parenting skills.[15,16,50-57] Such differences are found in nutrition, physical activity, tobacco and/or alcohol consumption, risk taking behaviours, hygiene. That indicates that differences in lifestyle could partially explain social inequalities in health, but researchers do not agree on their relative importance. Some regard differences in lifestyle as a sufficient explanation without further elaboration. Others regard them as contributory factors that in turn result from more fundamental causes.

Risk factors vary and operate differently for different socioeconomic groups.[44,58] Health compromising behaviours such as cigarette smoking, physical inactivity, poor diet, and substance abuse are closely related to both socioeconomic position (SEP) and health outcomes.[59-61] Epidemiologists have concluded that health and behaviour are influenced above all by social conditions.[62] For example, Blane et al.[63,64] reflect current thinking that a person's past social experiences become written into the physiology and pathology of their body. The social is literally embodied; and the body records the past. Similarly, Diez-Roux[65] (p.220) emphasises that "if context affects health it must somehow 'get into the body' and it ultimately operates through individual-level biochemical and psychological processes", as people are not 'blank slates' that can be moulded like clay. People's health bears the imprints of what positions they occupied from early life and currently occupy in the social hierarchy. Consequently, poorer conditions in early life cast long shadows forward over health in adult life.[66] Children in low socioeconomic status (SES) may produce a negative behavioural and psychosocial health dividend to be reaped in the future.[15] Davey Smith et al.[67,68] consider that socioeconomic and environmental factors become embodied and, through this biological embodiment, influence the health of people throughout their lives. And Brunner and Marmot[69] formulate models of pathways of the biological response to the social environment, suggesting that when people change their environment, their patterns of disease risk change, as do their behaviours.

Current research on the importance of social environments in relation to oral health is summed up by Sanders et al.[53] who state that to reduce social inequalities in adult oral health, efforts need to be directed to factors other than the dental behaviours of individuals. Rather than focusing on individuals alone, the approach needs to achieve a better balance of targeting both individual level factors and also the social environments in which health behaviours of individuals are developed and sustained.

So health related behaviours are an expression of the circumstances that condition and constrain an individual's behaviour. People respond to psychological stress and adverse circumstances by smoking, excessive alcohol consumption, comfort eating and risk taking.[70] Smoking, for example, is an activity engaged in by people in particular circumstances.[71-74] To understand why some people smoke and others do not requires knowledge of the activating circumstances.[75] Consequently, lifestyle, the clustering of behaviours, can be viewed as the manner in which social groups translate their objective situation into patterns of behaviour.[76,77] The propensity for risk behaviours to cluster indicates that behaviours are embedded in social environments and conditions in which people live.[78] Indeed, Blane[79, p. 432] argues that individual behaviours should be seen "as indicators of other factors which are more straightforwardly related to the social structure, and which are the true aetiological agents".

From an epidemiological perspective there are two patterns of health and behaviours that cast light on the psychosocial determinants of health behaviours. There is the universal finding that health inequalities in chronic disease mortality and morbidity and health behaviours are not found only between the rich and poor, or between 'the deprived' and 'everyone else'. They follow a social gradient. Health status and health related behaviours are related to socioeconomic status across the socioeconomic gradient in populations with relatively high socioeconomic status. The most advantaged have better health status than the less advantaged[80]. Leon et al.[81 (p.591)] declare: "Even in high income countries where there is little absolute poverty, there are fine and graduated inequalities in health status that span the full socioeconomic spectrum". Those in the higher ranks are healthier than those immediately below them. Social gradients in health, wherein health is better at each successive level of social position are consistently found for the majority of indicators in infancy, early childhood and adulthood.[21,22] What is more, the gradient exists for most kinds of ill health and causes of death and for most health related behaviours in industrialised populations.[23,82] Deaton[83, p.19] underlines that "the gradient across social classes in Britain in 1851 was markedly similar to that of a century and a half later, in spite of dramatic changes in the pattern of disease, so that even if policy is effective against particular diseases, it may have little effect on the gradient." The gradients in mortality and morbidity across socioeconomic classes appear to be relatively stable over long periods of time, even though the principal causes of death have changed considerably. This implies that there are underlying factors that influence susceptibility to a whole range of diseases.

Because the SES-health gradient is so enduring and general in the midst of diversity and change, SES-health researchers suggest that there is a generalized susceptibility to disease among those lower down the gradient.[84-87] Moreover, socio-economic differentials in health exist in all industrialised societies and occur throughout the social class scale, suggesting that there is not a threshold of absolute deprivation below which people are sicker, but a linear relationship between socio-economic circumstances and health[88]. Social position and economic and/or occupational disadvantage may be associated with generalized susceptibility to a wide range of diseases rather than with specific diseases and with specific dispositions to practice different health related behaviours (Figs. 3.3 and 3.4). It is apparent that a combination of factors - social, environmental, and individual - may be important and that to explain differentials in health; the cumulative effect of factors such as experiences from early life, health behaviours, and the environment in which people live and work may all contribute[89].

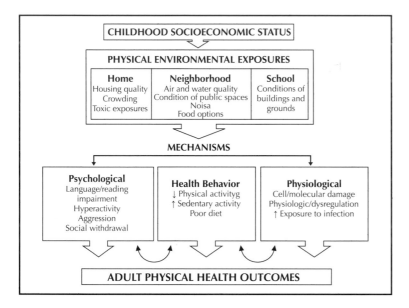

Fig. 3.3 – Examples of pathways that may link physical exposures associated with childhood and adolescent SES to adult health.[89]

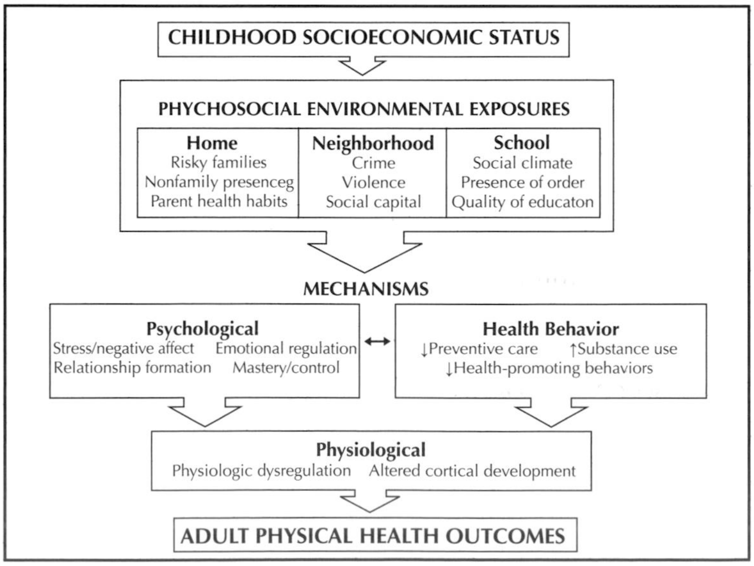

Fig. 3.4 – Examples of pathways that may link psychosocial exposures associated with childhood and adolescent SES to adult health.[89]

Surveys indicate that differences in lifestyle can only explain a small proportion of social inequalities in health. Material factors may act as a source of psychosocial stress, and psychosocial stress may influence health related behaviours, so each of them can influence health through specific biological factors. Adoption of health-threatening behaviours may be a response to material deprivation and stress, as "environments determine whether individuals take up tobacco, use alcohol, have poor diets, and engage in physical activity".[61] (p.38)

Policies and strategies to reduce inequalities and promote general and oral health

Strategies to improve health have oscillated between approaches relying on narrowly defined, technology-based medical/dental high-risk approaches and public health interventions, focused on tackling behaviour change through health education, or an understanding of health as a social phenomenon, requiring more complex forms of intersectoral policy action, and sometimes linked to a broader social justice agenda.[32,90,91]

Critics of health policy agree that health policies place too little emphasis on the social conditions that promote people's health and too much emphasis on personal responsibility and medical care for those at risk of disease.[11,92-95] Crawford[94, p. 663] points to "the emergence of an ideology which blames the individual for her or his illness and proposes that the individual should take more responsibility for her or his health". He argues that this ideology serves to divert attention from the social causation of diseases and to obscure the reality of class and the impact of social inequality on health. The critics therefore concluded that there was a case for "refocusing upstream" away from those individuals and groups who are mistakenly held responsible for their condition, toward a range of broader upstream political and economic forces.[11]

One of the most important insights in modern public health was put forward by Rose.[35, 96, 97] He proposes that "a large number of people exposed to a small risk may generate many more cases than a small number exposed to a high risk".[96] (p.37) This theorem has dramatic implications for public policies and resource allocation to improve the health of an entire population. With necessarily limited resources, large investments in questionably effective attempts to sustain a few high risk individuals leave little to promote the health of the majority. Appreciation of the continuum of risk suggests that small and perhaps even imperceptible improvements in everyone's health, including those at low risk, will yield greater overall gains for a society than very perceptible improvements in the level of health among a minority of high risk individuals. Moreover, as Rose points out, because the majority is usually at lower risk, they generate more cases than the small high risk group. Rose's critique of the high-risk strategy applies to dental disease. Batchelor and Sheiham,[37,98,99] in their refutation of the "80:20 dogma" that maintains that 80% of caries occurs in 20% of children, showed that approximately 90% of caries develops in the so-called low risk caries groups.

Based on the critical reassessments outlined above, Dahlgren and Whitehead[100-103] developed their model of the main determinants of health. The model makes clear that overarching societal factors operate through people's living and working conditions to influence health both directly and through health behaviour (Fig. 3.5).

Using the Dahlgren and Whitehead model, strategies can be developed at national, state and community levels or to classify specific interventions to capture their potential contribution to reducing inequalities in access to the determinants of good health (Fig. 3.6).

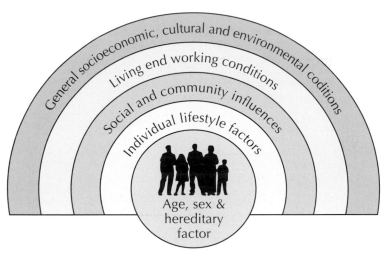

Fig. 3.5 – The main determinants of health.[100]

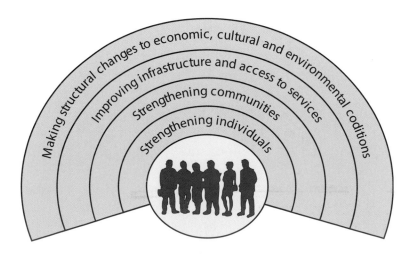

Fig. 3.6 – Policies and strategies to promote social equity in health.[104]

Subdivisions can be introduced into the category of 'individual risk factors' to separate behavioural factors (smoking, poor diet, oral and general hygiene practices, preventive health promoting practices including use of health facilities) and physiological factors (obesity, high blood pressure) or to distinguish between approaches favouring, for instance, drug-based interventions and behavioural interventions. As an analytical tool, the matrix could also serve as a stimulus for debate, to apply the matrix to specific policies to tease out divergences in perceptions of policy makers and the community.[105,106]

The WHO Commission on Social Determinants of Health - CSDH[32, 107] moved the agenda much further along. They recognized that existing health policies had failed to reduce inequities. The main groups of factors that have been identified as playing an important part in the explanation of health inequalities are material, psychosocial, and behavioural and/or biological factors. Social determinants of health are economic and social conditions that shape the health of individuals, communities, and jurisdiction as a whole. Social determinants of health also determine the extent to which a person possesses the physical, social, and personal resources to identify and achieve personal goals, satisfy needs of daily living, and cope with their environment. Some of the important social determinants of health include: early life factors or adversity in early life, low social status, education, employment and working conditions, relentless stress, food security and nutrition, addiction, gender, age, culture, neighbourhood and housing conditions, social networks or social exclusion, transportation, access to health care and an environment that promotes physical inactivity.

The WHO-CSDH used an important concept that corresponds to Graham's notion[30] of the social processes shaping the distribution of downstream social determinants. When referring to the more downstream factors, the CSDH use the term *intermediary determinants of health*. The structural determinants operate through a series of intermediary social factors or social determinants of health: "The social determinants of health inequities are causally antecedent to these intermediary determinants, which are linked, on the other side, to a set of individual-level influences, including health-related behaviours and physiological factors".[61, p. 35] The main categories of intermediary determinants of health are: material circumstances; psychosocial circumstances; behavioural and/or biological factors and the health system itself as a social determinant (Fig. 3.7).

Social-environmental or psychosocial circumstances include psychosocial stressors such as negative life events, job strain, stressful living circumstances and lack of social support and coping styles. Behavioural and biological factors include smoking, diet, alcohol consumption, and lack of physical exercise, which again can be either health protecting and enhancing, like exercise, or health damaging behaviours such as cigarette smoking and high sugars diets. Biological factors include genetic factors, and from the perspective of social determinants of health, age and gender distribution should be included.[61]

Graham[30,108] identified a spectrum ranging from remedying health disadvantages through narrowing health gaps to reducing health gradients. The first goal commits governments to improve the health of disadvantaged groups. The se-

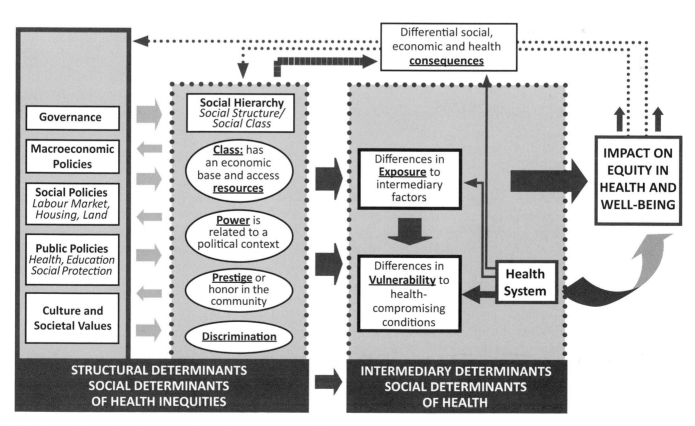

Fig. 3.7 – The role of intermediary determinants of health.

cond goal – to narrow health gaps – is more challenging as it requires a reversal of the trend towards widening health inequalities. To achieve it, the rate of health gain among the poorest groups needs to outstrip that achieved by the comparator group (typically defined as either the most advantaged group or the population as a whole). The goal of narrowing health gaps, like remedying health disadvantages, considers health inequalities as conditions which only those in disadvantaged circumstances are exposed. For that approach, strategies therefore focus solely on disadvantaged groups, seeking to improve their health in absolute terms; the more limited variant of the goal, and secondarily in relative terms. In contrast, the goal of reducing health gradients makes clear that health is unequally distributed not only between the poorest groups and the better-off majority but also across all socioeconomic groups.

For a broader concept of health inequalities that recognizes that health inequalities follow a social gradient, with the health gap increasing steadily with poorer social class, interventions must therefore reach more than the most di-

sadvantaged, socially excluded populations.[109] This wider framing of health inequalities demands a broader framing of policy goals known as "proportionate universalism".[32,61,110] Improving levels of health for the whole population requires a rate of health gain that is greatest for the poorest, progressively lower for better-off groups and lowest for those in the most advantaged circumstances. Differential rates of health improvement in turn require differential rates of improvement in the factors that promote good health.[106]

However, most interventions, both at the individual and community levels, remain focused on "downstream" tertiary treatments or one-on-one interventions directed at high-risk individuals. These efforts have their origins in the biomedical paradigm and risk factor epidemiology and the behavioural science research methods that serves as their handmaidens.[38] That prevailing paradigm is being challenged. We need to move beyond these "downstream" efforts towards a more appropriate whole population public health approach to health policy.[35]

There are three levels of public health interventions to improve health of the population:

1) Downstream efforts comprise treatments, rehabilitation, counselling and patient education for those already experiencing some disease and disability. This is the level which, while consuming most of the available resources, encompasses a very small segment of the general population;

2) Mid-stream prevention efforts to improve a population's health should involve two main areas: a) secondary prevention efforts which attempt to modify the risk levels of those individuals and groups who are very likely to experience some untoward outcome; b) primary prevention actions to encourage people not to commence risky health compromising behaviours that may increase their chances of experiencing a negative health event;

3) Even further upstream are healthy public policy interventions which include governmental, institutional, and organizational actions directed at entire populations which require adequate support through tax and fiscal structures, legal constraints and by reducing barriers to personal growth and making healthy choices easier and more harmful choices more difficult[111] and reimbursement mechanisms for those involved in health promotion and primary prevention.[38]

Although there are research studies on inequalities in health and numerous recommendations on interventions to reduce the inequalities, few interventions have been successful. Therefore it would be unrealistic to expect that a social determinants approach to reduce inequalities in oral health would be effective unless they adopt a linked strategy to reduce inequalities in general health, which is a multipronged approach to action on all determinants of health.[112] It will be important to consider a mix of strategies combining both upstream and downstream interventions. Graham[30,108] wisely mentions the importance of combined approaches, but maintaining the emphasis that the goal of reducing health gradients makes clear that health is unequally distributed not only between the poorest groups and the better-off majority but also across all socioeconomic groups. Therefore a population, rather high risk strategy focusing on disadvantaged groups should be adopted.[35,37,99] Such a strategy aims to change the slope of the gradient and thereby improve health for all.

The Health System and dental services as social determinants of health

Inadequate access to essential evidence based health services is one of the social determinants of social inequities in health. The concept of inequality and inequity in access to health care is captured by "the Inverse Care Law",[113] which says that the availability of good medical care tends to vary inversely with the need for it in the population served.

Therefore the role of the health system and services become particularly relevant through making good evidence–based quality care equitably accessible. In a comprehensive model, the health system itself should be viewed as an intermediary determinant. The health system can directly address differences in exposure and vulnerability not only by improving equitable access to care, but also in the promotion of intersectoral action to improve health status. The health system is capable of ensuring that health problems do not lead to a further deterioration of people's social status and should facilitate social reintegration of sick people.

The health system has at least three obligations in confronting inequity: (1) to ensure that resources are distributed between areas in proportion to their relative needs; (2) to respond appropriately to the health care needs of different social groups; (3) to take the lead in encouraging a wider and more strategic approach to developing healthy public policies at both the national and local level, to promote equity in health and social justice.[61,114,115]

Implications of policies on social determinants for Oral Health Promotion

The implications of the reports such as the WHO-CSDH and inequality for oral health are profound.[32,61] Oral health policy must focus much more attention on the social determinants of oral health and less on dental services. The social determinants are common to general and oral diseases.[116,117] Therefore, in the light of the CSDH's report there is an ethical human rights imperative for oral health planners to adopt and study and use a social determinants approach to promote oral health.[118]

Inequalities in oral health mirror those in general health[3]. The social gradient is consistently found for most common diseases, as well as oral diseases.[25,49,80,119-123] Social gradients in oral health persist over time and reflect the strong relationship between oral health and socioeconomic factors.[123] If social gradients in general and oral health are universal, then the determinants of the gradient needs to be addressed. Effective action to tackle oral health inequalities can only be developed when the underlying root causes of the problem are identified and understood. Clinical, and indeed much of modern epidemiological research, has concentrated on the individual "lifestyle" and biological risk factors.[124] Indeed, the dominant scientific approach in biomedical research has focused upon teasing out the molecular and genetic basis of disease at the micro level.[3] As oral diseases have risk factors in common with those of other chronic diseases there is a need for dental researchers to embed their research and policies with those working on the determinants of health inequa-lities. There is a major disconnect between research and policies to reduce inequalities in general health and dental research and oral health policies on inequalities in oral health.

In a critique of approaches used to improve oral health and reduce inequalities, Watt[3] concluded that a "radical reorientation" is required in oral disease prevention towards oral health promotion to achieve sustainable oral health improvements, and to reduce oral health inequalities, both between and within countries. The dominant oral health preventive model has evolved from the biomedical nature of dentistry, and an individual risk factor focus of much of clinical oral epidemiology. It is increasingly recognized that this approach alone will not be effective in achieving sustainable oral health improvements across the population, nor in reducing the oral health equity gap (Box 3.2). A paradigm shift is needed to one which addresses the underlying social determinants of oral health through a combination of complementary public health strategies.[2,9]

Box 3.2 – The limitations of the individual risk factor approach have been extensively reviewed. The reviews conclude that[2, 3, 116, 125-129]:

- This approach is ineffective and costly;
- It diverts limited resources away from upstream factors;
- "Lifestyle" interventions fail to acknowledge and address the underlying social determinants of health inequalities and are victim-blaming in nature;
- Many oral health education interventions lack a sound theoretical basis.

As stated above, a change in approach to prevent oral diseases and promote oral and general health is urgently required. The high-risk approach has dominated oral disease prevention as the inception of clinical prevention. This approach aims to focus attention on high-risk individuals. The high-risk approach is po-pular with both clinicians and health educators who espouse the behavioural origins of oral diseases. However, from a public health perspective, the approach has many limitations. The high-risk approach is palliative in nature. Action is not directed at the underlying causes of disease, so new high-risk individuals will therefore constantly emerge because the conditions creating disease have not been altered. Although extensive resources have been directed to investigating sophisticated means of identifying high--risk individuals, the predictive power of available screening tests are limited. In fact, one of the best available predictors of future caries is still past caries. Based upon Rose's original analysis of available approaches in preventive medicine, Baelum[130] have coined a useful expression, "sick teeth, sick individuals and sick populations". The widely used dominant high-risk approach that is popular among dental policy makers has demoted the more important population approach. In the population approach, "the causes of the causes" are addressed (Fig. 3.8). This more radical approach aims to address the underlying causes of disease across the whole population.[131,132]

A range of issues need to be addressed before significant progress is likely in reorienting dental public health research, practice and policy towards a social determinants model.[133-137] Among them are barriers such as the "lifestyle drift" – the tendency for policy to start off recognizing the need for action on upstream social determinants of health inequalities only to drift downstream to focus largely on individual lifestyle factors.[138] This emphasis on lifestyle factors distracts attention away from the determinants of the behaviours – the upstream causes of the causes. Therefore strategies should resist individualized victim-blaming lifestyle drift. Effective action to tackle oral health inequalities can only be developed when the underlying causes of the problem are identified and understood.

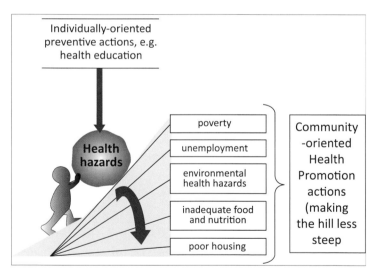

Fig. **3.8** – Health Promotion; Challenging the Sisyphus model that concentrates on the individual - Instead of focusing mainly on the individual and not making the health hazards load less, health promotion endeavours to make the hill less steep. "To make healthier choices the easier choices".

Public health research into the social determinants of health inequalities has identified causal pathways linking the biological, psychosocial, behavioural, environmental and political factors to health and disease outcomes is beginning to map out the social determinants of oral health inequalities. There is a need for closer collaboration and integration of dental public health activities with general health approaches. Building up suitable capacity among the dental public health workforce of personnel trained in a social determinants and population strategy framework is therefore a key priority.[128,129] A need also exists for better co-ordination of efforts, both within and between countries. In research, major gaps remain in the understanding of the social determinants of oral health and in particular of inequalities. The detailed nature and causal pathways linking biological, psychosocial, behavioural, environmental and political determinants of oral health inequalities need to be explored and researched in much greater depth. Rigorous, high-quality intervention studies need to be conducted and evaluated to identify effective measures to tackle oral health inequalities.

As the determinants of most non-communicable diseases are similar, so they have risk factors in common, it is logical and more efficient to integrate approaches to improve oral health with those directed at other major non-communicable diseases such as coronary heart disease, cancers, diabetes and obesity. Dental policy makers should stop using the vertical approach to prevention whereby each disease is treated in isolation from other diseases. Instead they should integrate their strategies with others who are using horizontal strategies.[139]

Frenk[140. p. 2] considers that "... it is not enough to develop health policies in the strict sectoral sense; we also need healthy policies that mobilize interventions from other sectors in order to pursue the social objective of better health." We must bridge the divide among three intellectual and programmatic traditions in public health. First, the social determinants of health; the second tradition has focused on specific interventions for specific disease categories - the so-called "vertical" approach to public health; lastly, the third tradition has taken a systemic or "horizontal" approach, seeking to modify the general structure and functioning of the set of organizations constituting the health system.

The Health Promotion Approach to reducing inequalities in oral health

Health promotion practice and policy is undergoing a radical change and is challenging the individualized health education model.[141] It has shifted the focus from behavioural change at the individual level that is orientated to separate diseases, to a health-oriented determinants approach, through the use of combinations of the five Ottawa Charter Action Areas.[142] There is convincing evidence that individualized health education approaches to prevent caries by dietary counselling or reinforcement of oral hygiene procedures in patients attending dental clinics are largely ineffective.[3,8,9] The effectiveness reviews highlight that most psychological theories of health behaviour changes used in oral health education largely ignore the fundamental importance of the social, environmental and political determinants of health. Systematic reviews on approaches used by dentists concluded that clinical prevention and health education approaches alone have been found to be relatively unsuccessful in achieving sustainable improvements in oral health (See Chapters 11 and 16).

A conceptual movement away from the traditional biomedical "downstream" and victim blaming approaches, to one addressing the "upstream" underlying social determinants of oral and general health is necessary.[8,143] Thus, there is a need for more supportive rather than judgemental approaches to oral health behaviour change. Oral health education programmes alone will have only a marginal impact and can indeed increase oral health inequalities. The poor effects of individualized approaches contrasts with more successful effects of environmental changes such as legislation to limit smoking, legislation and regulation on wearing seat belts and crash helmets, introducing regulations to get industry to change the composition of paediatric medicines by excluding sugars, developing guidelines on changing the composition of foods and drinks so that healthy choices are easier for people, government or community action to provide healthy low sugars and fats in meals in nursery and schools, and encouraging marketing low cost fluoride and anti-calculus toothpastes.

As the most common non communicable diseases such as obesity, coronary heart disease, cancers and dental caries and periodontal disease have major risk factors in common, the main strategy, and the one that requires considerably more dental research, is how to reduce the intake of sugars and increase fruit and vegetables consumption and reduce smoking.[144] That will require a shift in the emphasis of dental research to behavioural science and health promotion research to investigate methods of increasing health enhancing and reducing health-compromising behaviours.

Despite the declines in caries, in some communities there are sections of the population who have relatively high caries rates. The higher levels of caries in vulnerable groups suggest that they may be exposed to multiple risks and are likely to have other health problems. Prevention should therefore be reoriented to a broad community perspective which tackles the causes, the determinants of diseases, and makes healthy choices easier and unhealthy choices more difficult for most people.[143,145,146]

Tackling determinants and resulting behaviours requires an analysis of which approaches to use and what is the best strategy to apply. A rigorous exploration of the determinants of the major oral health problems would provide information that can be applied to improving oral health. It will also point to the greater importance of oral health promotion research agenda and policy strategies working in an effective global collaboration.[29]

The International Association for Dental Research (IADR) has set up a Global Oral Health Inequalities Task Group (GOHIRA) to review the shortcomings of present approaches to reduce oral diseases and inequalities, the importance of social determinants, and tied that to translational research needs and policies on implementation of strategies to reduce oral health inequalities.[110] The GOHIRA Task Group has synthesized current evidence to identify a five-year implementation and research agenda which should lead to improvements in global oral health. The recommendations and directions for change recommended by GOHIRA are outlined in Box 2.3.

Box 3.3 – The Key Points from the GOHIRA Review:

- The root causes of health inequalities are to be found in the social, economic and political mechanisms that give rise to a set of hierarchically ordered socioeconomic positions within society.
- Reducing health inequalities is a matter of fairness and social justice.
- There is a social gradient in health.
- Health inequalities result from social inequalities. Action on health inequalities requires action across all the social determinants of health.
- Focusing solely on the most disadvantaged will not reduce health inequalities sufficiently. To reduce the steepness of the social gradient in health, actions must be universal, but with a scale and intensity that is proportionate to the level of disadvantage. We call this proportionate universalism.
- Variation in determinants between groups suggests that health inequalities may not be unavoidable.
- A consistent equity-based approach to Social Determinants of Health (SDH) must ultimately lead to a gradients focus a proportionate universalism approach. However, strategies based on tackling health disadvantage, health gaps and gradients are not mutually exclusive. They can complement and build on each other.
- Arguably the single most significant lesson of the WHO Commission on Social Determinants of Health (CSDH) conceptual framework is that interventions and policies to reduce health inequities must not limit themselves to intermediary determinants, but must include policies specifically crafted to tackle underlying structural determinants: the social mechanisms that systematically produce an inequitable distribution of the determinants of health among population groups.
- To tackle structural as well as intermediary determinants requires intersectoral policy approaches.
- Interventions addressing intermediary determinants can improve average health indicators while leaving health inequities unchanged. For this reason, policy action on structural determinants is necessary.
- Intersectoral policymaking and implementation are crucial. This is because structural determinants can only be tackled through strategies that reach beyond the health sector.

Directions for Change:
- Shift emphasis away from individual to population determinants of oral health.
- Policies should be based on Proportionate Universalism.
- Tackle causes common to a number of chronic diseases - Common Risk/Health Factor Approach (CRHFA).
- Intersectoral policymaking and implementation are crucial.
- Integrate oral health into general health strategies.
- Act as advocates tackling the determinants of chronic diseases.
- Adopt a population rather than an individual strategy.
- Implement evidence based appropriate policies.

With particular reference to integrated action to reduce dental caries the Group determined that research should:[147]

a) Integrate health and oral health wherever possible, using common risk factors;

b) Be able to respond to and influence international developments in health, healthcare, and health payment systems as well as dental prevention and materials;

c) Exploit the potential for novel funding partnerships with industry and foundations;

d) More effective communication between and among the basic science, clinical science, and health promotion/public health research communities is needed.

For periodontal diseases, which constitute one of the major global oral health burdens, remaining a major cause of tooth loss in adults worldwide, the GOHIRA[148] propose twelve basic, translational, and applied research areas to address the issue of global periodontal health inequality.

In addition, considering the huge global inequalities that exist in all four oral mucosal infections identified as Global Oral Health Priorities: (a) HIV and associated viral, bacterial, and fungal infections; (b) tuberculosis; (c) NOMA; and (d) sexually transmitted diseases, it is imperative that this understanding be translated into affirmative action in lower- and middle-income countries to help oral health workers play their role in health teams for implementation of action programs, as these oral manifestations are largely associated with multisystem diseases.[149-152]

A short example of an approach and strategies to further reduce caries rates in groups with relatively high caries rates is presented here. Reducing caries in the high caries group is linked to reducing the rates in the majority of the child population at low risk.[37, 99] Why? Because the distribution of caries is a continuum; one cannot separate the high caries tail of the frequency distribution from the body of the populations' distribution. However, those in the high disease tail of the frequency distribution are usually in low socioeconomic posi-

tions or immigrant and refugee groups. These vulnerable groups may be exposed to numerous adverse social and economic conditions.[153-155] The changes in dental practice and approaches to prevention involve tackling the determinants of chronic diseases, including dental caries, and helping to "make healthy choices the easier choices and unhealthy choices more difficult"[111, 156], creating conditions for people to lead flourishing lives.[61]

There are significant changes in health promotion policy at international and national levels. The WHO-CSDH[32] provides convincing evidence that structural determinants and conditions of daily life are the major determinants of health and inequalities in health. The major conclusions of the CSDH are a wake-up call to all health professionals, including the oral health team. They herald a large shift in thinking about policies on promoting health. An environmental approach to disease prevention and health promotion is needed because many individually focused models of behaviour change have been relatively unsuccessful and persistence of the determinants would lead other people to adopt poor health behaviours and replace those who may have modified their behaviour following health education.[109,157,158] It is unreasonable to expect that people will change their behaviours when so many forces in the social, cultural and physical environment work against change.

On the other hand, if the social determinants of health are changed for the better, then there will be dramatic improvements in health equity between and within countries. Major contributions to improvement in oral health come from environmental influences, behavioural changes and, lastly, specific preventive and therapeutic measures.[159,160] Therefore greater emphasis must be placed on tackling the determinants of diseases – the environmental perspective, as poor social and economic circumstances affect health throughout life.[161] To change people's behaviours, change their environment. So, strategies to prevent oral disease should pay attention not only to the behaviour of individuals, but also to the environmental context within which people live.[162] Hence, the health pyramid suggested by Frieden[163] should be used to decide on priorities for action on health promotion and disease prevention (Fig. 3.9).

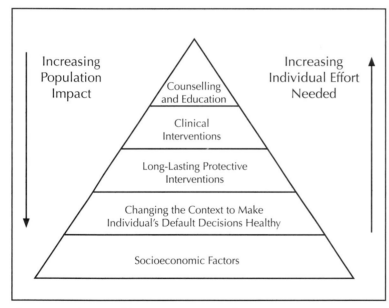

Fig. 3.9 – The Health Impact pyramid.[163]

Efforts to address socioeconomic determinants are given the highest priority followed by public health community-wide enabling measures interventions that change the context for health by making healthy choices the easier default decisions. Protective interventions with long-term benefits have higher priority than clinic-based prevention because an environment-based strategy offers greater scope for improvements in oral health than a strong commitment to individual dental care. In dental practice, however, even the best programs at the pyramid's higher levels achieve limited public health impact, largely because of their dependence on long-term individual's behaviour change. Therefore emphasis should be given to policies that make healthy choices the easier choices and health compromising choices more difficult and socially unacceptable.[111]

As dental interventions to reduce inequality are unlikely to focus on the socioeconomic determinants except to support political efforts to change the slope of the social gradient, the main priority for dental preventive interventions should be on collaborative integrated enabling research and policies that address the main proximal determinants of oral diseases: sugars, smoking, hygiene, risky behaviours and stress. The cornerstone of that approach is the Integrated Common Risk Factor Approach (CRFA).[116,127,133,164,165]

Specific policies for improving oral and dental health

The policies for improving oral health include efforts to get better health by reducing risks, promoting health and strengthening possibilities to cope with risk factors. There are a range of options to promote oral health. They are healthy public policies, legislation, regulation and fiscal measures and can all be utilized to promote oral health either at international, national and local levels. For example, at international level the WHO has published recommendations from expert committees on nutrition guidelines for a healthy diet.[166] Similarly the Health Promoting Schools (HPS) approach is recommended[167] as a strategy for promoting the health of young people. At national and local levels diet and nutrition and smoking guidelines should be used by nurseries, schools, hospitals and workplaces to create environments providing healthy food and drinks.[168]

There is a hierarchy of levels at which to intervene in a country. The highest is at national, regional and local levels, where government can legislate and regulate and implement fiscal measures, whereby health damaging products are taxed. Legislation includes no smoking policies, dietary guidelines banning sugary foods and drinks from nurseries and schools and requiring vegetables and salads and fruit in school meals. Dietary guidelines and policies on smoking can be backed up by media campaigns and school health education. The next level of priority is a Health Settings Strategy. The Health Settings Strategy is the main strategy for dental health personnel to work within. So it is ideal for the Directed Vulnerable Populations Strategy (DVPS) and the Integrated Common Risk Factor Approach (CRFA).

As with approaches by most other health professional groups, most dental efforts focus on the prevention of single diseases: caries, periodontal disease, oral cancer, and do not consider that determinants of oral diseases are common to a number of chronic diseases. Health promotion cannot and should not be compartmentalized to address problems and diseases of specific parts of the body. Probably, this is the main reason for the paucity of studies undertaken and minimal evidence of effectiveness of dentists and dental teams in

smoking prevention, smoking cessation, advice on alcohol consumption, diet counselling, advice on physical exercise, advice on skin cancer prevention and blood pressure monitoring.[169]

A new approach is needed. Until recently, the dominant approach to general health promotion has focused on actions to reduce specific diseases instead of directing policies to risk factors common to a number of diseases. The new approach is the CRFA where risk factors common to a number of major chronic diseases are tackled (Fig. 3.10).

That approach should be integrated with other sectors in horizontal programmes directed at improving general health and reducing non-communicable diseases. For example, it is imperative that dental planners collaborate with planners in other sectors to implement the WHO 2008-2013 Action Plan (Box 3.4), for the Global Strategy for the Prevention and Control of Noncommunicable Diseases using the CRFA.[170]

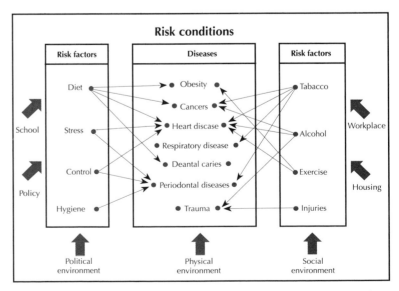

Fig. 3.10 – The Integrated Common Risk Factor Approach – CRFA[2].

Box 3.4 – The WHO Action Plan has six objectives:

1) To raise the priority accorded to noncommunicable disease in development work at global and national levels, and to integrate prevention and control of such diseases into policies across all government departments.

2) To establish and strengthen national policies and plans for the prevention and control of noncommunicable diseases.

3) To promote interventions to reduce the main shared modifiable risk factors for noncommunicable diseases: tobacco use, unhealthy diets, physical inactivity and harmful use of alcohol.

4) To promote research for the prevention and control of noncommunicable diseases.

5) To promote partnerships for the prevention and control of noncommunicable diseases, with interventions to reduce the main shared modifiable risk factors for noncommunicable diseases: tobacco use, unhealthy diets, physical inactivity and harmful use of alcohol.

6) To monitor noncommunicable diseases and their determinants and evaluate progress at the national, regional and global levels.

Integrating oral health in a CRFA is both logical and feasible. Risk factors common to major life threatening diseases like heart disease and cancer are best tackled on a broad front. The same risk factors affect oral diseases. Dentists should welcome the CRFA approach and develop strategies that fit in with general health promotion policies.[118]

There are three preventive strategies: two types of Risk Strategy and the Population Strategy (see Box 3.5). The two types of Risk Strategy are the High-Risk Strategy (HRS) and the Directed Vulnerable Populations Strategy (DVPS). In one kind of risk strategy, the HRS, individuals at risk are identified by screening. In the second kind of risk approach, the DVPS, vulnerable groups are identified by conventional oral health surveys, not by screening. A vulnerable population is defined by a higher measured exposure to a specific risk factor, being a subgroup or subpopulation who, because of shared social characteristics, is at higher risk of risks.[109] They may be people who share adverse social conditions such as living in a particular area that puts them at higher risk, or attending particular low socioeconomic schools with higher rates of caries, and, as is becoming more common in Europe, being from an immigrant group.

Box 3.5 – Preventive Strategies:

The Risk Strategy:
High-Risk Strategy (HRS), which seeks to identify individuals at high risk through screening and targeting them with evidence based interventions.
Directed Vulnerable Populations Strategy (DVPS), which protects sections of the population that share social characteristics that put them at higher risk of risks.
The Population Strategy:
Efforts are made to shift the risk distribution of the entire population to a more favourable level.

A major shortcoming of the HRS is that even if it were effective, the reductions in the overall number of new caries lesions in a population is very small because, according to Rose[35,96] the largest burden of ill health comes more from the many who are exposed to low inconspicuous risk than from the few who face an obvious problem, which is a finding supported in oral health studies.[37] Thus, risk differences between defined populations involve differences in the population distributions as a whole, rather than in the proportion of individuals with high risk.[171] In one dental study, when answering the question 'do low risk sub-groups develop more lesions than those with high caries levels', Batchelor and Sheiham[37] found that the majority of new lesions occurred in those children classified at lowest caries risk. Irrespective of the preventive regime adopted and the initial caries levels, children classified as "highest risk" contributed less than 6% of the total number of new caries lesions developing over a 4 year period. Hausen et al.[172] supported Batchelor and Sheiham's findings in their intervention study. Although at baseline 20% of Finnish children in the trial accounted for 80% of the DMF, over the three years of using a HRS intervention, a larger number of cavities developed in the 80% of low risk children than in the high-risk group 20% of children. These findings have important implications for deciding on which strategy to use. The Finnish trial shows that it is difficult, but not impossible, to help the high caries-risk individuals by measures that are normally applied in dental clinics. To further reduce caries among the high-risk children, the approach should be directed to the whole population or at vulnerable groups using a DVPS.

There is a growing consensus on the limitations of solely adopting a HRS in oral disease prevention. Another strategy is available. One that combines of both population and risk strategies.[9,36,173]

The Population Strategy (PS) is a radical approach as it is focused on the causes of the distribution; the determinants.[35] The PS controls the causes of the incidence of disease, whereas the HRS tries to protect and is palliative rather than radical. In the PS, efforts are made to shift the risk distribution and the frequency distribution of caries of the entire population to a more favourable level thereby decreasing the average risk of the population and the frequency distribution of disease and risk is moved to the left (Fig. 3.11).

Even a small decrease in the average level of a risk factor may result in a considerable reduction in the incidence of a health problem of the whole population. The PS can be applied nationally. However, when there are vulnerable groups or subsections of a population with high caries levels then the DVPS is applied. For the DVPS, although the group or district is selected as being at higher risk than elsewhere, the principles of the PS are used.

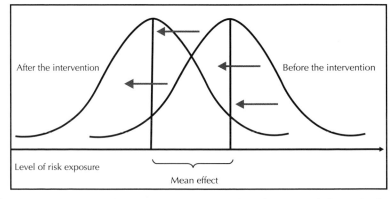

Fig. 3.11 – Population Strategy: the distribution of the whole population is shifted to the left.[35]

The pivotal factor used to determine the choice of preventive strategy is the axiom "that a large number of people exposed to a small risk may generate many more cases than a small number of people exposed to a high risk".[96, p.37] The more successful the PS, the less pronounced will be the so-called "tail" of the caries distribution curves which represents the so-called "high-risk subgroup", which some consider requires more individualized preventive and treatment programs. Where the high-risk subgroup fulfils the criteria for a vulnerable population then the DVPS is the strategy of choice. Table 3.1 identifies some interventions that have been, or can be, used in addressing oral health inequities.

The role of dentists

Most dental practitioner involvement in policy development will be as health advocates. Health advocacy is the actions of health professionals and others with perceived authority in health to influence decisions and actions of individuals, communities and government which influence health. Health advocacy involves educating senior government and community leaders and journalists - decision-makers in general, about specific issues and setting the agenda to obtain political decisions that improve health of the population. Health advocates place their skills at the disposal of the community - being on tap not on top.[127,174-176]

Table 3.1 – Interventions to reduce oral health inequities.[123]

Component	Social determinants and entry-points	Interventions to address oral health inequities
Socioeconomic context and position	• *Inequality of social structures and socioeconomic positions* • *Unequal distribution of resources and opportunities* • *Promoting equitable policies; and the availability of, and access to, resources* • *Infrastructure* • *Taxation and legislation*	• *Legislate local production of quality, affordable oral health products (e.g. toothpaste, toothbrushes)* • *Removal of taxes for oral health products* • *Placing oral health within the primary health care approach* • *Fair and equitable policies* • *Develop infrastructure for oral health services and population-based interventions*
Differential exposure	• *Water and sanitation* • *Fluorides and healthy food supply* • *Unhealthy environments* • *Lifestyles, beliefs, attitudes and health behaviours* • *Targeting settings and common risk factors* • *Social stigma of oral conditions*	• *Regulation on tobacco ban, fluoridation, better labelling, amount of fat, sugars and salt in foods and drinks, excess use of alcohol, advertising* • *Promote the use of mouth guards and safety helmets* • *Encourage interventions that adopt a common risk factor approach (tobacco, diet, alcohol, stress and personal hygiene)* • *Support healthy physical and psychosocial environments: e.g. roads (designs, lighting, traffic control, pedestrian facilities); living environments (physical, tackle overcrowding, etc.); schools; workplace; sanitation facilities and safe water supply* • *Encourage optimal exposure to fluorides: support implementation of fluoridation programmes (water, milk, salt and toothpaste) and, in some areas where necessary, defluoridation programmes*

Table 3.1 – Interventions to reduce oral health inequities[123]. (Continued)

		• *Promote oral health through general health prevention, health promotion and health education* • *Promote oral health through "healthy settings" initiatives (schools, workplace, cities and community-based establishments), and encourage them to be part of a larger network such as health-promoting schools networks*
Differential vulnerability	• *Poverty* • *Stress-induced responses to risk exposure* • *General health conditions* • *High-risk groups* • *Early life experiences* • *Access to oral health services, oral health products and protective options*	• *Greater availability of sugar-free alternatives and medicine* • *Support interventions and make tools available for breaking poverty and social inequities* • *Support measures that promote healthy eating and nutrition (e.g. healthy school dinners and healthy vending machines), and reduce amount of sugars, salt and fat in foods and drinks* • *Reorient oral health services, including capacity building and community-based oral health care provision to improve access and availability* • *Promote the availability of quality affordable oral health products (e.g. toothpaste, toothbrushes), subsidized oral health products and healthy foods and drinks* • *Regulate sale of harmful or unhealthy products to certain high-risk groups in certain settings* • *Promote oral health through chronic disease prevention, health promotion and health education* • *Integrate oral health into community, local, national and international health programmes* • *Work in collaboration across government departments and with local communities, other sectors, agencies, and nongovernmental and other organizations to promote oral health*
Differential health care outcomes	• *Uptake of oral health services* • *Inadequate oral health care provision and treatment options* • *High-risk groups*	• *Target resources that support disadvantaged or high-risk groups such as children, older people, people with HIV/AIDS, and people with oral cancer* • *Improve early detection of oral cancer and NOMA with timely treatment and referrals* • *Tobacco cessation services in dental practices* • *Include oral health in training of members of the primary health care team*
Differential consequences	• *Impact on quality of life* • *High personal, social and health service costs* • *Impact on other communities and social groupings* • *Social exclusion, stigma, effect on daily living*	• *Regulate sale of harmful or unhealthy products to certain high-risk groups in certain settings* • *Encourage healthy diets and moderate consumption of alcohol* • *Outreach oral health care towards vulnerable and poor population groups* • *Third-party payment systems reducing inequity in use of oral health service*

The objectives of dental planners should be to make healthy choices the easier choices. They should find which internal incentives promote enthusiasm for quality, economy and good patient service. Rational strategies for oral health promotion should incorporate policies to control the determinants of the distribution of oral diseases, establish goals and strategies on evidence-based oral health promotion.[177] Oral health promotion programmes will be enhanced by dentists establishing a national or local Oral Health Promotion Group or an Oral Health Action Team to ensure that oral health promoting strategies are incorporated into general health promotion plans. The oral health community must be "at the table" with other health professions and create opportunities for eliminating inequalities through collaborations of multiple sectors and institutions.[178]

References

1. Michie S, Abraham C. Health psychology in practice. Oxford: Blackwell Pub., and the British Psychological Society; 2004.

2. Watt RG. Strategies and approaches in oral disease prevention and health promotion. Bulletin of the World Health Organization. 2005; 83(9):711-718.

3. Watt RG. From victim blaming to upstream action: tackling the social determinants of oral health inequalities. Community Dentistry and Oral Epidemiology. 2007; 35(1):1-11.

4. Smedley BD, Syme SL. Promoting health: intervention strategies from social and behavioral research. American Journal of Health Promotion. 2001; 15(3):149-66.

5. National Research Council, Institute of Medicine. Promoting Health: Intervention Strategies from Social and Behavioral Research. Committee on Capitalizing on Social Science and Behavioral Research to Improve the Public's Health, Division of Health Promotion and Disease Prevention. Washington, DC: The National Academies Press; 2000.

6. Michie S, Jochelson K, Markham WA, Bridle C. Low-income groups and behaviour change interventions: a review of intervention content, effectiveness and theoretical frameworks. Journal of Epidemiology and Community Health. 2009; 63(8):610-22.

7. Michie S, Fixsen D, Grimshaw JM, Eccles MP. Specifying and reporting complex behaviour change interventions: the need for a scientific method. Implementation Science. 2009; 4:40.

8. Yevlahova D, Satur J. Models for individual oral health promotion and their effectiveness: a systematic review. Australian Dental Journal. 2009; 54(3):190-7.

9. Watt RG. Emerging theories into the social determinants of health: implications for oral health promotion. Community Dentistry and Oral Epidemiology. 2002; 30(4):241-247.

10. Freeman R, Ismail A. Assessing patients' health behaviours. Essential steps for motivating patients to adopt and maintain behaviours conducive to oral health. Monographs in Oral Science. 2009; 21:113-27.

11. McKinlay JB. A case for refocussing upstream – the political economy of illness. In: Enelow AJ, Henderson JB, editors. Applying behavioural science to cardiovascular risks, Proceedings of American Heart Association conference. Seattle, WA: American Heart Association; 1974. p. 7-17; republished in: Jaco EG (ed.). Patients, Physicians, and Illness: A Sourcebook in Behavioral Science and Health. New York: Free Press. 1979; pp.9-25.

12. Marmot M. Achieving health equity: from root causes to fair outcomes. The Lancet. 2007; 370(9593):1153-1163.

13. Rose G, Marmot MG. Social class and coronary heart disease. British Heart Journal. 1981; 45(1):13-9.

14. Davey Smith G, Bartley M, Blane D. The Black report on socioeconomic inequalities in health 10 years on. British Medical Journal. 1990; 301(6748):373-377.

15. Lynch JW, Kaplan GA, Salonen JT. Why do poor people behave poorly? Variation in adult health behaviours and psychosocial characteristics by stages of the socioeconomic lifecourse. Social Science and Medicine. 1997; 44(6):809-19.

16. Lantz PM, House JS, Lepkowski JM, Williams DR, Mero RP, Chen J. Socioeconomic factors, health behaviors, and mortality: results from a nationally representative prospective study of US adults. JAMA. 1998; 279(21):1703-8.

17. National Research Council. New Horizons in Health: An Integrative Approach. Board on Behavioral, Cognitive, and Sensory Sciences. Commission on Behavioral and Social Sciences and Education. Committee on Future Directions for Behavioral and Social Sciences Research at the National Institutes of Health. Washington, DC: National Academy Press. 2001.

18. Slama K. Background information for adopting a policy encouraging earmarked tobacco and alcohol taxes for the creation of health promotion foundations. Promotion & Education. 2006; 13(1):8-13.

19. Allegrante JP, Hanson DW, Sleet DA, Marks R. Ecological approaches to the prevention of unintentional injuries. Italian Journal of Public Health. 2010; 7(2):24-31.

20. Starfield B. Equity and health: a perspective on nonrandom distribution of health in the population. Revista Panamericana de Salud Publica. 2002; 12(6):384-7.

21. Starfield B, Riley AW, Witt WP, Robertson J. Social class gradients in health during adolescence. Journal of Epidemiology and Community Health. 2002; 56(5):354-61.

22. Starfield B, Robertson J, Riley AW. Social class gradients and health in childhood. Ambulatory Pediatric. 2002; 2(4):238-46.

23. Marmot M. The social pattern of health and disease. In: Blane D, Brunner E, Wilkinson R, editors. Health and social organization; towards a health policy for the twenty-first century. London: Routledge. 1996; p.42-67.

24. Leon D, Walt G, editors. Poverty, inequality and health: an international perspective. Oxford: Oxford University Press. 2000.

25. Sabbah W, Tsakos G, Chandola T, Sheiham A, Watt RG. Social gradients in oral and general health. Journal of Dental Research. 2007; 86(10):992-6.

26. WHO - World Health Organization. Closing the health inequalities gap: An international perspective. Copenhagen: The WHO European Office for Investment for Health and Development, with University of Dundee, and NHS - Health Scotland. 2005.

27. Krieger N. Epidemiology and the web of causation: has anyone seen the spider? Social Science and Medicine. 1994; 39(7):887-903.

28. Marmot M, (Chair). Fair Society, Healthy Lives (The Marmot Review): Strategic review of health inequalities in England post-2010. London: Marmot Review; 2010.

29. Marmot M, Bell R. Social determinants and dental health. Advances in Dental Research. 2011; 23(2):201-6.

30. Graham H. Social determinants and their unequal distribution: clarifying policy understandings. Milbank Quarterly. 2004; 82(1):101-124.

31. Centers for Disease Control and Prevention. CDC Health Disparities and Inequalities Report — United States, 2011. MMWR Morbidity and Mortality Weekly Report. 2011; 60(Supplement):113.

32. WHO - World Health Organization, Commission on Social Determinants of Health. Closing the gap in a generation: Health equity through action on the social determinants of health. Geneva: WHO. 2008.

33. Mikkonen J, Raphael D. Social Determinants of Health: The Canadian Facts. To-

ronto: York University School of Health Policy and Management. 2010.

34. McMichael AJ. The health of persons, populations, and planets: epidemiology comes full circle. Epidemiology. 1995; 6(6):633-635.

35. Rose G. Rose's Strategy of Preventive Medicine. New York: Oxford University Press. 2008.

36. Sheiham A, Joffe M. Public dental health strategies for identifying and controlling dental caries in high and low risk populations. In: Johnson NW, editor. Risk markers for oral diseases. Cambridge: Cambridge University Press. 1992; p.445-481.

37. Batchelor P, Sheiham A. The limitations of a 'high-risk' approach for the prevention of dental caries. Community Dentistry and Oral Epidemiology. 2002; 30(4):302-312.

38. McKinlay JB. Paradigmatic obstacles to improving the health of populations - implications for health policy. Salud Publica Mexico. 1998; 40(4):369-79.

39. Farmer P. Social inequalities and emerging infectious diseases. Emerging Infectious Diseases. 1996; 2(4):259-269.

40. Farmer P, editor. Infections and inequalities: the modern plagues. Berkeley and Los Angeles: University of California Press. 2001.

41. McKinlay JB, Marceau LD. A tale of 3 tails. American Journal of Public Health. 1999; 89(3):295-298.

42. Graham H, Kelly MP. Health inequalities: concepts, frameworks and policy. NHS and Health Development Agency, briefing paper. Available at: http://www.nice.org.uk/niceMedia/pdf/health_inequalities_policy_graham.pdf. Accessed: nov 2011.

43. Frank JW. Why "population health"? Canadian Journal of Public Health. 1995; 86(3):162-164.

44. Marmot MG, Wilkinson RG. Social determinants of health. New York: Oxford University Press. 2006.

45. Marmot M. Health in an unequal world. The Lancet. 2006; 368(9552):2081-2094.

46. Petticrew M, Tugwell P, Kristjansson E, Oliver S, Ueffing E, Welch V. Damned if you do, damned if you don't: subgroup analysis and equity. Journal of Epidemiology and Community Health. 2011.

47. Tugwell P, Robinson V, Morris E. Mapping global health inequalities: challenges and opportunities. Availabe from: http://escholarship.org/uc/item/2f11d67c. Access: nov 2011.

48. Tugwell P, Petticrew M, Kristjansson E, Welch V, Ueffing E, Waters E, et al. Assessing equity in systematic reviews: realising the recommendations of the Commission on Social Determinants of Health. British Medical Journal. 2010; 341:c4739.

49. Sanders AE. Social Determinants of Oral Health: conditions linked to socioeconomic inequalities in oral health and in the Australian population. AIHW cat. no. POH 7. Canberra: Australian Institute of Health and Welfare (Population Oral Health Series No. 7). 2007.

50. Petersen PE. Social inequalities in dental health. Towards a theoretical explanation. Community Dentistry and Oral Epidemiology. 1990; 18(3):153-8.

51. Pine CM, Adair PM, Nicoll AD, Burnside G, Petersen PE, Beighton D, et al. International comparisons of health inequalities in childhood dental caries. Community Dental Health. 2004; 21(1 Suppl):121-30.

52. Sanders AE, Spencer AJ, Stewart JF. Clustering of risk behaviours for oral and general health. Community Dental Health. 2005; 22(3):133-40.

53. Sanders AE, Spencer AJ, Slade GD. Evaluating the role of dental behaviour in oral health inequalities. Community Dentistry and Oral Epidemiology. 2006; 34(1):71-79.

54. Scarborough P, Allender S, Rayner M, Goldacre M. An index of unhealthy lifestyle is associated with coronary heart disease mortality rates for small areas in England after adjustment for deprivation. Health and Place. 2011; 17(2):691-5.

55. Stringhini S, Dugravot A, Shipley M, Goldberg M, Zins M, Kivimaki M, et al. Health behaviours, socioeconomic status, and mortality: further analyses of the British Whitehall II and the French

GAZEL prospective cohorts. PLoS Medicine. 2011; 8(2):e1000419.

56. Nyberg G, Sundblom E, Norman A, Elinder LS. A healthy school start - parental support to promote healthy dietary habits and physical activity in children: design and evaluation of a cluster-randomised intervention. BMC Public Health. 2011; 11:185.

57. Ruijsbroek A, Wijga AH, Kerkhof M, Koppelman GH, Smit HA, Droomers M. The development of socio-economic health differences in childhood: results of the Dutch longitudinal PIAMA birth cohort. BMC Public Health. 2011; 11:225.

58. Marmot M. The causes of the causes. Health Services Journal. 2009; 119(6152):12.

59. Jarvis MJ, Wardle J, Waller J, Owen L. Prevalence of hardcore smoking in England, and associated attitudes and beliefs: cross sectional study. British Medical Journal. 2003; 326(7398):1061.

60. Wardle J, Jarvis MJ, Steggles N, Sutton S, Williamson S, Farrimond H, et al. Socioeconomic disparities in cancer-risk behaviors in adolescence: baseline results from the Health and Behaviour in Teenagers Study (HABITS). Preventive Medicine. 2003; 36(6):721-30.

61. WHO - World Health Organization. Commission on Social Determinants of Health. A Conceptual Framework for Action on the Social Determinants of Health. Discussion paper for the Commission on Social Determinants of Health - Last version. Geneva: WHO. 2007.

62. Sabbah W, Tsakos G, Sheiham A, Watt RG. The role of health-related behaviors in the socioeconomic disparities in oral health. Social Science and Medicine. 2009; 68(2):298-303.

63. Blane D. Health inequality and public policy: one year on from the Acheson report. Journal of Epidemiology and Community Health. 1999; 53(12):748.

64. Blane D, Berney L, Smith GD, Gunnell DJ, Holland P. Reconstructing the life course: health during early old age in a follow-up study based on the Boyd Orr cohort. Public Health. 1999; 113(3):117-24.

65. Diez-Roux AV. Bringing context back into epidemiology: variables and fallacies in multilevel analysis. American Journal of Public Health. 1998; 88(2):216-222.

66. Graham H, Power C. Childhood disadvantage and health inequalities: a framework for policy based on lifecourse research. Child: Care, Health and Development. 2004; 30(6):671-8.

67. Davey Smith G. Health inequalities: lifecourse approaches. Southampton: Policy Press. 2000.

68. Davey Smith G, Leary S, Ness A, Lawlor DA. Challenges and novel approaches in the epidemiological study of early life influences on later disease. Advances in Experimental Medicine and Biology. 2009; 646:1-14.

69. Brunner E, Marmot M. Social organisation, stress, and health. In: Marmot M, Wilkinson RG, editors. Social determinants of health. 1st ed. Oxford, New York: Oxford University Press. 1999; p.17-43.

70. Elstad JI. The psycho-social perspective on social inequalities in health. Sociology of Health & Illness. 1998; 20(5):598-618.

71. Evans RG, Barer ML, Marmor TR, editors. Why are some people healthy and others not? The determinants of health of populations. 1st ed. New York: Aldine de Gruyter. 1994.

72. Evans RG, Stoddart GL. Producing health, consuming health care. Social Science and Medicine. 1990; 31(12):1347-1363.

73. Evans RG, Stoddart GL. Consuming Research, Producing Policy? American Journal of Public Health. 2003; 93(3):371-379.

74. Lavis JN. Ideas at the margin or marginalized ideas? Nonmedical determinants of health in Canada. Health Affairs. 2002; 21(2):107-112.

75. Griesbach D, Amos A, Currie C. Adolescent smoking and family structure in Europe. Social Science and Medicine. 2003; 56(1):41-52.

76. Dean K. Conceptual, theoretical and methodological issues in self-care research. Social Science and Medicine 1989;29(2):117-123.

77. Dean K. Self-care components of lifestyles: The importance of gender, attitudes and the social situation. Social Science and Medicine. 1989; 29(2):137-152.

78. Ma J, Betts NM, Hampl JS. Clustering of lifestyle behaviors: the relationship between cigarette smoking, alcohol consumption, and dietary intake. American Journal of Health Promotion. 2000; 15(2):107-117.

79. Blane D. An assessment of the Black Report's explanations of health inequalities. Sociology of Health & Illness. 1985; 7(3):423-445.

80. Adler NE, Ostrove JM. Socioeconomic status and health: what we know and what we don't. Annals of the New York Academy of Science. 1999; 896:3-15.

81. Leon DA, Walt G, Gilson L. International perspectives on health inequalities and policy. British Medical Journal. 2001; 322(7286):591-594.

82. Marmot M, Wilkinson RG, editors. Social determinants of health. 1st ed. Oxford, New York: Oxford University Press. 1999.

83. Deaton A. Policy implications of the gradient of health and wealth. Health Affairs (Millwood). 2002; 21(2):13-30.

84. Cassel J. The contribution of the social environment to host resistance. American Journal of Epidemiology. 1976; 104(2):107-123.

85. Marmot MG, Shipley MJ, Rose G. Inequalities in death - specific explanations of a general pattern? Lancet. 1984; 1(8384):1003-6.

86. Susser MW, Watson W, Hopper K. Sociology in Medicine. New York: Oxford University Press. 1985.

87. Syme SL, Berkman LF. Social class, susceptibility and sickness. American Journal of Epidemiology. 1976; 104(1):1-8.

88. Macintyre S. Understanding the social patterning of health: the role of the social sciences. Journal of Public Health Medicine. 1994; 16(1):53-59.

89. Cohen S, Janicki-Deverts D, Chen E, Matthews KA. Childhood socioeconomic status and adult health. Annals of the New York Academy of Sciences. 2010; 1186(1):37-55.

90. Blas E, Kurup AS, editors. Equity, social determinants and public health programmes. Geneva: World Health Organization. 2010.

91. Blas E, Sommerfeld J, Kurup AS, editors. Social determinants approaches to public health: from concept to practice. Geneva: World Health Organization, Department of Ethics, Equity, Trade, and Human Rights Health (ETH). 2011.

92. Illich I. Limits to medicine. Medical Nemesis: the expropriation of health. London: Marion Boyars. 1995.

93. Navarro V. Social class, political power and the state and their implications in medicine. Social Science and Medicine. 1976; 10(9-10):437-57.

94. Crawford R. You are dangerous to your health: the ideology and politics of victim blaming. International Journal of Health Services. 1977; 7(4):663-680.

95. McKeown T. The role of medicine: dream, mirage, or nemesis? 1st ed. Princeton, New Jersey: Princeton University Press. 1979.

96. Rose G. Sick individuals an sick populations. International Journal of Epidemiology. 1985; 14(1):32-38.

97. Rose G. The strategy of preventive medicine. 1st ed. Oxford, New York, Tokyo: Oxford University Press. 1993.

98. Batchelor PA, Sheiham A. Grouping of tooth surfaces by susceptibility to caries: a study in 5-16 year-old children. BMC Oral Health. 2004; 4(1):2.

99. Batchelor PA, Sheiham A. The distribution of burden of dental caries in schoolchildren: a critique of the high-risk caries prevention strategy for populations. BMC Oral Health. 2006; 6(3):1-22.

100. Dahlgren G, Whitehead M. Tackling inequalities in health: What can we learn from what has been tried? Working paper prepared for the King's Fund International Seminar on Tackling Inequalities in Health. London: Ditchely Park, Oxford: King's Fund. 1993.

101. Dahlgren G, Whitehead M. European strategies for tackling social inequities in health: Levelling up Part 2. Copenhagen: WHO Regional Office for Europe. 2006.

102. Whitehead M. A typology of actions to tackle social inequalities in health. Journal of Epidemiology and Community Health. 2007; 61(6):473-478.

103. Whitehead M, Dahlgren G. Concepts and principles for tackling social inequities in health: Levelling up Part 1. Copenhagen: WHO Regional Office for Europe. 2006.

104. Dahlgren G, Whitehead M. Policies and strategies to promote social equity in health. Copenhagen: WHO/Regional Office for Europe. 1992.

105. Graham H, editor. Understanding health inequalities. York: Open University Press. 2009.

106. Graham H. Health inequalities, social determinants and public health policy. Policy & Politics 2009;37(4):463-479.

107. WHO - World Health Organization, World Conference on Social Determinants of Health. Rio Political Declaration on Social Determinants of Health. Rio de Janeiro: WHO. 2011.

108. Graham H. Tackling inequalities in health in England: remedying health disadvantages, narrowing health gaps or reducing health gradients? Journal of Social Policy. 2004; 33(1):115-131.

109. Frohlich KL, Potvin L. Transcending the known in public health practice: The inequality paradox: The population approach and vulnerable populations. American Journal of Public Health. 2008; 98(2):216-221.

110. Sheiham A, Alexander D, Cohen L, Marinho V, Moyses S, Petersen PE, et al. Global oral health inequalities: task group - implementation and delivery of oral health strategies. Advances in Dental Research. 2011; 23(2):259-67.

111. Milio N. Making healthy public policy; developing the science by learning the art: an ecological framework for policy studies. Health Promotion. 1987; 2(3):263-74.

112. Ruffin J. The science of eliminating health disparities: embracing a new paradigm. American Journal of Public Health. 2010; 100(S1):S8-9.

113. Hart JT. The inverse care law. Lancet. 1971; 1(7696):405-12.

114. Starfield B. Primary care: balancing health needs, services, and technology. New York: Oxford University Press. 1998.

115. Starfield B. Basic concepts in population health and health care. Journal of Epidemiology and Community Health. 2001; 55(7):452-4.

116. Sheiham A, Watt RG. The common risk factor approach: a rational basis for promoting oral health. Community Dentistry and Oral Epidemiology. 2000; 28(6):399-406.

117. Sheiham A. Oral health, general health and quality of life. Bulletin of the World Health Organization. 2005; 83(9):644.

118. Sheiham A. Closing the gap in a generation: health equity through action on the social determinants of health. A report of the WHO Commission on Social Determinants of Health (CSDH) 2008. Community Dental Health. 2009; 26(1):2-3.

119. Adler NE, Rehkopf DH. U.S. disparities in health: descriptions, causes, and mechanisms. Annual Review of Public Health. 2008; 29:235-52.

120. Adler NE, Boyce T, Chesney MA, Cohen S, Folkman S, Kahn RL, et al. Socioeconomic status and health. The challenge of the gradient. The American Psychologist. 1994; 49(1):15-24.

121. Sanders AE, Slade GD. Deficits in perceptions of oral health relative to general health in populations. Journal of Public Health Dentistry. 2006; 66(4):255-62.

122. Sanders AE, Slade GD, Turrell G, John Spencer A, Marcenes W. The shape of the socioeconomic-oral health gradient: implications for theoretical explanations. Community Dentistry and Oral Epidemiology. 2006; 34(4):310-319.

123. Kwan S, Petersen PE. Oral health: equity and social determinants. In: Blas E, Kurup AS, editors. Equity, social determinants and public health programmes. Geneva: World Health Organization. 2010; p.159-176.

124. Petersen PE, Kwan S. Evaluation of community-based oral health promotion and oral disease prevention - WHO recommendations for improved evidence in

public health practice. Community Dental Health. 2004; 21(4 Suppl):319-29.

125. Eriksen HM, Dimitrov V. Ecology of oral health: a complexity perspective. European Journal of Oral Science. 2003; 111(4):285-290.

126. Eriksen HM, Dimitrov V. The human mouth: oral functions in a social complexity perspective. Acta Odontologica Scandinava. 2003; 61(3):172-7.

127. Sheiham A. Improving oral health for all: focusing on determinants and conditions. Health Education Journal. 2000; 59(4):351-363.

128. Sheiham A. Public health approaches to promoting dental health. Journal of Public Health. 2001; 9(2):100-111.

129. Newton JT, Bower EJ. The social determinants of oral health: new approaches to conceptualizing and researching complex causal networks. Community Dentistry and Oral Epidemiology. 2005; 33(1):25-34.

130. Baelum V, Lopez R. Periodontal epidemiology: towards social science or molecular biology? Community Dentistry and Oral Epidemiology. 2004; 32(4):239-49.

131. Bambra C, Gibson M, Sowden A, Wright K, Whitehead M, Petticrew M. Tackling the wider social determinants of health and health inequalities: evidence from systematic reviews. Journal of Epidemiology and Community Health. 2010; 64(4):284-91.

132. Bambra C, Smith KE, Garthwaite K, Joyce KE, Hunter DJ. A labour of Sisyphus? Public policy and health inequalities research from the Black and Acheson Reports to the Marmot Review. Journal of Epidemiology and Community Health. 2011; 65(5):399-406.

133. Petersen PE. Challenges to improvement of oral health in the 21st century - the approach of the WHO Global Oral Health Programme. International Dental Journal. 2004; 54(6 Suppl 1):329-43.

134. Petersen PE. Priorities for research for oral health in the 21st century - the approach of the WHO Global Oral Health Programme. Community Dental Health. 2005; 22(2):71-4.

135. Petersen PE. The burden of oral disease: challenges to improving oral health in the 21st century. Bulletin of the World Health Organization. 2005; 83(1):3.

136. Petersen PE. Global policy for improvement of oral health in the 21st century - implications to oral health research of World Health Assembly 2007, World Health Organization. Community Dentistry and Oral Epidemiology. 2009; 37(1):1-8.

137. Petersen PE, Kwan S. Equity, social determinants and public health programmes - the case of oral health. Community Dentistry and Oral Epidemiology. 2011.

138. Popay J, Whitehead M, Hunter DJ. Injustice is killing people on a large scale - but what is to be done about it? Journal of Public Health. 2010; 32(2):148-149.

139. Frenk J. Reinventing primary health care: the need for systems integration. Lancet. 2009; 374(9684):170-3.

140. Frenk J. Bridging the divide: Comprehensive reform to improve health in Mexico. Nairobi, Kenya: Commission on Social Determinants of Health. 2006.

141. Fisher-Owens SA, Gansky SA, Platt LJ, Weintraub JA, Soobader M-J, Bramlett MD, et al. Influences on Children's Oral Health: A Conceptual Model. Pediatrics. 2007; 120(3):e510-e520.

142. Tang K-C, Beaglehole R, O'Byrne D. Policy and partnership for health promotion action — addressing the determinants of health. Bulletin of the World Health Organization. 2005; 83(12):884-885.

143. Baelum V. Dentistry and population approaches for preventing dental diseases. Journal of Dentistry. 2011.

144. Tsakos G, Herrick K, Sheiham A, Watt RG. Edentulism and fruit and vegetable intake in low-income adults. Journal of Dental Research. 2010; 89(5):462-7.

145. Moysés SJ, Sheiham A. O papel dos profissionais de saúde bucal na promoção de saúde. In: Buischi YdP, editor. Promoção de saúde bucal na clínica odontológica. 1st ed. São Paulo: Artes Médicas/APCD. 2000; p.23-37.

146. Moysés ST, Watt R. Promoção de saúde bucal: definições. In: Buischi YdP, edi-

tor. Promoção de saúde bucal na clínica odontológica. 1st ed. São Paulo: Artes Médicas/APCD. 2000; p.1-22.

147. Pitts N, Amaechi B, Niederman R, Acevedo AM, Vianna R, Ganss C, et al. Global oral health inequalities: dental caries task group-research agenda. Advances in Dental Research. 2011; 23(2):211-20.

148. Jin LJ, Armitage GC, Klinge B, Lang NP, Tonetti M, Williams RC. Global oral health inequalities: task group - periodontal disease. Advances in Dental Research. 2011; 23(2):221-6.

149. Shiboski C, Hodgson T, Challacombe SJ. Overview and research agenda arising from the Sixth World Workshop on Oral Health and Disease in AIDS. Advances in Dental Research. 2011; 23(1):7-9.

150. Challacombe S, Coogan M, Williams D, Greenspan J. Overview and research agenda arising from the 5th World Workshop on Oral Health and Disease in AIDS. Advances in Dental Research. 2006; 19(1):5-9.

151. Challacombe S, Chidzonga M, Glick M, Hodgson T, Magalhaes M, Shiboski C, et al. Global oral health inequalities: oral infections-challenges and approaches. Advances in Dental Research. 2011; 23(2):227-36.

152. Challacombe SJ, Coogan MM, Williams DM. Overview of the Fourth International Workshop on the Oral Manifestations of HIV Infection. Oral Diseases. 2002; 8 Suppl 2:9-14.

153. Pattussi MP, Marcenes W, Croucher R, Sheiham A. Social deprivation, income inequality, social cohesion and dental caries in Brazilian school children. Social Science and Medicine. 2001; 53(7):915-925.

154. Thomson WM, Poulton R, Milne BJ, Caspi A, Broughton JR, Ayers KM. Socioeconomic inequalities in oral health in childhood and adulthood in a birth cohort. Community Dentistry and Oral Epidemiology. 2004; 32(5):345-353.

155. Matlin A, Walmsley D. Some are more equal than others. British Dental Journal. 2010; 209(6):261.

156. Milio NR. Healthy nations: creating a new ecology of public policy for health. Canadian Journal of Public Health. 1985; 76 Suppl 1:79-87.

157. McKinlay JB. The promotion of health through planned sociopolitical change: challenges for research and policy. Social Science and Medicine. 1993; 36(2):109-117.

158. Syme SL. To prevent disease: the need for a new approach. In: Blane D, Brunner E, Wilkinson RG, editors. Health And Social Organization. Towards a Health Policy for the 21st Century. London: Routledge. 1996; p.21-31.

159. Moyses SJ, Moyses ST, McCarthy M, Sheiham A. Intra-urban differentials in child dental trauma in relation to healthy cities policies in Curitiba, Brazil. Health & Place. 2006; 12(1):48-64.

160. Moysés ST, Moysés SJ, Watt RG, Sheiham A. Associations between health promoting schools policies on some indicators of oral health. Health Promotion International. 2003; 18(3):209-218.

161. Wilkinson R, Marmot M, editors. Social determinants of health: the solid facts. 2nd ed. Copenhagen: Centre for Urban Health, World Health Organisation, Regional Office for Europe. 2003.

162. WHO - World Health Organization. Milestones in health promotion: statements from global conferences. Geneva: WHO. 2009.

163. Frieden TR. A framework for public health action: the health impact pyramid. American Journal of Public Health. 2010; 100(4):590-5.

164. Moysés SJ, Sheiham A. Saúde bucal coletiva: personagens, autores ou... Pirandello de novo? In: Kriger L, editor. Promoção de saúde bucal: paradigma, ciência, humanização. 3ª ed. São Paulo: Artes Médicas. 2003; p.387-442.

165. Baelum V, van Palenstein Helderman W, Hugoson A, Yee R, Fejerskov O. A global perspective on changes in the burden of caries and periodontitis: implications for dentistry. Journal of Oral Rehabilitation. 2007; 34(12):872-906; discussion 940.

166. WHO - World Health Organization. CINDI dietary guide. In. Copenhagen: WHO Regional Office for Europe. 2000; p.32.

167. WHO - World Health Organization. WHO's Global School Health Initia-

tive: Health Promoting Schools; a healthy setting for living, learning and working. Geneva: WHO; 1998 1998. Report No.: WHO/HPR/HEP/98.4.

168. WHO - World Health Organization, UNESCO. Local action: creating Health Promoting Schools. Available: www.who.int/hpr/archive/gshi/docs/index.html; Access: Oct 2010.

169. Dyer TA, Robinson PG. General health promotion in general dental practice - The involvement of the dental team Part 1: A review of the evidence of effectiveness of brief public health interventions. British Dental Journal. 2006; 200(12):679-685.

170. WHO - World Health Organization. 2008-2013 action plan for the global strategy for the prevention and control of noncommunicable diseases : prevent and control cardiovascular diseases, cancers, chronic respiratory diseases and diabetes. Geneva: WHO. 2008.

171. Chor D, Faerstein E. An epidemiological approach to health promotion: the ideas of Geoffrey Rose. Cadernos de Saúde Pública. 2000; 16(1):241-244.

172. Hausen H, Karkkainen S, Seppa L. Application of the high-risk strategy to control dental caries. Community Dentistry and Oral Epidemiology. 2000; 28:26 - 34.

173. Burt BA. Concepts of risk in dental public health. Community Dentistry and Oral Epidemiology. 2005; 33(4):240-247.

174. Shilton T. Health promotion competencies: providing a road map for health promotion to assume a prominent role in global health. Global Health Promotion. 2009; 16(2):42-6.

175. Scriven A, Speller V. Global issues and challenges beyond Ottawa: the way forward. Promotion & Education. 2007; 14(4):194-8, 255-9, 269-73.

176. Wallerstein N. What is the evidence on effectiveness of empowerment to improve health? Copenhagen: WHO Regional Office for Europe -Health Evidence Network Report. 2006.

177. Bronkhorst EM, Truin GJ, Batchelor P, Sheiham A. Health through oral health; guidelines for planning and monitoring for oral health care: a critical comment on the WHO model. Journal of Public Health Dentistry. 1991; 51(4):223-7.

178. Garcia I, Tabak LA. Global oral health inequalities: the view from a research funder. Advances in Dent Research. 2011; 23(2):207-10.

Chapter 4

The Determinants of Oral Health-Related Behaviours; Clustering of Behaviours

Georgios Tsakos
Saeed Alzahrani

The importance of behaviours for health and well-being of populations is well established.[1] There is conclusive evidence of increased morbidity and mortality risks associated with different detrimental behaviours, such as smoking, unhealthy diet, physical inactivity and excessive alcohol consumption.[2-7]

Although it is simpler to study behaviours one at a time, behaviours do not occur singly. Children usually have a number of health related behaviours. For example, while it is easier to think only about the risk of smoking, smokers tend to also adopt other health-compromising behaviours while they may also follow a few health promoting behaviours. Therefore this chapter focuses on the clustering of oral health related behaviours among adolescents, as it is important to look at the combined effects of multiple behaviours on health. In addition, we will also pay particular attention to the broader determinants of clustering of behaviours to gain insights that can be useful for shaping and targeting health promotion interventions.

What is clustering of health-related behaviours?

Behavioural clustering is when two or more behaviours, such as smoking, alcohol, diet patterns, hygiene practices, co-occur in the same person.

Why focus on clustering and why among adolescents?

Clustering is important because the co-occurrence of multiple health-compromising behaviours is associated with increased risk of chronic diseases, cancer and cardiovascular disease.[8] The increased risk is the result of accumulation and combination of their individual detrimental effects on health.[8-10] That highlights that their combination is much more detrimental than their individual effects. In adults, studies show that clustering of smoking, alcohol intake, physical inactivity and insufficient fruit and vegetable intake, four well-established behavioural markers, is associated with four times higher mortality risk[11] and more than a two-fold difference in incidence of strokes.[12]

Behavioural patterns of adulthood are primarily shaped during childhood, and in particular adolescence. For example, adopting a healthy eating habit in adolescence, such as consumption of adequate amount of fruits and vegetables, is likely to track into adulthood.[13-15] Similarly, tooth brushing behaviour is developed in childhood[16] and then follows standard lifecourse trajectories throughout later adolescence and adulthood.[17] Starting smoking during adolescence is a good predictor of continuing this detrimental habit for many more years into adulthood.[18] Acknowledging that adolescence is a crucial period developmentally, Lawlor et al.[19] suggested that risk behaviours should be improved during adolescence. As a result, understanding how health-related behaviours relate to one another in adolescents has important implications throughout the life course.

How do health-related behaviours interrelate?

Many studies report on the interrelationships between different behaviours. These studies looked at different numbers and combinations of behaviours, thereby providing an extensive but patchy picture of the interrelations. Let's take a look, for example, at key behaviours in adolescence and see how they do interrelate. We will start from behaviours related to healthy eating, and then move to oral hygiene, physical activity, physical fighting, and smoking. All these have a considerable effect on the health of adolescents. But do they happen in isolation?

Adequate fruit consumption and reduced sugar consumption are basic elements of a healthy diet. Higher fruit intake is associated with increased physical activity[20-22] and with lower rates of smoking and alcohol consumption.[23] In terms of dietary behaviours, lower fruit intake coincides with higher consumption of sweets and soft drinks and saturated fat.[23-25]

Focussing on oral hygiene, tooth brushing is significantly associated with different health-related behaviours. Regular or occasional smokers tend to brush their teeth less frequently[26] and this inverse association between smoking and tooth brushing also occurs in adolescents.[27] Moreover, oral and general hygiene are interrelated; adolescents that brushed their teeth were more likely to shower more often or change underwear frequently.[28] And adolescents that had breakfast on weekdays were more likely to undertake more frequent tooth brushing.[29]

Apart from the aforementioned association with fruits and vegetables consumption,[20-22] physical activity is linked with healthy eating in general,[30] while physical inactivity is associated with sedentary lifestyles.[31] On the "negative" aspect of physical behaviours, physical fighting is a reliable predictor of multiple risk behaviours[32, 33] and has been associated with carrying weapons and injury,[34] as well as with substance abuse.[35]

The most widely used health behavioural marker is smoking. Indeed, smoking is viewed by many as a 'gateway' to other detrimental behaviours like drug use.[36] Furthermore, smokers are at an increased risk of drinking alcohol and taking illicit drugs.[37,38] Compared to non-smokers, smokers had less favourable eating habits[39] and significantly higher intakes of energy, saturated fat, cholesterol, and alcohol and lower intakes of polyunsaturated fat, vitamins C, E, and dietary fibre.[23] And smoking was also associated with lower levels of physical activity, for example undertaking less exercise.[40]

Despite these associations between different behaviours, most research has focused on one or a few behaviours at a time, thereby limiting understanding of the inter-relationships between different health-related behaviours.[41] The few studies that have considered multiple behaviours, have looked at their interrelationship to assess whether they are uni-dimensional, bi-dimensional or multidimensional.

A uni-dimensional approach of the interrelationship between health-related behaviours suggests a consistent pattern across all health-related behaviours. So, people would be expected to act in the same manner towards all health-related behaviours[42] and there would be similar motivations for the different behaviours. If true, this could be helpful because the explanation for any one behaviour would explain other behaviours in general. However, there is no empirical support for the uni-dimensionality of the interrelating behaviours.[43]

Dimensions of Behavioural Interrelationships
Uni-dimensional: one consistent pattern covers all health-related behaviours
Bi-dimensional: two distinct patterns; health-compromising versus health-enhancing behaviours
Multi-dimensional: different patterns, potential variationthroughout life course

---

However, studies have shown a common behavioural dimension for the interrelationship of health-compromising behaviours among adolescents. A study showed a positive correlation between problem drinking, marijuana use, delinquent-type behaviour and sexual intercourse,[44] another study concluded that adolescent drinking, drug use, risky driving and delinquency are interrelated.[45] This evidence guided the thinking that there was a 'syndrome of problem behaviour in adolescence' or that at least these "problem behaviours" formed a discrete behavioural dimension.[46] This concept completely neglects the presence of non-harmful health-enhancing behaviours, and therefore indicates that a bi-dimensional or multi-dimensional interrelationship of health behaviours is more likely.

Langlie[47] postulated a hypothesis for the bi-dimensionality of health behaviours. She showed that preventive behaviours were not independent from each other and suggested two dimensions of health-related behaviours; the "direct" and the "indirect" behavioural risk factors. Nutbeam et al.[48] also postulated a two-dimensional structure of health-related behaviours that distinguished health-enhancing from health-compromising behaviours that was empirically supported by further studies on adolescents.[49]

Roysamb et al.[50] went a step further and reported a multidimensional model of behavioural interrelations in adolescents. This incorporated the basic division of the bi-dimensional model into health-enhancing and health-compromising behaviours but also showed that not all behaviours can be appropriately grouped under these two broad categories. Instead, they suggested a model consisting of three groups: "high action", "addiction" and "protection" behaviours. A multidimensional approach had already been suggested Williams and Wechsler[51] and Terre et al.[52] had indicated that patterns of behavioural interrelationships may vary at different developmental stages of life. Furthermore, a systematic review of 34 studies on types of positive health behaviours and factors related to behaviours for people aged 12-24 years concluded that relationships between health-related behaviours during adolescence are multidimensional and complex.[53] Therefore, the interrelationships between health-related behaviours of adolescents and adults seem to be best conceptualized as multidimensional. Multidimensionality assumes that certain health behaviours tend to cluster.[42,49,54] Therefore, it is important to ascertain the composition of clustering patterns of multiple health-related behaviours.

Clustering patterns

There are a number of different clustering patterns of health-related behaviours among adolescent populations (Table 4.1). There were positive associations between a range of health-compromising behaviours (unhealthy weight loss, substance abuse, suicide risk, delinquency, and sexual activity) in adolescents at different stages of development (early, middle, and late adolescence) and from different ethnic backgrounds.[55] The study assessed associations between two behaviours at a time. The strongest associations were between substance abuse and delinquency, substance abuse and suicide risk, substance abuse and sexual activity, and between suicide risk and delinquency. An important pioneer study among adolescents 12-17 years of age showed pairwise associations for different high-risk behaviours (smoking, binge drinking, driving under the influence of alcohol, riding a car with a drunk driver, non-use safety belts and non-use oral contraceptives) but did not look at clustering patterns of multiple health-compromising behaviours.[56] Analysis of a large national sample of US adolescents indicated that a number of health-risk behaviours tended to co-occur.[57] Overall, relatively few adolescents engaged in two or more of these behaviours, but the clustering was more prevalent among males and adolescents not attending school.

Wiefferink et al.[58] conducted a comprehensive systematic review of studies published between 1995 and 2003 to identify the clustering of four health-related behaviours: smoking, alcohol abuse, safe sex and healthy nutrition, and their determinants in adolescents (10-18 years). They found that smoking, alcohol abuse and sexual experience clustered. Most studies provided clear evidence that smoking and alcohol abuse clustered and there was also evidence that sexual experience clustered with smoking. Furthermore, only one study identified three patterns of clusters involving dietary behaviours. The largest cluster was adolescents who ate healthily but did not smoke or drink alcohol (50% of sample). The second cluster (20%) was adolescents who ate unhealthily, smoked and drank alcohol. The third cluster (30%) was adolescents who ate unhealthily but did not smoke or drink alcohol. In contrast to the majority of previous studies that focused solely on health-compromising behaviours, Kremers et al.[59] examined clustering of energy-related behaviours (consumption of energy-dense snacks, intake of high-fat sandwich, fruit consumption, using active transport and physical activity) among Dutch adolescents. Fruit consumption was positively associated with physical activity, and snacking behaviour was positively associated with high-fat sandwich fillings. However, this study was confined to associations of two behaviours at a time, thereby not addressing multiple behaviour clustering.

Using a large sample of Australian adolescents, Lawlor et al.[19] examined the extent of clustering of smoking, extensive TV viewing, overweight, and high blood pressure. Extensive television watching was considered as a marker of physical inactivity, while overweight and high blood pressure may not be behaviours in their own right but are markers of dietary and physical activity behaviours. All these factors are related to an increased risk for cardiovascular disease. A different focus was introduced by Viner et al.[60] in a study of adolescents in East London in UK. They looked

at the count of basic health-compromising behaviours (smoking, drinking alcohol and drugs use) and showed that only about 1% reported all three risk behaviours, 3% had two and 11% had one. Clearly, this population had good behavioural patterns, though there were still important variations by age, sex, ethnicity and social support, but not by socioeconomic status.

Bartlett et al.[61] used the US National Longitudinal Study of Adolescent Health to examine clusters of problematic behaviours (lying, stealing, fighting, using a weapon against another person, public disruption, lack of birth control use, having multiple sex partners, having sex under the influence of drugs or alcohol, property destruction, being loud/rowdy, running away, skipping school, and alcohol or marijuana use) at two times. Behaviours clustered in three distinct patterns: 1) a "normal" cluster, 2) a "problematic" cluster, and 3) a "deviant" behaviours cluster. The "normal" cluster included adolescents not commonly engaging in excessively risky behaviours, though they still reported significant alcohol use, being loud and rowdy in public, and lying to their parents. The "problematic" and "deviant" clusters included adolescents with a more risky behavioural pattern, with the latter group reporting worse rates. The key behaviours that distinguished between the "normal" and the "problematic" cluster referred to lack of use of birth control and having multiple sex partners, whereas selling drugs and weapon use distinguished the "deviant" cluster from others.

Using data from a national survey of 10-17 year-olds in Canada, Alamian and Paradis[62] that risk behaviours (alcohol drinking, tobacco smoking, sedentary lifestyle and high body mass index) clustered in multiple combinations;

they identified 32 different clustering patterns. Older and socioeconomically deprived adolescents had higher levels of risk behaviours clustering. A study among Dutch adolescents included a wide variety of health-compromising (alcohol consumption, smoking, illegal drug use, unsafe sex, physical inactivity, skipping breakfast, not eating fruits and vegetables, poor sleep, unlawful traffic) and delinquency behaviours (vandalism, violence and crime against property) and showed two clusters for adolescents aged 12-15 years and three clusters for those aged 16-18 years[63]. Similarly, a national sample of US adolescents aged 12-14 years could be categorised into four groups in terms of the co-occurrence of risky behaviours (delinquency, drinking alcohol, smoking, drug use, sexual behaviour and physical inactivity): a high risk group (i.e. adolescents undertaking many risky behaviours), a low risk group.[64]

More recently, a study in eight European cities assessed clustering patterns of physical activity, sedentary and dietary habits and identified five clusters: an "unhealthy" cluster (all health-compromising behaviours), a "sedentary" cluster, one characterised by poor quality diet and physical inactivity, one with good quality diet and physical inactivity, and a "healthy" cluster.[65] A recent study on a representative sample of Saudi Arabian male adolescents in Riyadh used different methodologies to assess clustering of six health-related behaviours (intake of fruits, intake of sweets, tooth brushing, physical activity, smoking, and physical fighting). Using hierarchical agglomerative cluster analysis, the study suggested two broad and stable clusters: one consisted of low fruit consumption, infrequent tooth brushing and low physical activity, and another included high sweets consumption, smoking and physical fighting. These six behaviours clustered in different patterns, but most patterns with a high clustering ratio included smoking, which seemed to act as "gateway" behaviour in terms of predicting further clustering.[66]

In summary, despite looking at different types of health-related behaviours and employing different analytical methodologies, studies have shown that health-related behaviours are significantly associated and also tend to cluster in multiple patterns or groups among adolescents. Now that we have shown the existence and extent of clustering, it is important to draw our attention to the factors that determine behavioural clustering among adolescents.

Table 4.1 – Studies on clustering of multiple health-related behaviours among adolescents.

Authors, date	Age (years)	Type of behaviours	Types of patterns
Neumark-Sztainer et al.[55]	11-21	Unhealthy weight loss, substance abuse, suicide risk, delinquency, and sexual activity.	Positive association between all behaviours
Petridou et al.[56]	12-17	Smoking, binge drinking, driving under the influence of alcohol, riding a car with a drunk driver, non-use of safety belts and non-use of oral contraceptives.	Pairwise associations

Table 4.1 – Studies on clustering of multiple health-related behaviours among adolescents. (Continue)

Brener and Collins[57]	12-17	Seat belt use, weapon carrying, tobacco, alcohol, drug use, and sexual behaviour.	Clustering of two or more risk behaviours: non-prevalent
Kremers et al.[59]	12-18	Energy related behaviours: consumption of energy-dense snacks, the use of high-fat sandwich fillings, fruit consumption, active transport and physical activity during leisure time.	Low levels of fruit and vegetable consumption clustered with low levels of physical activity
Bartlett et al.[61]	11-21	Wide range of problematic behaviours	Three clusters: 1) normal, 2) problem, and 3) deviant.
Lawlor et al.[19]	14	Coronary heart diseases risk factors: smoking, high level of watching TV, overweight, and high blood pressure.	Risk factors clustered; 10% reported three or four risk factors.
Viner, et al.[60]	11-14	Smoking, drinking alcohol, and drugs use	Low prevalence of clustering
Wiefferink et al.[58]	10-18	Smoking, alcohol abuse, safe sex and healthy nutrition	Clusters: Smoking and alcohol abuse; + sexual experience.
Alamian and Paradis[62]	10-17	Physical inactivity, sedentary behaviour, tobacco smoking, alcohol drinking and high body mass index.	Clustered in many patterns[32]
Van Nieuwenhuijzen et al.[89]	12-18	Wide range of health-compromising and delinquency behaviours	Several interrelated clusters
Hair et al.[64]	12-14	Delinquency, drinking alcohol, smoking, drug use, sexual behaviour and physical activity	Four groups: high risk, low risk, and two moderate risk groups
Ottevaere et al.[65]	12-18	Physical activity, sedentary and dietary habits	Five clusters
Alzahrani[66]	13-14 17-19	Intake of fruit, intake of sweets, physical activity, tooth brushing, smoking and physical fighting.	Two broad clusters among both younger and older adolescents. More than 60 clustering patterns; smoking as a "gateway".

Which factors determine behavioural clustering?

Different factors determine clustering of health-related behaviours. Demographic, socioeconomic and psychosocial factors are the main determinants of clustering and they are briefly explored here (Table 4.2).

Determinants of clustering - Demographic factors

Age is a strong determinant of behavioural clustering among adolescents, as it is an indirect marker of the different stages of development in adolescence. First, the prevalence of health-compromising behaviours increases with age.[67]

Younger adolescents have a healthier behavioural pattern than older counterparts,[61] though there is evidence for the contrary as well.[89] More importantly, the clustering of multiple health-compromising behaviours increases with adolescents' age.[21,55-57,60,63,66,68,69]

There are sex differences in the behavioural patterns of adolescents. Boys tend to have higher levels of health-compromising behaviours clustering than girls.[55,57,64,70-72] Bartlett et al.[61] categorised adolescents into "normal", "problem" and "deviant" behavioural clusters and found that the former primarily consisted of females while in the "deviant behaviours" cluster boys outnumbered girls by three times. However, some studies report either no sex differences in clustering[19,73] or worse patterns for girls.[74]

Family structure and characteristics affect behavioural clustering and patterns of adolescents. In general, adolescents from families that had both parents had a better behavioural pattern, with more healthy behaviours, than one parent families who instead had higher levels of clustering of health-compromising behaviours.[58,60,64,68] Furthermore, unfavourable behavioural pattern of parents, such as smoking or low intake of fruits and vegetables, is a good marker of adolescent health-compromising behaviours clustering,[21,68] while greater parental supervision and support was associated with lower probability of unhealthy behaviours clustering.[75]

Determinants of clustering – Socioeconomic position

Most, but not all, studies on the relationship between socioeconomic position and clustering of health-compromising behaviours in adolescence have reported significant inverse associations. Compared to adolescents in higher socioeconomic groups, lower socioeconomic position is related to a higher prevalence of clustering of multiple risk factors.[56,76,77] And this has been shown for different aspects of socioeconomic position, such as education, income, social class and affluence.

Attending school was protective against engaging in multiple risk behaviours.[57] Adolescents from lower educated families tended to have more risky behaviours,[56,66] while post-secondary school parental education level was indicative of lower probability of accumulated health-compromising behaviours among adolescents.[68] Similar inverse associations were also shown in relation to family income[19] and socioeconomic status.[61] Adolescents from affluent families were more likely to follow good behavioural patterns (e.g. frequent tooth brushing, regular exercise, receive preventive services) and less likely to smoke frequently compared with those from less affluent families.[27]

However, the associations between adolescents' health-related behaviours and their socioeconomic position are not as strong as among adults,[58,78] while others have even shown non-significant results.[60] A systematic review showed there is no clear influence of socioeconomic status on adolescents' behavioural clustering, as some studies found an inverse association but others did not.[58]

Determinants of clustering – Psychosocial factors

"Psychosocial" is an umbrella term that covers a wide range of factors that could be described as being at the interaction between social and psychological factors, in a way looking at how the social environment affects an individual's psychology or behaviour. By definition, psychosocial factors are expected to be closely linked to behavioural patterns. Therefore it is essential to consider them as potential determinants of behavioural clustering. This chapter can only briefly review the literature on some psychosocial factors (such as self-esteem, future orientation, life satisfaction, and social relationships and support) that have been examined in relation to behavioural patterns and clustering among adolescents.

A systematic review of the relevant literature showed that self-esteem was positively associated with practicing safe sex, eating healthily, non-smoking, and low alcohol use,[58] while a more recent study showed that adolescents with high self-esteem were less likely to have multiple behavioural risk factors.[68] Most importantly, this has long term effects as low self-esteem in childhood and preadolescence is associated with multiple health-compromising behaviours in adolescence.[79]

Adolescents with better future orientation, namely those that had more positive plans about their future, were less likely to use drugs, drink alcohol and have frequent alcohol problems,[80] while they also tended to brush their teeth more frequently.[81] Life satisfaction, a person's global assessment of his/her life, is another important psychosocial factor and has been described as a significant predictor of suicidal ideas in adolescents.[82] Low perceived life satisfaction was significantly associated with smoking, marijuana use and alcohol use,[83] as well as weapon carrying, getting injured and physical fighting.[84] A study among Saudi Arabian adolescents showed that life satisfaction was significantly negatively associated with clustering of health-compromising behaviours after adjusting for age and parental education level.[66]

Adolescents' behaviours can be influenced by their peers.[85,86] On the one hand, peer pressure may be responsible for embarking on health-compromising behaviours;[87,88] adolescents whose peers smoked or drank alcohol had themselves higher probability for undertaking risky behaviours, such as substance abuse[89] and health-compromising behavioural clustering.[68] And the number of evening meetings with friends was positively associated with the clustering of health-compromising behaviours after adjusting for age and parental education level.[66] However, peer relationships and support can also have a beneficial effect. For example, high levels of social and family support were linked to a lower level of risky behaviours clustering.[60] Furthermore, adolescents who had frequent evening meetings with friends were more likely to undertake physical activity.[25] And healthy behaviours of their peers and parents were associated with their own healthy behaviours clustering.[58]

In summary, behavioural patterns and clustering of adolescents are affected by different demographic factors and socioeconomic position, while there is also evidence about their psychosocial determinants. While more research is needed on the determinants of behavioural clustering, it is important to draw the current evidence together and look at the implications for public health action.

Table 4.2 – Key determinants of clustering of multiple health-related behaviours among adolescents.

Determinants	Associations with clustering (direction)	Authors, date
Age	Health-compromising behaviours (positive)	Neumark-Sztainer et al.,1996; Petridou et al., 1997; Berner & Collins, 1998;Takakura et al., 2001; Bartlett et al, 2005; Sanchez et al., 2007; van Nieuwenhuijzen et al., 2009; Alamian & Paradis, 2009b; Alzahrani, 2012
Gender	Higher clustering of risky behaviours among males	Raitakari et al., 1995; Neumark-Sztainer et al.,1996; Burk et al., 1997; Zweig et al., 2002; Ohene et al., 2005; Viner et al., 2006; van Nieuwenhuijzen et al., 2009
Family structure (Two-parents families)	Risky behaviours (negative)	Family structure (Two-parents families) Risky behaviours (negative) Wiefferink et al., 2006; Viner et al., 2006; Alamian & Paradis, 2009b; Hair et al., 2009
Socioeconomic Position (Family income; Family affluence; Education)	Risky behaviours (negative)	Raitakari et al., 1995; Petridou et al., 1997; Brener and Collins, 1998; Lawlor et al., 2005; Bartlett et al., 2005; Poortinga, 2007; de Vries et al., 2008 Alamian & Paradis, 2009b; Park et al., 2010; Alzahrani, 2012
Family support	Risky behaviours (negative)	Viner et al., 2006
Self-esteem	Risky behaviours (negative)	Wiefferink et al., 2006; Alamian & Paradis, 2009b
Peer relationships	Health-compromising behaviours (varies)	Negative: Viner et al., 2006; Positive: Alamian & Paradis, 2009b; Alzahrani 2012
Life satisfaction	Health-compromising behaviours (negative)	Alzahrani 2012

What are the implications of findings for public health policy?

Most studies among adolescents focused on a single behaviour or looked at associations between two health-related behaviours. In this chapter, we have shown that this is not the complete picture. Health behaviours tend to cluster and they do so in a variety of patterns. As clustering of multiple health-compromising behaviours has a cumulative or synergistic negative effect on health, it is important to gain better understanding about how behaviours relate to one another in adolescents.

The patterns of clustering for different health-related behaviours should be used to design appropriate and tailored health promotion programmes. Importantly, interventions focussing on multiple behaviours have potentially greater impact on public health than single behaviour interventions.[90,91] Building on the existing focus of health promotion towards a common risk factor approach whereby a few behavioural risk factors are responsible for different diseases (see Chapter 7), this chapter showed that these common risk factors tend to cluster in some people. And this clustering should be considered by health promotion programmes, such as the one on Health Promoting Schools[92] (see Chapter 20), using multifaceted strategies to tackle clusters of health-compromising behaviours rather than focussing on single risk behaviours separately. Public health interventions may also use knowledge from clustering patterns and target "gateway" behaviours such as smoking, as these behaviours are indicators of clustering with other risk behaviours. Behavioural patterns initiated during childhood and adolescence track into adulthood,[13,15] therefore health promotion interventions to alter behaviours should primarily focus on adolescence in order to maximise long-term benefits of following healthy behavioural patterns. To change behaviours one needs to change the environment,[93] so interventions should promote protective environments and enable healthy community actions (see Chapter 8). Studies on health-compromising behavioural clustering among adolescents indicate that lower socioeconomic position groups are more affected, and there is also some evidence in relation to psychosocial determinants. Therefore, a social determinants upstream approach to formulate and target public health interventions has potential to address the common underlying determinants of risk behaviours clustering.

References

1. Aaro LE, Laberg JC, Wold B (1995). Health Behaviors Among Adolescents - Towards A Hypothesis of 2 Dimensions. Health Educ Res. 10(1):83-93.

2. Alamian A, Paradis G (2009a). Clustering of chronic disease behavioral risk factors in Canadian children and adolescents. Prev Med. 48(5):493-499.

3. Alamian A, Paradis G (2009b). Correlates of Multiple Chronic Disease Behavioral Risk Factors in Canadian Children and Adolescents. Am J Epidemiol. 170(10):1279-1289.

4. Alzahrani S (2012). Clustering of health-related behaviours among Saudi Arabian adolescents (PhD Thesis). University College London (UCL).

5. Astrom A (2004). Stability of oral health-related behaviour in a Norwegian cohort between the ages of 15 and 23years. Community Dent Oral Epidemiol. 32(5):354-362.

6. Atkins D, Clancy C (2004). Multiple risk factors interventions: Are we up to the challenge? Am J Prev Med. 27(Supplement 1):102-103.

7. Bartlett R, Holditch-Davis D, Belyea M (2005). Clusters of problem behaviors in adolescents. Res Nurs Health. 28(3):230-239.

8. Bender D, Losel F (1997). Protective and risk effects of peer relations and social support on antisocial behaviour in adolescents from multi-problem milieus. Journal of Adolescence. 20(6):661-678.

9. Biddle SJ, Gorely T, Stensel DJ (2004). Health-enhancing physical activity and sedentary behaviour in children and adolescents. Journal of Sports Sciences. 22(8):679-701.

10. Blair SN, Jacobs DR, Jr., Powell KE (1985). Relationships between exercise or physical activity and other health behaviors. Public Health Rep. 100(2):172-180.

11. Brener ND, Collins JL (1998). Co-occurrence of health-risk behaviors among adolescents in the United States. J Adolesc Health. 22(3):209-213.

12. Breslow L, Enstrom JE (1980). Persistence of health habits and their relationship to mortality. Prev Med. 9(4):469-483.

13. Burke V, Milligan RA, Beilin LJ, Dunbar D, Spencer M, Balde E et al. (1997). Clustering of health-related behaviors among 18-year-old Australians. Prev Med. 26(5):724-733.

14. CDC (2004). The Health Consequences of Smoking: a Report of the Surgeon General. Washington, DC, US: Department of Health and Human Services, Center for Disease Control and Prevention.

15. Coulson NS, Eiser C, Eiser JR (1997). Diet, smoking and exercise: interrelationships between adolescent health behaviours. Child Care Health Dev. 23(3):207-216.

16. Critchley JA, Capewell S (2003). Mortality Risk Reduction Associated With Smoking Cessation in Patients With Coronary Heart Disease. JAMA. 290(1):86-97.

17. Currie C, Gabhainn SN, Godeau E, Roberts C, Smith R, Currie D et al. (2008). Inequalities in young people's health, HBSC international report from 2005/2006 survey. Copenhagen, Denmark: WHO Regoinal Office For Europe.

18. Currie C, Roberts C, Morgan A, Smith R, Settertobulte W, Samdal O et al. (2004). Young people's health in context. Health Behaviour in School-Aged Childern (HBSC) study: international report from the 2001/2002 survey. Copenhagen: WHO Regional Office for Europe.

19. Dallongeville J, Marecaux N, Fruchart JC, Amouyel P (1998). Cigarette smoking is associated with unhealthy patterns of nutrient intake: a meta-analysis. J Nutr. 128(9):1450-1457.

20. Danaei G, Ding EL, Mozaffarian D, Taylor B, Rehm JA, Murray CJL et al. (2009). The Preventable Causes of Death in the United States: Comparative Risk Assessment of Dietary, Lifestyle, and Metabolic Risk Factors. PLoS Med. 6(4):e1000058.

21. de Vries H, van 't Riet J, Spigt M, Metsemakers J, van den Akker M, Vermunt JK et al. (2008). Clusters of lifestyle behaviors: Results from the Dutch SMILE study. Prev Med. 46(3):203-208.

22. del Carmen M, Alcon G, Pedersen J, Maria A, Gonzalez C (2002). Greenlandic family structure and communication with parents: influence on schoolchildren's drinking behaviour. Int J Circumpolar Health. 61:319-331.

23. Donovan JE, Jessor R (1985). Structure of problem behavior in adolescence and young adulthood. J Consult Clin Psychol. 53(6):890-904.

24. Dorri M, Sheiham A, Watt RG (2009). Relationship between general hygiene behaviours and oral hygiene behaviours in Iranian adolescents. Eur J Oral Sci. 117(4):407-412.

25. Dorri M, Sheiham A, Watt RG (2011). The relationship among educational achievement, career aspiration, and oral hygiene behaviours in Iranian adolescents. Eur J Oral Sci. 119(1):48-54.

26. Duncan SC, Duncan TE, Hops H (1998). Progressions of Alcohol, Cigarette, and Marijuana Use in Adolescence. J Behav Med. 21(4):375-388.

27. Ezzati M, Lopez AD (2003). Estimates of global mortality attributable to smoking in 2000. The Lancet. 362(9387):847-852.

28. Faeh D, Viswanathan B, Chiolero A, Warren W, Bovet P (2006). Clustering of smoking, alcohol drinking and cannabis use in adolescents in a rapidly developing country. BMC Public Health. 6:169.

29. Grufman M, Berg-Kelly K (1997). Physical fighting and associated health behaviours among Swedish adolescents. Acta Paediatr. 86(1):77-81.

30. Hair EC, Park MJ, Ling TJ, Moore KA (2009). Risky Behaviors in Late Adolescence: Co-occurrence, Predictors, and Consequences. J Adolesc Health. 45(3):253-261.

31. Hanson MD, Chen E (2007). Socioeconomic Status and Health Behaviors in Adolescence: A Review of the Literature. J Behav Med. 30(3):263-285.

32. Harada S, Akhter R, Kurita K, Mori M, Hoshikoshi M, Tamashiro H et al. (2005). Relationships between lifestyle and dental health behaviors in a rural population in Japan. Community Dent Oral Epidemiol. 33(1):17-24.

33. Hays R, Stacy AW, DiMatteo MR (1984). Covariation among health-related behaviors. Addictive Behaviors. 9(3):315-318.

34. Holman CD, English DR, Milne E, Winter MG (1996). Meta-analysis of alcohol and all-cause mortality: a validation of NHMRC recommendations. Med J Aust. 164(3):141-145.

35. Honkala E, Rajala M, Rlmpela M (1981). Oral hygiene habits among adolescents in Finland. Community Dent Oral Epidemiol. 9(2):61-68.

36. Hyun SP, Karen GS, Eun HJ, Hyun YK (2006). Predictors of Suicidal Ideation Among High School Students by Gender in South Korea. J Sch Health. 76:181-188.

37. Kandel D, Yamaguchi K, Chen K (1992). Stages of Progression in Drug Involvement from Adolescence to Adulthood: Further Evidence for the Gateway Theory. Journal of Studies on Alcohol. 53:447-457.

38. Katzmarzyk PT, Janssen I, Ardern CI (2003). Physical inactivity, excess adiposity and premature mortality. Obesity Reviews. 4(4):257-290.

39. Kelder SH, Perry CL, Klepp KI, Lytle LL (1994). Longitudinal tracking of adolescent smoking, physical activity, and food choice behaviors. Am J Public Health. 84(7):1121-1126.

40. Khaw KT, Wareham N, Bingham S, Welch A, Luben R, Day N (2008). Combined Impact of Health Behaviours and Mortality in Men and Women: The EPIC-Norfolk Prospective Population Study. PLoS Med. 5(1):e12.

41. Kivimaki M, Lawlor DA, Davey SG, Kouvonen A, Virtanen M, Elovainio M et al. (2007). Socioeconomic position, co-occurrence of behavior-related risk factors, and coronary heart disease: the Finnish Public Sector study. Am J Public Health. 97(5):874-879.

42. Kremers SPJ, De Bruijn GJ, Schaalma H, Brug J (2004). Clustering of energy balance-related behaviours and their intrapersonal determinants. Psychology & Health. 19(5):595-606.

43. Kuntsche EN, Gmel G (2004). Emotional wellbeing and violence among social and solitary risky single occasion drinkers in adolescence. Addiction. 99(3):331-339.

44. Langlie JK (1979). Interrelationships among preventive health behaviors: a test of competing hypotheses. Public Health Rep. 94(3):216-225.

45. Lawlor DA, O'Callaghan MJ, Mamun AA, Williams GM, Bor W, Najman JM (2005). Socioeconomic Position, Cognitive Function, and Clustering of Cardiovascular Risk Factors in Adolescence: Findings From the Mater University Study of Pregnancy and Its Outcomes. Psychosom Med. 67(6):862-868.

46. Levin KA, Currie C (2010). Adolescent toothbrushing and the home environment: sociodemographic factors, family relationships and mealtime routines and disorganisation. Community Dent Oral Epidemiol. 38(1):10-18.

47. Lien N, Lytle LA, Klepp KI (2001). Stability in Consumption of Fruit, Vegetables, and Sugary Foods in a Cohort from Age 14 to Age 21. Prev Med. 33(3): 217-226.

48. Lundborg P (2006). Having the wrong friends? Peer effects in adolescent substance use. Journal of Health Economics. 25(2):214-233.

49. McGee R, Williams S (2000). Does low self-esteem predict health compromising behaviours among adolescents? J Adolesc Health. 23(5):569-582.

50. McVicar D (2011). Estimates of peer effects in adolescent smoking across twenty six European Countries. Soc Sci Med. 73(8):1186-1193.

51. Meng L, Maskarinec G, Lee J, Kolonel LN (1999). Lifestyle Factors and Chronic Diseases: Application of a Composite Risk Index. Prev Med. 29(4):296-304.

52. Mikkila V, Rasanen L, Raitakari OT, Pietinen P, Viikari J (2005). Consistent dietary patterns identified from childhood to adulthood: the cardiovascular risk in Young Finns Study. Br J Nutr. 93(6):923-931.

53. Milio N (1986). Promoting health through public policy. Ottawa: Canadian Public Health Association.

54. Mistry R, McCarthy WJ, Yancey AK, Lu Y, Patel M (2009). Resilience and patterns of health risk behaviors in California adolescents. Prev Med. 48(3):291-297.

55. Mokdad AH, Marks JS, Stroup DF, Gerberding JL (2004). Actual Causes of Death in the United States, 2000. JAMA. 291(10):1238-1245.

56. Murray C, Lopez A (1997). Global mortality, disability, and the contribution of risk factors: Global Burden of Disease Study. The Lancet. 349(9063):1436-1442.

57. Myint PK, Luben RN, Wareham NJ, Bingham SA, Khaw KT (2009). Combined effect of health behaviours and risk of first ever stroke in 20040 men and women over 11 years' follow-up in Norfolk cohort of European Prospective Investigation of Cancer (EPIC Norfolk): prospective population study. BMJ. 2009(338):b349.

58. Neumark-Sztainer D, Story M, French S, Cassuto N, Jacobs DR, Jr., Resnick MD (1996). Patterns of health-compromising behaviors among Minnesota adolescents: sociodemographic variations. Am J Public Health. 86(11):1599-1606.

59. Nutbeam D, Aaro L, Wold B (1991). The lifestyle concept and health education with young people. Results from a WHO international survey. World Health Stat Q 44(2):55-61.

60. Ohene SA, Ireland M, Blum RW (2005). The clustering of risk behaviors among Caribbean youth. Matern Child Health J. 9(1):91-100.

61. Ottevaere C, Huybrechts I, Benser J, De Bourdeaudhuij I, Cuenca-Garcia M, Dallongeville J et al. (2011). Clustering patterns of physical activity, sedentary and dietary behavior among European adolescents: The HELENA study. BMC Public Health. 11(1):328-338.

62. Park Y, Patton L, Kim H (2010). Clustering of Oral and General Health Risk Behaviors in Korean Adolescents: A National Representative Sample. J Adolesc Health. 47(3):277-281.

63. Pate RR, Heath GW, Dowda M, Trost SG (1996). Associations between physical activity and other health behaviors in a representative sample of US adolescents. Am J Public Health. 86(11):1577-1581.

64. Pate RR, Pratt M, Blair SN, Haskell WL, Macera CA, Bouchard C et al. (1995). Physical Activity and Public Health: A Recommendation From the Centers for Disease Control and Prevention and the American College of Sports Medicine. JAMA. 273(5):402-407.

65. Patterson RE, Haines PS, Popkin BM (1994). Health lifestyle patterns of U.S. adults. Prev Med. 23(4):453-460.

66. Pearson N, Atkin A, Biddle S, Gorely T, Edwardson C (2009). Patterns of adolescent physical activity and dietary behaviours. Int J Behav Nutr Phys Act. 2009(6):34.

67. Petridou E, Zavitsanos X, Dessypris N, Frangakis C, Mandyla M, Doxiadis S et al. (1997). Adolescents in high-risk trajectory: clustering of risky behavior and the origins of socioeconomic health differentials. Prev Med. 26(2):215-219.

68. Pickett W, Craig W, Harel Y, Cunningham J, Simpson K, Molcho M et al. (2005). Cross-national Study of Fighting and Weapon Carrying as Determinants of Adolescent Injury. Pediatrics. 116(6):e855-e863.

69. Pierce JP, Gilpin E (1996). How long will today's new adolescent smoker be addicted to cigarettes? Am J Public Health. 86(2):253-256.

70. Pronk NP, Anderson LH, Crain AL, Martinson BC, O'Connor PJ, Sherwood NE et al. (2004). Meeting recommendations for multiple healthy lifestyle factors. Prevalence, clustering, and predictors among adolescent, adult, and senior health plan members. Am J Prev Med. 27(2 Suppl):25-33.

71. Raitakari OT, Leino M, Rakkonen K, Porkka KV, Taimela S, Rasanen L et al. (1995). Clustering of risk habits in young adults. The Cardiovascular Risk in Young Finns Study. Am J Epidemiol. 142(1):36-44.

72. Rhee D, Yun S, Khang Y (2007). Co-Occurrence of Problem Behaviors in South Korean Adolescents: Findings from Korea Youth Panel Survey. Journal of Adolescent Health. 40(2):195-197.

73. Robbins RN, Bryan A (2004). Relationships Between Future Orientation, Impulsive Sensation Seeking, and Risk Behavior Among Adjudicated Adolescents. J Adolesc Health. 19(4):428-445.

74. Roysamb E, Rse J, Kraft P (1997). On the structure and dimensionality of health-related behaviour in adolescents. Psychology & Health. 12(4):437-452.

75. Sallis JF, Prochaska JJ, Taylor WC (2000). A review of correlates of physical activity of children and adolescents. Medi-

cine & Science in Sports & Exercise. 32(5):963-975.

76. Sanchez A, Norman GJ, Sallis JF, Calfas KJ, Cella J, Patrick K (2007). Patterns and Correlates of Physical Activity and Nutrition Behaviors in Adolescents. Am J Prev Med. 32(2):124-130.

77. Schuit AJ, van Loon AJ, Tijhuis M, Ocke M (2002). Clustering of lifestyle risk factors in a general adult population. Prev Med. 35(3):219-224.

78. Settertobulte W, Matos M (2004). Peers. In: Young people's health in context: international report from the HBSC 2001/2002 survey. Currie C, Roberts C, Morgan A, Smith R, Settertobulte W, Samdal O et al., editors. Copenhagen: WHO Regional Office for Europe. pp.34-41.

79. Sheiham A, Watt RG (2000). The Common Risk Factor Approach: a rational basis for promoting oral health. Community Dent Oral Epidemiol. 28(6):399-406.

80. Sosin DM, Koepsell TD, Rivara FP, Mercy JA (1995). Fighting as a marker for multiple problem behaviors in adolescents. J Adolesc Health. 16(3):209-215.

81. Spear HJ, Kulbok PA (2001). Adolescent health behaviors and related factors: a review. Public Health Nurs. 18(2):82-93.

82. Stefansdottir IK, Vilhjalmsson R (2007). Dimensions of health-related lifestyle in young adulthood: results from a national population survey. Scand J Caring Sci. 21(3):321-328.

83. Takakura M, Nagayama T, Sakihara S, Willcox C (2001). Patterns of Health-Risk Behavior Among Japanese High School Students. J Sch Health. 71(1):23-29.

84. Tapp JT, Goldenthal P (1982). A factor analytic study of health habits. Prev Med. 11(6):724-728.

85. Taylor RS, Brown A, Ebrahim S, Jolliffe J, Noorani H, Rees K et al. (2004). Exercise-based rehabilitation for patients with coronary heart disease: systematic review and meta-analysis of randomized controlled trials (abstract). Am J Med. 116(10):682-692.

86. Terre L, Drabman RS, Meydrech EF (1990). Relationships among children's health-related behaviors: a multivariate, developmental perspective. Prev Med. 19(2):134-146.

87. Torabi MR, Bailey WJ, Majd-Jabbari M (1993). Cigarette Smoking as a Predictor of Alcohol and Other Drug Use by Children and Adolescents: Evidence of the "Gateway Drug Effect". J Sch Health. 63(7):302-306.

88. Valois RF, Zullig KJ, Huebner ES, Drane JW (2001). Relationship between life satisfaction and violent behaviours among adolescents. Am J Health Behav.

89. van Nieuwenhuijzen M, Junger M, Velderman MK, Wiefferink KH, Paulussen TWGM, Hox J et al. (2009). Clustering of health-compromising behavior and delinquency in adolescents and adults in the Dutch population. Prev Med. 48(6):572-578.

90. Viner RM, Haines MM, Head JA, Bhui K, Taylor S, Stansfeld SA et al. (2006). Variations in associations of health risk behaviors among ethnic minority early adolescents. J Adolesc Health. 38(1):55. e15-55.e23.

91. Vingilis E, Adlaf E (1990). The structure of problem behaviour among Ontario high school students: a confirmatory-factor analysis. Health Educ Res. 5(2):151-160.

92. Watt RG, Sheiham A (2012). Integrating the Common Risk Factor Approach into a Social Determinants Framework. Community Dent Oral Epidemiol (Accepted for Publication).

93. WHO (1998). Health Promoting Schools: a healthy setting for living, learning and working. Geneva: World Health Organisation.

94. WHO (2000). The World Health Report 2000. Geneva: World Health Organisation.

95. WHO (2003). Diet, nutrition and the prevention of chronic diseases. Report of the joint WHO/FAO Expert Consultation on Diet, Nutrition and the Prevention of Chronic Diseases. Geneva: World Health Organisation.

96. WHO (2008). WHO Report On the Global Tobacco Epidemic-The MPOWER package. Geneva: World Health Organisation.

97. WHO (2009). Global health risks: mortility and burden of disease attributable to selected major risks. Geneva: World Health Organisation.

98. Wiefferink CH, Peters L, Hoekstra F, Dam GT, Buijs GJ, Paulussen TG (2006). Clustering of health-related behaviors and their determinants: possible consequences for school health interventions. Prev Sci. 7(2):127-149.

99. Williams AF, Wechsler H (1972). Interrelationship of preventive actions in health and other areas. Health Serv Rep. 87(10):969-976.

100. Zullig KJ, Valois RF, Huebner ES, Oeltmann JE, Drane JW (2001). Relationship between perceived life satisfaction and adolescents' substance abuse. Journal of Adolescent Health. 29(4):279-288.

Chapter 5

Development of Behaviours and Habits Conducive to Oral Health

Claides Abegg
Ruth Freeman

Introduction

This chapter is about health behaviours. It will explore the literature which illustrates people's health behaviours and will provide explanatory models as a means of understanding behaviour and behaviour change. Therefore factors related to the development of behaviours conducive to oral health and models of behaviour and behaviour change will be described. Health behaviours are conceptualised as behaviours related to health that play an important role in the general and oral health of children and adults and which are beneficial to health at each stage of an individual's health life course.

The development of health and oral health-related behaviours

The development of health and oral health-related behaviours has been shown to be affected by three groups of factors:

- Demographic factors: gender, socioeconomic status, age.
- Environmental and structural factors: environments that enable or inhibit behaviour change; structures that increase or reduce access to health resources such as social capital.
- Psycho-social factors: socialization – influence from social and peer-groups; social norms; daily routines including working and family life and social support.

While these factors are known to affect the adoption of actions advantageous to health, in order to have a clear understanding of their specific roles it is necessary to divide them into their component parts.

Demographic factors *Gender*

Differences have been shown to exist between men and women in relation to the adoption of preventive health behaviours. Women adopt more health-related behaviours and access medical preventive and therapeutic services than men.[1] For instance, Watt and Sheiham,[2] showed that a higher number of female compared with male adolescents attempted to reduce their dietary fat intake. Besides, women brush their teeth and use dental floss more often than men.[3-9] Possible explanations for these differences between the genders may be associated with the woman's role with the society, related to socio-cultural and socio-psychological factors,[1] and the pressure that society exerts on women to make them attractive to men. The importance of health-related behaviours at the expense of health-directed behaviours is thus observed with girls being more concerned about their appearance than the boys.[10]

Socioeconomic status

The evidence of the association between oral health-related behaviours and socioeconomic status abounds in the literature.[6] There is evidence of a social class gradient in oral hygiene behaviours among adolescents and young adults with those from higher compared to lower socioeconomic groups and people who lived in the urban areas rather than rural areas having greater adherence with oral hygiene routines.[3,9,11,12] Abegg[7] showed that the social class gradient in oral hygiene persisted into adulthood; higher socioeconomic category brushed their teeth more often and used dental floss more often than lower socioeconomic adults.

Similarly, Watt and Sheiham[2] found differences between adolescents from high and low socioeconomic categories in relation to the change to a healthier diet. Those adolescents from a high socioeconomic category took into consideration educational leaflets about diet, a higher availability of healthy food, and will power. Adolescents from low socioeconomic category did not consider that these factors were important.

Social and economic conditions may be facilitators or limit the adoption and adherence of health-related habits. The choices and the access to information and education of people with low purchasing power are usually more restricted and may make it difficult to adopt behaviours conducive to health. For example, in the case of dental floss use, the economic factor can be a powerful conditioner because it is an expensive item, not accessible to a large proportion of the population. In the same way, adherence with healthier diet regimes has cost implications for low income groups.

The life course, socialization and the establishment of health behaviours

The process of development of attitudes and behaviours in related to health along the life course is called a "health career" or "life-course in relation to health".[13] A health career offers to the health professional "the description of the ways by which a person's attitudes develop along the time in relation to health."[14] The main factors that influence over the health career in the different phases of life can be seen in figure 5.1.[14,15]

A health career begins in infancy. The influence of parental values, family norms, and social environment affect the behaviours of individuals and are relevant to the promotion of a child's oral health. Parents play a fundamental role in the creation of habits conducive to their child's health.

Fig. 5.1 – Factors that influence people's behaviour at different stages of life.

Childhood	Primary socialization	- Influence of family environment - Little personal control on the behaviour
Adolescence	Secondary socialization	- Development of personal and individual identity - Strong influence from peer groups and people considered as models - Time of rebellion and experiments - Change of role and responsibilities
Adult life	Tertiary socialization	- Routine nature of daily life - Role of parents and bigger responsibilities - Higher access to resources for some (high socioeconomic class)
Mature life Older age	Tertiary socialization	- Potentially less control on the behaviours - Differences between generations: different values - Different expectations in relation to health an quality of life

Children learn and adopt behaviours and habits during childhood by the process of socialization. Socialization is a process of transmission of values, such as routines, knowledge, attitudes, considered of significance to survival by people and the community.[13] It is a continuous experience during the whole life course and for purposes of description it is usually divided into primary, secondary, and tertiary socialization.[14]

Primary socialization begins in the earliest phases of the childhood and is the most important period when family health values and essential social norms are experienced for the first time. The parents' influence, especially the mother's allows, the process of internalization of behaviours, attitudes and beliefs to occur.[16] Primary socialization allows children to identify themselves with the parents' behaviour with parents acting as role models. The parent's attitudes, perceptions and adherence with health and oral health-related behaviours will consequently influence the child's attitudes, perceptions and routines.

At the start of life, mothers play a central role caring for their child's body and educating the child to tooth brush and to wash their hands and face acting as a prototype for future self-care.[16,18,19] In general, children do not like their face, hands and teeth to be washed and in early life this is done by parents[14]. With physical growth and manual dexterity, children will want to copy their parents and wash their own bodies and the teeth. Thus, by the means of copying, children acquire their parent's health values and with constant repetition and praise, this value becomes a habit.

> A child raised in a family environment where oral health care is valued will become an adult who will value oral health.[17]

At the end of the first year of life, the majority of the children have started to take solid foods. It is in this phase that standards of sugar intake are established.[20] Gradually, as children become older they start to adapt family's dietary standards or household rules which is an important step as children' take ownership of their own health actions. Adaptation of parental rules allows children to incorporate parental behaviours into their own oral health and dietary routines.[21,22] For children this stage is not without danger since perceived "good" behaviours will be rewarded and perceived "bad" actions will result in punishment. Nevertheless, it is through the caring, nurturing and educative processes during primary socialization that children develop their set of health rules based upon those of the family.

Secondary socialization merges with primary socialization and it is during this stage of life, the factors that influence the children's behaviour are outside of the family circle as the child establishes relationships outside of the home. Behaviours developed as a result of primary socialization will undergo a process of modification being affected by the beliefs and values of friends and others attending school.[13] Bateman[23] summarized the factors that influence children during secondary socialization. This included the parents; friends and school mates; the reference group, (e.g. celebrities); advertisements of dental products in the media and oral health education at schools and by dental staff in clinics and practices.

In primary education classroom friends and teachers act as role-models for general behaviours and actions related to health and oral health. In later years, adolescent's toothbrushing behaviours become more susceptible to the influence of friends than parents and dental care professionals.[21] Koivusilta et al.[24] have shown how the adoption of health and oral health-related behaviours are altered through adolescence. They have proposed that in early adolescence health behaviours are affected by friends and in later adolescence there is a tendency to return to traditional or family health-related behaviours. While Dorri et al.[25] observed that toothbrushing frequency increased in accordance with the quantity and quality of peer social networks, Koivusilta et al.[24] suggested that by 16-years, adolescents' health oral health-related behaviours have become established.

Beyond the influence of friends is the effect of the reference group. Consequently, the media plays an important role in secondary socialization and might be considered an opinion maker for the population playing an important role in health-related attitude and behaviour formation. The media may affect negatively oral health and health by the promotion of harmful items, such as energy-dense but nutritionally poor snacks but may also have positive influence as observed in the promotion of the use of fluoride toothpaste.[26] This has been observed in the increased consumption of fluoride toothpaste, and its marked impact on the reduction of dental caries prevalence.[26]

> Along the life-course, health education is obtained from various sources; the home, the school, the work place, and the media all of which influence the development of oral health--related attitudes and behaviours related to health.

Tertiary socialization occurs through out adult life. It is related to the acquisition of new health-related habits and changes in health behaviours. Tertiary socialization is influenced by three factors: professionalization, health education, and social norms.[14] Professionalization is associated with a change of values related to the health of people who become health professionals and is linked to professional education being influenced by teachers and colleagues. The acquisition of professional knowledge has been shown to influence the student's oral health-related behaviours.[14] Moreover, the acknowledgement of the health professional by the society as someone who has considerable evidence-based health knowledge, provides legitimacy to provide counselling on health which will influence attitudes and behaviours of society and hence influence social norms (see: Structural and environmental factors).

Routines

During the socialization process children learn behaviours that are integrated into daily routines. Parental health-related behaviours are internalized and as mentioned above through a tortuous process become accepted as the individual's daily routine. Consequently they are not easily changed. In adulthood they form a major part of daily activities and have the character of inflexible routines.[27]

The link between oral health-related behaviours and routines has been described in different studies. Graham[28] showed that on a day-to-day level, much health-related behaviour exists at a routine level. Croucher[29] in a study with British adults found that tooth cle-

aning was part of routines which were placed in a sequence of activities, timings and location. Tooth cleaning pattern formed "a stable and tightly organized system", and had to be fitted into daily activities, where there are competing demands derived from different lifestyles. The relationship between routines of daily activities and oral hygiene behaviour was investigated in Brazilian adults. Subjects with high routines and less flexibility of daily activities were more likely to clean their teeth less frequently compared to subjects with low routines of daily activities. In addition, those who had more flexibility in their working hours brushed their teeth and used dental floss with a higher frequency, and had a lower dental plaque level.[30]

It may be concluded that the organization of everyday life plays an important role in health-related behaviour. Adherence with recommended health behaviours is greater when they are integrated into routines without additional effort and costs.

Structural and environmental factors

Oral health-related behaviours are also affected by cultural and societal forces including concepts of social capital and exclusion. Individuals tend to see themselves belonging to a specific social group, and this is dependent on social factors, such as occupation, education, income and ethnicity. Their health-related behaviours will reflect their s ocio-economic status, their position in the social structure and the environment in which they reside.[19,31]

Social norms, therefore, play a dominant role on people's behaviours and are defined as beliefs and values common to the society where the individuals live and interact. Social norms define behaviours of a social group and being accepted as "normal" provide social cohesion and group identity.[18] The role of social capital upon health-related behaviours is linked with social cohesion and groups identity. Central to social capital are community capacity building and trusting social networks within groups (bonding social capital) and between groups (bridging social capital) which enable people to access health resources. Integral to accessing health resources and adherence with health behaviour advice are the mutually trusting networks between the community and health professionals (linking social capital). Moore et al.[32] have shown that trust in health professionals is an essential predictor of health service use and so, those with poor social capital with poor social networks will experience exclusion from health resources with the subsequent effects upon their health and health-related behaviours.

Among the several factors associated with health-related actions, it is useful to mention the importance of health education. Appropriate and evidence-based information about habits that lead to oral health is essential for oral health promotion. Parents are the main influence in the creation of children's habits that lead to health. Therefore, it is very important that they have evidence-based information on tooth-brushing, the use of fluoride and diet, especially regarding sugars intake.

Besides information, it is essential that people's personal means and abilities to adopt health-conducive behaviours are considered. For example, financial resources to buy toothbrushes and toothpastes are essential.

The development of the ability to properly use a toothbrush and toothpaste depends mainly on the parents. The recommendations are that they help their children to toothbrush until they are seven years old.

The significance of environments or social spaces supportive to health in the behaviours related to health promotion is widely acknowledged and is discussed in Chapter 5 of this book.

Models of health and oral health-related behaviours

Several models involving psychological factors have been proposed to provide a cogent understanding of health and oral health behaviours. The models described in this next section have been extensively examined in an effort to understand action that lead to health promotion. In this section, the most frequently used models will be described in relation to oral health promotion.

Health Locus of Control

Health Locus of Control is a derivation of the concept of localized control conceived by Rotter's social learning theory.[33] In this model, we try to understand how much the individuals believe that the events that happen to them, for example, having health or becoming sick, depends on their own efforts and ability, or that they are the result of external factors, such as luck, chance, or destiny. Individuals that believe that they have control over what happens to them are called inners, while those who believe that what happens to them is related to chance or destiny and do not perceive their control over what happens to them are called externals. The external factors have been divided in two dimensions: powerful other's control, when the individual believes that his or her health depends on people with power over his or her life, like doctors and dentists, and those who chance control, related to random factors, to chance.[34]

Odman et al.[35] did not find any significant relationship between the health locus of control and the improvement of abilities in oral hygiene or in the reduction of dental plaque. A study that investigated if the health locus of control would serve to anticipate people's response to a dental plaque control programme concluded that people could be classified into two groups.[36] The first group included individuals who perceived their susceptibility to diseases by influence of strong external factors, or who believed that the susceptibility could be controlled by their own actions. The second group included individuals who considered that the susceptibility to diseases was influenced by luck. The important point is that only the members of the first group had a more positive response to the regimen and plaque control. Children whose mothers had an external control over health showed higher risk of caries when compared to children whose mothers had an internal control of health.[37]

Theory of Reasoned Action

The Theory of Reasoned Action developed by Ajzen and Fishbein[38] postulates that the behaviour is predicted by the intention of the person to accomplish it or not. The intention of adopting certain kind of behaviour is related to two important factors: the subjective norm and the attitude in relation to the behaviour. The subjective norm means that the individuals perceive the desire of other people that they behave in a certain specific way. The attitude is related to the beliefs about the behaviour's consequences, together with the evaluation of the importance of them.[34]

Some applications of the Theory of Reasoned Action have been used on family planning, weight loss, physical exercise, patient's satisfaction, immunization, and hypertension and oral health. Such studies showed that the intention of adopting a certain behaviour always allows previewing its accomplishment, especially when time is short and the intention is clearly defined.[39] In dentistry, the Theory of Reasoned Action has been tested to study the habit of tooth brushing, the intention to use dental floss,[23,40] and search for dental care.[41] In one study, the Theory of Reasoned Action did not explain what affects tooth brushing behaviour.[23] In another study, there was a relationship between intention and behaviour.[40] Overall the Theory of Reasoned Action has been criticized for assuming a simple causal structure, the intention previewing the behaviour, and the attitudes completely mediating the effects of cognition over intention.[34]

Health Belief Model

The Health Belief Model[42,43] considers that the individuals will adopt a preventive behaviour if they feel susceptible to the disease, if the disease is identified as sufficiently severe to affect any aspect of their life style and if they believe that their action can help to overcome the disease or to be more important than any cost involved with it. The initiative to act can be caused by a 'trigger' like the individual perception of the person or by reading about issues related to health.[39] Janz and Becker[43] in a study review about the Health Belief Model and preventive oral behaviours, concluded that for each one of the beliefs in health there was another study or studies that did not achieve the expected correlation. For example, the Health Belief Model was not able to predict the behaviour of children in relation to dental visits,[44] participation in preventive programmes,[45] or the adherence to home mouth washes.[46.47.48]

There is no consistency in results of empirical studies using the Health Belief Model. On the other hand, the most favourable results are found in retrospective studies, suggesting that, past behaviour predicts the present and future behaviours. Health-related behaviours, such as tooth brushing and dental floss use, are not consequences of beliefs in health. They are most likely to be associated with hygiene and grooming. These habitual behaviours are so automatic that rational considerations on risks and cost/benefit do not modify them.[49]

Self-efficacy

Self-efficacy was initially described by Bandura.[50.51] Since then it has been used in several studies about health-related behaviour. Self-efficacy is the trust that the individual has that a certain behaviour can be adopted or modified, and that he or she can evaluate how much he or she is able to control his or her own behaviour in certain situations.[52]

Self-efficacy sees the change of behaviour as dependent on the ability of the personal perception to deal with stress and annoyance and to mobilize oneself to achieve the proposed objectives. This affects the intention of changing risk behaviours, the effort made to reach that purpose, and the determination to continue trying, in spite of barriers that may undermine the motivation.[53]

Schwarzer,[53] in a review about health behaviours, showed that self-efficacy is a good prognosis of change and of the intention to change behaviour. On the intention to use and the real behaviour of dental floss use. On the intention of joining to the prevention of the consequences of breast cancer and to the breast self-examination. On the intention of using and the use of contraceptives. Several studies have shown a relationship between self-efficacy and healthy behaviour and it is therefore useful in health promotion.[34]

Salutogenic Model

The salutogenic model, proposed by Antonovsky postulates that concentrating on resources and the ability of people to create health is more appropriate than focusing on understanding disease, because the factors that promote health are different from those that pose a risk for the occurrence of disease (Antonovsky.[54,55] The main construct of the Salutogenic model is the Sense of Coherence (SOC).

The SOC expresses how confident individuals are that they are capable of understanding and dealing with their daily experiences, enabling them to apply general resistance resources (GRRs). These GRRs can be identified in the immediate and the distant environment of people, including coping strategies, social support, religion, cultural identity and preventive health orientation. An individual´s sense of coherence consists of three dimensions, comprehensibility (cognitive), manageability (behavioural) and meaningfulness (motivational). (Antonovsky[55]). Individuals and communities with higher SOC are more capable to cope with stressors which are considered a standard feature of humans. Therefore, they have higher ability to maintain and improve their health and well-being and are more motivated to adopt healthy behaviors, even in unfavorable circumstances.

According to the literature, SOC is an important resource to promote health which reinforces individual's capacity of resistance and develops a positive meaning of health.[56,57]

The Sense of Coherence has been associated to several health outcomes and to health-related behaviours such as physical acitivity[58] and type of diet.[59] In one of the first studies investigating the relationship between the Sense of Coherence Scale and oral health behaviours,[60] observed that adolescents with higher SOC were more likely to make preventive dental visits than those with lower SOC. A higher SOC was also associated with visiting the dentist regularly in adults.[61,62]

Some studies have also demonstrated that the Sense of Coherence is associated with tooth brushing behaviour. A lower toothbrushing frequency and quality was described in Finish youths and adults with lower level of SOC.[63,64]

The theoretical approach of the Sense of Coherence Scale is in line with the principles of the Otawa Charter[65] which advocates the importance of personal and social development, and enhancing life skills. In this way, individuals and communities will have increased options to exercise more control over their health and to make choices conducive to health.

Models of behaviour change

The relationship between health education and increased knowledge is well known and remains the mainstay of public health awareness programmes. With regard to the evidence-base, studies to change oral health-related behaviours solely by means of health education have resulted in short term changes in behaviours.[66,67,68] Schou and Locker,[69] in a systematic review about the efficacy of oral health education showed that the biggest gains obtained by these programmes were in oral health-related knowledge and attitudes; but not behaviour change. The tendency for health education programmes to focus on knowledge, rather than on values or community needs was felt to be due to using oversimplified models for changing health behaviours which relied on educational models of behaviour change. Health promotion interventions, however, which are successful, rely on alternative strategies. At the centre of these behaviour change models is the appreciation that it is difficult for people to change. Therefore this section will describe two health change models which are client-centred and have been used to assist people to change their health and oral-health behaviours. They are the Stages of change or the Trans-Theoretical Model (TTM) and motivational interviewing.

Trans-Theoretical Model of behaviour change[70]

The TTM provides a strategy to tailor the health promotion to the client's needs while acknowledges competing life priorities. One of its strengths is that it recognizes and allows for relapsing behaviour and the redirection of action. In the TTM adherence with health-related behaviours is an evolving 'process' in which the health professional acts 'facilitator'. The TTM has five basic stages (Fig. 5.2):

The first two stages Pre-contemplation & Contemplation. These two phases include the time when an individual is becoming aware of her health and the potential benefits of changing behaviour. At this time they are not ready to change but are becoming aware of the alternatives available to them to assist them to change. These phases include information gathering, and working through feelings about making changes before making any decisions so that the intervention is tailored to the individual's needs.[71] The preparation phase improves self-awareness, self-image, and increases self-efficacy with clients being supported and prepared for action. During action and maintenance stages the benefits of changing outweigh the 'costs' with specific health goals being identified. The relapse, stage occurs when [or if] maintenance strategies breakdown and previous behaviours

resumed. Relapse is common, particularly where the behaviours are complex and difficult to sustain. This reinforces the need for tailoring and realistic goals which are achievable.

Motivational interviewing (MI)[72]

Behaviour change is a complex process, and is dependent on whether or not patients are ready to change. The identification of the individual's competing life priorities and their state of readiness to change allows a tailored approach to health behaviour change to be realized. In this client-centred model of behaviour change the individual has ownership of the decision to change. The steps in MI promote empowerment and adherence with behaviours for health. The first step in MI is to identify the health behaviour to be modified. In some instances this will be just one behaviour e.g. inter-dental cleaning, in others the patient may have a selection of behaviours to change e.g. cariogenic snacks or drinks. The choice of behaviour to change belongs with the client. The second step is to assess readiness to change which is critical. People may be unsure (ambivalent), ready or not ready to change. Within MI it through understanding ambivalence that allows readiness to change be identified and negotiations to occur to enable behaviour change (Fig. 5.3).

A systematic review with meta-analysis of studies that have investigated behaviour change has shown that that changes in health-related behaviours occur when interventions are tailored to the needs of people.[71] Moreover when behaviours become integrated into daily routines they become automatic and are incorporated into an individual's lifestyle.

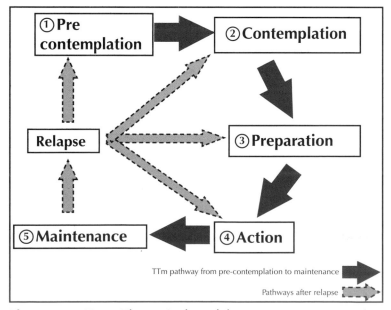

Figure 5.2 – Trans-Theoretical model.

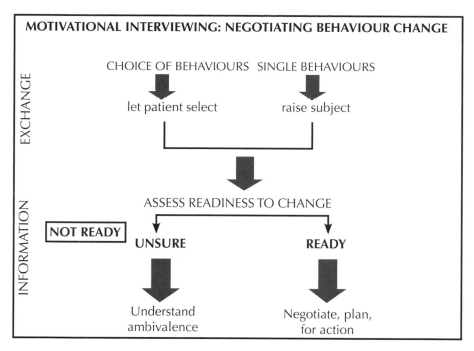

Figure 5.3 – Motivational Interviewing.

Conclusions

The development of health-related behaviours is complex and dynamic changing as individuals progress through their life-course. Demographic factors are known to influence health-related behaviours. Primary and secondary socialization which occurs during childhood and adolescence directly influences the formation of behaviours. In this period, the parent's role is pivotal. At adult life, during tertiary socialization, a wider range of social, environmental, and psychological factors influence people's behaviours. Changes of health-related behaviours in adult life are associated with changes in the social context in which people live and their established social relationships. Social capital theory suggests that trusting social relationships favour changes in health-related behaviours. New friends, a new job, and moving to another address are all known to affect people's health-related behaviours.[27,59]

It is the interaction of these factors that determines an individual's health-related behaviours.

Health-related behaviours are difficult to change. Health behaviour models that combine the developmental factors provide a theoretical and explanatory basis for the understanding of health-related behaviours. Models of behaviour change emphasise the importance of tailoring the intervention to the individuals' needs while providing social support during the initial process of change

The formation of health-related behaviours begins in childhood and is essential for both general and oral health of individuals for their whole life. A knowledge of factors that influence and how people may be supported to adopt health-related behaviours is essential for dental health professionals, since it is their task to help children and parents and those responsible for planning oral health and health promotion.

References

1. Kandrack MA. Gender differences in health related behaviour: some unanswered questions. Social Science and Medicine. 1991; 32:579-90.

2. Watt RG, Sheiham A. Dietary patterns and changes in inner city adolescents. Journal of. Human Nutrition and Dietetics. 1996; 9:451-61.

3. Murtuomaa H. Toothbrushing in Finland. Community Dent Oral Epidemiol. 1979; 7:185-90.

4. Nyyssonen V, Honkala E. Toothbrushing frequency in four consecutive studies of Finnish adolescents. J Clin Periodont. 1984a; 11:682-8.

5. Nyyssonen V, Honkala, E. Oral hygiene status and habitual toothbrushing in children. Journal of Dentistry for Children. 1984b; 4:285-8.

6. Gift HC. Current utilization patterns of oral hygiene practices: state-of-the science review. In: Löe H, Kleinman DV(eds.). Dental plaque control measures and oral hygiene practices. Oxford: IRL. 1986; p.285-8.

7. Abegg C. Hábitos de hygiene bucal de adultos porto-alegrenses. Revista de Saúde Pública. 1997; 31(6):586-93.

8. Honkala E, Freeman R. Oral higiene behaviour and periodontal status in European adolescents: an overview. Community Dent Oral Epidemiol. 1988; 16:194-8.

9. Todd J, Lader D. Adult dental heath-dental 1988: United Kingdom. London: HMSO. 1991.

10. Hodge HC. Factors associated with toothbrushing behaviour. [Ph.D Thesis], University of Manchester. 1979.

11. Rise J, Haugejorden O, Wold B, Aarö LE. Distribution of dental health behaviours in Nordic schoolchildren. Community Dent Oral Epidemiol. 1991a; 19:9-13.

12. Rise J, Aarö LE. Determinants of dental health behaviours in Nordic schoolchildren. Community Denti Oral Epidemiol. 1991b; 19:14-9.

13. Tones BK. Socialisation, Health Career and the Health Education of Schoolchild. J.Int Health Educ. 1979;17(1):23-8.

14. Freeman R. The determinants of dental health attitudes and behaviours. British Dent J. 1999; 187(1):15-8.

15. Croucher R, Watt R. Health Behaviour Change. Personal communication. M.A. in Public Health. University of London. 1994.

16. Blinkhorn AS. Toothbrushing as part of primary socialization. [PhD Thesis], Manchester, Department of Preventive Dentistry, University of Manchester. 1976.

17. Gift HC. Social factors in oral health promotion. In: Schou L, Blinkhorn AS, (eds). Oral Health Promotion. Oxford: Oxford Medical Publications. 1993; p.65-98.

18. Baric L, Blinkhorn SA. & MacArthur. A health education approach to nutrition and dental health education. J Prec Dent. 1974; 1:11-23.

19. Rayner JF, Cohen LK. A position on school dental health education. J Prev Dent. 1974; 1:11-23.

20. Honkala E. Oral health promotion with children and adolescents. In: Schou, L. and Blinkhorn, A. (eds). Oral Health Promotion. Oxford: Oxford University. 1993; p.169-87.

21. Freeman R, Whelton H, Gibson B. Toothbrushing rules: power dynamics and toothbrushing in children. Social Science and Dentistry. 2010; 1(1):37-47.

22. Freeman R, Ekins R, Oliver M. Doing Best for Children: An emerging grounded theory of parents' policing strategies to regulate between meal snacking. Grounded Theory Review. 2005; 4(3):59-80.

23. Bateman P. Understanding and predicting toothbrushing behavior in adolescents. MSc. (PhD Thesis) Department of Community Dental Helth, London Hospital Medical College. 1985.

24. Koivusilta L, Honkala S, Honkala E. Rimpelä A. Toothbrushing as Part of the Adolescent Lifestyle Predicts Education Level. J Dent Res. 2003; 82(5):361-366.

25. Dorri M, Sheiham A, Watt RG. Relationship between general hygiene behaiuuviours and oral hygiene behaviours in Iranian adolescents. European Journal of Oral Sciences. 2009; 117:407-412.

26. Drowner MC. The role of oral health promotion in oral health policy. In: Schou L, Blinkhorn AS. Oral Health Promotion. Oxford: Oxford Medical Publications. 1993; p.121-41.

27. Cullen IG, Phelps E. Diary techniques and problems of urban life. Joint Unit for Planning Research, University College London. 1975.

28. Graham H. Women health and the family. Brighton: Harvester. 1984.

29. Croucher R, Lay perspectives on oral hygiene performance: their use in hypothesis development. Community Dent Health. 1994; 11:105-10.

30. Abegg C, Croucher R, Marcenes WS. Sheiham A. How do routines of daily activities and flexibility of daily activities affect tooth-cleaning behavior? J of Public Health Dent. 2000; 154-58.

31. Jacob MC, Plamping D. The practice of primary dental care. London: Wright. 1989.

32. Moore S, Bockenholt U, Daniel M, Frohlich K, Kestens Y, Richard L. Social capital and core network ties: a validation of individual-level social capital measures and their association with extra and intra-neighbourhood ties and self rated health. Health & Place. 2011; 17:536-544.

33. Rotter JB, Chance J, Phares EJ. Applications of a social-learning theory. New York: Holt, Rinehart and Winston. 1972.

34. Soogard AJ. Theories and models of health behavior. In: Shou L, Blinkhorn AS, (eds.) Oral Health Promotion. Oxford: Oxford University. 1993; p.25-64.

35. Odman PA, Lange AL, Bakdash MB. Utilization of locus of control in the predictions of patient's oral hygiene performance. J Clin Periodontology. 1984; 11, 367-72.

36. Galgut PN, Waite IM. Todd-Pokropek A, Barnby GJ. The relationship between the multidimensional health locus of control and the performance of subjects on a preventive periodontal programme. J Clin Periodont. 1987; 14:171-6.

37. Reisine S, Litt M. Social and psychological theories and their use for dental practice. Int Dent J. 1993; 43:279-87.

38. Ajzen I, Fishbein M. Understanding Attitudes and Predicting Social Behavior. Prentice-Hall, Englewood Cliffs, NJ. 1980.

39. Mullen PD, Hersey JC, Iverson DC. Health behavioural models compared. Social Science and Medicine. 1987; 24:973-81.

40. McCaul KD, O'Neill HK, Glasgow RE. Predicting the performance of dental hygiene behaviours: an examination of the Fishbein and Ajzen model and self-efficacy expectations. J Applied Soc Psychol. 1988; 18:118-28.

41. Hoogstraten J, De Haan W, Ter Horst G. Stimulating the demand for dental care: an application of Ajzen and Fishbein's theory of reasoned action. European J Soc Psychol. 1985; 15:401-14.

42. Haefner DP. The health belief model and preventive dental behaviour. In: Becker, M (ed.). The health belief model and personal health behaviour. Thorofare: Charles B. Slack. 1974.

43. Janz NK, Becker MH. The health Belief Model: a decade later. Health Education Quarterly. 1984; 11:1-47.

44. Kegeles S. Why people seek dental care: a test of a conceptual formulation. J Human Behaviour. 1963; 4:166-173.

45. Weisenberg M, Kegeles S, Lünd A. Children's health beliefs and acceptance of a dental preventive activity. J Health and Social Behavior. 1980; 21:59-74.

46. Kegeles S, Lünd AK. Acceptance by children of a daily home mouthrinse program. Social Science and Medicine. 1978; 12, 199-210.

47. Kegeles S, Lünd AK. Adolescent's health beliefs and acceptance of a novel preventive dental activity: replication and extension. Health Education Quarterly. 1982; 98:192-208.

48. Kegeles S, Lünd AK. Adolescent's health beliefs and acceptance of a novel preventive dental activity: a further note. Social Science and Medicine. 1984; 19:978-982.

49. Ingleheart MS, Tedesco LA. The role of the family in preventing oral diseases, In: Cohen LK, Gift HC. (eds.) Disease Prevention and Oral Health Promotion. Copenhagen: Munksgaard. 1995; p.271-92.

50. Bandura, A. Self-efficacy: towards a unifying theory of bahaviour change. Psychological Review. 1977; 84:191-215.

51. Bandura A. Social foundations of thought and action. Englewood Cliffs: Prentice Hall. 1986.

52. Ogden J. Psycosocial theory and the creation of the risk self. Social Science and Medicine. 1995; 40:409-15.

53. Schwarzer R. Self-efficacy in the adoption and maitenance of health behaviours: theoretical approaches and a new model. In: Schwarzer R, (ed.) Self efficacy: thought control of action. Washington: Hemisphere. 1992; p.217-243.

54. Antonovsky A. Health, stress and coping. San Francisco: Jossey-Bass; 1979. Antonovsky A. Unraveling the mystery of health – how people manage stress and stay well. London: Jossey- Bass. 1987.

55. Eriksson M, Lindström B. Antonovsky's sense of coherence scale and relation with health: a systematic review. J Epidemiol Community Health. 2006; 60:376-81.

56. Silva NA, Mendonça MHM, Vettore MV. A salutogenic approach to oral health promotion. Cad. Saúde Pública. 2008; 24(4):521-30.

57. Kuuppelomaki M, Utriainen P. A 3 year follow-up study of health care student's sense of coherence and related smoking, drinking and physical exercise factors. International Journal of Nursing Studies. 2003; 40(4):383-8.

58. Lindmark U, Stegmayr B, Nilsson B, Lindhal B, Johansson I. Food selection associated with sense of coherence in adults. Nutrition Journal. 2005; 28(4):4-9.

59. Freire MCM, Sheiham A, Hardy RA. Adolescents' sense of coherence, oral health status, and oral health-related behaviours. Community Dentistry and Oral Epidemiology. 2001; 29(3):204-12.

60. Savolainen J, Knuuttila M, Suominen-Taipale L, Martelin T, Nordblad A, Niskanen M, et al. A strong sense of coherence promotes regular dental attendance in adults. Community Dent Health. 2004; 21(4):271-76.

61. Bernabé E, Kivimäki M, Tsakos G, Suominen-Taipale L, Nordblad A, Sovalainen J, et al. The relationship among sense of coherence, socio-economic status, and oral health-related behaviours among Finnish dentate adults. European Journal of Oral Sciences. 2009; 117(4):413-18.

62. Savolainen J, Suominen-Taipale L, Uutela A, Martelin T, Niskanen M, Knuuttila M. Sense of coherence as a determinants of toothbrushing frequency and level of oral hygiene. Journal of Periodontology. 2005; 76(6):1006-12.

63. Bernabé E, Watt RG, Sheiham A, Suominen-Taipale L, Nordblad A, Savolainen J, et al. The influence of sense of coherence on the relationship between childhood socioeconomic status and adult oral health-related behaviours. Community Dent Oral Epidemiology. 2009; 37(5):57-65.

64. WHO. The Otawa Charter for Health Promotion 1986. [homepage on the Internet]. [cited 19 September 2011] Available from: www.who.int/hpr/NPH/docs/ottawa_charter_hp

65. Schou, L. Active-involvement principle in dental health education. Community Dent Oral Epidemiol. 1985; 13: 128-32.

66. Kiyak HA, Mulligan K. Behavioural research relate to oral hygiene practices: state-of-the-science review. In: Loe, H. Kleinman DV, (eds.). Dental Plaque Control Measures and Oral Hygiene Practices. Oxford: IRL. 1986; p.225-37

67. Kay EJ, Locker D. Is dental health education effective? A systematic review of current evidence. Community Dent Oral Epidemiol. 1996; 24:231-35.

68. Schou L, Locker D. A review of the effectiveness of health education and health promotion. Dutch Centre for Health Promotion and Health Education. 1994;4:7-31.

69. Prochanska JO, DiClemente CC. Stages and processes of self change of smoking: toward an integrative model of change. Journal of Consulting and Clinical Psychology. 1983; 51(3):390-395.

70. Wanyonyi KL, Themessl-Hubber M, Humphris G, Freeman R. A systematic review and meta-analysis of face-to-face communication of tailored health messages: Implications for practice. Patient Education and Counseling. (2011). In press.

71. Rollnick S, Mason P, Butler C. Health behaviors change: a guide for practitioners. London: Churchill Livingstone. 2000.

Chapter 6

Preventive Strategies: Concepts and Principles of Health Promotion

Vibeke Baelum
Richard G. Watt

Introduction

Traditionally, societies look to their health care sector when concerns arise over population ill-health.[8] However, the tools available to health professionals are insufficient to bring about sustainable improvements of population health. Many dental professionals do indeed engage in oral disease prevention, but this is generally limited to chair side preventive activities. Their activities are based on the common notion that dental caries, gingivitis and periodontitis are all behavioural diseases shaped by individual lifestyles. This approach disregards the broader social determinants of lifestyles. The behaviour of any given individual reflects cultural norms, expectations, and the opportunities arising from the circumstances in which they are born, grow, live, work and age.[8] These contextual circumstances are socio-economically determined and structurally maintained, and their effects reach way above their influences as individual attributes (Fig. 6.1).

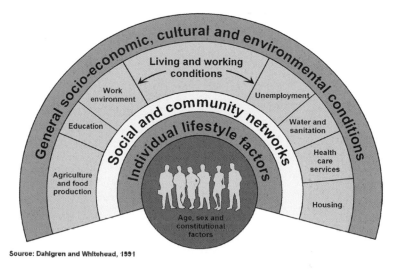

Source: Dahlgren and Whitehead, 1991

Fig. 6.1 – The determinants of population health.

Examples of such contextual factors are many and varied, as shown in figures 6.2 to 6.5. Shopkeepers usually prefer to display sweets and confectionary near the check-out counters where people queue for payment (Fig. 6.2). The reason is that this is the best way to sell more of these non-essential commodities. People who live in the favela shown in figure 6.3 are exposed to a social and physical environment that is not conducive to good health. If your neighbourhood is characterized by the shops shown in figure 6.4, you are much more likely to have a high intake of fast-food meals. These are high in fat and sugars, and low in proteins, dietary fibres, vitamins and essential nutrients, and increase the risk of many diseases, including dental caries (Fig. 6.5). While it is common to urge people with a high intake of fast-food meals (or other unhealthy behaviours) to change their lifestyle this approach is de-contextualised and ignores the very powerful forces involved in the production, distribution, sale and consumption[26] of the commodities. Using smoking as an example, Nancy Krieger[26] characterized a cigarette not only as the well-known commodity that has profoundly deleterious biological and addictive effects on the human body when smoked and promotes increasing social gradients in health but also, and simultaneously, as an extremely profitable commercial product whose production, distribution and sale generates profits along the whole range from landowners over manufacturers to retailers up to government (Box 6.1). This characterization is based on the eco-social perspective[25] on population health, which holds that both the material substances themselves (the physical or biological risks that are biologically embodied) as well as the political economy, societal structures and social relations inherent in their production must be considered if we are to make sustainable public health progress. The cigarette characterization provided by Krieger can be adapted to suit most of the commodities that push people in the direction of unhealthy habits such as those involving smoking, excessive alcohol consumption, poor dietary practices and sedentary lifestyles, and the fast-food meal characterization might read as shown in the box (Box 6.2).

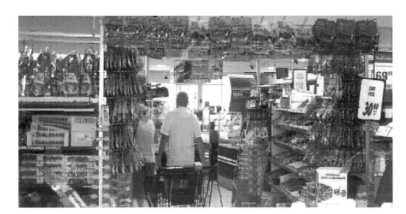

Fig. 6.2 – The check-out counter area of a grocery store is dominated by sweets and confectionaries.

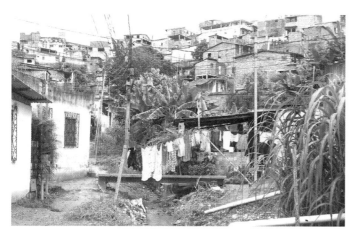

Fig. 6.3 – A Brazilian favela – environment is not conducive to good health.

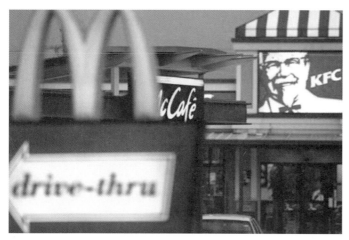

Fig. 6.4 – Down the fast-food lane.

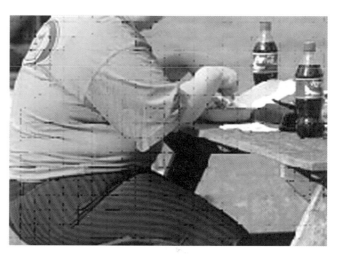

Fig. 6.5 – Enjoying a fast-food meal.

Box 6.1 – A cigarette is and simultaneously.

> - A combustible mass of tobacco leaves and additives whose burning smoke transports psychoactive and addictive chemicals (e.g., nicotine) and carcinogens deep down the respiratory tract to the innermost parts of the lung and its alveolar capillaries, thereby increasing risk of cancer, cardiovascular and pulmonary disease, and other smoking-related ailments
> - A highly profitable product whose production, distribution, advertisement, and consumption involves relentless corporate marketing (including manipulation of ideologies involving freedom, class, gender, sexuality and race/ethnicity and targeting of marginalized groups), government regulation and taxation, tobacco farmers and workers, landownership, trade agreements, and international treaties

Box 6.2 – A fast-food meal is and simultaneously.

> - A high-fat, high-carb mass of nutrients with a high glycemic index whose ingestion promotes excess caloric intake and demotes intake of sufficient dietary fibres and essential nutrients such as vitamins, thereby increasing the risk of diabetes, cardiovascular disease and other diet-related ailments
> - A highly profitable product, whose production, distribution, advertisement, and consumption involves relentless corporate marketing (including targeting of marginalized groups), government regulation and taxation, farmers and workers, trade agreements and international treaties

Effective approaches to the prevention and control of oral diseases must be aligned with this causal view. We cannot expect to make progress unless we consider the whole range of policies, structures and events that are conducive to population exposure to health risks. Unfortunately, the ethos and philosophy of the health professions, including medicine and dentistry, is focused to a downstream, patient-centred, curative and rehabilitative approach to diseases. This is illustrated for dentistry in figure 6.6. While rehabilitative services are needed to care for those who have already suffered the consequences of oral diseases, they do not influence the incidence of disease and therefore do not improve population oral health.

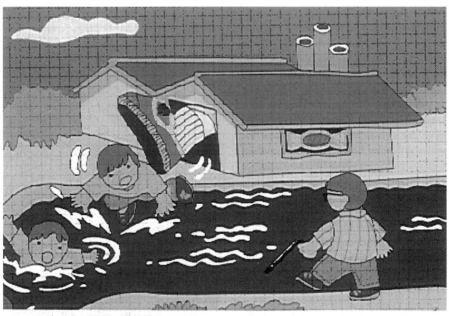
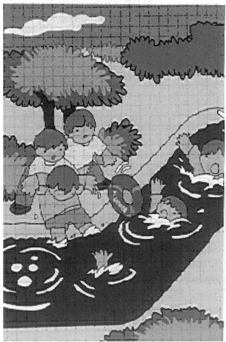
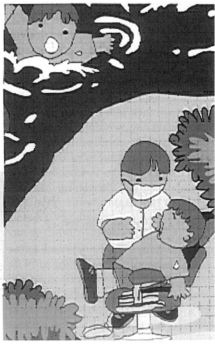

Fig. 6.6 – Upstream the confectionary industry is pushing people into the caries stream. Midstream dental professionals try to prevent people from drowning by throwing fluoride life-belts at them, and downstream the chair-side dentist is resuscitating the fortunate ones.

Preventive strategies – battling disease

In a seminal paper, Geoffrey Rose[41] pointed out the usefulness of distinguishing two kinds of etiological questions. Noting that the determinants of disease incidence in a population are not necessarily the same as the causes of disease in single individuals, Rose suggested a similar distinction between the individual and the population-based applied to preventive strategies.

Prevention for individuals – the high-risk strategy

The high-risk strategy is based on the use of screening to detect individuals at high risk to disease. Although those identified probably thought they were well, they are brought to understand that they are in effect patients who must be treated for their risks. The high-risk strategy seeks to achieve a truncation of the risk distribution (Fig. 6.7), such that disease risks above certain threshold values are eliminated.

In his book The Strategy of Preventive Medicine, Geoffrey Rose[42] lists a number of reasons why the high-risk strategy is intuitively appealing (Box 6.3). In the high-risk strategy, intervention is restricted to those individuals who as a consequence of the screening results now perceive themselves as having a problem. Intervention therefore makes sense to both the health professional and to the patient. Since low-risk individuals are not interfered with, resources are used in a cost-effective way, and the hassles are avoided of urging preventive actions on the majority of low-risk people who have limited prospect of benefit.

Implementation of a high-risk preventive strategy has important prerequisites (Box 6.4). First, and foremost, the strategy involves screening for risk. In some settings screening may be quite straightforward, e.g., the midwife's APGAR scoring of the newborn baby, but in many other settings the relevant

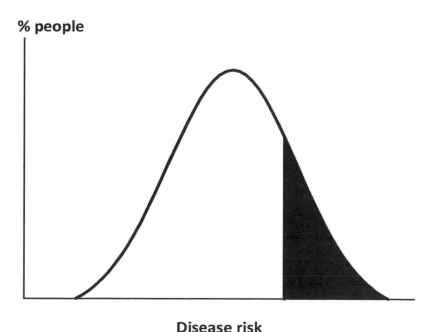

% people

Disease risk

Fig. 6.7 – Truncation of the risk distribution in the high-risk preventive strategy.

Box 6.3 – Advantages of the high-risk strategy.

- Intervention is appropriate to the individual
- No interference with those not at special risk
- Readily accommodated within the ethos, philosophy and organization of health care
- Cost-effective use of resources
- Selectivity improves the benefit-to-risk ratio

Box 6.4 – Prerequisites for the high-risk strategy.

- Existence of intervention that is effective and safe
- Existence of intervention that is acceptable and will be complied with
- Existence of a screening method that is acceptable and will elicit a high degree of response
- Reasonable total costs of preventing one disease event to the health services
- Reasonable total costs, in physical, social and emotional terms, to participants of preventing one disease events

screening procedures may be difficult and expensive. Often, the evidence for the intervention is based on efficacy studies, i.e., randomized controlled clinical trials carried out under ideal conditions. However, these studies do not provide the necessary evidence for the effectiveness of, and compliance with, the intervention when applied under average condition over a period of many years. These shortcomings lead to the one of the principle limitations of the high-risk strategy, problems of feasibility and costs (Box 6.5). The behavioural inadequacy of the high-risk strategy stems from the idea that only the high-risk subject, not their peers or social environment, needs to change. It is unreasonable to expect people to behave substantially different from their peers. A more appropriate approach would be to seek a change in the behavioural norms and the circumstances facilitating behaviours. As previously alluded to, the identification of high--risk in a non-diseased subject alters this person's status to that of a patient,

whereby prevention becomes medicalized. Screening methods tend to be imperfect, which may have serious consequences for the person wrongly deemed at high-risk, just as the real high-risk persons may falsely feel exonerated if the screening test is negative.

If using the high-risk strategy, one should bear in mind that this strategy does not target the causes of risk. This means that new high-risk subjects will continue to emerge, and the results of the high-risk strategy will therefore be palliative and temporary only. The fundamental problem in focusing only on those at high risk was epitomized in the iceberg metaphor coined by Rose[42] (Box 6.6).

The perhaps most serious limitation of the high-risk strategy is that its contribution to the overall control of disease may be rather small. This originates from the fact that low risk does not mean absence of risk. Rose[42] thus noted that a large number of people exposed to a small risk may generate many more cases than a small number exposed to a high

Box 6.5 – Limitations of the high-risk strategy.

- Problems of feasibility and costs
- Behaviourally inadequate
- Prevention becomes medicalized
- Success is only palliative and temporary
- Poor ability to predict the future of individuals
- Contribution to overall control of disease may be small

Box 6.6 – Rose's iceberg Metaphor.

"..... the mild can be the father of the severe. The visible tip of the iceberg of disease can be neither understood nor properly controlled if it is thought to constitute the entire problem"

risk. Batchelor and Sheiham[4] demonstrated this problem with the high-risk strategy for the prevention of dental caries. A child's past caries experience is the best predictor of their future caries experience,[15,16] but most of the new caries lesions developed among those children who, on the basis of past caries experience, were classified as being at the lowest risk.[4]

Even though the high-risk strategy for prevention has been described as a 'targeted rescue operation for the vulnerable individual',[42] examples do exist of successful high-risk strategies in the field of oral health. Hausen and co-workers conducted a community trial of a caries controlling regimen in a Finnish low caries population screened for the presence of active initial caries lesions.[17] Caries-active children were randomized into an intervention group and a control group. In the intervention group all caries preventive activities were carried out by trained dental hygienists, and the children were seen by a dentist only if a caries lesion requiring filling was ob-

served by the dental hygienist. Children in the control group were seen by dentists and received the treatments normally provided in the public dental clinics. The intervention was very comprehensive and included counselling focused to the child's oral hygiene and dietary practices; and toothbrushes, fluoride toothpaste, fluoride and xylitol lozenges distributed for free. Most importantly, all active caries lesions in the intervention group were treated non-operatively using fluoride and chlorhexidine varnishes and professional cleaning until the lesions appeared to be reversed. After 3.4 yr the caries increment at the cavity level (ΔD3MFS) in the intervention and control groups was 2.56 and 4.60, respectively, showing a significant reduction in the caries increment in the intervention group of this overall low caries population.[17]

When balancing the costs of the program against the effect,[19,20] it was found that the program was cost-effective and that cost-effectiveness could even be further improved if the intervention was left in the hands of dental nurses.[19] Clearly, this program benefited from an already existing infrastructure in the form of a public dental health care program for children, just as the distribution of dental caries in the Finnish child population is so skewed that a high-risk approach could be justified. Moreover, it should be borne in mind that this high-risk approach, despite being cost-effective in a Finnish scenario, is likely to be way too costly in countries with low health budgets available.

Prevention for populations – the population strategy

The causes of disease incidence in a population are found in the determinants of the population average.[41] While the high-risk strategy essentially segregates the high-risk individuals from the rest of their society, the population strategy is based on the notion that a reduced population average risk will bring about much larger benefits. The reasons for this are shown in figure 6.8. The curve to the right hand side shows the distribution of risk in the population before a population preventive strategy has been implemented, while the curve to the left hand side shows the distribution of risk some years after the strategy has been fully rolled out in the population. The 'high-risk' group, delineated by the vertical dashed line, is just the upper tail of the continuous distribution of risk in the population. When we shift the whole risk distribution to the left, we will not only have considerably reduced the size of the 'high-risk' group but we will also have generated preventive benefit corresponding to the black area (Fig. 6.8).

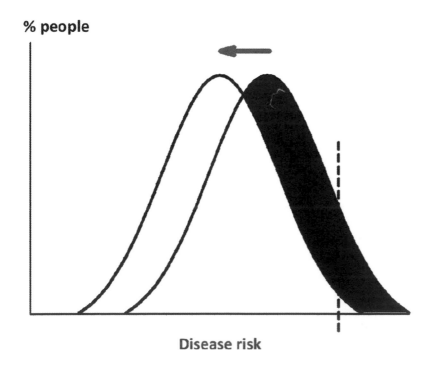

% people

Disease risk

Fig. 6.8 – The population strategy seeks to move the entire risk distribution towards lower risks.

The population strategy for prevention has important strengths (Box 6.7), because it is more radical and addresses the root causes of risk, whereby the risks of the whole population are shifted towards lower risks. A small reduction in the risk average will have marked impact on disease frequency in the population. The strategy is behaviourally appropriate because it does not segregate people according to their risk and does not expect a minority to behave differently from the remainder of the population.

The limitations of the population strategy (Box 6.8) depend on the nature of the intervention. McLaren[33] distinguishes between interventions that are agentic and interventions that are structural (Box 6.9). If the intervention is agentic and seeks to motivate people to change their behaviour, for example though health educational campaigns targeting the dietary, drinking, smoking and exercise habits, it is well known that the results may be disappointing since people's motivation for change may be quite poor. This is because most people are unlikely to perceive an immediate and tangible benefit of changing their health related behaviour. Even though smokers are well aware that smoking is a documented strong risk factor for a plethora of serious threats to both their own health and longevity and that of their surroundings, they often continue smoking.

Health professionals may also lack motivation, in part because of the low rate of success of health education, and in part because the ethos and philosophy of medicine and dentistry make it difficult for these health professionals to see health and disease as anything but a problem for single individuals.

Box 6.7 – Strengths of the population strategy.

- It is radical
- It is powerful
- It is appropriate

Box 6.8 – Limitations of the population strategy.

- Acceptability – people
- May increase health disparities
- Acceptability – health professionals
- Feasibility – government, industry
- Cost and safety issues

Box 6.9 – Interventions can be:

- Agentic – the intervention directly targets behavioural changes in individuals
- Structural – the intervention targets the circumstances and conditions in which behaviours occur

Agentic interventions tend to result in a differential uptake of the intervention, whereby they may lead to increased social inequalities in health. The 'innovators' and 'early adopter's in the population tend to have the necessary economic and social resources for readily changing,[33] while 'late adopters', who typically belong to less resourceful socioeconomic strata, perceive more barriers to change. This is the mechanism that has made some criticize the population strategy for increasing the social disparities in health.[13] Studies of agentic interventions targeting oral hygiene or dietary practices can be summarized as showing that effects on oral hygiene levels, if present, are small and transient.[21-24,48,51] People's knowledge and awareness of oral health problems and methods for their prevention may be improved but the improvements observed during short trial periods do not translate into sustained oral hygiene or dietary improvements in the longer term. Importantly, there are indications that dental health education programs may serve to increase the inequality in the distribution of oral diseases.[44] However, as McLaren[33] showed, population prevention need not be associated with increasing social gradients if structural interventions are implemented.

Structural prevention – a population strategy

The main distinction between the agentic population strategy and the structural population strategy for prevention is that the former directly targets individual behaviour (e.g., through health education and behavioural campaigns), whereas in structural strategies the target is the conditions and circumstances leading to unhealthy behaviours or undesired health consequences.

We are all familiar with a number of structural preventive strategies, e.g., restrictions on food advertising targeting young children, reductions in the salt, fat and sugar contents of convenience foods and taxation on tobacco and alcohol products as a disincentive to their purchase. Speed limits exemplify a structural strategy to prevent road accidents, and people will be punished if they are caught breaking them. A structural preventive strategy that is likely to have wide consequences for health is the ban on smoking in public spaces such as work places, bars and restaurants, since it puts a limit to the places where smoking can occur. Only recently, the city of New York expanded the smoking ban to also include all city parks and city beaches,[18] and in Iceland a proposal has recently been made to take cigarettes out of the usual kiosks and supermarkets and make them available only in pharmacies, where they may be obtained only on the basis of a prescription from their physician.[37] If adopted this strategy has a huge potential for the prevention of the uptake of smoking.

The best known example of a structural population strategy within the field of oral health is the artificial fluoridation of drinking water to prevent dental caries. This intervention has even been declared a top-ten public health achievement of the 20th century in the United States[7]. Even so, this strategy is useful for illustrating one of the safety limitations that may apply with population strategies. Artificial water fluoridation was introduced in many places during the 1940's-1960's following Dean's studies,[9-11] which showed an inverse relationship between drinking fluoridated water and the average caries experience of children. When the water fluoridation programs were implemented dental caries was a huge problem in many populations. However, since the 1960's a considerable caries decline has been observed among children in many countries,[29] and considerable proportions of contemporary child populations now have a D3MFT of.[05,36] While it might be tempting to suggest that this results from the water fluoridation, the decline has been observed in non-fluoridated communities and has continued in previously water fluoridated areas after the cessation of fluoridation.[27,28] Ingestion of fluoride during early childhood causes dental fluorosis;[12] the prevalence of which has been found to increase both in fluoridated and non-fluoridated communities.[43,45] It is therefore not surprising that concerns over what may be termed 'mass medication' and the risk of dental fluorosis associated with water fluoridation,[31] combined with the increasing availability of fluorides from other sources, notably toothpastes, have led to the discontinuation of water fluoridation programs in several places.[31]

In general the methods and means of the structural preventive strategy include legislation, regulation, taxation, and pricing. It is therefore clear that the political level is critical to the implementation of structural preventive strategies for change. Widespread changes in the population's behaviours will cause a whole range of spill-over effects because the production, distribution, and sale of commodities and services will change in response to the changed consumption patterns. This may necessitate the involvement of national and local government, civil society and local communities, businesses, global forums and international agencies[8] in the implementation of structural preventive strategies.

Amalgamating high-risk and population strategies

Preventive strategies have been devised, which amalgamates the characteristics of the high-risk and the population strategy. In one approach, 'vulnerable' population groups are targeted because they - by virtue of their position in the social strata - are exposed to contextual conditions that distinguish them from the rest of the population. The distinguishing social characteristics may involve factors such as ethnicity, minority status and poverty. These vulnerable groups share social characteristics that put them at higher risk of risks, i.e., they have a greater than average risk exposure.[13] It is important to understand that these population groups may not necessarily be at high-risk with respect to any single risk factor, but their average risk exposure is higher than for the remainder of the population.

Another amalgamated strategy is geographic targeting, where interventions are targeted to areas with a known high concentration of high-risk subjects.[6] This approach has been used with success in preventing approximal caries in medium and high risk areas.[47] Targeting 'vulnerable' populations or geographic areas where high-risk groups live has the advantage that screening tests are not needed. Tailored structural interventions can be targeted at these population groups to improve the physical and social environments conducive to good health.

Battling disease or promoting health?

So far, we have mainly considered health risks and the prevention of disease.

This reflects the tools of health professionals since we tend to define the health problems and their solutions to fit with the ethos and philosophy of our professions. We should always bear in mind that as health professionals we are equipped with a limited set of tools, and these may not be the best means for achieving healthy populations. The essence of this problem was elegantly captured by Maslow,[30] who phrased Maslow's Hammer (Box 6.10). Within each of our health professions we tend to concentrate our efforts on the diseases or the solutions that constitute the domain of our profession. In oral health care we are inclined to treat the mouth as if it was separate from the rest of the body. We see a high snacking frequency as a problem for the development of dental caries, and largely ignore the effect on body weight because that is not our domain. When faced with oral health problems we tend to suggest downstream solutions targeted to single individuals because these are the solutions available in our preventive armamentarium. We focus on oral hygiene; largely ignoring that toothbrushing is an integral part of body hygiene, which is carried out for the sake of freshness and appearance more than for dental health reasons. In many circumstances we might fruitfully look to the industry to see how they manage to sell a number of unhealthy habits using the associations to youth, beauty, success, and bright white smiles (Fig. 6.9). If unhealthy habits can be 'marketed' this way, it should indeed be possible to promote healthy habits using the same connotations.

Box 6.10 – Maslows hammer.

".. it is tempting, if the only tool you have is a hammer, to treat everything as if it were a nail"

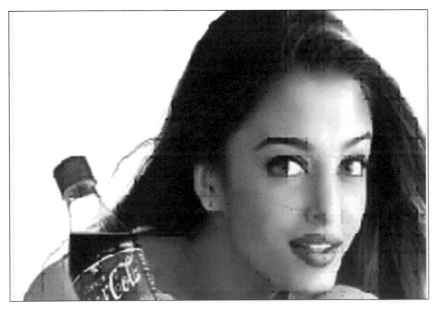

Fig. 6.9 – Associating high-sugar containing sodas with youth, beauty, health and bright white smile.

Health promotion

Health promotion is a key element in population health. Whereas prevention focuses on reducing diseases and their risks, health promotion focuses on enhancing the chances of staying healthy by changing the conditions and ways of living. In health promotion, as laid down in the 1986 Ottawa Charter,[1] (Box 6.11) focus is on the process of enabling people and communities to increase control over, and to improve, their health. The intervention strategies for health promotion place much greater emphasis on the importance of the political, economical, structural and social determinants of population health.[34,39] Unlike traditional individual-oriented prevention, health promotion is truly concerned with the upstream determinants of health and disease. The essence of health promotion can be expressed in the phrase "make the healthy choices the easier choices" (Box 6.12).[35]

Box 6.11 – Ottawa charter (1986) health promotion action means.

- **Build healthy public policy**

  Health promotion goes beyond health care. It puts health on the agenda of policy makers in all sectors and at all levels, directing them to be aware of the health consequences of their decisions and to accept their responsibilities for health.

- **Create supportive environments**

  Our societies are complex and interrelated. Health cannot be separated from other goals. The inextricable links between people and their environment constitutes the basis for a socio-ecological approach to health.

- **Strengthen community action**

  Health promotion works through concrete and effective community action in setting priorities, making decisions, planning strategies and implementing them to achieve better health.

- **Develop personal skills**

  Health promotion supports personal and social development through providing information, education for health and enhancing life skills.

- **Reorient health services**

  The responsibility for health promotion in health services is shared among individuals, community groups, health professionals, health service institutions and governments

Box 6.12 – Health promotion philosophy.

Make the healthy choices the easier choices
through
Healthy public policies

The strategies for intervention in health promotion are based on an ecological model for health-related behaviours (Box 6.13), which sees mass behaviour as a reflection of factors operating at different levels,[34,39] ranging from the individual level over the social and contextual level to the structural level involving government and international bodies.

Realizing that the global context for health promotion has changed dramatically since the 1986 Ottawa charter[1] was formulated; an addendum was made in 2005 to take the effects of globalization into account. The Bangkok Charter for Health Promotion in a Globalized World[2] is rooted in a concern for the health effects of increasing inequalities within and between countries, global environmental change, new patterns of consumption and communication, commercialization and urbanization (Box 6.14). This charter therefore calls for action at four levels: The international, the national, in local communities and civil society, and in the corporate sector. The Bangkok charter emphasises the need for strong political action, broad participation, and sustained advocacy, and the charter further underlines the importance of controlling the upstream determinants of health and disease.

Box 6.13 – Ecological model for health promotion.

- **Individual factors:** Knowledge, attitudes, skills, self- concept, development history
- **Interpersonal processes:** Formal and informal social network, social support system, family, work group, friendship network
- **Institutional factors:** Social institutions with organizational characteristics and formal rules and regulations
- **Community factors:** Relationships among organizations, institutions and informal networks within defined boundaries
- **Public policy:** Local, state, national and international laws and policies

Box 6.14 – Bangkok charter.[2]

- **Health promotion should be made: Central to the global development agenda**
  Governments and international bodies must act to curb the harmful effects of:
  Trade, Products, Services and Marketing Strategies
- **A core responsibility for all of government**
  Local, regional and national governments must prioritize investments in health; provide sustainable financing for health promotion; and make the health consequences explicit of policies and legislation
- **A key focus of communities and civil society**
  They often lead in initiating, shaping and undertaking health promotion, and they should have the rights, resources and opportunities to amplify and sustain their contributions. Civil society needs to exercise its power in the marketplace by giving preference to the goods and services of companies that show social responsibility.
- **A requirement for good corporate practice**
  The private sector is responsible for Health and safety in the workplace, for health promotion among employees, and they should comply with national and international agreements that promote and protect health. Ethical and responsible business practices and fair trade commitment exemplify good corporate practice

From intent to practice in health promotion

Readers with a health professional background may wonder how the very commendable statements of intent that are laid down in the health promotion charters can be brought into action. As expressed in the Bangkok charter, health promotion activities typically originate in local communities and civil society. It is from this level and platform that the public health professional associations can use their knowledge and political strength to campaign for healthy policies to be implemented at the political and corporate level. Moreover, the knowledge and practical experience of public health professionals may be instrumental in ensuring knowledge transfer and helping to build the capacity for health promotion in the community.

The essence of health promotion is enabling individuals and communities to achieve health through the creation of a supportive environment where the healthy choices are the easy choices. The principles underpinning health promotion (Box 6.15) include empowerment, community participation, taking an holistic view, working in an intersectoral manner, equity focused, using evidence based approaches and implementing multi-strategy interventions[50].

Box 6.15 – Principles of oral health promotion.

- **Empowerment**
  Enable individuals and communities to exert more control over the determinants of their oral health
- **Participation**
  Stakeholders should be actively engaged in all stages of planning, implementing and evaluating interventions
- **Holistic**
  Focus on broad common determinants of oral and general health
- **Intersectoral**
  Oral health should be on the agenda of all relevant agencies and sectors to ensure joint strategic partnership working
- **Equity**
  Focus on ways to reduce oral health inequalities and social gradients
- **Evidence based**
  Use existing knowledge on what works to promote effective interventions
- **Sustainable**
  Aim to achieve long term improvements in oral health that are maintained and secure
- **Multi-strategy**
  Use a combination of complementary health promotion strategies such as healthy public policies, community development and environmental change to promote oral health
- **Evaluation**
  Ensure health promotion strategies are evaluated using appropriate methods and measures

Oral health promotion

Most Western high-income countries are characterized by oral health care systems based on highly developed services chiefly provided by licensed dental practitioners. Although the status as a profession should entail a "strong sense of social purpose",[14] the actual strength of dental professional's sense of social purpose has been questioned. Renshaw[38] noted that the "influence of the businessman in dentistry has been growing alarmingly and will have to be curbed if we are to retain the public's approval for what we do". Tomar & Cohen[49] concluded that if it is a goal of society to ensure optimal health of the population attention should be directed to the public health system. Such may be difficult to achieve in the high-income countries where attempts to change the oral health care system are likely to be met by "substantial barriers if not open hostility"[49] and be opposed by the professionals, including the dentists[40]. In his review of the "paradigmatic obstacles" to improving the health of populations McKinlay[32] identified the currently dominant biomedical paradigm as a key cause of ineffective and unjust health policies. The biomedical paradigm diverts the limited resources to the curative and rehabilitative services, blames the victims by focusing on individual lifestyle, produces a lifestyle approach to health policies and de-contextualizes the culturally generated and structurally maintained risk behaviors. A similar observation was made by Rose[41] who noted that a major obstacle to overcome in disease prevention "is the enormous difficulty for medical personnel to see health as a population issue and not merely as a problem for individuals".

In the low- and middle income countries the dental profession may not yet have gained a sufficient stronghold as a liberal trade, and it is therefore most likely in these settings that the opportunity exists to avoid repeating many of the curative and rehabilitative mistakes that continue to be made in the high-income countries.[3]

These low- and middle income countries may take advantage of the opportunity to set priorities using a population-based common risk factor approach.[46] It is well-known that there is a tremendous overlap of the risk factors for oral diseases with the risk factors for other chronic diseases. Policies and interventions based on the common risk factor approach are therefore potentially far more beneficial than isolated, disease specific interventions. Adopting such an approach also carries the advantage of a much wider range of interventions. Importantly, interventions may be implemented that address the threats to population health at levels that are beyond the scope and expertise of health professionals,[49] whether dental or medical. Hence, public health interventions to improve the health of the population may range from the downstream patient-centered curative and rehabilitative rescue operation (Fig. 6.6), which is in the realms of the health professionals, to the upstream public policy approach to healthy lifestyles targeting common risk factors, i.e., structural prevention (Fig. 6.10). At the midstream level preventive approaches may be implemented, in which attempts are made to modify risk among individuals or groups of particularly high risk (high risk and vulnerable population approaches). Other interventions at the midstream level include the agentic preventive population approaches. Interventions are needed at all levels, but a much more balanced distribution of efforts and re-sources along the whole range of public health interventions is clearly required[32] if appropriate, evidence-based, effective, cost-effective, sustainable, equitable, universal, comprehensive and ethical delivery of health care is a goal (Box 6.16). As is, most of the already li-mited resources are typically spent on the downstream curative approaches, which serve only a fraction of the population in the middle- and low-income countries, and are grossly ineffective in addressing population health.

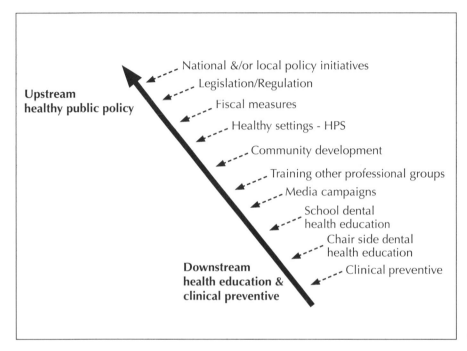

Upstream healthy public policy

National &/or local policy initiatives
Legislation/Regulation
Fiscal measures
Healthy settings - HPS
Community development
Training other professional groups
Media campaigns
School dental health education
Chair side dental health education
Clinical preventive

Downstream health education & clinical preventive

Fig. 6.10 – Upstream/downstream: options for oral disease prevention.

Box 6.16 – The ideal oral health care system is:

- Integrated with general health care
- Emphasizing health promotion and disease prevention
- Monitors population oral health status and needs
- Evidence-based
- Effective
- Cost-effective
- Sustainable
- Equitable
- Universal
- Comprehensive
- Ethical
- Continuously assessing quality and assuring
- Culturally competent
- Empowering individuals and communities

Concluding remarks

In many settings the health care sector is deeply ingrained in a biomedical paradigm that poses important obstacles to population health.[32] Many health care providers are professionals whose actions are not primarily governed by concerns for the health of the public at large.[41] The political level is therefore critical for implementation of strategies for change, since action on the social determinants of health must involve the whole of government, civil society and local communities, businesses, global forums and international agencies.[8] A tremendous commitment and political will on the part of the public and their elected officials is required to align existing health care systems with the attributes of an ideal system, i.e. on that is integrated, based on health promotion and prevention, monitored, evidence-based, effective, cost-effective, sustainable, equitable, universal, comprehensive, ethical, quality assessed, culturally competent and empowering individuals and communities.[49]

References

1. Anonymous. Ottawa charter for health promotion. Can J Public Health. 1986; 77:425-30.

2. The Bangkok Charter for Health Promotion in a Globalized World. 2005 [cited 2011 Jul 1];Available from: URL: http://www.who.int/healthpromotion/conferences/6gchp/bangkok_charter/en/

3. Baelum V, van Palenstein HW, Hugoson A, Yee R, Fejerskov O. A global perspective on changes in the burden of caries and periodontitis: implications for dentistry. J Oral Rehabil. 2007; 34:872-906.

4. Batchelor P, Sheiham A. The distribution of burden of dental caries in schoolchildren: a critique of the high risk caries prevention strategy for populations. BMC Oral Health. 2006; 6:3.

5. Brown LJ, Kingman A, Brunelle JA, Selwitz RH. Most US schoolchildren are caries-free in their permanent teeth - this is no myth. Public Health Rep. 1995; 110:531-3.

6. Burt BA. Concepts of risk in dental public health. Community Dent Oral Epidemiol. 2005; 33:240-7.

7. CDC. Ten great public health achievements - United States, 1900-1999. MMWR Morb Mortal Wkly Rep. 1999; 48:241-3.

8. CSDH. Closing the gap in a generation. Health equity through action on the social determinants of health. Final report of the Commission on Social Determinants of Health. Geneva: World Health Organization. 2008.

9. Dean HT, Arnold FAJr, Elvove E. Domestic water and dental caries. V. Additional studies of the relation of fluoride domestic waters to dental caries experience in 4,425 while children aged 12-14 years of 13 cities in 4 states. Public Health Rep. 1942; 57:1155-79.

10. Dean HT, Jay P, Arnold FAJr, Elvove E. Domestic water and dental caries. II. A study of 2,832 white children aged 12-14 years, of eight suburban Chicago communities, including L. acidophilus studies of 1,761 children. Public Health Rep. 1941; 56:761-92.

11. Dean HT, Jay P, Arnold FAJr, McClure FJ, Elvove E. Domestic water and dental caries, including certain aspects of oral L. acidophilus. Public Health Rep. 1939; 54:862-88.

12. Fejerskov O, Manji F, Baelum V. The nature and mechanisms of dental fluorosis in man. J Dent Res. 1990; 69(spec):692-700.

13. Frohlich KL, Potvin L. Transcending the known in public health practice: the inequality paradox: the population ap-

proach and vulnerable populations. Am J Public Health. 2008; 98:216-21.

14. Gelbier S. 125 years of developments in dentistry, 1880-2005. Part 2: law and the dental profession. Br Dent J. 2005; 199:470-3.

15. Hausen H. Caries prediction - state of the art. Community Dent Oral Epidemiol. 1997; 25:87-96.

16. Hausen H. Caries prediction. In: Fejerskov O, Kidd E, editors. Dental caries - the disease and its clinical management. 2nd ed. Oxford: Blackwell Munksgaard. 2008; 527-42.

17. Hausen H, Seppä L, Poutanen R, Niinimaa A, Lahti S, Kärkkäinen S, Pietilä I. Noninvasive control of dental caries in children with active initial lesions. A randomized clinical trial. Caries Res. 2007; 41:384-91.

18. Hernandez JC. Smoking ban for beaches and parks is approved. NY Times. 2011 Feb 3.

19. Hietasalo P, Seppä L, Lahti S, Niinimaa A, Kallio J, Aronen P, Sintonen H, Hausen H. Cost-effectiveness of an experimental caries-control regimen in a 3.4-yr randomized clinical trial among 11-12-yr-old Finnish schoolchildren. Eur J Oral Sci. 2009; 117:728-33.

20. Hietasalo P, Seppä L, Niinimaa A, Kallio J, Lahti S, Hausen H. Post-trial costs, clinical outcomes, and dental service utilization after a randomized controlled clinical trial for caries control among Finnish adolescents. Eur J Oral Sci. 2010; 118:265-9.

21. Kallio PJ. Health promotion and behavioral approaches in the prevention of periodontal disease in children and adolescents. Periodontol. 2000-2001; 26:135-45.

22. Kay E, Locker D. A systematic review of the effectiveness of health promotion aimed at improving oral health. Community Dent Health. 1998; 15:132-44.

23. Kay EJ, Locker D. Is dental health education effective? A systematic review of current evidence. Community Dent Oral Epidemiol. 1996; 24:231-5.

24. Kay EJ, Locker D. Oral health promotion and caries prevention. Prim Dent Care. 1999; 6:35-7.

25. Krieger N. Theories for social epidemiology in the 21st century: an ecosocial perspective. Int J Epidemiol. 2001; 30:668-77.

26. Krieger N. Proximal, distal, and the politics of causation: what's level got to do with it? Am J Public Health. 2008; 98:221-30.

27. Künzel W, Fischer T. Caries prevalence after cessation of water fluoridation in La Salud, Cuba. Caries Res. 2000; 34:20-5.

28. Künzel W, Fischer T, Lorenz R, Brühmann S. Decline of caries prevalence after the cessation of water fluoridation in the former East Germany. Community Dent Oral Epidemiol. 2000; 28:382-9.

29. Marthaler TM. Changes in dental caries 1953-2003. Caries Res. 2004; 38:173-81.

30. Maslow HA. Acquiring knowledge of a person as a task for the scientist. In: The psychology of science: a reconnaissance. Maurice Bassett Publishing. 1966.

31. McDonagh M, Whiting P, Bradley M, Cooper J, Sutton A, Chestnutt I, Misso K, Wilson P, Treasure E, Kleijnen J. A systematic review of public water fluoridation. University of York: NHS Centre for Reviews and Dissemination. 2000.

32. McKinlay JB. Paradigmatic obstacles to improving the health of populations-implications for health policy. Salud Publica Mex. 1998; 40:369-79.

33. McLaren L, McIntyre L, Kirkpatrick S. Rose's population strategy of prevention need not increase social inequalities in health. Int J Epidemiol. 2010; 39:372-7.

34. McLeroy KR, Bibeau D, Steckler A, Glanz K. An ecological perspective on health promotion programs. Health Educ Q. 1988; 15:351-77.

35. Milio N. Promoting health through public policy. Ottawa: Canadian Public Health Association. 1986.

36. Poulsen S, Pedersen MM. Dental caries in Danish children: 1988-2001. Eur J Paediatr Dent. 2002; 4:195-8.

37. Powell N. Iceland proposes cigarette prescriptions. The Globe and Mail. 2011 Jul 11.

38. Renshaw J. After the first 125 years of the BDJ where might clinical dentistry be heading? Br Dent J. 2005; 199:331-7.

39. Richard L, Gauvin L, Raine K. Ecological models revisited: their uses and evolution in health promotion over two decades. Annu Rev Public Health. 2011; 32:307-26.

40. Riordan PJ. Can organised dental care for children be both good and cheap? Community Dent Oral Epidemiol. 1997; 25:119-25.

41. Rose G. Sick individuals and sick populations. Int J Epidemiol. 1985; 14:32-8.

42. Rose G. The strategy of preventive medicine. Oxford: Oxford University Press. 1992.

43. Rozier RG. The prevalence and severity of enamel fluorosis in North American children. J Public Health Dent. 1999; 59:239-46.

44. Schou L, Wight C. Does dental health education affect inequalities in dental health? Community Dent Health. 1994; 11:97-100.

45. Selwitz RH, Nowjack-Raymer RE, Kingman A, Driscoll WS. Dental caries and dental fluorosis among schoolchildren who were lifelong residents of communities having either low or optimal levels of fluoride in drinking water. J Public Health Dent. 1998; 58:28-35.

46. Sheiham A, Watt RG. The common risk factor approach: a rational basis for promoting oral health. Community Dent Oral Epidemiol. 2000; 28:399-406.

47. Sköld UM, Petersson LG, Lith A, Birhhed D. Effect of school-based fluoride varnish programmes on approximal caries in adolescents from different caries risk areas. Caries Res. 2005; 39:273-9.

48. Sprod AJ, Anderson R, Treasure ET. Effective oral health promotion: literature review. Cardiff: Dental Public Health Unit, Health Promotion Wales. 1996.

49. Tomar SL, Cohen LK. Attributes of an ideal oral health care system. J Public Health Dent. 2010; 70 Suppl 1:S6-S14.

50. Watt RG. From victim blaming to upstream action: tackling the social determinants of oral health inequalities. Community Dent Oral Epidemiol. 2007; 35:1-11.

51. Watt RG, Marinho VC. Does oral health promotion improve oral hygiene and gingival health? Periodontol. 2000-2005; 37:35-47.

Chapter 7

A Social Determinants, Integrated Common Risk Factor Approach (CRFA) to Promoting Oral Health and Reducing Oral Health Inequalities

Aubrey Sheiham
Richard G Watt

Introduction

Most dental approaches to prevention focus on single diseases; dental caries, periodontal disease and oral cancer, and do not give sufficient attention to the fact that the determinants of oral diseases are common to a number of other chronic diseases. As the main behavoural risk factors, such as diet, smoking, alcohol consumption and stress, affect numerous diseases, health promotion cannot, and should not, be compartmentalized to address diseases of specific parts of the body. A broader approach is needed. Until recently, the dominant approaches to general health promotion focused on actions to reduce specific diseases, instead of directing policies to risk factors common to a number of diseases. An alternative public health approach is the common risk factor approach (CRFA) where risk factors common to a number of major chronic diseases are tackled.[1,2]

Box 7.1 – The key concept underlying the integrated common risk factor approach.

The key concept underlying the integrated common risk factor approach is that promoting general health by controlling a small number of important risk factors, should have a major impact on a number of common chronic diseases, including oral conditions, at a lower cost than narrow disease specific approaches.

This chapter will outline the basis for the CRFA and how the concept has been expanded and adopted by international bodies, such as the WHO, and by policy makers concerned about promoting health and preventing non-communicable diseases. The strategies to implement the CRFA for promoting oral health will be described in a number of the other chapters in this book.

Understanding behavioural domains

The majority of strategies to prevent dental diseases have used an individualized, high-risk strategy[3]. Such approaches are based on inadequate theories that do not take into account the motivations of people to change their health related behaviours and thereby their health and wellbeing. Unless we understand the nature of the behaviours that need to be changed, it is very unlikely that our interventions will be maximally effective. Sound theories are needed to explain and predict health behaviours and to design and evaluate interventions. The components of the theories should be well elaborated so that we can better understand what actually drives behaviour change. The reasons for basing interventions on good theory is that interventions are likely to be more effective if they are based on a sound understanding of the causal determinants, namely, the mechanisms of behaviour change. Second, theory can be tested only if those interventions and evaluations are based on sound concepts that are clearly specified. Most importantly, theory-based interventions facilitate an understanding of what works and thus form a basis for developing better theories that apply in different populations, contexts and for various behaviours.[4,5] An example of the inadequate theories used by dentists and dental educators is that five preventive dental behaviours that are targeted to be changed are grouped together. Instead, key specific behaviours should be identified to understand the motivations for each of the behaviours. They may need different approaches as they have differing mechanisms. For example, the five most important behaviours related to oral health, diet, hygiene, dental attendance, smoking and use of fluorides come from significantly different behavioural domains. Diet is related to nourishment and what is good or bad to eat, hygiene to concern about dirt and infection, cleanliness and social acceptability, and dental attendance is related to attitudes to health professionals and dentists and the trust in dental professional's ability to improve their oral health. Attitudes to use of fluorides are related to views about political interventions, such as mass medication in the case of water fluoridation, and about effectiveness of medicinal preparations where topical fluorides are concerned. So, grouping the five dentally related behaviours together and adopting similar approaches for all of them, is unlikely to be very successful (see Chapter 16). Moreover, individuals may simultaneously hold both negative and positive attitudes to one or more of the behaviours, independent of each other.[6] Such attitudinal ambivalence may account for some of the variance in health behaviours.[7,8]

Box 7.2 – Understanding the underlying influences and determinants of behaviours.

> It is essential that we understand the underlying influences and determinants of behaviours. A variety of health related behaviours are important to oral health. Dental professionals, oral health promoters and policy makers need to acknowledge the diverse influences and motivations for these different behaviours. Failure to do this will impede efforts to promote sustained behaviour change.

In addition to the aforementioned shortcomings of theory, the separation psychologically of the mouth – the compartmentalization – from the rest of body when practicing dental prevention, are further examples of the poor theoretical basis for dental strategies. People do not think there is a diet that is not good for teeth, and another diet that is not good for survival and health in general. They think of a diet that is nourishing and enjoyable and that is good for health in general.

Moving beyond a behavioural domain to social determinants approach

The original concept of the CRFA was based on recommendations from the WHO that encouraged an integrated approach to chronic disease prevention.[9,10] In 2000, the CRFA concept was further developed and applied to oral health, with an emphasis on directing action at the shared risk factors for chronic diseases, and that includes numerous oral conditions.[1] The common risk factor approach (CRFA) has been widely accepted and endorsed globally by dental policy makers, dental researchers and oral health promoters.[11-18] The CRFA has formed the theoretical basis for the closer integration of oral and general health strategies.[19] Integration is the extent, pattern, and rate of adoption and eventual assimilation of health interventions into each of the critical functions of a health system.[20] Integration can occur at different levels of the health system - local, district, regional or national, depending on the prevailing governance arrangements.[21,22]

The theoretical focus and interpretation of the CRFA outlined by Sheiham and Watt[1] placed much attention on oral health related behaviours and not enough on the broader social determinants of behaviours. A reason for this was the recognition that the dental profession worked in such isolation from other health groups that, by at least adopting an integrated behavioural approach, would be a major step forwards. The behavioural focus of the CRFA has however partially hindered progress in tackling oral health inequalities by placing too much attention on oral health related behaviours and not enough on the social determinants of behaviours.[2] A sounder analysis indicates that people's behaviours are determined to a large extent by social determinants (Fig. 7.1), as outlined in Chapter 3 in this book and by Watt and Sheiham.[2] Recent developments and important reports on determinants of health and inequalities in health emphasize the importance of psychosocial and economic and political determinants of health and disease.[23,24] (see Chapter 3) The WHO Commission on Social Determinants of Health (CSDH) social determinants of health framework outlined in figure 7.1 identifies the social determinants of health and the social determinants of health and inequities in health; shows how major determinants relate to each other; clarifies the mechanisms by which social determinants generate health inequities and provides a framework for evaluating which SDH are the most important to address.[24] The model shows that a person's socioeconomic position affects their health, but that this effect is not direct. The framework attributes much importance to the socioeconomic-political context and indicates that social position determines health through intermediary determinants. Intermediary determinants such as behaviours and psychosocial, biological factors are influenced by social position that is in turn strongly affected by the socioeconomic and political context.[24]

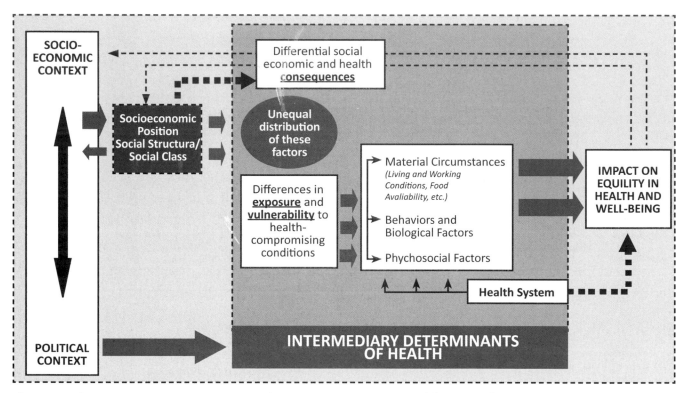

Fig. 7.1 – The WHO Commission on Social Determinants conceptual framework.[24]

People live in social, political, and economic systems that shape behaviours and access to resources they need to maintain good health.[24-29] Behaviours are linked to the conditions in which people are born, grow, live, work and age. That broader perspective requires an expansion of concepts relating to the CRFA as there is a need to refocus health promotion approaches to change behaviours so that the approaches incorporate concurrent interventions at multiple levels; individual, family, community, and society.[30] Failure to focus on environmental determinants explains why behavioural preventive interventions in dental settings are relatively ineffective in changing long-term oral health behaviours (see Chapter 3).[31-33] To permanently change individual behaviours, particular relevant aspects of the environments and social structures need to be changed because health behaviours are shaped by environments. The importance of the psychosocial and social environmental influences on oral conditions was therefore emphasized more in a later development of the CRFA.[2,28] Dental policy should not focus only on individual behavioural factors and ignore the broader social determinants. The effects of the social environment on health behaviours are related to how individuals with varying personal propensities, vulnerabilities and capabilities interact with other individuals and with their social and economic environments.

Box 7.3 – Importance of shared broader social determinants of chronic diseases and health inequalities.

The CRFA should not be too narrowly focused only on the shared behavioural risks for chronic diseases. Recognition also needs to focus on the shared broader social determinants of chronic diseases and health inequalities. Behaviours are patterned by the social environments in which people are born, grow, live, work and age.

A common risk factor approach - an integrated approach

The original CRFA paper by Sheiham and Watt[1] outlined the theoretical and epidemiological basis for an integrated approach for promoting oral health. The immediate main proximal causes of the major dental diseases, caries and periodontal disease are diet, dirt (plaque) and smoking. Oral mucosal lesions, oral cancer, temporomandibular joint dysfunction and pain are related to tobacco, alcohol and stress and trauma to teeth to accidents (Fig. 7.2). As these causes are common to a number of other chronic diseases commonly referred to as non-communicable diseases (NCDs) such as cardiovascular diseases, cancers, diabetes and oral diseases[17-19,34,] it is rational to use a common risk factor approach (CRFA) than one directed at specific diseases. Emphasis was therefore placed upon directing action at shared behavioural risks common to many chronic conditions, namely, unhealthy diets, tobacco use, alcohol misuse, poor hygiene and lack of physical activity, rather than the traditional disease specific approaches.

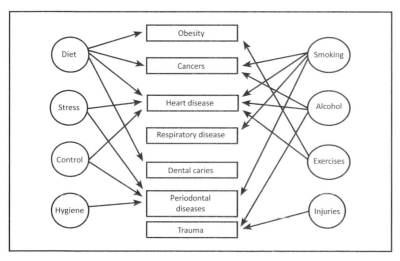

Fig. 7.2 – The Common Risk Factor Approach; Risk Factors common to a number of chronic diseases.[1]

The role of shared psychosocial influences such as stress and perceived control in the aetiology of chronic diseases, and most importantly, the underlying influence of the wider social environment on oral health inequalities was highlighted. The importance of the psychosocial and social environmental influences on oral conditions was further elaborated in a subsequent development of the CRFA (Fig. 7.3).[28]

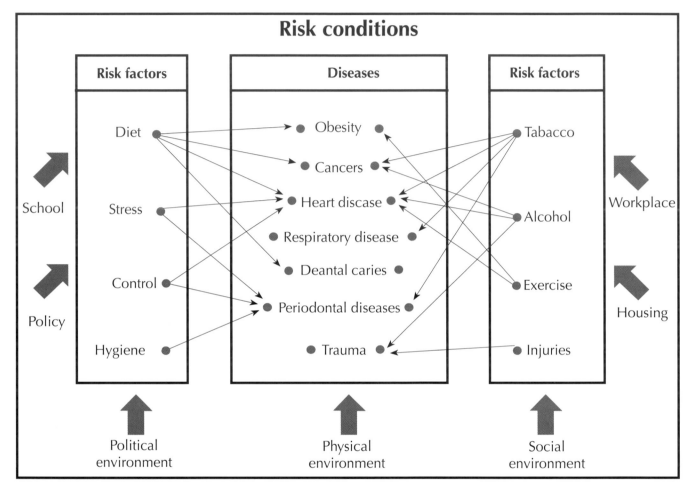

Fig. 7.3 – Expanded CRFA approach including social determinants.[28]

The CRFA was expanded to the Common Risk/Health Factor Approach (CRHFA) to include health factors thereby drawing attention to health promoting behaviours and not only to risk factors. Because that term CRHFA is not widely used, the term CRFA assumes the inclusion of health promoting factors. The Common Risk/Health Factor Approach distinguishes between actions aimed at reducing "risk factors" and actions promoting "health factors". This integrated strategy includes efforts to improve health by reducing risks, promoting health and strengthening possibilities to cope with 'given' risk factors and to promote factors that enhance health. A major benefit of the Common Risk/Health Factor Approach is the focus on improving health conditions in general for the whole population and for groups at high risk, thereby reducing social inequities.

The key concept underlying the integrated common risk approach is that promoting general health by controlling a small number of risk factors, will exert a favourable major effect, not only on a single disease, but simultaneously on several diseases, at a lower cost, greater efficiency and effectiveness than disease specific approaches.[18] For example, a CRFA preventive strategy to reduce obesity by changing the diet and reducing smoking is likely to affect rates of caries and periodontal disease and oral cancers. Savings in time and money may be made by coordinating the work done by various specialist groups and organizations. Moreover, decision-makers and individuals will be more likely to be influenced by approaches directed at preventing heart diseases, obesity, stroke, cancers, diabetes, as well as dental caries and oral cancer than if disease-specific recommendations for oral diseases are made alone.

The epidemiological basis for CRFA

The main non-communicable diseases, cardiovascular diseases, cancers, chronic respiratory diseases, diabetes and oral diseases account for 60% of deaths globally, killing millions of people each year.[34,35] Eighty percent of those deaths occur in low and middle income countries where the toll is disproportionate during the prime productive years; youth and middle age. According to the World Economic Forum's 2009 report, non-communicable diseases are among the most severe threats to global economic development, more likely to be realized and potentially more detrimental than fiscal crises or natural disasters. Increasingly, such diseases are also linked to poverty and socioeconomic inequalities and are

no longer "diseases of affluence." "Because of their multiple interacting causes and complications, as well as their lifelong nature, non-communicable diseases challenge current paradigms of health care organization and delivery."[35]

Oral diseases are important non-communicable diseases with a significant impact on overall health and wellbeing. As stated earlier, non-communicable diseases have common causes. The CRFA is based on epidemiological findings linking shared distal and proximal risk factors to chronic non-communicable diseases. The same unhealthy diet affects the incidence of heart diseases, cancers and oral diseases.[36] The WHO Assembly stated that "The common major risk factors for chronic diseases are the same for men and women in all regions: unhealthy diet, physical inactivity, and tobacco and alcohol use. A diet high in non-milk extrinsic sugars, saturated fats and salt and low in complex carbohydrate and/or fibre and foods high in antioxidants such as fruit, vegetables and cereal products is highly likely to cause non-communicable diseases".[37] Moreover, stress and low control, alcohol, environmental hygiene, injuries and a sedentary lifestyle contribute to a number of chronic diseases. Therefore, because the life threatening non-communicable diseases are of wide scale concern to policy makers and the public, working with food policy strategists to change a poor diet is more likely to be accepted and succeed than one which only stresses control of sugars for caries reduction. Particularly, as caries is not viewed as life threatening and the dental profession has conveyed, the idea put forward by members of the dental profession to policy makers that fluoride and toothbrushing will be sufficient to control the incidence of caries is highly contentious. Similarly, tobacco smoking affects heart disease and respiratory diseases as well as oral diseases. Therefore, programmes to reduce smoking will result in "killing two birds with one stone". Trauma to teeth affects about one in five children. Preventing tooth trauma requires a broadly based strategy to prevent accidents, especially those affecting the head.[38-72]

Clustering of risk factors

Clustering is the co-occurrence of a number of characteristics in one individual (see Chapter 4). Overall risk factor patterns in populations include behavioural and demographic characteristics. The main risk factors for the major chronic diseases frequently cluster in the same individuals. Excessive alcohol consumption and smoking commonly go together. People who smoke are more likely to eat a diet high in fats and sugars and low in fibre, polyunsaturated fatty acids, fruit and nutrient rich foods containing Vitamin A, C and E, take less exercise and drink more alcohol than non-smokers. Indeed the higher rate of cancer in smokers may be affected by their lower intake of nutrients with antioxidant properties and their higher heart disease rates to lower intakes of polyunsaturated fatty acids.

The clustering of risk factors in individuals and groups, particularly those at the lower levels of the social gradient suggests that preventive approaches should be directed at clusters of risk factors common to a number of diseases and the social structures which influence individual's health risks.[73-78] The clustering of behaviours can be viewed as the way in which social groups "translate their objective situation into patterns of behaviour".[79] Experience "gets under the skin".[80,81] Indeed the propensity for risk behaviours to cluster in certain groups indicates that behaviours are determined by social environments and conditions in which people live.[82]

Social environments that influence behaviours and create health inequalities

Social conditions are important in shaping individual health behaviours encompassed in the CRFA, because environments and early developmental influences shape people's psychological outlooks, such as their views about their futures as well as their feelings of control over their lives and environments.

Box 7.4 – Importance of targeting at-risk populations rather than the specific behaviours of high risk individuals.

> The clustering of health behaviours highlights the common determinants of different behaviours and of the importance of targeting at-risk populations rather than the specific behaviours of high risk individuals.

Box 7.5 – The drivers of social inequality and the social gradient in health.

> Social conditions are also the main drivers for health inequalities and the social gradient in health outcomes. The social gradient is not always smooth. For example, the most disadvantaged may suffer a disproportionate burden of ill health compared to all other groups along the social gradient as they experience the accumulation of different forms of social disadvantage.

"People benefit from high status not only because it is less stressful to be on top but also because being there leads to benefits that translate into better health. Knowledge about risk and protective factors and the wherewithal to act on it, leads to socioeconomic differences in smoking, exercise, diet, seat-belt use, screening and so on".[83] On the other hand people on the lower rungs of the social gradient ladder have increased exposure to environmental health hazards, less sense of control, chronic and acute stress in life and school and stress of prejudice.[84-87] Such factors lead to greater future discounting, lower self-esteem and poorer social relationships and social support.[80]

Health related behaviours are an expression of the circumstances that condition and constrain people's behaviours. People respond to psychological stress and adverse social circumstances by smoking, excessive alcohol consumption, comfort eating and risk taking. Therefore we repeatedly stress in this chapter that health status and behaviours are determined above all by social conditions.[79] Poor early social conditions "cast long shadows" over health in later adult life.[88-91] Children living in low socioeconomic conditions may "produce a negative behavioural and psychosocial health dividend to be reaped in the future."[92] Adverse social conditions and negative life events become literally biologically embodied. Patterns of behaviours and diseases therefore act as markers of social disadvantage.

The effects of the social environment on health behaviours are related to how individuals of different socioeconomic statuses with varying personal propensities, vulnerabilities and capabilities interact with each other and with others, and their social and economic environments. The resultant patterns of health promoting or health compromising behaviours are related to personal vulnerabilities and capabilities, and control over resources and access to information.

The report of the WHO Commission on the Social Determinants of Health[24] outlines how the major determinants relate to each other and the mechanisms involved in generating inequalities in population health. The key components of the CSDH framework include the socio-political context, structural determinants and socioeconomic position, and intermediary determinants (Fig. 7.4).[91,93] The WHO uses the term "structural determinants" to refer to the interplay between the socioeconomic and political context, structural mechanisms and processes generating social hierarchy and the resulting socioeconomic position of individuals. The final element of the CSDH framework is termed the intermediary determinants.

Socioeconomic position influences health through these specific intermediary factors such as neighbourhood, schools and housing conditions; psychological circumstances and also behavioural and biological factors. The behavioural factors include those common risk factors in the CRFA. The unequal distribution of the intermediary factors is associated with differentials in exposure and vulnerability to health compromising conditions, as well as with different consequences of ill health, constitutes the fundamental mechanism through which socioeconomic position generates health inequalities.[91,92] The model also includes the health care system as a social determinant of health through recognition of the role of health services in influencing health inequalities.

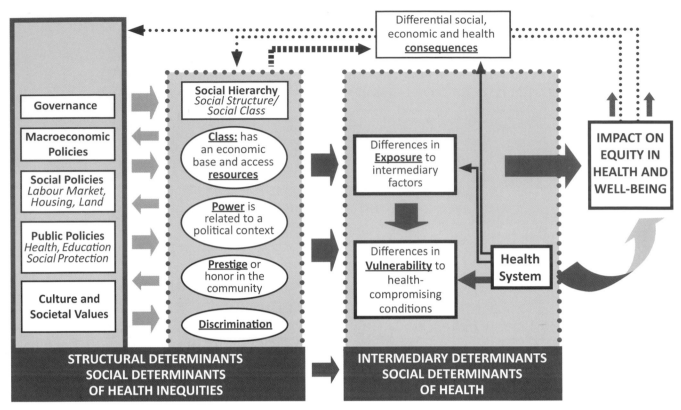

Fig. 7.4 – The WHO CSDH social determinants model.[91,93]

The socio-political context, structural determinants and socioeconomic position, and intermediary determinants are grouped as Upstream, Midstream and Downstream in the model by Turrell, Oldenburg and McGuffog.[94] They also consider health behaviours as Midstream intermediate level factors (Fig. 7.5).

Applying the MEME (Multiple Exposures – Multiple Effects) model

Many scientists, policy-makers and international and national bodies recognize that health is determined by multiple factors, including factors that shape the conditions in which people are born, grow, live, work, and age.[24] Policies and programmes that have not been recognized as re-

lated to health, are now known or thought to have important health consequences.[95] For example, public health has been linked to housing policies that determine the quality and location of housing developments, to transportation policies that affect availability of public transportation, to agricultural policies that influence the availability of various types of affordable foods. The recognition that health is shaped by a broad array of factors emphasizes the importance of understanding the health consequences of decision-making. In fact, it is argued that major improvements in public health cannot be achieved without considering the root causes of ill health; the causes of the causes. An example of how multiple factors affect health is the MEME model (Multiple Exposures — Multiple Effects) (Fig. 7.6).[96]

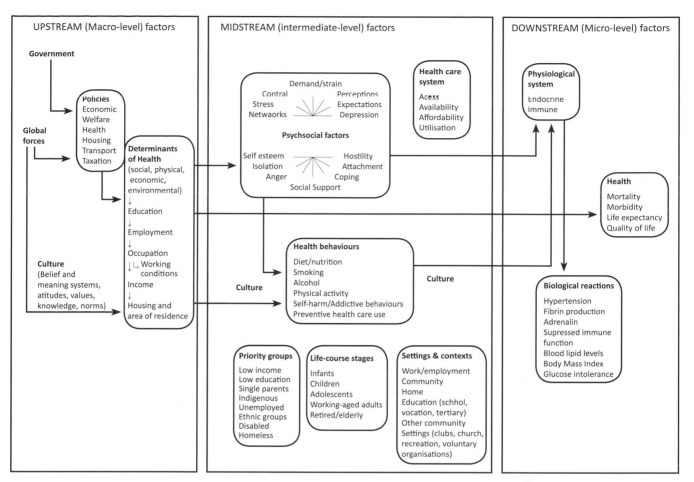

Fig. 7.5 – A framework of socioeconomic determinants of health.[93]

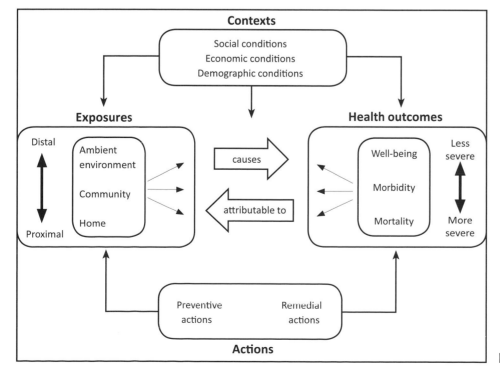

Fig. 7.6 – The MEME model.[96]

The MEME model emphasizes the divergent, multiple links between exposure and health effects. "On the environmental side, it recognizes a spectrum of exposures, from more proximal to more distal, which can occur in a number of different settings – in the case of children, in the home, the community and the wider, ambient environment. On the health side it recognizes that effects may be expressed in different ways, and at different levels of severity (e.g. as morbidity or mortality). In addition, it recognizes that both exposures and health outcomes may be affected by more remote, contextual factors, such as social conditions, demographics and economic development that influence the susceptibility of the population to environmental health effects." Actions are taken either to remediate disease or, preventatively, to avoid it by reducing exposures in the environment. "In the longer term, actions may also be targeted at the underlying factors - for example, by trying to alleviate poverty or enhance development."[96]

Policy Implications of Using a Common Risk Factor Approach

Focusing solely on changing oral health behaviours is a relatively ineffective strategy for tackling oral health inequalities. Future oral health policy needs to focus upon the structural determinants – the political and economic drivers in society that influence behaviours. Action principally on the structural determinants is the responsibility of national policy makers and professional organisations. However the development of individual, local and regional policies can be directed at the intermediary determinants of oral health – the local circumstances and proximal causes of oral diseases. Oral health policies focusing on the intermediary determinants can focus on developing supportive oral health environments in a variety of local settings such as schools, colleges, hospitals, workplaces and care organisations. Of particular importance is to consider how such a policy agenda can be implemented in pre-school settings to ensure that a supportive early life environment is created. Legislative, regulatory and fiscal policies and controls can be implemented to promote and maintain oral health through creating supportive local environments as outlined in the Ottawa Charter and the Marmot Review.[95,97] Fundamental to the success of this policy agenda is the need for effective integration of oral health with general health approaches and intersectoral working across relevant sectors. Community participation is also an essential element of oral health policy ensuring that people gain more more control over their lives as well as to creating environments that make healthier choices the easier choices and health compromising behaviours more difficult.

A radical shift in the preventive approach to promote oral health is urgently needed. The isolated, compartmentalized and individualistically focused approach, may improve the health of some individuals but is unlikely to effectively promote the community's oral health or reduce inequalities in health. The common risk factor approach implemented through a comprehensive health promotion strategy based upon the principles of the Ottawa Charter is more likely to be effective than the present theoretically flawed methods.[5,28,29] Sustainable change will be achieved by focusing actions on the common underlying determinants of health, in partnership with a range of other agencies and the community. Such an approach is dependent upon implementing a complementary range of strategies including health education, policy development, community action and legislation.

Central to promoting health using the CRFA is the important principle of focusing on 'horizontal' rather than 'vertical' programmes and on the whole population rather than on disease-specific at-risk groups. Many community programmes have shifted from vertical programmes that address specific diseases, towards a more horizontal and diagonal approach, thus enlarging their scope to cover more than one non-communicable disease.[98-100]

Box 7.6 – Two approaches for an equity oriented health policy.

> There are basically two approaches for an equity oriented health policy;
> - Focusing on actions to reduce specific diseases, or
> - On specific risk factors and public policies aimed at improving health conditions in general and among those at particular risk.

Three strategies may be used based upon the causes of common chronic diseases.

- Most chronic diseases have a multifactorial causation. In that case, integrated action may be taken against a number of risk factors related to one or more diseases.[18]
- Second, if one risk factor affects several diseases, the strategy may be integrated across disease boundaries.

- The third approach overlaps with the first. Here some of the risk factors cluster and occur mainly in groups of people. Changing one of the factors may influence the other health compromising behaviours. For example, smoking, heavy drinking and poor diet cluster in the same people (see Chapter 4). Changing their smoking behaviour may affect other behaviours.

Box 6.7 – Health promotion strategic framework.

> - Focus upon common underlying determinants of health avoiding a victim blaming approach.
> - Community participation rather than professionally dominated activities.
> - Emphasis on addressing health inequalities to achieve sustainable improvements in oral health.
> - Working in partnership across sectors and disciplines adopt a range of complementary public health policies rather than individually focused health education.

The 1994 Institute of Medicine (IOM)[101] report on prevention research, proposed a new framework for classifying prevention based on Gordon's[103] operational classification of disease prevention. The 1994 IOM report, emphasized the importance of putting prevention into a broader context. A context which includes not only treatment but also maintenance interventions when continued care is indicated.[101] The IOM model divided the continuum of services into three parts: prevention, treatment, and maintenance (Fig. 7.7). The prevention category was divided into three classifications; universal, selective and indicated prevention. The features of maintenance were "(1) the patient's compliance with long-term treatment to reduce relapse and recurrence and (2) the provision of after-care services to the patient, including rehabilitation".[101]

The rationale for targeting a type of intervention either universally or to a high-risk subgroup was that the potential benefit was substantially higher than the cost and the risk of negative effects. Weisz, Sandler, Durlak, and Anton[103] added a relatively new concept to the

three levels of prevention strategies in the IOM report, namely, "health promotion/positive development". They clearly separate prevention and treatment. "Health Promotion/Positive Development Strategies target an entire population with the goal of enhancing strengths so as to reduce the risk of later problem outcomes and/or to increase prospects for positive development."[103]

Another classification for prevention originally developed in the field of obesity proposes three different approaches (see Box 7.9).

Box 7.9 – Another classification for prevention.

- Universal prevention,
- Targeted Selective Interventions and
- Targeted Indicated prevention strategies

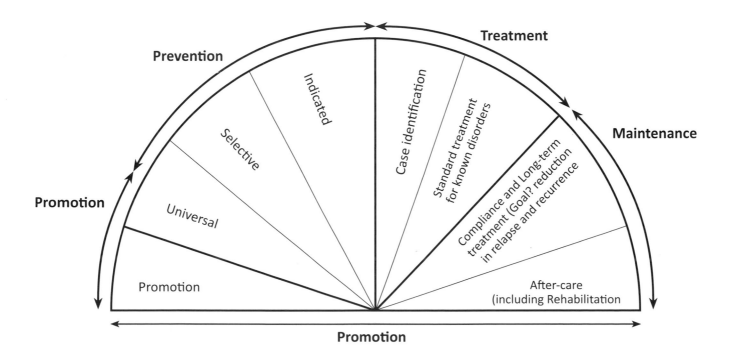

Fig. 7.7 – Continuum of Care Protractor; health intervention spectrum. Different levels of prevention are distinguished by the level of risk of disorder/distress in various populations groups. Adapted from.[101]

Levels of prevention measures

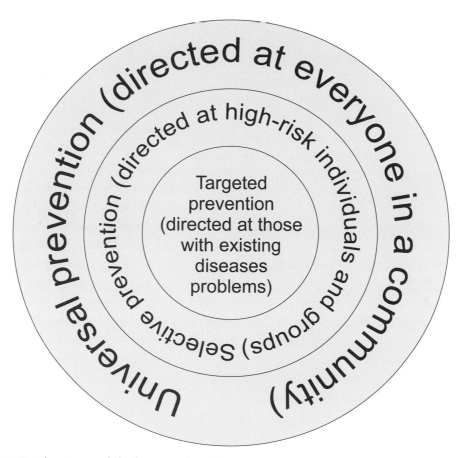

Figu. 7.8 – The WHO Obesity model of prevention.[104]

Universal prevention, is based on a total population approach, whereas selective and the two targeted prevention strategies are directed at high-risk groups. [104,105] As for obesity, dental caries is related to "normal physiology within a pathological environment".[47] Thus all interventions should aim to create environments that facilitate and promote behavioural changes in terms of diet are important for the prevention of dental caries as well as other chronic conditions, such as obesity. That is a good example of the application of the CRFA. A population-level strategy or, to use Gordon's classification, a universal measure may be more optimal and cost-effective than interventions targeted further downstream at the individual level. Acting on the most upstream level of determinants of health typically means the level of national policy. This may help shift national norms and values that lead to the passage, adoption, and ultimately, success of the relevant legislation. Alternately, upstream policy interventions may also refer to modifying the broader, social determinants of health, such as income, through the provision of earned income tax credits and minimum wage increases and better universal education systems.

For example, a universal preventive measure for oral diseases should include the provision of general advice to policy makers and the public to introduce policies to encourage the consumption a diet low in extrinsic sugars accompanied by a regulatory policy requiring food labeling. A selective intervention could include a programme focusing on diet and behavioral changes for high risk individuals who consume sugars frequently and do not regularly use a fluoridated toothpaste. An indicated preventive measure might include fluoride varnish for those diagnosed as having non-cavitated white spot caries lesions.

Universal Prevention

A Universal Prevention Strategy is directed at the entire population (national, local community, school, and neighborhood). Universal prevention programs are delivered to large groups without any prior screening for risk. The entire population is assessed as at-risk and capable of benefiting from prevention programmes. They are designed to address risk factors in entire populations of children without attempting to detect those at elevated risk. For example, schools-wide interventions creates positive school environments. This is a proactive approach replaces the need to develop individual interventions for many students who engage in similar inappropriate behaviours. These strategies are considered to be "primary prevention" in that they build the capacity of the school to provide a safe environment for all children and to more effectively implement selective and indicated interventions;

All members of the population share the same general risk for all diseases and as outlined earlier in this chapter, those risk factors are common to a number of chronic diseases. Many members of the population are at risk of onset of some health compromising behaviours, although the risk may vary greatly among individuals.

Targeted Selective Interventions

Targeted Selective Interventions are used with groups who require more than universal strategies but less than intensive individualized interventions. It targets groups identified because they share significant risk factors. They are applied only when the individual is a member of a subgroup whose risk of disease is above average. The purpose of selective or targeted interventions is to support children who are at-risk for or are beginning to exhibit signs of health compromising behaviours. Such interventions can be offered in small group settings for children exhibiting similar behaviours. These interventions are considered to be "secondary prevention." and are the more traditional population oriented public health education interventions targeted toward the high-risk segments of the population. Selective prevention strategies target subsets of the total population by virtue of their membership of a particular segment of the population that is considered to be at risk for oral diseases. It targets the entire subgroup regardless of the degree of risk of any individuals in the group because the subgroup as a whole is at higher risk than the general population. An individual's personal risk is not specifically assessed or identified and is based solely on a presumption given his or her membership in the at-risk subgroup. Risk groups may be identified on the basis of psychological, social, or environmental risk factors known to be associated with oral and general diseases. For example, children of poorer parents, or students who are failing academically. Targeted subgroups may be defined by age, sex, family history, place of residence such as low-income neighborhoods.

Selective interventions are most appropriate if their cost is moderate and if the risk of negative effects is minimal or nonexistent.

Targeted Indicated prevention strategies

Targeted Indicated Prevention Strategies are applicable to persons who, on examination, manifest a risk factor, condition, or abnormality that identifies them individually as being at high risk for the future development of a disease. This type of intervention, usually provided in the context of clinical practice, deals only with individuals diagnosed with a disease, not with the nameless statistical subset of a population as in selective preventive measures. Indicated prevention strategies are designed to prevent the onset of health compromising behaviours in individuals. Indicated prevention strategies targets individuals who are exhibiting health compromising behaviours or consequences of them. The strategies are designed to prevent the onset of health compromising behaviours and oral diseases in individuals. Indicated prevention approaches are used for individuals who exhibit risk factors that increase their chances of developing a problem. Indicated prevention programmes address risk factors associated with the individual. Less emphasis is placed on assessing or addressing environmental influences, such as community values. Individuals can be referred to indicated prevention programmes by parents, teachers, school counselors, school nurses.

Four approaches to promoting health; generic individual approach, targeted individual approach, generic community approach and a targeted community approach

Visram and Drinkwater[106] have proposed four approaches to promoting health; generic individual approach, targeted individual approach, generic community approach and a targeted community approach (Box 7.10) (Fig. 7.9).[106]

The approaches are similar to those proposed by the IOM and Weisz et al.[101,103] All of the four approaches should be applied, but priority should be given to the generic community and targeted community approaches. The four approaches recommended by Visram and Drinkwater[106] are similar to the approaches that Sheiham and Watt recommended, based on the concepts put forward by Rose. Because the categories outlined by Visram and Drinkwater include a role for the individual dentists, their categorization can be incorporated into the High-Risk Strategy (HRS) outlined below.

Based on the concepts outlined above, Sheiham has recommended three preventive strategies: two types of Risk Strategy and the Population Strategy (see Box 7.11)[107]. The two types of Risk Strategy are the High-Risk Strategy (HRS) and the Directed Vulnerable Populations Strategy (DVPS). In one kind of risk strategy, the HRS, individuals at risk are identified by screening. In the second kind of risk approach, the DVPS, vulnerable groups are identified by conventional oral health surveys, not by screening. A vulnerable population is defined by a higher measured exposure to a specific risk factor, being a subgroup or subpopulation who, because of shared social characteristics, is at higher risk of risks[108]. They are people sharing adverse social conditions that puts them at higher risk, or they may attend particular schools with higher rates of caries.

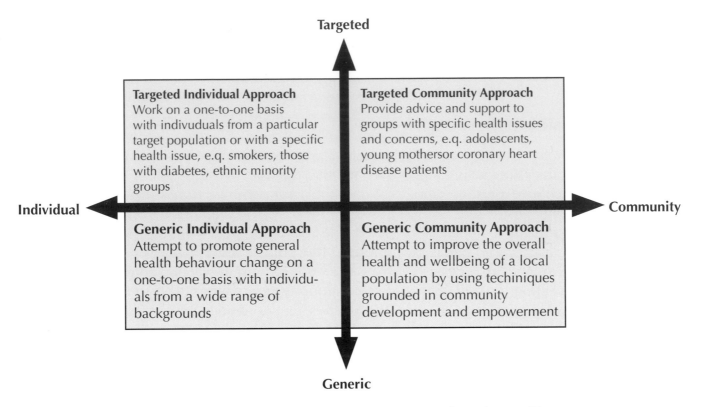

Fig. 7.9 – Four categories of good practice recommended by Visram and Drinkwater.[106]

Box 7.10 – Four categories of good practice.[106]

1) A generic individual approach
Health educators will employ this approach and attempt to improve the health of their local population by promoting health behaviour change with individuals on a one-to-one basis. They also direct people to preventative and other services. Health educators using this approach usually undergo training, including psychology-based methods in behaviour change.

2) A targeted individual approach
This approach involves targeting people from specific groups within the community or with particular health issues, and working with them on a one-to-one basis to improve their health and wellbeing.

3) A generic community approach
This approach attempts to improve the overall health and wellbeing of the wider community, rather than focusing on any specific issue or group. This can be done by community development programmes, designed to enable people to take part in and shape initiatives and decisions that affect the health of individuals and communities. They are grounded in community empowerment and give individuals an opportunity to develop their skills.

4) A targeted community approach
This category includes projects taking a community development approach to tackle a specific health issue and/or focusing on a specific target group within the local population.

Box 7.11 – Three strategies for prevention and health promotion.

Preventive Strategies:
Two Risk Strategies:
High-Risk Strategy (HRS), which seeks to identify individuals at high risk using screening and targeting them with evidence based interventions.
Directed Vulnerable Populations Strategy (DVPS), which protects sections of the population that share social characteristics that put them at higher risk of risks.
The Population Strategy:
Efforts are made to shift the risk distribution of the entire population to a more favourable level.

A major shortcoming of the HRS is that even if it were effective (see Chapter 3). The intervention trial shows that it is difficult, to help high caries-risk individuals by measures that are normally applied in dental clinics. To further reduce caries among the high-risk children, the approach should be directed to the whole population or at vulnerable groups using a DVPS.

Policies for tackling oral diseases and reducing oral health inequalities

The policy for reducing dental diseases includes efforts to improve health by reducing risks, promoting health and strengthening possibilities to cope with risk factors. There are a range of options to promote oral health mainly based on the Ottawa Declaration.[95] They are healthy public policies, legislation, regulation and fiscal measures and can all be utilized to promote oral health either at international, national and local levels. There is a hierarchy of levels at which to intervene in a country. The highest is at national and local levels. National and local government can legislate and regulate and implement fiscal measures, whereby health damaging products are taxed. Legislation includes dietary guidelines banning sugary foods and drinks from nurseries and schools and requiring vegetables and salads and fruit in school meals. Dietary guidelines can be backed up by media campaigns and school health education. The next level of priority is a Health Settings Strategy. The Health Settings Strategy is the main strategy for dental health personnel to work within. So it is ideal for the Targeted Community Approach[106] and the CRFA.

The Settings Approach

The basis for the settings approach is that certain places or settings are more appropriate for promoting health of people at different stages of their lives. A settings approach locates public health action in social, cultural and physical places in which children live, learn and play. This approach has been applied to health promoting schools and healthy localities.

Some key settings cover the bulk of the general population. These in turn fit within the wider settings of the city, district and village. The settings are the Educational Setting, Healthy Cities, The Workplace Setting, Healthy Locality, The Recreation Setting, Healthy Villages, Family Setting, Healthcare Setting. The grid below illustrates a range of activities that can be used to decide which settings may be appropriate and for a target group (Fig. 7.10).

Settings	Groups Toddlers	Preschool	Children	Teens	Young adults	Adults	Older adults
MCH clinics	√						
Nurseries	√	√					
Schools			√	√			
Work					√	√	
Community		√		√	√	√	√
Practices	√	√	√	√	√	√	√

Fig. 7.10 – The Settings Approach. Targeting groups at various stages of the lifecourse in the most appropriate settings.

Examples of the CRFA and Health Promotion Strategies Populations Strategy

Food policy

The CRFA uses a holistic nutrition programme which aims to improve the overall nutritional status of school children. Such an approach, if successful, will not only reduce calorie dense non--milk extrinsic sugars (NMES) consumption and hence improve oral health, but will also improve the overall quality of preschool children's diet and thereby promote their growth and future development.[4] The CRFA approach recognizes the importance of influencing key groups such as food producers, manufacturers and government departments because a range of sectors are involved in the 'food chain', all of whom have a potential role to play in changing diets. Health education forms only one component part of the overall programme and can be targeted at a range of influential partners and professionals, not only the public. The approach should include efforts to improve health by reducing risks, promoting health and strengthening possibilities to cope with 'given' risk factors – creating supportive environments reducing the negative effects of certain risk factors and facilitating behaviour changes.

Here are some examples of national and local actions to promote oral health.

National level

- National strategies on diet and physical activities;
- National food and agriculture policies: pricing, food programmes, push and pull mechanisms;
- National dietary and physical activities guidelines;
- Food standards for pre-school nurseries/schools: Support food and nutrient standards for school meals, and other foods and drinks provided in schools;
- Public sector catering
- Information environment: health claims, marketing, advertising, labelling;

- Advertising: Support regulation on content and timing of television adverts promoting children's foods and drinks;
- Food labelling: Encourage tighter legislation on food labeling;
- Building prevention into health services;
- Encourage greater availability of sugar-free paediatric medicines;
- Support removal of value added tax and other taxes on fluoride toothpastes.

Examples of the oral health aspects of the abovementioned policies are:

Tackling Early Childhood Caries (ECC)

An oral health promotion approach to prevent Early Childhood Caries should be directed at eliminating or reducing refined sugars from paediatric medicines and baby drinks. Such an approach makes health promoting choices easier for mothers. The following strategies can be used:

- dental public health personnel should encourage Government to introduce legislation forbidding the addition of sugars to all prescribed paediatric medicines, and if possible over the counter paediatric medicines, such as cough mixtures.
- Sugars in baby foods and drinks. Because of the increased concern about early exposure to sugars and nutrient dilution, overweight and dental caries, alliances of groups concerned about maternity and child health should put pressure on manufacturers to reduce sugars in baby foods and drinks.

- Dietary guidelines for nurseries and carers. As part of general regulations regarding nurseries and training of professional carers, dietary guidelines have been formulated which must be adhered to by nurseries.[109]

Local level

- Support development of local infant feeding policies including breastfeeding.
- Develop oral health and nutrition policies in preschools and nurseries.
- Encourage nurseries and schools to provide healthy snacks and drinks.
- Encourage schools to become part of the Health Promoting Schools Network.[110,111]
- Have Nutritional Standards for school meals.
- Soft drink interventions at schools. Prevent the sale of sugars containing soft drinks in and near schools.
- Change food culture within schools.
- Improve quality of products sold in school tuck shops and vending machines.
- Have set meals in primary schools rather than cash cafeterias.
- Encourage sales of subsidized fluoride toothpastes through community clinics and health visitors.

Health promoting schools and nurseries (HPS)

The World Health Assembly of WHO urges governments "to promote oral health in schools, aiming at developing healthy lifestyles and self care practices in children"[37] (see Chapter 19). The preschool nursery and school are attractive settings for health promotion, for it provides a way of reaching a many children and young people. The WHO Health Promoting Schools (HPS) programme offers a sound approach to tackling the problem of dental caries. The approach focuses on the influence of the social and physical environment on health.[111,112]

The HPS approach aims to improve health for the total school population by developing supportive environments conducive to the promotion of health. The HPS concept embraces the principles that health of individuals can be advanced by both health education in taught curriculum, and schools providing a supportive and safe physical and social environment conductive to making healthy choices. A HPS can be characterized as a school constantly strengthening its capacity as a healthy setting for living, learning and working. All the HPS activities depend upon collaborative working between staff, students, parents, education authorities, local government and health professionals. In addition, through the interaction with external environments and alliances with local community, school health promotion can be improved, and can positively influence the community in which pupil's health choices are made.

The HPS concept has been introduced worldwide as an important strategy that provides opportunities to tackle health inequalities in society, not only of young people but also of the population at large. Of particular relevance to oral health promotion would be nutrition, smoking and accident prevention policies. Students should be provided with a range of food choices within schools including nutritional options. Such initiatives recognize the importance of increasing the availability of cheap and appealing nutritious foods and drinks within school canteens, tuck shops and vending machines.

Applying the CRFA in schools using the Targeted Community Approach involves the following steps:

- Identify schools with a high prevalence of overweight children or children with high caries levels.
- Assess the determinants and evidence for effective interventions.
- Assist in creating environments supporting health and are essential for preventing chronic diseases including caries using a CRFA. That involves policies on healthy eating and applying national guidelines on restricting high fat, high sugars, high salt foods and beverages and offering healthy alternatives.
- Collaboration and strong partnerships are key to preventing chronic diseases, including caries.
- Evaluation of strategies to understand what works.

The evaluation of the oral health aspects of Health Promoting Schools policies indicate that marked improvements in oral health can be achieved. In Brazil food policies in state nurseries in a very deprived region not only substantially reduced sugars consumption and improved the nutritional quality of the diet but also successfully reduced caries increments over a one year period.[109] Health promoting schools not only had reduced levels of caries but had lower levels of traumatic dental injuries.[113,114]

The role of dentists in working towards a CRFA

Most dental practitioner involvement in policy development to apply the broader CRFA that incorporate tackling the social determinants of health will be as health advocates. Health advocacy is the actions of health professionals and others with perceived authority in health to influence decisions and actions of individuals, communities and government which influence health. Health advocacy involves educating senior government and community leaders and journalists - decision-makers in general, about specific issues and setting the agenda to obtain political decisions that improve health of the population. Health advocates place their skills at the disposal of the community - being on tap not on top.

The objective of planners of dental care should be to make healthy choices the easier choices. They should find which internal incentives promote enthusiasm for quality, economy and good patient service. Rational strategies for oral health promotion should incorporate policies to control the determinants of the distribution of oral diseases, establish goals and strategies on evidence-based oral health promotion. Oral health promotion programmes will be enhanced by dentists establishing a national or local Oral Health Promotion Group or a Oral Health Action Team to ensure that oral health promoting strategies are incorporated into general health promotion plans. Integrating oral health in a CRFA is both logical and feasible. Risk factors common to major life threatening diseases like heart disease and cancer are best tackled on a broad front. The same risk factors affect oral diseases. Dentists should welcome the CRFA approach and develop strategies that fit in with general health promotion policies.

Recently, a related health care concept - personalized medicine - has emerged. It can also be applied to dentistry. The adjectives "predictive," "preventive," and "preemptive" are frequently attached to this concept,[11,115] suggesting that prediction based on early information about an individual can lead to the avoidance of disorder; namely, secondary prevention. This concept can be applied to prevention and preemption of oral disorders. The concept of personalized medicine/dentistry is a dimension of indicated prevention, but as only one component of a broader spectrum of needed approaches.

Conclusions

Traditional clinical preventive approaches that narrowly focus on dental diseases in isolation from other areas of public health are ineffective at reducing oral health inequalities, very costly and fail to achieve sustainable changes in oral health. The CRFA provides the theoretical and practical basis for integrating oral health into general health improvement strategies. Future oral health promotion strategies implemented at local, regional or national levels should focus on the shared behavioural, psychosocial and environmental factors that determine chronic diseases, including oral conditions, and are the causes of health inequalities. The approaches should tackle the upstream determinants of health,[24,118] because to change behaviours it is essential to change the environments where people live. In addition, policy makers should make healthy choices the easier choices and unhealthy choices more difficult.[119]

References

1. Sheiham A, Watt RG. The Common Risk Factor Approach: a rational basis for promoting oral health. Community Dent Oral Epidemiol. 2000; 28:399-406.
2. Watt RG, Sheiham A. Integrating the Common Risk Factor Approach into a Social Determinants framework. 2012 Submitted.
3. Batchelor P, Sheiham A. The limitations of a 'high risk' approach for the prevention of dental caries. Community Dent Oral Epidemiol. 2002; 30:302-312.
4. Michie S, Designing and implementing behaviour change interventions to improve population health. Journal of Health Services Research & Policy. 2008; 13(Suppl 3):64-69.
5. Michie S, Johnston M, Francis J, Hardeman W, Eccles M. From theory to intervention: Mapping theoretically derived behavioural determinants to behaviour change techniques. Applied Psychology. 2008; 57(4):660-680
6. Armitage CJ, Conner M. Efficacy of the theory of planned behaviour: a meta analytic review. Br J Social Psychology. 2001; 40:471-499.
7. Conner M, Sparks P, Povey R, James R, Sheperd R, Armitage CJ. Moderator effects of attitudinal ambivalence on attitude–behaviour relationships. European J Social Psychology. 2002; 32:705-708.
8. Conner M, Povey R, Sparks P, James R, Sheperd R. Moderating role of attitudinal ambivalence within the theory of planned behaviour. British Journal of Social Psychology. 2003; 42:75-94.
9. World Health Organization. Risk factors and comprehensive control of chronic diseases. Report ICP/CVD 020(2), Geneva: World Health Organization. 1980.
10. Grabauskas V. Integrated programme for community health in noncommunicable disease (Interhealth). In: Leparski E, editor. The prevention of non-communicable diseases: experiences and prospects. World Health Organization Regional Office for Europe, Copenhagen. 1987; 285-310.
11. Petersen PE. The World Oral Health Report 2003: continuous improvement of oral health in the 21st century - the approach of the WHO Global Oral Health Programme. Community Dent Oral Epidemiol. 2003; 31(Suppl.1):3-24.
12. Petersen PE. Priorities for research for oral health in the 21st Century - the approach of the WHO Global Oral Health Programme. Community Dent Health. 2005; 22:71-4.
13. Petersen PE. Global research challenges for oral health. Global Forum Update Res Health. 2005; 2:181-4.
14. Petersen PE. Global policy for improvement of oral health in the 21st century – implications to oral health research of World Health Assembly 2007, World Health Organization. Community Dent Oral Epidemiol. 2009; 37:1-8.
15. Petersen PE, Kwan S. The 7th WHO Global Conference on Health Promotion - towards integration of oral health (Nairobi, Kenya 2009). Community Dental Health. (Supplement 1) 2010; 27:129-136.
16. Kwan S, Petersen PE. Oral health: equity and social determinants. In: Equity, social determinants and public health programmes. Edited by Erik Blas and Anand Sivasankara Kurup. Geneva: World Health Organization. 2010. pp.159-176. http://whqlibdoc.who.int/publications/2010/9789241563970_eng.pdf
17. Williams DM. Global oral health inequalities: The research agenda. Adv Dent Res. 2011; 23:198-200.
18. Sheiham A, Alexander D, Cohen L, Marinho V, Moysés S, Petersen PE, et al. Global Oral Health Inequalities: Task Group – Implementation and Delivery of Oral Health Strategies. Advances in Dental Research. 2011; 23:259-267.
19. World Health Organization. Global strategy for the prevention and control of noncommunicable diseases. Geneva: World Health Organization. 2000.
20. Atun RA, Menabde N. Health systems and systems thinking. In: Coker R, Atun RA, McKee M, editors. Health systems and communicable disease control. Buckingham: Open University Press.

2008. http://www.euro.who.int/Document/E91946.pdf

21. Atun R, Bennett S, Duran A. When do vertical (stand-alone) programmes have a place in health systems? Copenhagen: World Health Organization. 2008.

22. Atun R, de Jongh T, Secci F, Ohiri K, Adeyi O. Integration of targeted health interventions into health systems: a conceptual framework for analysis. Health Policy and Planning. 2010; 25:104-111.

23. World Health Organization, Europe. Health 21: The health for all framework for the WHO European region, Copenhagen: WHO Regional Office for Europe. 1999.

24. World Health Organization. Closing the gap in a generation. Health equity through action on social determinants of health. Commission on Social Determinants of Health Final Report. Geneva: World Health Organization. 2008. http://www.who.int/social_determinants/thecommission/finalreport/en/index.html

25. World Health Organization. Preventing chronic diseases: A vital investment. Geneva: World Health Organization. 2005. http://www.who.int/chp/chronic_disease_report/en.http://www.euro.who.int/InformationSources/Publications/Catalogue/20020808_2

26. World Health Organization. Closing the Health Inequalities Gap: An International Perspective. (Iain K Crombie, Linda Irvine Lawrence, Elliot Hilary Wallace). Copenhagen: WHO Regional Office for Europe. 2005. http://www.who.int/social_determinants/resources/closing_h_inequalities_gap.pdf

27. World Health Organization. Equity, social determinants and public health programmes. Edited by Erik Blas and Anand Sivasankara Kurup. Geneva: World Health Organization. 2010. http://whqlibdoc.who.int/publications/2010/9789241563970_eng.pdf

28. Watt RG. Strategies and approaches in oral disease prevention and health promotion. Bull World Health Organ. 2005; 83:711-718.

29. Watt RG. From victim blaming to upstream action; tackling the social determinants of oral health inequalities. Community Dent Oral Epidemiol. 2007; 35:1-11.

30. Institute of Medicine. Committee on Health and Behavior. Health and behavior: The interplay of biological, behavioral, and societal influences. Washington DC: National Academy of Sciences. 2000. http://www.nap.edu/openbook/0309070309/

31. Yevlahova D, Satur J. Models for individual oral health promotion and their effectiveness: a systematic review. Australian Dental Journal. 2009; 54:190-197.

32. Freeman R, Ismail A. Assessing patients' health behaviours. Essential steps for motivating patients to adopt and maintain behaviours conducive to oral health. 2009; 21:113-27.

33. Rogers JG. Evidence-based oral health promotion resource. Melbourne; Prevention and Population Health Branch, Government of Victoria, Department of Health. 2011. http://www.health.vic.gov.au/healthpromotion/evidence_res/evidence_index.htm

34. World Health Organization. 2008-2013 Action Plan for the Global Strategy for the Prevention and Control of Noncommunicable Diseases: prevent and control cardiovascular diseases, cancers, chronic respiratory diseases and diabetes. Geneva: World Health Organization. 2008. http://whqlibdoc.who.int/publications/2009/9789241597418_eng.pdf

35. Narayan KM, Ali MK, Koplan JP. Global noncommunicable diseases - where worlds meet. N Eng J Med. 2010; 363:1196-8.

36. World Health Organization. Diet, nutrition, and the prevention of chronic diseases. Technical Report Series No 916. Geneva: World Health Organization. 2003. http://whqlibdoc.who.int/trs/WHO_TRS_916.pdf

37. World Health Organization. Oral health: action plan for promotion and integrated disease prevention. Sixtieth World Health Assembly WHA60.17 Agenda

item 12.9 23 May 2007. http://apps.who.int/gb/ebwha/pdf_files/WHA60/A60_16-en.pdf

38. Burt BA, Pai S. Sugar consumption and caries risk: a systematic review. J Dent Educ. 2001; 65:1017-23.

39. Moynihan P, Lingström P, Rugg-Gunn AJ, Birkhed D. The role of dietary control. In: Fejerskov O, Kidd EAM, editors. Dental Caries. The disease and its clinical management, 3rd edn. Copenhagen: Blackwell Munksgaard. 2003; 222-244.

40. Sheiham A. Why free sugars consumption should be below 15 kg per person per year in industrialised countries: the dental evidence. Br Dent J. 1991; 171:63-65.

41. Sheiham A. Dietary effects on dental diseases. Public Health Nutr 2001;4:569-?

42. Moynihan, P.J., Dietary advice in dental practice. British Dental Journal. 2002; 193: 563-8.

43. Moynihan P, Petersen PE. Diet, nutrition and prevention of dental diseases. Public Health Nutrition. 2004; 7(1A):201-26.

44. Liese AD, Schulz M, Fang F, Wolever TMS, D'Agostino RB Jr, Sparks KC, Mayer-Davis EJ. Dietary glycemic index and glycemic load, carbohydrate and fiber intake, and measures of insulin sensitivity, secretion, and adiposity in the Insulin Resistance Atherosclerosis Study. Diabetes Care. 2005; 28:2832-2838.

45. World Health Organization. Redefining obesity and its treatment. Geneva: World Health Organization. 2000. http://www.wpro.who.int/NR/rdonlyres/0A35147B-B1D5-45A6-9FF2-F7D86608A4DE/0/Redefiningobesity.pdf

46. World Health Organization. Obesity: preventing and managing the global epidemic. Report of WHO consultation. World Health Organization, Technical Report Series 894. Geneva, Switzerland. 2000.

47. Egger G, Swinburn B. An ecological approach to the obesity pandemic. Br Med J. 1997; 315:477-480.

48. Pavia M, Pileggi C, Nobile CG, Angelillo IF. Association between fruit and vegetable consumption and oral cancer; a meta-analysis of observational studies. Am J Clin Nutr. 2006; 83:1126-1134.

49. Royal College of Physicians of London. Smoking or health? London: Pitman Medical Publishing. 1977.

50. World Health Organization. Global strategy on diet, physical activity and health. Geneva: World Health Organization. 2004. http://www.who.int/dietphysicalactivity/strategy/eb11344/strategy_english_web.pdf

51. Peto R, Lopez A, Boreham J, Thun M, Health C, Doll R. Mortality from smoking worldwide. Br Med Bull. 1996; 67:51-56.

52. Jarvis, M, Wardle J. Social patterning of individual health behaviours: the case of cigarette smoking. In: Marmot M, Wilkinson R. editors. Social determinants of health. Oxford: Oxford University Press. 2006; pp.224-337.

53. Kinane DF, Chestnutt IG. Smoking and periodontal disease. Crit Rev Oral Biol Med. 2000; 11:356-365.

54. Rivera-Hidalgo F. Smoking and periodontal disease. Periodontology. 2000-2003; 32(1):50-58.

55. Znaor A, Brennan P, Gajalakshmi V, Mathew A, Shanta V, Varghese C, et al. Independent and combined effects of tobacco smoking, chewing and alcohol habits on the risk of oral, pharyngeal and esophageal cancers in Indian men. Int J Cancer. 2003; 105:681-686.

56. Warnakulasuriya S. Food, nutrition and oral cancer. In: Food constituents and oral health. Wilson M, editor. Oxford: Woodhead Publishing Limited. 2003; pp.273-295.

57. Johnson NW, Warnakulasuriya S, Gupta PC, Dimba E, Chindia M, Otoh EC, et al. Global Oral Health Inequalities in Incidence and Outcomes for Oral Cancer: Causes and Solutions. Adv Dent Res. 2011; 23:237-246.

58. Lubin JH, Gaudet MM, Olshan AF, Kelsey K, Boffetta P, Brennan P, et al. Body mass index, cigarette smoking, and alcohol consumption and cancers of the oral cavity, pharynx, and larynx: modeling odds ratios in pooled case-control data. Am J Epidemiol. 2010; 171:1250-1261.

59. World Cancer Research Fund/American Institute for Cancer Research. Food, nutrition and physical activity and prevention of cancer. A global perspective. Washington, DC: AIRC. 2007.

60. World Health Organization. Global Status Report: alcohol policy. Geneva: World Health Organization. 2004. http://www.who.int/substance_abuse/publications/en/global_status_report_alcohol_policy_overview.pdf

61. Rehm J, Room R, Monteiro M, Gmel G, Graham K, Rehn N, et al. Alcohol as a Risk Factor for Global Burden of Disease. Eur Addict Res. 2003;9:157-164.

62. Andreasson S, Brandt L. Mortality and morbidity related to alcohol. Alcohol-alcohol. 1997; 32:173-178.

63. McMurran M. Alcohol and violence. Child Abuse Review. 1999; 8(4):215-296.

64. World Health Organization. WHO facts on Youth violence and alcohol. Geneva: World Health Organization. 2006. http://www.who.int/violence_injury_prevention/violence/world_report/factsheets/fs_youth.pdf

65. Marmot MG., Fuhrer R, Ettner SL, Marks NF, Bumpass L, Ryff CD. Contribution of Psychosocial Factors to Socioeconomic Differences in Health. The Milbank Quarterly. 1998; 76(3):403-448.

66. Sheiham A, Nicolau B. Evaluation of social and psychological factors in periodontal disease. Periodontology. 2000-2005; 39:118-131.

67. Marcenes WS, Sheiham A. The relationship between work stress and oral health status. Social Sciences in Medicine. 1992; 35:151-1520.

68. Hugo FN, Hilgert JB, Bozzetti MC, Bandeira D R, Goncxalves TR, Pawlowski J, de Sousa MdaLR. Chronic Stress, Depression, and Cortisol Levels as Risk Indicators of Elevated Plaque and Gingivitis Levels in Individuals Aged 50 Years and Older. J Periodonto. 2006; 77:1008-1014.

69. Rehm J, Room R, Graham K, Monteiro M, Gmel G, Sempos CT. The relationship of average volume of alcohol consumption and patterns of drinking to burden of disease: an overview. Addiction. 2003; 98(9):1209-1228.

70. Krug EG et al., eds. World report on violence and health. Geneva: World Health Organization. 2002. http://whqlibdoc.who.int/publications/2002/9241545615_eng.pdf

71. Dorri M, Sheiham A, Watt RG. Relationship between general hygiene behaviours and oral hygiene behaviours in Iranian adolescents. Eur J Oral Sci. 2009; 117:407-12.

72. Haskell WL, Lee I-M, Pate RR, Powell KE, Blair SN., Franklin B. A, et al. Physical Activity and Public Health: Updated Recommendation for Adults from the American College of Sports Medicine and the American Heart Association. Medicine & Science in Sports & Exercise. 2007; 39(8):1423-1434.

73. Wiefferink CH, Peters L, Hoekstra F, Dam GT, Buijs GJ, Paulussen TG. Clustering of health-related behaviors and their determinants: possible consequences for school health interventions. Prev Sci. 2006; 7(2):127-149.

74. Sanders AE, Spencer AJ, Stewart JF. Clustering of risk behaviours for oral and general health. Community Dent Health. 2005; 22(3):133-40.

75. Ma J, Betts N M., and Hampl JS. Clustering of Lifestyle Behaviors: The Relationship Between Cigarette Smoking, Alcohol Consumption, and Dietary Intake. American J Health Promotion. 2000; 15(2):107-117.

76. Langlie, JK. Interrelationships among preventive health behaviors: A test of competing hypotheses. Public Health Reports. 1979; 94(3):216-225.

77. Rajala M, Honkala, E, Rimpelä M, Lammi S. Toothbrushing in relation to other health habits in Finland. Community Dentistry and Oral Epidemiology. 1980; 8:106-113.

78. Paavola M, Vartiainen E, Haukkala A. Smoking, alcohol use, and physical activity: A 13-year longitudinal study ranging from adolescence to adulthood. Journal of Adolescent Health. 2004; 35:238-244.

79. Link BG, Phelan JC. Social Conditions As Fundamental Causes of Disease. J Health and Social Behavior. 1995; 35 (Extra Issue): 80-94.

80. Hertzman C, Boyce T. How Experience Gets Under the Skin to Create Gradients in Developmental Health. Annual Review of Public Health. 2010; 31:329-347.

81. Irwin LG, Siddiqi A, Hertzman C. The equalizing power of early child development: from the commission on social determinants of health to action. Child Health and Education. 2010; 2(1):3-18.

82. Link BG, Northridge ME, Phelan JC, Ganz ML. Social epidemiology and the fundamental cause concept: on the structuring of effective cancer screens by socioeconomic status. Milbank Quarterly. 1998; 76(3):375-402.

83. Graham H. Socioeconomic inequalities in health in the UK: Evidence on patterns and determinants. A short report for the Disability Rights Commission. Lancaster University: Institute for Health Research, September 2004 http://www.leeds.ac.uk/disability-studies/archiveuk/graham/socioeconomic_inequalities.pdf

84. Banks J, Marmot M, Oldfield Z, Smith JP. The SES health gradient on both sides of the Atlantic. NBER Working Paper Series. Working Paper 12674. November 2006. Available from: http://www.nber.org/papers/w12674.pdf

85. Lopez R, Fernandez O, Baelum V. Social gradients in periodontal disease among adolescents. Community Dent Oral Epidemiol. 2006; 34:184-196.

86. Marmot MG, Rose G, Shipley M, Hamilton PJS. Employment grade and coronary heart disease in British civil servants. Journal of Epidemiology and Community Health. 1978; 32:244-249.

87. Wilkinson RG. Unhealthy Societies. The Affliction of Inequality. London: Routledge. 1996.

88. Graham H. Social Determinants and Their Unequal Distribution: Clarifying Policy Understandings. The Milbank Quarterly. 2004; 82(1):101-124.

89. Link BG, Phelan JC. "Fundamental Sources of Health Inequalities." In: Policy Challenges in Modern Health Care, D. Mechanic editor, L.B. Rogut, D.C. 71-84. 2005.

90. Phelan, JC, Link, BG, Diez-Roux A, Kawachi I, Levin B. Fundamental Causes of Social Inequalities in Mortality: A Test of the Theory. Journal of Health and Social Behavior. 2004; 45:265-28.

91. Solar O, Irwin A. A conceptual framework for action on the social determinants of health. Social determinants of health discussion. Paper 2 (Policy and Practice). Geneva: World Health Organization, 2010. http://whqlibdoc.who.int/publications/2010/9789241500852_eng.pdf

92. Lynch JW, Kaplan GA, Salonen JT. Why do poor people behave poorly? Variation in adult health behaviours and psychosocial characteristics by stages of the socioeconomic lifecourse. Soc Sci Med. 1997; 44:809–19.

93. World Health Organization. Commission on Social Determinants of Health. A Conceptual Framework for Action on the Social Determinants of Health. Discussion paper for the Commission on Social Determinants of Health - Last version. Geneva: World Health Organisation. 2007.

94. Turrell G, Oldenburg B, McGuffog I, Dent R Socioeconomic determinants of health: towards a national research program and a policy and intervention agenda. Queensland University of Technology, School of Public Health, Ausinfo, Canberra. 1999. http://eprints.qut.edu.au/585/1/turrell_health_inequalities.pdf

95. World Health Organisation. Ottawa Charter for Health Promotion. 1986. http://www.who.int/hpr/NPH/docs/ottawa_charter_hp.pdf

96. World Health Organization. Making a difference: indicators to improve children's environmental health: prepared by David Briggs. Geneva; World Health Organization. 2003. http://www.who.int/phe/children/en/cehindicsum.pdf

97. The Marmot Review. Fair Society, Healthy Lives. The Marmot Review. Strategic Review of Health Inequalities post-2010. http://www.marmotreview.org/AssetLibrary/pdfs/Reports/FairSocietyHealthyLivesExecSummary.pdf

98. Frenk J. Bridging the divide: Comprehensive reform to improve health in Mexico. Nairobi, Kenya: Commission on Social Determinants of Health. 2006.

99. Frenk J. Reinventing primary health care: the need for systems integration. Lancet. 2009; 374(9684):170-3.

100. Frenk J. A New Vision for Health Systems in the 21st Century: Investing in People. World Bank. Education of Health professionals for the 21st century: A Global Independent Commission. Washington, D. C. March 7, 2011. http://siteresources.worldbank.org/HEALTHNUTRITIONANDPOPULATION/Resources/281627-1114107818507/1011070-1299526333144/030711JFrenkLancetReportWB.pdf

101. Institute of Medicine Report. Reducing Risks for Mental Disorders: Frontiers for Preventive Intervention Research. Mrazek PJ, Haggerty RJ. Editors. Committee on Prevention of Mental Disorders, Institute of Medicine. The Washington DC: National Acadamies Press. 1994.

102. Gordon R. An operational classification of disease prevention. In: Steinberg JA, Silverman MM. editors, Preventing mental disorders. Rockville, MD: Department of Health and Human Services. 1987; pp.20-26.

103. Weisz J, Sandler I, Durlak J, Anton B. Promoting and protecting youth mental health through evidence-based prevention and treatment. American Psychologist. 2005; 60(6):628-648.

104. World Health Organization. Redefining obesity and its treatment. Geneva: World Health Organization, 2000. http://www.wpro.who.int/NR/rdonlyres/0A35147B-B1D5-45A6-9FF2-F7D86608A4DE/0/Redefiningobesity.pdf

105. World Health Organisation. Obesity: preventing and managing the global epidemic.Report of WHO consultation. World Health Organization, Technical Report Series 894. Geneva, Switzerland: WHO. 2000.

106. Visram S, Drinkwater C. Health Trainers. A Review of the Evidence. Primary Care Development Centre, Kielder House, Coach Lane Campus West, Northumbria University, Newcastle-upon-Tyne, NE7 7XA. Available from: www.pcdc.org.uk. August 2005.

107. Sheiham A. Strategies for further reductions in dental caries: applying the common risk factor approach and directed vulnerable populations strategy. In: Splieth Ch. H. Revolutions in Paediatric Dentistry". Quintessence Publishing. Chapter 6. 2011.

108. Frohlich KL, Potvin L. Transcending the known in public health practice: The inequality paradox: The population approach and vulnerable populations. American Journal of Public Health. 2008; 98(2):216-221.

109. Rodrigues C, Watt R, Sheiham A. The effects of dietary guidelines on sugar intake in 3 year olds attending nurseries. Health Promotion Int. 1999; 14:329-335.

110. Focusing Resources on Effective School Health (FRESH). A FRESH Start to Improving the Quality and Equity of Education, 2008. http://www.freshschools.org/Pages/default.aspx. Accessed October 2011.

111. World Health Organization. Health Promoting Schools; a healthy setting for living, learning and working. Geneva: World Health Organization. 1998.

112. World Health Organization. Oral Health Promotion: An Essential Element of a Health-Promoting School. WHO Information Series on School Health. 2003 http://new.paho.org/hq/dmdocuments/2009/OH_st_sch.pdf

113. Moyses S, Moyses S, Watt RG, Sheiham A. The impact of health promoting schools policies on the oral health status of 12 year olds. Health Promot Int. 2003; 18:209-218.

114. Malikaew P, Watt RG, Sheiham A. Association between school environments and traumatic dental injuries. Oral Health Preventive Dent. 2003; 4:255-266.

115. Zerhouni EA. The promise of personalized medicine. NIH Medline Plus. 2006. http://www.nih.gov/about/director/interviews/NLMmagazinewinter2007.pdf

116. Insel TR. From prevention to preemption: A paradigm shift in psychiatry. Psychiatric Times. 2008. http://www.psychiatrictimes.com/display/article/10168/1171240.

117. Insel TR, Young LJ. The neurobiology of attachment. Nature Reviews Neuroscience. 2001; 2(2):129-136.

118. McKinlay JB. The promotion of health through planned sociopolitical change: challenges for research and policy. Soc Sci Med. 1993; 36:109-117.

119. Milio N. Making healthy public policy. Health Promotion. 1988; 2:263-27.

Chapter 8

Promoting Oral Health by Creating Healthy Environments and Using the Common Risk Factor Approach

Samuel Jorge Moysés
Simone Tetu Moysés
Aubrey Sheiham

Introduction

Major improvements in public health cannot be achieved without considering the root causes of ill health; the causes of the causes. Health is determined by multiple factors, including factors that shape the conditions in which people are born, grow, live, work, and age. Upstream determinants, the features of the social and physical environment such as socioeconomic status, influence individual behaviours, disease and health. Higher organizational levels influence lower levels in hierarchically organized biological systems.[1] Campbell said that "all processes at the lower levels of a hierarchy are restrained by and act in conformity at the laws of the higher levels." Intermediate-level factors are also influenced by higher levels of organization. Some models of the deter-

minants, such as the model proposed by Dahlgren and Whitehead,[2] consider that there are strong links between levels of health determinants (Fig. 8.1). Such models suggest how intervening at one level will affect factors downstream from that level.

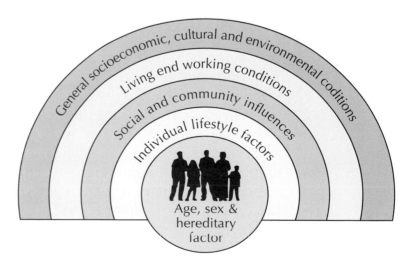

Fig. 8.1 – Social determinant model.

The US Task Force on Community Preventive Services[3] concluded that access to societal resources such as the standard of living, social institutions, political and economic structures, and the built environment are the key determinants of health. The socially embedded conditions that affect health were grouped into six key areas:

- neighborhood living conditions;
- opportunities for learning and capacity for development;
- employment opportunities and community development;
- prevailing norms, customs, and processes;
- social cohesion, civic engagement, and collective efficacy; and
- health promotion, disease prevention, and healthcare opportunities.

Neighbourhoods and communities are obvious important upstream determinants of health. Social environments affects health by enabling positive behaviours, making healthy choices the easy ones, or by negatively influencing emotional and behavioural states.[4]

Health promotion is an important component of public policies. The WHO definition of health promotion[5] accepts that structural elements (physical/social environment) are central to any strategy of health promotion because individual lifestyle and behaviours are moulded by the environment. The Institute of Medicine Report[6] stated that 'It is unreasonable to expect that people will change their behaviour easily when so many forces in the social, cultural, and physical environment conspire against such change.

Therefore, environmental approaches to alter factors that negatively influence health focus on identification and reduction of risk behaviours associated with morbidity and premature deaths, and on the structural elements that determine them. Health promotion therefore involves legislative and fiscal measures, such as safe seatbelts in cars and soft surfaces in children's playgrounds, higher taxes for cigarettes and alcohol, and social measures such guidelines on food, sanitation and housing. This chapter discusses strategies for creating environments favourable to health and outlines implications for oral health promotion of children. Initially, conceptual and practical fields of this strategy will be briefly highlighted. Next, influences of social and environmental factors in particular will be reviewed as determinants for general and oral health. Key elements of evidence about the effects of environmental measures on health will be outlined. Finally, some examples of environmental approaches to promote oral health will be presented.

Importance of healthy environments

Creating healthy environments has a very high priority for action in health promotion (Box 8.1).[7-14] The term "environment" incorporates not only the "physical or natural" dimension that defines the dynamic relationship between people and their life space, but also cultural, social, political, and economic dimensions of this relationship.

Healthy environments enable people to acquire more control over their own health by creating social and physical contexts and social relations favourable to health and human development. Promoting health, therefore, requires that local people and organizations play a pivotal role in the planning of social environments that support health promoting choices, and make explicit the political commitment to sustainable

Box 8.1 – Fields of action in health promotion.

- Healthy public policies – to stimulate all policy makers, within and outside of the health sector, with the explicit concern with health and equity in all fields of public policies with an impact on health, making the healthy choices the easier ones.
- Establishment of favourable environments to health - to develop health promotion actions in social spaces, creating life and working conditions that lead to health and well being.
- Strengthening of community action – health can only be warranted and sustained when the community acquires control over its health.
- Development of personal abilities – health promotion stimulates the personal development by means of the access to health information and education, developing in the individuals or groups the necessary competencies and abilities so that they are apt to make healthy choices.
- Reorientation of health services – to encourage health services to have as a basis new paradigms of health, aimed to the prevention and health promotion.

human development and the reduction of social and health inequalities.

Children need safe, healthy, supporting, nurturing, caring, and responsive living environments.[15] The nurturant qualities of the environments where children grow up, live, and learn matter the most for their development. The environments that are responsible for fostering these nurturant conditions for children range from the intimate realm of the family, the local community, where they study and play, to the broader socioeconomic context shaped by governments, international agencies, and civil society that determine their access to resources for maintenance of life and the guarantee the right to better health and citizenship. These environments and their characteristics are the determinants of early childhood development. In turn, early childhood development is a determinant of health, wellbeing, and learning skills across the lifecourse.[16,17]

Social and environmental factors as determinants of health

Some people still believe that health of children is basically a matter of kee-

ping them well fed, clean, and preventing them from becoming sick. However, health involves dimensions much wider than hygiene or "absence of diseases". It also involves physical health: it is necessary to feel well and healthy; mental and emotional health: it is necessary to be happy and balanced, and able to use efficiently one's mind and body; social health, besides individual health: children need to live in cooperative environments where they are respected. They should have access to appropriate learning opportunities. In addition, everyone should have equal rights and opportunities.

Promoting the health of children, therefore, highlights the fundamental need to recognize wider determinants of health. Theoretical models explaining health determinants that reinforce the interrelation and interdependence between social and cultural factors, on one hand, and environmental, structural, and material ones, on the other hand, have directly influenced public health actions towards the child population in the past decades.[2,18]

The contemporary discussion about inequalities in health has also emphasized the influence of social, economic, and environmental conditions on health, including oral health.[14,19] There is good evidence that children living in low socioeconomic conditions have a higher prevalence of dental caries.[20-24] In Brazil, a country with large socio-economic differences, many studies have confirmed the effects of socio-environmental conditions on the prevalence of dental caries, dental trauma and pain in children and adolescents.[25-33]

Other broader determinants may also influence patterns of health and disease of children. Moysés[34] showed how intra-urban differences in public policy implementation in some low income regions in the city of Curitiba affected oral health in children. Oral health depended on the micro areas where the children lived, characterized by different levels of implementation of public policies in fields like education, health, food, and housing.

Social gradients play an important in inequalities in general and oral health.[35] Bueno et al.,[36] when exploring trends in some Millennium Development Goals and oral health outcomes in 49 cities in Southern Brazil, demonstrated the impact of local socioeconomic and socioenvironmental status on inequalities in human development, mother and child health, and children's dental caries. They concluded that inequalities in oral health will only be reduced with an effective, appropriate and sustainable intersectoral health promotion policy, which must focus on the broad determinants of health.

Promoting the health of children, therefore, involves expanding actions beyond individual behaviours. This means recognizing that environmental conditions may differentially affect health, and behaviours of children. The relationship between the child and the environment are characterized by cycles of interacting influences, in which physical and social characteristics of the closer environments where they develop, including the family, the school, and the community, directly influence their health, as their own individual and group actions in these environments modify their ability to achieve health.[37,38]

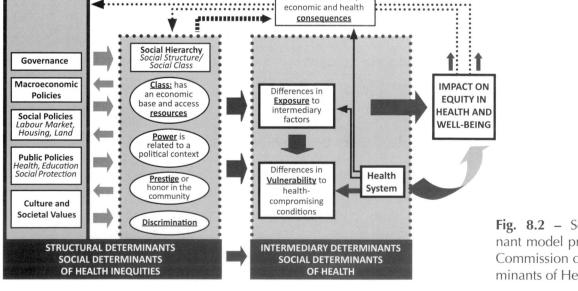

Fig. 8.2 – Social determinant model proposed by the Commission of Social Determinants of Health.[15]

The role of the family environment

Children with limited protection are more vulnerable and are more likely to have poor health, including oral health.[39] In modern societies the family assumes a fundamental role for the individual's survival by the protection and maintenance of their needs, by transmitting ethical principles, habits and behaviours, establishing links of security and trust.[40] Therefore, the family is considered a powerful social force to promote physical and emotional well-being, to prevent and control diseases. Family influences affect, cognitive, and behavioural responses that are directly related to general and oral health promotion. Fear, values, and the importance related to appropriate dental care, beliefs about oral health and how people establish and maintain self care, oral hygiene habits, and a healthy diet are some examples of practices forged within the family.[41]

The way families support or promote health among children is influenced by several family functions, abilities, and structural characteristics. A house with two parents, instead of only one, household division of tasks, methods of raising children, and the employment of the mother are considered important characteristics related to health and health behaviour of children.[42,43] Family can also be an important source of social support to its members, when it creates the necessary environment for a healthy life, increasing confidence, creating opportunities of access to learning, resources, equipment and time that facilitates health practices, and provides the necessary information for healthier choices. The social context of the family that determines circumstances where family and environment interact is crucial for the support forged in the family. Lifecourse socioeconomic status influencing the accumulation of risk and social mobility of the family, for example, may have an impact on oral health.[17] So, the establishment of public policies focused on the support to the nuclear family should be an important strategy for the health promotion of children.

Social networks and social support

Social networks and social support are particularly important in the context of material deprivation to give support to mechanisms of control over certain determinants of health and disease.[44] The social support created in the environments where children live becomes essential for promoting their health. The support provided by people from the family, or important people at school, or in the community, may encourage children to assume healthy behaviours. Social support may also influence health through increasing perceptions of control over the environment, reinforcing self-confidence, and that improves well being. On the other hand, a "buffering" effect of social support may act when the support of another person may moderate the impact of the stressor agents, helping the person to control consequences of stress, and thereby enhance or maintain health.[45] Therefore, social support can be an important enabling factor for health.[46] In this way, actions for strengthening interpersonal relationships such as towards controlling violence in the school, for example, may have an important impact on children's health.

Environments and health related behaviours

Social and material factors affect health and health related behaviours (see Chapter 3). Therefore, efforts to improve health need to pay more attention to addressing the upstream environmental determinants of health and health related behaviours. Health promotion policy should recognize that to change behaviours, one needs to change those aspects of environments that determined the behaviours. An environmental approach to disease prevention and health promotion is needed because even if the intervention was successful for some, the persistence of the adverse determinants would lead other people to adopt poor health behaviours and replace those who may have modified their behaviour following health education.[47-50] If all that health services does is to rescue people from the river downstream without making the river shallower and easier to cross, namely, changing the environment, then more people will fall into the river because the conditions are unchanged (See Chapter 3). Theories on the importance of environment are based on the premise that it is the environment that influences behaviour. Choices go beyond individual volition.[51] People are unlikely to change their behaviours when so many forces in the social, cultural and physical environment work against change. So, strategies to prevent diseases should pay more attention to the environmental context within which people live as well as the behaviours of individuals.[52] Therefore, rather than focusing on individuals alone, it is necessary to target both the social environments and individual level factors in which health behaviours of individuals are developed and sustained.[49]

As stated earlier, behavioural decisions are rooted in people's social and economic circumstances. Childhood deprivation, the stress of poverty, overcrowding, living in a run-down area, feeling powerless, do not give people hope and feelings of control over their lives and the resources that enables them to successfully make changes in behaviour. People born at the upper end of the social gradient into more advantageous situations find it easier to adopt healthy lifestyles and limit unhealthy behaviours. Interventions to reduce inequalities in health must therefore tackle the macro environmental factors and the physical and social environment, as well as adverse health behaviours and access to health care.[53] Policy makers should broaden their perspective to the analysis of the specific aspects of environments that give rise to the exposures that shape individual-level as well as group-level behaviours rather than looking for relationships between exposures to a single or small number of specific risk factors and diseases[54-57] An important factor that has limited epidemiology's ability to examine the causes of disease in populations is the "individualization" of epidemiology; the notion that the risk of disease depends exclusively on individual-level characteristics.[55] Diez-Roux extends her criticism to the behavioural model of disease whereby choices and behaviours of individuals are isolated from their social contexts.

Sociologists have stressed the importance of how 'places' 'locales' that structure peoples' lives and affect behaviour and concepts of risk.[55,57-59] These environmental determinants of health and behaviour are undisputed, but adequate mechanisms of how particular places stimulate certain behaviours are contentious. So, lifestyle, the clustering of behaviours, can be viewed as the "manner in which social groups translate their objective situation into patterns of behaviour".[60] Understanding why poorer people behave poorly[61] requires recognition that specific behaviours occur in certain social contexts. Decontextualizing behaviour from their setting obscures their social determinants and encourages "blaming the victims" of inequality for their unhealthy lifestyles.[61] Social environments with few basic resources such as access to healthy foods, safe housing, jobs, decent schools, supportive social networks, access to health care and other public and private goods and service, those with the highest public health risks for chronic diseases and high mortality rates.[62,63] Understanding why this happens requires recognition of the fact that individuals and communities interact with their physical and social environments and that influences their health related behaviours.[64] Conceptualizing

health as a product, in part, of social conditions, facilitates the identification of relationships between social determinants and health outcomes that may be amenable to community and primary dental care health promotion interventions.[65]

Environments, especially social contexts, place constraints on opportunities and choices, as well as enabling people to make healthy choices.[64] Healthy choices are not always the easier ones for those lower down the social gradient and they consequently find it more difficult to change their behaviours. Robustly consistent findings in differing societies suggest some universal human responses to particular environments. Why, universally, do people behave in similar ways in certain environments? People interact dynamically with their environments both being changed by it and changing it.

A plausible theory of what elements of environments influence behaviours is the 'fundamental social cause hypothesis'.[66]

"The social environment influences behaviour by shaping norms, enforcing patterns of social control, providing environmental opportunities to engage in particular behaviours and reducing or producing stress, for which engaging in specific behaviours might be an effective short-term coping strategy".[64]

Fundamental social cause hypothesis

The theory has four features:
- Social conditions influence multiple disease outcomes;
- It affects these disease outcomes through multiple risk factors;
- The association between the fundamental cause and mortality is reproduced over time via the replacement of intervening mechanisms;

- The "essential feature of fundamental social causes is that they involve access to resources that can be used to avoid risks or to minimize the consequences of disease once it occurs".[66,67]

Link and Phelan[66,68] regard the key feature of fundamental social causes to be that health advantages enjoyed by higher socioeconomic status people is in their greater access to and effective utilization of resources such as money, knowledge, power, prestige, and beneficial social connections. They consider that social conditions are important in shaping individual health behaviours because resources shape access to health-relevant circumstances, "contextualizing risk factors". Resources affect access to the physical and social, such as neighborhoods, occupations, and social networks. "People benefit from high status not only because it is less stressful to be on top but also because being there leads to benefits that translate into better health. Knowledge about risk and protective factors, and the wherewithal to act on it, leads to socioeconomic differences in smoking, exercise, diet, seat-belt use, screening, and so on".[69] On the other hand, persons on the lower rungs of the social gradient ladder have increased exposure to a broad range of environmental and psychosocial factors related to health, exposure to occupational and environmental health hazards, less sense of control, chronic and acute stress in life and work, stress of racism, class prejudice, greater discounting of the future, lower self-esteem and poorer social relationships and social supports (social capital). That suggests that socioeconomic differences in health and health behaviours arise because those with more resources, usually those in higher socioeconomic positions, having better health, is that they have access to more health promoting facilities, environments, foods, and are better able to take advantage of new knowledge about health, have more access to interventions, and have grown up in environments that foster good health.

The "fundamental cause explanation" argues that those with more resources are more able to change their behaviours when information on their adverse effects becomes available.[70] For example, in the decades since the governmental reports on the harmfulness of smoking, groups with more resources have been less likely to initiate as well as more likely to quit smoking.[71] Social resources that are instrumental in providing advantage are not limited to economic advantage, but extend to social capital and human capital, such as education.[71] Indeed, all health related behaviours, with the exception of alcohol consumption, are significantly related to education level.

Similarly, Macintyre, Maciver and Sooman[72] suggest that there are five broad ways in which socioeconomic factors might influence health and behaviours of people living in disadvantaged areas:

- Physical features of the environment;
- The effect of the domestic and working environment in the local area;
- The provision of services including health and social care, and educational quality;
- Socio-cultural features of neighbourhoods;
- The reputation of an area that may affect psychological health and morale.

So, lifestyle can be viewed as the 'manner in which social groups translate their objective situation into patterns of behaviour'.[72] Lifesyle is and expression of the social and cultural circumstances that condition and constrain behaviour in addition to the personal decisions the individual may make. That view of how lifestyle are generated shifts the focus of health promotion from individuals to populations and to disease-causing conditions, including physical and social conditions, such as the groups to which they belong, the neighborhoods where they live, the organization of workplaces and policies we create to order our lives.

In summary, the establishment of health promoting environments for all has a very high priority for action in health promotion. Therefore it is vital to consider the health promoting public policies related to environment.

Influences of social environmental policies on children's health

Healthy public policies have been defined as all general policies developed by governments and public institutions, emphasizing propositions and actions that aim at social change. They highlight a series of related activities which can enhance the health and human development of the population.[73,74]

The Ottawa Charter states that healthy public policies can be seen as part of the health promotion proposals, explicit in the Healthy Cities project,[75] and in the Adelaide Declaration about health promotion and healthy public policies, sponsored by the World Health Organization.[76] Although based on the same grounds that guide the health promotion paradigm, healthy public policies involves a greater orientation towards public health, social justice, and the structural changes in society, avoiding the tendency of "victim blaming" and high-risk approach, which is more probable to arise with strategies that focus only on individuals and their lifestyles.[77,78] So, it is necessary that public policies address the root causes of health and disease, tackling social determinants and the environment, taking into account the principles of the common risk factor approach in a multidisciplinary and intersectoral approach.[79,80]

A broad perspective of healthy policies in the communities reinforces human development as central to achieve health, and links communities, environment and economy that requires a socially equitable, ecological sustainable, and a liveable built environment society.[74] Such policies must encompass actions to promote community conviviality, based on social cohesion and social solidarity, and a sufficient level of economic activity to ensure that basic needs for all are met.

Therefore, levels of implementation of community healthy public policy can be a marker for community factors related to children's health. For example, comprehensive health promotion policies for children could focus on recreational equipment and leisure areas; quality, safety and supportive day care centres and schools; condition of the streets; environmental protection, with adequate use of water; and the kinds of foods that are easily available and affordable.

As discussed before, the evidence that material conditions are associated with health is very strong.[55] It was also discussed the importance of social capital – the cohesiveness and trust in their communities and the social groups and networks to which they belong.

There is also a direct causal relationship between the level of structural and environmental development of a geo-populational area and oral health. For example, there are clear relationships between traumatic injuries, including dento-facial trauma and the levels of deprivation of a neighbourhood.[81] Trauma in adults and children is related to factors that are external to the home environment, including traffic accidents and urban violence.[82-85] However, traumatic accidents in children point to how important are the internal home environment or factors immediately associated to the places where children spend the major part of their daily life, like day care centres, schools, or the residential area (see Chapter 15).[28,33,86-88]

Recent Brazilian studies have demonstrated associations between the Human Development Index (HDI) of states and municipalities, and other measures of social and environmental policies, and dental caries experience in children.[36,89,90] The HDI is a good measure of the social and environmental conditions in which people live, using indicators of income, education, and life expectancy to reflect opportunities for a decent life, the access to knowledge, and the healthiness of the place. The findings of these studies indicate that oral health or disease may reflect the same determinant for quality of life in general, as other outcomes related to human development followed the same pattern of oral health.

The inclusion of socio-environmental factors as explanations for the oral health of populations has lead to interesting insights. For example, the study by Gratrix and Holloway,[91] generated important inferences about the approach to the social determinants of health. They correlated levels of oral disease and community characteristics related to health in contrasting neighbourhoods. They adopted an ecologic approach. The communities with high levels of caries had a lower percentage of babies with normal birth weight; lower percentages of children with updated immunization, and more children born to separated couples. Communities with a high prevalence of caries also tended to wean babies early, they used more nursing bottles and commercial baby foods for longer. The parents in the communities with a high prevalence of caries had a higher proportion of social and financial problems and participated

less in Parents and Teacher's Associations. Their children had lower levels of school attendance and punctuality and a record of bad behaviour and higher intake of sweets after school hours. The previous correlations must be interpreted taking into account the hierarchy of determinants, sothat they do not generate any confusion of causal chains. Nevertheless, oral health professionals should not be intimidated by the finding that phenomena in the mouth may be excellent "markers" of stressors, biologic, and social events, such as poverty, poor nutrition, low school performance, or family disruptions.

Socio-environmental factors frequently are the primary concern and the responsibility of local and state public health institutions. The WHO recognize that community social environmental factors that affect oral health include the process of adding fluoride to the water supply and to toothpastes, policies related to tobacco, alcohol and drugs, preventive oral care subsidized by public and free access, healthy diet, environmental surveillance, and public education for health.[92-95] More general environmental factors include the economic context, relative wealth, political participation, social level of tension and violence.

The study of Moysés[96] analysing the impact of public policies in communities environments in Curitiba, Brazil, showed the influence socio-environmental factors have on oral health and support findings outlined above, namely:

- Healthy public policy interventions in the fields of sanitation, education, housing, integral care for the preschool child, and nutrition, affected standards of oral health. Socio-environmental components, measured at the group level and focusing on healthy public policies and social cohesion, explained variations in oral health, beyond individual variables.

- Associations existed between "public policies/social cohesion" and the prevalence of caries-free individuals.

- There were intra-urban differences in oral health and indicators of implementation of healthy public policies. The oral health status depended on the kind of micro-areas where the children lived, and areas which received unequal public attention.

- Deprivation in its broader sense, which included deprivation of public policies and social cohesion in the community in which one lives, was associated to an increased risk of oral diseases. The inequalities between micro-areas may have been increased by the difference in implementation of governmental interventions. It is probable that there has been a social benefit, in relation to the "indirect income" about the domestic economies, provided by subsidising of services like day care centres, education, housing, and nutrition in the best micro-areas.

- In particular, the study pointed to the benefits that healthy public interventions can generate for oral health, but also indicated the need that these policies be directed to the whole urban population, avoiding the larger social inequalities between areas of the same city.

The expansion of boundaries: strengthening of community actions to promote the general and oral health of children

The Surgeon General's Report on Oral Health in America,[97] acknowled-

ged the new dimensions to be considered in respect of oral health, namely the close relation between oral and general health. Marmot,[19,98] based on the recommendations of the WHO Commission on Social Determinants of Health, suggested that actions to tackle inequalities in oral health must address the "causes of the causes", by improving living conditions, specially for children and mothers, creating opportunities for the development of capacities, and creating and developing healthy and sustainable places and communities. All these perspectives create an auspicious environment for the renewed action, with challenges and opportunities for dentistry in a new relationship with global society.

These new recommendations in official documents, set new objectives for oral health, with an emphasis on the socio-environmental determinants of health. The new objectives confront the socioeconomic factors that generate inequalities, creating national policies and regional/local programmes for the consumption of healthy foods, the prevention of violence and trauma, school and community-based programmes, the fight against smoking and the use of toxic substances, the improvement of access and the quality of health care, the monitoring of workplaces, and the safety in transport and on public streets.

This thinking on the value of more general community and environmental factors, points to new perceptions about the characteristics of the health-disease process, as well as the means to organize oral health care. In Denmark, for example, where they investigated standards of care in 141 municipal services (71% of all services in the country), it was concluded that the changes to the dental services should consider the more intensive use of population-based activities and a larger use of auxiliary personnel.[99] That shows there is a movement in favour of community based actions. Similarly, in Australia, a study points to the need to implement community approaches aimed at reducing social inequalities and removing economic, cultural and access barriers.[100] In Finland, there is concern about the epidemiologic polarization in levels of health and oral health in children; many children are caries-free, but a small percentage still have a great burden of oral disease. Studies that try to understand family factors associated with the phenomenon of the polarization illustrate that the caries experience in five-year--old children was significantly associated with the mother's irregular habits of hygiene, with the annual occurrence of new caries in parents, with the intake of sugar from 18 months of age, and with the low age of the mothers.[101] Findings like these throw new light on the understanding of phenomena that cannot be solved by conventional clinical dental practice.

For the new standards of prevention and care to be implemented requires population-based approaches and involvement of families and communities. It is essential for families and communities to be provided with evidence on the new technologies for processing of relevant information. For this reason, the systematic critical reviews of the literature, and the practice of health policies based on evidence, offer the synthesis of the effects of several measures of health promotion. They will certainly promote new standards of decision making that affects health. As an example of these processes of knowledge analysis, the studies by Kay and Locker,[102,103] show, for example that the use of fluoride continues to be effective in caries prevention, that campaigns in the media aimed at education for health are not effective, and that more knowledge, or access to information, does not necessarily reflect changes of attitudes and behaviour of people (see Chapter 11).

The persistence of unacceptable levels of dental disease in some groups suggests that current approaches to prevention and health promotion should be reoriented and highlights the need for a broad community perspective which tackles the causes of the causes, the determinants of diseases, and makes healthy choices easier and unhealthy choices more difficult for most people. Tackling determinants and the behaviours requires an analysis of which approaches to use and what is the best strategy to apply.

Integrating prevention and health promotion approaches

The changes in dental practice and approaches to prevention and health promotion that are recommended involve tackling the determinants of chronic diseases, including dental caries, using the Common Risk Factor Approach Outlined in Chapter 3, and helping to 'make healthy choices the easier choices and unhealthy choices more difficult'.[104] There are at least two approaches and three strategies to use in promoting health (see Chapter 6). An individual focus approach directs attention to changing people's behaviours to lower disease risk. Systematic reviews demonstrate that the effectiveness of long-term behavioral change in dental patients is poor (see Chapter 5).

The second health promotion approach involves an environmental perspective. An environmental approach to disease prevention and health promotion is needed because many individually focused models of behaviour change have been unsuccessful. The persistence of the determinants would lead to other people to adopt poor health behaviours and replace those people who may have modified their behaviour following health education[48,50] Major contributions to improvement in oral health can come from environmental influences, behavioural changes and, lastly, specific preventive and therapeutic measures. Therefore, greater emphasis must be placed on tackling the determinants of diseases – the environmental perspective. To change people's behaviours requires a change in their environment. So, strategies to prevent disease and improve health should pay attention not only to the behaviour of individuals, but also to the environmental context within which people live. Therefore, when deciding on priorities for prevention and health promotion, community-wide measures should have higher priority than clinic-based prevention because an environment-based strategy offers greater hope of improvements in dental health than a heavy commitment to individual health care.

There are three preventive/health promotion strategies: two types of Risk Strategy and the Population Strategy (see Chapter 6) (Box 8.2). The two types of Risk Strategy are the High-Risk Strategy (HRS) and the Directed Vulnerable Populations Strategy (DVPS). In one kind of risk strategy, the HRS, individuals at risk are identified by screening. In the second kind of risk approach, the Directed Vulnerable Populations Strategy, vulnerable groups are identified by conventional dental surveys, not by screening. A vulnerable population "…is defined by a higher measured exposure to a specific risk factor. All individuals in a population at risk show a higher risk exposure. A vulnerable population is a subgroup or subpopulation who, because of shared social characteristics, is at higher risk of risks".[50] They may be people who share adverse social and environmental conditions such as living in a particular area that puts them at higher risk, or attending particular low socio-economic schools with higher rates of diseases.

Box 8.2 – Preventive and health promotion strategies.

- The Risk Strategy:
- **1. High-Risk Strategy (HRS),** which seeks to identify individuals at high risk through screening and targeting them with evidence based interventions.
- **2. Directed Vulnerable Populations Strategy (DVPS)** protects sections of the population that share social characteristics that put them at higher risk of risks.
- *The Population Strategy:* Efforts are made to shift the risk distribution of the entire population to a more favourable level.

A major shortcoming of the HRS is that even it were effective, which as yet it has not been shown to be, the reductions in the overall number of new fraction of disease in a population is very small because the largest burden of ill health comes more from the many who are exposed to low inconspicuous risk than from the few who face an obvious problem.[105] A finding supported in dental studies. In one dental study about dental caries, Batchelor and Sheiham[106] found that "the majority of new lesions occurred in those children classified at lowest caries risk. Irrespective of the preventive regime adopted and the initial caries levels, children classified as 'highest risk' contributed less than 6% of the total number of new caries lesions developing over a 4 year period." Hausen et al.[107] supported Batchelor and Sheiham's findings in their intervention study. Although at baseline 20% of Finnish children in the trial accounted for 80% of the DMF, over the three years of using a HRS intervention, a larger number of cavities developed in the 80% of low risk children than in the high-risk group 20% of children. These findings have important implications for deciding on which strategy to use. The Finnish trial shows that it is difficult, but not impossible, to help the high caries-risk individuals by measures applied at clinics. To further reduce caries among the high-risk children, the approach should be directed to the whole population or at vulnerable groups using a Directed Vulnerable Populations Strategy.

So it is apparent that the High Risk Strategy for preventing caries, and periodontal disease, has several drawbacks, and if relied upon exclusively cannot be expected to make a major impact on oral health in populations nor reduce caries levels in those at high risk. There is a growing consensus on the limitations of solely adopting a HRS in oral disease prevention. Another strategy is available. One that combines both population and risk strategies.

The alternative to the HRS is the Population Strategy (PS). The PS is a radical approach in that it is focused on the causes of the distribution, the determinants.[108] The PS controls the causes of the incidence of disease, whereas the HRS tries to protect and is palliative. In the PS efforts are made to shift the risk distribution and the frequency distribution of caries of the entire population to a more favorable level thereby decreasing the average risk of the population and the frequency distribution of disease and risk is moved to the left. Even a small decrease in the average level of a risk factor may result in a considerable reduction in the incidence of a health problem of the whole population. The PS should be applied nationally. However, when there are vulnerable groups or subgroups of a population with high caries levels then the Directed Vulnerable Population Strategy (DVPS) is applied. For that strategy, although the group or district is selected as being at higher risk than elsewhere, the principles of the population strategy are used.

The DVPS can be directed at a designated neighborhood or group of the total population who have a higher level of dental diseases than other groups in the population. This DVPS might for example be used for programmes in a particular health district, school or locality. The DVPS is complementary to a PS as it uses most of the methods of the PS but DVPS directs the approach to a vulnerable group, or subsections of a population. A DVPS ensures that vulnerable populations share the benefits of a PS. In addition, a DVPS addresses most of the multiple determinants and risks that the vulnerable populations are exposed to. Most importantly, the DVPS is sensitive to their particular social and environmental conditions.

The pivotal factor used to determine the choice of health promotion strategy is the fundamental axiom "that a large number of people exposed to a small risk may generate many more cases than a small number of people exposed to a high risk". The largest "... burden of ill health comes more from the many who are exposed to low inconspicuous risk than from the few who face an obvious problem".[108] The more successful the population strategy, the less pronounced will be the so--called 'tail' of the caries distribution curves which represents the so-called 'high-risk subgroup'. That subgroup is frequently considered to require more individualized preventive and treatment programs. Where the high-risk subgroup fulfils the criteria for a vulnerable population then the DVPS is the strategy of choice.

The Settings Approach

The healthy settings approach reoriented thinking away from an approach to health based on health services, toward one emphasizing the role of other sectors and associated agencies in the promotion of health by influencing upstream determinants.[109] Taking a settings approach to health promotion means addressing the contexts within which people live, work, and play, and increase the likelihood of success because it offers opportunities to situate practice in these contexts.[110]

The basis for the settings approach is that certain places or settings are more appropriate than others for promoting health of people at different stages of their lives. The concept of a 'setting' is fundamental to theory and practice in health promotion. A settings approach locates public health action in social, cultural and physical places in which children live, learn and play.

During the last decades, many global and local movements towards building healthy environments, such as WHO's Healthy Cities and Health Promoting Schools programmes, has contributed to urban policy change in different contexts.[111] Some key settings cover the bulk of the general population and children. These in turn fit within the wider settings of the city, district and village. The settings are the Healthy Cities, Healthy Villages, Healthy Locality, Educational Settings, The Recreation Setting, The Family Setting, The Healthcare Setting.

The matrix below illustrates a range of health promotion activities whereby planners can make decisions on which setting is best for a particular group for the Directed Vulnerable Population Strategies and the Common Risk Factor Approach (Fig. 8.3 and 8.4).[112]

This chapter aimed to provide a review of the justification for using settings and environments that prevent the development of a number of childhood conditions using a Common Risk Factor Approach. The conditions are overweight, obesity and caries. They have risk factors in common. Environmental approaches in disease prevention deal with social and technical-material conditions of daily living, as those conditions significantly influence health behavior. Strategies that focus on the obesogenic environment are considered increasingly important in the prevention of obesity in children and adolescents. They can be applied at different levels such as schools and communities. These interventions should aim to improve the availability of healthy foods and physical activity facilities, by provision of healthy meals and foods in schools, restaurants, and stores and by price reductions of healthy foods (see Chapter 12). Physical activity can be supported by creating attractive green spaces and playgrounds in schools and cities, improving sidewalk networks and a supportive pedestrian environment, and implementing walk-to-school projects. On a national level, policies and legislation can support changes in the social and situational environments, relating to catering in schools or television advertising.

ACTIVITIES	SETTINGS					TARGET GROUP					
	Community	Education	Primary care	Regional/National projects	Work place	Pre-school	Young people	Adults	Older people	Disalded groups	Professionals
Education											
Legistation											
Regulation											
Fiscal											
Organization change											
Community development											
Reorientation of health system											

Fig. 8.3 – Health promoting activities, settings, and target group.

SETTINGS	GROUPS						
	Toddlers	Pre-school	Primary	Teenagers	Young adults	Adults	Older people
Maternal and Child Health							
Clinics							
Nurseries							
Schools							
Work							
Community							
Practices							

Fig. 8.4 – Settings and groups for health promotion.

Building policies for reducing dental caries in vulnerable groups

There are two factors that need to be taken into consideration for reducing caries levels: diet and fluorides. The main focus should be on strategies to improve diet as that fits well into the CRFA (see Chapter 12), with a focus on Directed Vulnerable Population Strategies (DVPS). Healthy eating contributes to overall well-being and is a cornerstone in the prevention of a number of conditions including heart disease, diabetes, high blood pressure, stroke, cancer and dental caries. Eating behaviours adopted during childhood are likely to be maintained into adulthood, underscoring the importance of encouraging healthy eating as early in life as possible. Planners are concerned about the high levels of consumption of energy dense low nutrition foods and beverages that are high in refined non-milk extrinsic sugars. Such diets are common among low income and vulnerable groups who have relatively high levels of caries and childhood obesity. The major lifestyle related risk behaviours for Non Communicable Diseases (NCDs) are unhealthy diets, smoking, excessive alcohol and lack of physical exercise. The burden to society of NCDs comes mainly from a combination of these behaviours rather than any single one. Central to this strategy is recognizing that a number of NCDs share common risk behaviours and should be dealt with integrated programmes aimed at all relevant groups.

The policy for reducing dental caries includes efforts to improve health by reducing risks, promoting health and strengthening possibilities to cope with risk factors. There are a range of options to promote oral health. They are healthy public policies, legislation, regulation and fiscal measures and can all be utilized to promote oral health either at international, national and local levels.[8] At international level, the WHO have published recommendations from expert committees on nutrition guidelines for a healthy diet.[113,114] Similarly the Health Promoting Schools (HPS) approach is recommended by WHO as a strategy for promoting the health of young people (see Chapter 19). At national and local levels diet and nutrition and oral health guidelines are used by institutions such as nurseries, schools, hospitals and workplaces to create environments providing healthy food and drinks. There is a hierarchy of levels at which to intervene in a country. The highest is at national and local levels. National and local government can legislate and regulate and implement fiscal measures, whereby health damaging products are taxed. Legislation includes dietary guidelines banning chocolates, crisps and sugary foods and drinks from nurseries and schools and requiring vegetables and salads and fruit to be part of the school meal. Dietary guidelines can be backed up by media campaigns and school health education. The next level of priority is Health Settings Strategy, that helps to identify settings, vulnerable groups, and partners that can be involved on oral health promotion actions focused on the establishment of opportunities for healthy diet.

Examples of the CRFA and the Directed Vulnerable Populations Strategy (DVPS) in practice

Food policy

The CRFA uses a holistic nutrition programme which aims to improve the overall nutritional status of school children. Such an approach, if successful, will not only reduce calorie dense non-milk extrinsic sugars (NMES) consumption and hence improve oral health, but will also improve the overall quality of preschool children's diet and thereby promote their growth and future development. A principle is rather than focus attention mainly on the consumers of food, the CRFA approach recognizes the importance of influencing key groups such as food producers, manufacturers and government departments because a range of sectors are involved in the 'food chain', all of whom have a potential role to play in changing diets. Health education forms only one component part of the overall programme and can be targeted at a range of influential partners and professionals, not only the public (Figs. 8.3 and 8.4). Other complementary actions can address cost and access issues in relation to food. The approach should include efforts to improve health by reducing risks, promoting health and strengthening possibilities to cope with 'given' risk factors – creating supportive environments reducing the negative effects of certain risk factors and facilitating behaviour changes.

In some countries dietary guidelines and food policies in nurseries and schools have not only substantially reduced sugars consumption and improved the nutritional quality of the diet but have also successfully reduced caries increments.[115] Similar food policy guidelines have been introduced for residential homes for older people.

Here are some examples of local and national DVPS actions to promote oral health.

National level

- Support food and nutrient standards for school meals, and other foods and drinks sold in schools.
- Support regulation on content and timing of television adverts promoting children's foods and drinks.
- Encourage tighter legislation on food labeling and food claims on products.
- Encourage greater availability of sugar-free paediatric medicines.
- Support removal of value added tax and other taxes on fluoride toothpastes.

Examples of the oral health aspects of the abovementioned policies are:

Tackling Early Childhood Caries (ECC). The conventional approach to reducing ECC was through education of parents and carers. Whilst some success has been reported for these time-consuming measures, an oral health promotion approach should be directed at eliminating or reducing refined sugars from paediatric medicines and baby drinks makes health promoting choices easier for hard pressed mothers, many who are single parents and poor. The following strategies were used:
- A group consisting of representatives of paediatrics, paedodontics, dental public health and the pharmaceu-

tical industry submitted a report to Government which lead to a law forbidding the addition of sugars to all prescribed paediatric medicines.
- Sugars in baby foods and drinks. Because of the increased awareness of the links between early exposure to sugars and nutrient dilution, overweight and dental caries, maternity alliances have put pressure on manufacturers to reduce sugars in baby foods and drinks. Manufacturers have responded to consumer pressure and reduced the sugars and the pH of their drinks.
- Dietary guidelines for nurseries and carers. As part of general regulations regarding nurseries and training of professional carers, dietary guidelines have been formulated which must be adhered to by nurseries.[115,116]

Local level

- Support development of local infant feeding policies and ensure oral health messages are included.
- Develop oral health and nutrition policies in preschools and nurseries.
- Encourage nurseries and schools to provide subsidies on healthy snacks and drinks.
- Encourage schools to become part of the Health Promoting Schools Network
- Encourage sales of subsidized fluoride toothpastes through community clinics and health visitors.

Health promoting schools and nurseries (See Chapters 18 and 19)

A resolution on oral health at the 60th World Health Assembly of WHO in 2007, urges governments 'to promote oral health in schools, aiming at developing healthy lifestyles and self care practices in children'.[117] By implementing the WHO recommendations, reduced morbidity, improved growth, and improved educational outcomes can be achieved. The preschool nursery and school are attractive settings for health promotion, for it provides a way of reaching a large proportion of children and young people, and brings with it a team of professional educators. The WHO Health Promoting Schools (HPS) programme offers a sound approach to tackling the problem of dental caries. Such an approach focuses upon the influence of the social and physical environment on health. The concept of the HPS places emphasis upon developing a range of complementary policies and actions to promote the health and well being of students, staff and the wider community involved in the school.

The HPS approach aims to improve health for the total school population by developing supportive environments conducive to the promotion of health offers opportunities for, and requires commitments to, the provision of safe and health enhancing social and physical environment. The health promoting school concept embraces the principles that the health of individuals can be advanced by both the provision of health education in taught curriculum, and schools providing a supportive and safe physical and social environment conductive to making healthy choices. In addition, through the interaction with external environments and alliances with local community, school health promotion can be improved, and can positively influence the community in which pupil's health choices are made. Among the list of components and checkpoints that could be used as indicators of health promoting schools[118] are some environmental aspects:

- The physical environment of the school, including buildings, grounds, equipment for both indoor and outdoor activities, and areas surrounding the school.

- The school social environment, as a combination of the relationships among staff, students, and between staff and students. It is considered that this element can be influenced by the relationship between parents and the school and all in the community whom provide role models for students and staff by the attitudes and values they display in their social environment.

- *Community* relationship, included the connections between the school and the student's families and key local groups who support and promote health.

The HPS concept has been spread worldwide as an important strategy that provides opportunities to tackle health inequalities in society, not only of young people but also of the population at large. Of particular relevance to oral health promotion would be nutrition, smoking and accident prevention policies. In addition, efforts such as the Schools Meals Campaign and School Nutrition Action Groups (SNAG).[119] are initiatives that aim to provide students with a range of food choices within schools including nutritional options. Such initiatives recognize the importance of increasing the availability of cheap and appealing nutritious foods and drinks within school canteens, tuck shops and vending machines.

Applying the CRFA in schools using the Directed Vulnerable Population Strategy involves the following steps:

- Identify schools with a high prevalence of overweight children and children with high caries levels.

- Assess the determinants and evidence for effective interventions.
- Create environments that support health and are essential for preventing chronic diseases including caries. That involves policies on healthy eating and applying national guidelines on restricting high fat, high sugars, high salt foods and beverages and offering healthy alternatives.
- Collaboration and strong partnerships are key to preventing chronic diseases, including caries.
- Evaluation of strategies to understand what works.

The evaluation of the oral health aspects of HPS indicate that marked improvements in oral health can be achieved. In Brazil food policies in state nurseries in a very deprived region not only substantially reduced sugars consumption and improved the nutritional quality of the diet but also successfully reduced caries increments over a one year period.[115] Health promoting schools not only had reduced levels of caries but had lower levels of traumatic dental injuries.[25,120]

Another example of an intersectoral CRFA based on 'Focusing Resources on Effective School Health' (Fresh) that was applied to decrease caries in a very high caries population in elementary schools in the Philippines is the 'Fit for School' (FIT) essential health care package (see Chapter 19).[121]

The role of dental professionals

Most dental professional involvement in policy development will be as health advocates. Health advocacy involves educating senior government and community leaders and journalists - decision-makers in general, about specific issues and setting the agenda to obtain political decisions that improve health of the population. Health advocates place their skills at the disposal of the community - being on tap not on top.

The objective of planners of dental care should be to make healthy choices the easier choices. They should find which internal incentives promote enthusiasm for quality, economy and good service. Rational strategies for oral health promotion should incorporate policies to control the determinants of the distribution of oral diseases, establish goals and strategies on evidence-based oral health promotion. Oral health promotion programmes will be enhanced by dentists establishing a local Oral Health Promotion Group or a Oral Health Action Team to ensure that oral health promoting strategies are incorporated into general health promotion plans. Integrating oral health in a CRFA is both logical and feasible. Oral health policy should welcome the CRFA approach and develop strategies that fit in with general health promotion policies.

Conclusions

There is substantial evidence of the significance of the role played by environmental factors in the determination of oral diseases in children. The link between environment and behaviours is very strong. Therefore, policies to promote health promoting behaviours and discourage health compromising behaviours should focus attention on environments. In line with the Ottawa Declaration which states that "Health promotion is the process of enabling people to increase control over, and to improve, their health" individuals or groups must be able to realize aspirations, to satisfy needs, and to change or cope with the environment. To do that there is a need to Create Supportive Environments. Environments should create "The inextricable links between people and their environment constitutes the basis for a socioecological approach to health. The overall guiding principle for the world, nations, regions and communities alike, is the need to encourage reciprocal maintenance - to take care of each other, our communities and our natural environment".[8]

To change behaviours policy makers need to change the environment. The establishment of health promoting environments is frequently linked to wider public policies that try to affect determinants of health. Public policies created to promote health of children in different social spaces, such as their homes, the day care centres and the school may encourage socially oriented practices that highlight the possibilities of positive actions along the life course, starting in infancy.

References

1. Campbell D. 'Downward Causation' in Hierarchically Organized Biological Systems. In: Ayala F, Dobzhansky T, editors. Studies in the Philosophy of Biology:Reductionism and Related Problems: University of California Press. 1974; p.180.

2. Dahlgren G, Whitehead M. Policies and strategies to promote social equity in health. Copenhagen: WHO/Regional Office for Europe. 1992.

3. Anderson LM, Scrimshaw SC, Fullilove MT, Fielding JE. Task Force on Community Preventive Services. The Community Guide's model for linking the social environment to health. Am J Prev Med. 2003; 24(3S):12-20.

4. Kubzansky LD, Kawachi I. Affective States and Health. In: Berkman LF, Kawachi I, editors. Social Epidemiology. New York: Oxford University Press. 2000; p.213-41.

5. WHO - World Health Organization. Ottawa Charter for Health Promotion. Health Promotion. 1987; 1(4):iii-v.

6. National Academy of Science. Promoting Health: Intervention Strategies from Social and Behavioral Research. Institute of Medicine Report. Washington: National Academy Press; 2000 [cited 2000 06/02/2012]; Available from: http://iom.edu/Reports/2000/Promoting-Health-Intervention-Strategies-from-Social-and-Behavioral-Research.aspx.

7. WHO - World Health Organization. Health for All by the Year 2000. Geneva: WHO. 1977.

8. WHO - World Health Organization. The Ottawa charter for Health Promotion. Geneve: WHO; 1986 [Acessado em 12/09/2006]; Available from: Available at: https://www.who.int/healthpromotion/conferences/previous/ottawa/en/.

9. WHO - World Health Organization, editor. Supportive Environments for Health. Third International Conference on Health Promotion; 1991 9-15 June 1991; Sundsvall, Sweden: WHO, United Nations Environment Programme, The Nordic Council of Ministers.

10. WHO - World Health Organization. WHO Commission on Health and Environment: Report of the panel on urbanization. Geneva: World Health Organization. 1992. Report No.: WHO/EHE/92.5.

11. WHO - World Health Organization. World Oral Health Promotion Conference. FDI World. 1997; July/August: 1113-4.

12. WHO - World Health Organization, editor. Fifth Global Conference for Health Promotion 2000 5-9 June; Mexico: Available at: https://www.who.int/hpr/conference/products/Conferencereport/conferencereport.html.

13. WHO - World Health Organization. Bangkok charter for health promotion in the a globalized world. Geneve: WHO; 2005 [Acessado em 13/03/2007]; Available at: https://www.who.int/healthpromotion/conferences/en/.

14. WHO - World Health Organization. Commission on Social Determinants of Health. A Conceptual Framework for Action on the Social Determinants of Health. Discussion paper for the Commission on Social Determinants of Health - Last version. Geneva: WHO. 2007.

15. WHO - World Health Organization, Commission on Social Determinants of Health. Closing the gap in a generation: Health equity through action on the social determinants of health. Geneva: WHO. 2008.

16. Siddiqi A, Irwin LG, Hertzman C. Total Environment Assessment Model for Early Child Development. Evidence Report. Vancouver: Human Early Learning Partnership. 2007.

17. Peres MA, Peres KG, Thompson WM, Broadbent JM, Gigante DP, Horta BL. The influence of family income trajectories from birth to adulthood on adult oral health: findings from the 1982 Pelotas birth cohort. American Journal of Public Health. 2011; 101(4):730-6.

18. WHO, Comission of Social Determinants of Health. Closing the gap in a generation: health equity through action on the social determinants of health. Final Report of the Commission on Social Determinants of Health. Geneva: World Health Organization. 2008.

19. Marmot M, Bell R. Social determinants and dental health. Advances in Dental Research. 2011 May; 23(2):201-6.

20. Mendes LGA, Biazevic MGH, Michel-Crosato E, Mendes MOA. Dental caries and associated factors among Brazilian adolescents: a longitudinal study. Brazilian Journal of Oral Sience. 2008; 7(26):1614-9.

21. Levin KA, Davies CA, Topping GV, Assaf AV, Pitts NB. Inequalities in dental caries of 5-year-old children in Scotland, 1993-2003. Eur J Public Health. 2009; 19(3):337-42.

22. Plutzer K, Keirse M. Incidence and prevention of early childhood caries in one- and two-parent families. Child Care Health Dev. 2011; 37(1):5-10.

23. Gatou T, Kounari HK, Mamai-Homata E. Dental caries prevalence and treatment needs of 5- to 12-year-old children in relation to area-based income and immigrant background in Greece. Int Dent J. 2011; 61(3):144-51.

24. Da Rosa P, Nicolau B, Brodeur JM, Benigeri M, Bedos C, Rousseau MC. Associations between school deprivation indices and oral health status. Community Dent Oral Epidemiol. 2011 Jun; 39(3):213-20.

25. Moysés ST, Moysés SJ, Watt RG, Sheiham A. Associations between health promoting schools policies on some indicators of oral health. Health Promotion International. 2003; 18(3):209-18.

26. Goes PS, Watt R, Hardy RG, Sheiham A. The prevalence and severity of dental pain in 14-15 year old Brazilian schoolchildren. Community Dent Health. 2007 Dec; 24(4):217-24.

27. Borges CM, Cascaes AM, Fischer TK, Boing AF, Peres MA, Peres KG. Dor nos dentes e gengivas e fatores associados em adolescentes brasileiros: análise do inquérito nacional de saúde bucal SB-Brasil 2002-2003. Cadernos de Saúde Pública. 2008; 24(8):1825-34.

28. Moyses ST, Camilotti AG, Vetorello M, Moyses SJ. Spatial analysis of dental trauma in 12-year-old schoolchildren in Curitiba, Brazil. Dental Traumatology. 2008 Aug; 24(4):449-53.

29. Gabardo MC, da Silva WJ, Moyses ST, Moyses SJ. Water fluoridation as a marker for sociodental inequalities. Community Dentistry and Oral Epidemiology. 2008 Apr; 36(2):103-7.

30. Peres K, Peres M, Araujo C, Menezes A, Hallal P. Social and dental status along the life course and oral health impacts in adolescents: a population-based birth cohort. Health and Quality of Life Outcomes. 2009; 7(1):95.

31. Noro LRA, Roncalli AG, Mendes Júnior FIR, Lima KC. Incidência de cárie dentária em adolescentes em município do Nordeste brasileiro, 2006. Cadernos de Saúde Pública. 2009; 25(4):783-90.

32. Jorge KO, Moysés SJ, Ferreira EFe, Ramos-Jorge ML, Zarzar PMPdA. Prevalence and factors associated to dental trauma in infants 1-3 years of age. Dental Traumatology. 2009; 25(2):185-9.

33. Carvalho M, Moyses S, Bueno R, Shimakura S, Moyses S. A geographical population analysis of dental trauma in school-children aged 12 and 15 in the city of Curitiba-Brazil. BMC Health Services Research. 2010; 10(203):1-8.

34. Moysés SJ. Oral health and healthy cities: an analysis of intra-urban differentials in oral health outcomes in relation to "healthy cities" policies in Curitiba, Brazil [PhD Thesis]. London: University College London. 2000.

35. Sabbah W, Tsakos G, Chandola T, Sheiham A, Watt RG. Social gradients in oral and general health. Journal of Dental Research. 2007 Oct; 86(10):992-6.

36. Bueno RE, Moysés SJ, Moysés ST. Millennium development goals and oral health in cities in southern Brazil. Community Dentistry and Oral Epidemiology. 2010; 38(3):197-205.

37. Stokols D. Translating social ecological theory into guidelines for community health promotion. American Journal of Health Promotion. 1996; 10(4):282-98.

38. Stokols D, Allen J, Bellingham RL. The social ecology of health promotion: implications for research and practice. American Journal of Health Promotion. 1996; 10(4):247-51.

39. Mattheus DJ. Vulnerability related to oral health in early childhood: a concept analysis. J Adv Nurs. 2010; 66(9):2116-25.

40. Baptista MN. Suporte familiar e violência. In: Romaro RA, Capitão CG, editors. As faces da violência. São Paulo: Vetor. 2007; p.69-100.

41. Inglehart MR, Tedesco LA. The role of the family in preventing oral diseases. In: Cohen LK, Gift HC, editors. Disease prevention and oral health promotion; socio-dental sciences in action. Copenhagen: Munksgaard. 1995; p.271-305.

42. Pratt L. The support functions of the family. In: Badura B, Kickbusch I, editors. Health promotion research; towards a new social epidemiology. Copenhagen: WHO/Europe. 1991; p.229-50.

43. Wadsworth M. Early life. In: Marmot M, Wilkinson RG, editors. Social determinants of health. Oxford: Oxford University Press. 1999; p.44-63.

44. Rogers A, Popay J, Williams G, Latham M. Inequalities in health and health promotion: insights from the qualitative research literature. 1st ed. London: Health Education Authority. 1997.

45. Stansfeld SA. Social support and social cohesion. In: Marmot M, Wilkinson RG, editors. Social determinants of health. 1st ed. Oxford, New York: Oxford University Press. 1999; p.155-78.

46. Baldani MH, Mendes YB, Lawder JA, Lara APd, Rodrigues MM, Antunes JL. Inequalities in dental services utilization among Brazilian low-income children: the role of individual determinants. J Public Health Dent. 2011; 71(1):46-53.

47. McKinlay JB. The promotion of health through planned sociopolitical change: challenges for research and policy. Social Science and Medicine. 1993; 36(2):109-17.

48. Syme SL. To prevent disease: the need for a new approach. In: Blane D, Brunner E, Wilkinson RG, editors. Health And Social Organization Towards a Health Policy for the 21st Century. London: Routledge. 1996; p.21-31.

49. Sanders AE, Spencer AJ, Slade GD. Evaluating the role of dental behaviour in oral health inequalities. Community Dentistry and Oral Epidemiology. 2006 Feb; 34(1):71-9.

50. Frohlich KL, Potvin L. Transcending the known in public health practice: The inequality paradox: The population approach and vulnerable populations. American Journal of Public Health. 2008 February 1, 2008; 98(2):216-21.

51. Slama K. Background information for adopting a policy encouraging earmarked tobacco and alcohol taxes for the creation of health promotion foundations. Promotion & Education. 2006 March 1, 2006; 13(1):8-13.

52. WHO - World Health Organization. Milestones in health promotion: statements from global conferences. Geneva: WHO. 2009.

53. WHO - World Health Organization. Closing the health inequalities gap: An international perspective. Copenhagen: The WHO European Office for Investment for Health and Development, with

University of Dundee, and NHS - Health Scotland. 2005.

54. Korff MV, Koepsell T, Curry S, Diehr P. Multi-level analysis in epidemiologic research on health behaviours and outcomes. American Journal of Epidemiology. 1992; 135(10):1077-82.

55. Diez-Roux AV. Bringing context back into epidemiology: variables and fallacies in multilevel analysis. American Journal of Public Health. 1998 February 1, 1998; 88(2):216-22.

56. Anderson L, Fullilove M, Scrimshaw S, Fielding J, Normand J, Zaza S, et al. A Framework for Evidenced-Based Reviews of Interventions for Supportive Social Environments. Ann NY Acad Sci. 1999 January 1, 1999; 896(1):487-9.

57. Galea S, Vlahov D, Sisco S. The second annual international conference on urban health. October 15-18, 2003. J Urban Health. 2003 Sep; 80(3 Suppl 1):II1-II2.

58. Popay J, Williams G, Thomas C, Gatrell A. Theorising inequalities in health: the place of lay knowledge. In: Bartley M, Blane D, Smith GD, editors. The sociology of health inequalities. 1st ed. Oxford, UK and Malden, USA: Blackwell Publishers Ltd. 1998; p.59-83.

59. Bartley M, Blane D, Smith GD, editors. The sociology of health inequalities. 1st ed. Oxford, UK and Malden, USA: Blackwell Publishers Ltd. 1998.

60. Dean K. Issues in the development of health promotion indicators. Health Promotion International. 1988 January 1, 1988; 3(1):13-21.

61. Lynch J, Kaplan GA, Salonen R, Salonen JT. Socioeconomic status and progression of carotid atherosclerosis. Prospective evidence from the Kuopio Ischemic Heart Disease Risk Factor Study. Arterioscler Thromb Vasc Biol. 1997 Mar; 17(3):513-9.

62. Evans RG, Barer ML, Marmor TR, editors. Why are some people healthy and others not? The determinants of health of populations. 1st ed. New York: Aldine de Gruyter. 1994.

63. Daniels N, Kennedy B, Kawachi I. Is inequality bad for our health? Boston: Beacon Press. 2000.

64. USA, Institute of Medicine. Health and behavior: the interplay of biological, behavioral, and societal influences. Washington: National Academy Press. 2001.

65. Task Force on Community Preventive Services. Recommendations to Promote Healthy Social Environments. American Journal of Preventive Medicine. 2003; 24(3S):21-4.

66. Link BG, Phelan JC. Social Conditions as Fundamental Causes of Disease. Journal of Health and Social Behavior. 1995(extra issue):80-94.

67. Phelan JC, Link B, Diez-Roux A, Kawachi I, Levin B. Fundamental Causes of Social Inequalities in Mortality: A Test of the Theory. Journal of Health & Social Behavior. 2004; (45):265-85.

68. Link BG, Phelan JC. Mckeown and the idea that social conditions are the fundamental causes of disease. American Journal of Public Health. 2002; 92(5):730-2.

69. Link BG, Northridge ME, Phelan J, Ganz ML. Social epidemiology and the fundamental cause concept: On the structuring of effective cancer screens by socioeconomic status. The Milbank Quarterly. 1998; 76(3):375-402.

70. Link BG. Social conditions as fundamental causes of disease. Journal of Health and Social Behavior. 1995(Extra Issue):80-94.

71. Ensminger ME, Smith KC, Juon HS, Pearson JL, Robertson JA. Women, smoking, and social disadvantage over the life course: A longitudinal study of African American women. Drug and Alcohol Dependence. 2009; (104):34-41.

72. Macintyre S, Maciver S, Sooman A. Area, class and health: should we be focusing on places or people? Journal of Social Policy. 1993; 22(2):213-34.

73. Walt G. Health policy: an introduction to process and power. 1st ed. Johannesburg, London, New Jersey: Witwatersrand University Press and Zed Books. 1994.

74. Hancock T, Gibson R. Healthy, sustainable communities. Alternatives Journal [serial on the Internet]. 1996; (20): Available from: http://findarticles.com/p/articles/mi_hb6685/is_n2_v22/ai_n28666871/?tag=content;col1.

75. WHO - World Health Organization. Healthy Cities project. A guide to assessing

healthy cities. Copenhagen: FADL, WHO Healthy Cities1988. Report No.: Paper # 3.

76. WHO - World Health Organization. The Adelaide recommendations: healthy public policy. Health Promotion. 1988; 3(2):183-6.

77. Joffe M, Sutcliffe J. Developing policies for a healthy environment. Health Promotion International. 1997; 12(2):169-73.

78. Price C, Tsouros A, editors. Our cities, our future: policies and actions plans for health and sustainable development. 1st ed. Copenhagen: WHO Healthy Cities Project Office. 1996.

79. Kwan S, Petersen PE. Oral health: equity and social determinants. In: Blas E, Kurup AS, editors. Equity, social determinants and public health programmes. Geneva: World Health Organization. 2010; p.159-76.

80. Sheiham A, Alexander D, Cohen L, Marinho V, Moyses S, Petersen PE, et al. Global oral health inequalities: task group - implementation and delivery of oral health strategies. Advances in Dental Research. 2011 May; 23(2):259-67.

81. Pattussi MP, Hardy R, Sheiham A. Neighborhood social capital and dental injuries in Brazilian adolescents. American Journal of Public Health. 2006 Aug; 96(8):1462-8.

82. Rezende FMC, Gaujac C, Rocha AC, Peres MPSM. Estudo prospectivo do trauma dento-alveolar no Hospital das Clínicas da Faculdade de Medicina da Universidade de São Paulo. Clinics [online]. 2007; 62(2):133-8.

83. Lin S, Levin L, Goldman S, Peleg K. Dento-alveolar and maxillofacial injuries: a 5-year multi-center study. Part 1: general vs facial and dental trauma. Dental Traumatology. 2008 Feb; 24(1):53-5.

84. Guedes OA, Alencar AHGd, Lopes LG, Pécora JD, Estrela C. A retrospective study of traumatic dental injuries in a Brazilian dental urgency service. Braz Dent J. 2010; 21(2):153-7.

85. Glendor U. Aetiology and risk factors related to traumatic dental injuries--a review of the literature. Dent Traumatol. 2009; 25(1):19-31.

86. Moyses ST, Moyses SJ, Watt RG, Sheiham A. Associations between health promoting schools' policies and indicators of oral health in Brazil. Health Promot Int. 2003; 18(3):209-18.

87. Ramos-Jorge ML, Tataounoff J, Correa-Faria P, Alcantara CE, Ramos-Jorge J, Marques LS. Non-accidental collision followed by dental trauma: associated factors. Dent Traumatol. 2011; 27(6):442-5.

88. Rosa PD, Nicolau B, Brodeur JM, Benigeri M, Bedos C, Rousseau MC. Associations between school deprivation indices and oral health status. Community Dent Oral Epidemiol. 2011; 39(3):213-20.

89. Moysés SJ. Desigualdades em saúde bucal e desenvolvimento humano: um ensaio em preto, branco e alguns tons de cinza. Rev Bras Odontol Saúde Coletiva. 2000; 1(1):7-17.

90. Antunes JL, Peres MA, Mello TRdC, Waldman EA. Multilevel assessment of determinants of dental caries experience in Brazil. Community Dent Oral Epidemiol. 2006; 34(2):146-52.

91. Gatrix D, Holloway PJ. Factors of deprivation associated with dental caries in young children. Community Dental Health. 1994; 11:66-70.

92. WHO - World Health Organization. Oral health care systems: an International Collaborative Study. In: Arnlijot HA, Barmes DE, Cohen K, Hunter PVB, II S, editors. 1st ed. Geneva: Quintessence Publishing Company Ltd. 1985.

93. Petersen PE. World Health Organization global policy for improvement of oral health - World Health Assembly 2007. Int Dent J. 2008 Jun; 58(3):115-21.

94. Petersen PE. Global policy for improvement of oral health in the 21st century - implications to oral health research of World Health Assembly 2007, World Health Organization. Community Dentistry and Oral Epidemiology. 2009 Feb; 37(1):1-8.

95. Petersen PE. Improvement of global oral health - the leadership role of the World Health Organization. Community Dental Health. 2010 Dec; 27(4):194-8.

96. Moyses SJ, Moyses ST, McCarthy M, Sheiham A. Intra-urban differentials in child dental trauma in relation to healthy cities policies in Curitiba, Brazil. Health & Place. 2006; 12(1):48-64.

97. USA, HHS. Oral health in America: a Report of the Surgeon General. Rockville, MD: HHS, National Institutes of Health, National Institute of Dental and Craniofacila Research. 2000.

98. Marmot M, (Chair). Fair Society, Healthy Lives (The Marmot Review): Strategic review of health inequalities in England post-2010. London: Marmot Review. 2010.

99. Petersen PE, Torres AM. Preventive oral health care and health promotion provided for children and adolescents by the Municipal Dental Health Service in Denmark. Int J Paediatr Dent. 1999 Jun; 9(2):81-91.

100. Choo A, Delac DM, Messer LB. Oral hygiene measures and promotion: review and considerations. Australian Dental Journal. 2001; 46(3):166-73.

101. Mattila ML, Rautava P, Sillanpää M, Paunio P. Caries in five-year-old children and associations with family-related factors. Journal of Dental Research. 2000; 79(3):875-81.

102. Kay EJ, Locker D. Is dental health education effective? A systematic review of current evidence. Community Dent Oral Epidemiol. 1996 Aug; 24(4):231-5.

103. Kay E, Locker D. A systematic review of the effectiveness of health promotion aimed at improving oral health. Community Dentistry and Oral Epidemiology. 1998;15(3):132-44.

104. Milio N. Promoting health through public policy. Philadelphia: F.A. Davis Company. 1983.

105. Rose G. The strategy of preventive medicine. 1st ed. Oxford, New York, Tokyo: Oxford University Press. 1993.

106. Batchelor P, Sheiham A. The limitations of a 'high-risk' approach for the prevention of dental caries. Community Dentistry and Oral Epidemiology. 2002; 30(4):302-12.

107. Hausen H, Karkkainen S, Seppa L. Application of the high-risk strategy to control dental caries. Community Dentistry and Oral Epidemiology. 2000; 28:26-34.

108. Rose G. Rose's Strategy of Preventive Medicine. New York: Oxford University Press. 2008.

109. Barten F, Mitlin D, Mulholland C, Hardoy A, Stern R. Integrated Approaches to Address the Social Determinants of Health for Reducing Health Inequity. Journal of Urban Health: Bulletin of the New York Academy of Medicine. 2007; 84(1):i164-i73.

110. Poland B, Krupa G, McCall D. Settings for Health Promotion: An Analytic Framework to Guide Intervention Design and Implementation. Health Promot Pract. 2009; October 10(4):505-16.

111. Naerssen T, Barten F. Healthy Cities in Developing Countries. Lessons to be Learned. Saarbrucken: Verlag fur Entwicklungspolitik: NICCOS. 2002.

112. Daly B, Fuller S. Strengthening oral health promotion in the commissioning process. Lancashire. 1996.

113. WHO - World Health Organization. Global strategy on diet, physical activity and health. Paris: WHO. 2004.

114. WHO. Global network of institutions for scientific advice on nutrition: Report of the first meeting, 11-12 March 2010. Geneva: WHO. 2010.

115. Rodrigues CS, Sheiham A. The relationships between dietary guidelines, sugar intake and caries in primary teeth in low income Brazilian 3-year-olds: a longitudinal study. Int J Paediatr Dent. 2000 Mar; 10(1):47-55.

116. Watt RG, Dykes J, Sheiham A. Preschool children's consumption of drinks: implications for dental health. Community Dent Health. 2000 Mar; 17(1):8-13.

117. WHO. Oral health: action plan for promotion and integrated disease prevention. 2007.

118. WHO, Office W-WPR. Regional guidelines; development of health promoting schools - a framework for action. Manila: WHO. 1996.

119. Health Education Trust. School Nutrition Action Groups (SNAG). HET; 2011 [cited 2012 4 Februery].Available from: http://www.healthedtrust.com/pages/snag.htm

120. Malikaew P, Watt RG, Sheiham A. Associations between school environments and childhood traumatic dental injuries. Oral Health Prev Dent. 2003; 1(4):255-66.

121. Monse B, Naliponguit E, Belizario V, Benzian H, Helderman WPv. Essential health care package for children--the 'Fit for School' program in the Philippines. Int Dent J. 2010; 60(2):85-93.

Chapter 9

Evidence-based Dentistry

Valéria Coelho Catão Marinho
Richard Niederman

Introduction

Evidence-based dentistry (EBD) is the integration of the current best clinical evidence, with clinical judgment, and patient values and circumstances to improve health. This chapter presents an approach for rapidly identifying and rapidly evaluating the current best clinical evidence to determine whether this clinical evidence is valid, important, and can be implemented in practice.

To accomplish this the chapter presents a description of the steps involved in the process, and illustrates the steps with an example.

The perspective used throughout the chapter is that of the oral health care professional whether serving individual patients or populations. It is therefore applicable to patients, clinicians, academic institutions, organizations, and governments.

Evidence-based Dentistry – Core concepts and developments

The concept of evidence-based clinical practice was introduced into dentistry more than 15 years ago by Derek Richards and Alan Lawrence with the publication in 1995 of the manifesto describing EBD[1] and the setting up of the Centre for Evidence-based Dentistry at Oxford University in England (www.cebd.org/). It evolved from Evidence-based Medicine (EBM), a concept that came into general awareness in 1992 with the publication of a seminal paper by a clinical epidemiology group at McMaster University in Canada.[2] EBM evolved as an explicit way to teach the practice of medicine in which the clinicians become aware of the evidence in support of their clinical practice, and of the strength of that evidence, through a self-directed and problem-based approach to learning.

Professor David Sackett, a pioneer in the field, defined EBM as "the conscientious, explicit and judicious use of current best evidence in making decisions about the care of individual patients; it is about integrating clinical expertise and patients' preferences, with the best available evidence from research".[3] The American Dental Association (ADA) also defines EBD in this way (http://ebd.ada.org/) (Box 9.1). There are three main elements to the concept (Fig. 9.1):

- Best clinical trial evidence, which is clinically relevant;
- Clinical expertise, which means the ability to use clinical skills and past experience to identify each patient's health state and diagnosis, their individual risks and benefits for potential interventions;
- The patients' personal values and expectations, their preference, concerns and needs.

The EBD approach is applicable at all levels, by anyone who needs to make decisions about health care (eg: patients, clinicians, academic institutions, organizations, and governments).

But why is EBD receiving so much attention?

In almost every country, all areas of health care are facing similar challenges in coping with: technological innovations; an overload of unfiltered information, with a fraction of new knowledge being both adequately tested and important enough; the absence of open, comprehensive access to good information relevant to patient's well-being; increased public demand for better care; and shortages of financial resources (Box 9.2).

In dentistry, as in other specialties, the traditionally favoured sources of knowledge are unsystematic observations from clinical experience and an understanding of the basic mechanisms of disease. However, with an increased awareness of the gaps between scientific evidence and health care practice, standard practice and expert opinion have become less and less reliable as a basis for making clinical decisions. Because of this, 40 years ago, in his seminal monograph Effectiveness and Efficiency, Archie Cochrane (1909-1988), a British epidemiologist and pioneer in the field of evaluation of medical interventions, raised questions about the most commonly used therapies and procedures. He was concerned about the degree to which medical practice was based on robust research, since a large proportion of practice had not been well evaluated.[4] This concern was quantitatively demonstrated in a U.S. Institute of Medicine report "To Err is Human". This report indicated that each day, in the U.S., the equivalent of a airplane full of people dies due to medical error (50,000 people per year).[5]

Dental practitioners find that life-long learning is a challenge. With relatively little training in research methods, an internet-linked twenty-four-hour-per-day, seven-day-per-week information society, and clinical information and technology that continuously evolve, how can anyone keep up? Bastian and collea-

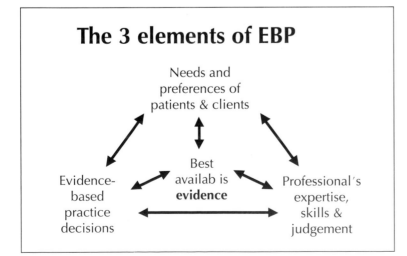

The 3 elements of EBP

Needs and preferences of patients & clients

Evidence-based practice decisions

Best availab is **evidence**

Professional's expertise, skills & judgement

Fig. 9.1 – The three elements of evidence-based dental practice.

gues[6] highlighted this problem in a recent paper, where they pointed out that keeping up with information in health care has never been easy, when 75 controlled trials and 11 systematic reviews are published each day and a plateau in growth has not yet been reached. Estimates for oral health indicate that with more than 500 clinical trials per year in each clinical specialty, to stay current one would theoretically need to identify, obtain, read, and evaluate more than one article per day 365 days per year, a Herculean task.[7]

Meanwhile, patients demanding better quality care want dentists and clinicians who know, rather than believe, that a prescribed treatment works best; and governments, health authorities and insurers need a good basis for making informed decisions about resource allocation during an era in which health care costs are escalating fast.

It is because of its potential to address the issues of information overload and mal distribution that evidence-based practice has gained prominence. The approach has spread rapidly to various areas of health care and many different countries, and has been embraced by several representative medical and dental bodies worldwide.

The inauguration of the Cochrane Collaboration in 1993, in response to Archie Cochrane's plea to the medical professional to organise a "critical summary, by speciality or subspecialty, adapted periodically, of all relevant randomised controlled trials",[8] was a milestone in the development of evidence-based practice. The international work of the Cochrane Collaboration (http://www.cochrane.org/), and the work of the Cochrane Oral Health Group (http://www.ohg.cochrane.org/) in dentistry, has been crucial for the increasing adoption and dissemination of evidence-based practice in health care. This is because it identifies the best clinical research of effectiveness – randomised controlled trials (RCTs) - and summarises the relevant evidence in high quality up-to-date systematic reviews (Cochrane reviews). This process makes reliable evidence accessible to facilitate its translation into sound health care practice and better services for patients/populations.

Box 9.1 – Definition of Evidence-based Dentistry (EBD).

EBD is an approach to oral healthcare that requires the judicious integration of systematic assessments of clinically relevant scientific evidence, relating to the patient's oral and medical condition and history, with the dentist's clinical expertise and the patient's treatment needs and preferences (http://ebd.ada.org/).

Box 9.2 – Main drivers for the growth of EBD.

- Science and technology innovations; overwhelming generation of health care information
- Health professionals, more aware of the gaps between scientific evidence and health care practice, want to upgrade their knowledge base routinely
- Consumers are expecting higher quality care and better communication about the rationale behind treatment decisions
- Government/Health Authorities need to make informed decisions on allocation of resources

Evidence-based dentistry – Principles for practice

An evidence-based approach to oral health involves directly incorporating the current best clinical evidence in decision making. This contrasts with the traditional, but insufficient information sources, which may not provide either the current or the best evidence. There are several reasons to be cautious when following the traditional approaches to clinical decision making:

- The information derived from ones own clinical experience or from an understanding of patho-physiological principles can be misleading and usually overestimates efficacy and can lead to erroneous conclusions.[9]
- The information derived from expert or peer opinion, which usually coincides with standard practice, often lags far behind valid evidence and is frequently inconsistent with it.[10]
- Most importantly, traditional textbooks are useful as conceptual information sources. However, as sources of synthesised information they are only as up-to-date as their most recent reference, and most lack a systematic approach to evidence surveillance, summarisation, and citation.[11]

Although the skills and resources needed to follow the EBD approach are somewhat new, the principles – or core ideas are not (Box 9.3). All dental practitioners consult the literature at least occasionally after identifying questions about new products for diagnosis, prevention, or therapy, and use their clinical expertise to apply these findings in their practice, and monitor the impact of changes in their practice. However, it

is the ability to: systematically frame the problem into an answerable question; efficiently identify the best information available (and conversely avoid getting the wrong material); evaluate this information for validity and clinical importance; apply the up-to-date information in patient care; and evaluate the clinical impact, that supports the process of becoming an evidence-based clinical practice. Furthermore, in contrast with the traditional model of dental practice, with EBD, the methods by which an evidence-based conclusion has been reached are made transparent and in this way anyone involved is in a position of evaluating the validity and usefulness of the conclusions. EBD should therefore give dentists greater confidence in the basis of clinical decisions.

There is always some uncertainty about the benefits and potential adverse effects associated with decisions on diagnosis, prognosis, prevention, treatment, and the economics of health care. Evidence-based dentistry encompasses all these situations and can transform the way health care providers deal with them in a clear and efficient fashion. The application of this approach to solve the uncertainties on the effectiveness of treatment best demonstrates the benefits of an evidence-based approach to care.

Evidence-based dentistry – How it works in practice

The evidence-based approach to decision making involves four steps (Box 9.4). The first step is designing a well-structured question based on a clinical problem of interest. To illustrate we will start by presenting a clinical dilemma in preventive dentistry, in the field of caries prevention:

Box 9.3 – Main Ideas underlying the practice of EBD.

- Oral health care decisions should be based on the best available evidence from research
- The patients' oral health problem, rather than habits or protocols, determines the type of evidence to be sought
- Identifying and evaluating the best evidence requires mastering search skills and means using epidemiological and biostatistical ways of thinking
- Conclusions derived from critically appraising the evidence are useful only if put into action in managing patients' conditions
- The impact on practice should be constantly evaluated

Box 9.4 –Stages in evidence-based clinical practice.

Step 1 - Define the clinical problem and produce a focused question
Step 2 - Search the literature and select relevant study(s)
Step 3 - Appraise the best evidence available
Step 4 - Apply the useful findings to solve the clinical problem

Suppose you are deciding whether to apply pit and fissure sealants once or providing fluoride varnishes at regular intervals to newly erupted permanent molars to avoid occlusal caries in children taking part in a school-based caries preventive program.

In the following sections, the four-step method of evidence-based health care is applied to answer this clinical problem. A detailed description of each step can be found in a number of published papers and textbooks.[12-15] An explicit and simple framework to convey key information is provided to show how the process can be workable in dental practice. Relevant methodological developments and the tools available to facilitate the use of the approach in dental practice are also gradually introduced in this context.

Turning a clinical problem into an answerable question and defining the information required to resolve it

Pertinent and focused questions in dental practice that initiate the evidence-based approach are normally structured in terms of the Patient/Population(P), Intervention or Exposure (I/E), Comparison (C), and outcome (O). The framework that breaks the clinical question into these 4 components is known by the acronym PICO/PECO. Using this structure we can then ask specifically: "In this patient/population, what are the likely effects of this intervention/exposure (compared with an alternative procedure), on this outcome"?

Going back to the example, we can formally structure the question using this framework (Table 9.1): "In children with newly erupted molars (the patient population), will placement of pit and fissure sealants (the intervention), when compared with fluoride varnish applications (the comparison), result in fewer caries? (the outcome of interest)".

The clinical question can be articulated identically using the PICO/PECO framework for issues around diagnosis, prognosis, therapy, iatrogenic harm or quality of care. Carefully articulating an answerable question in this format provides two benefits: it ensures that everyone understands the issue, and it foreshadows step two — searching for the best evidence pertaining to the question. (The current best evidence depends entirely on the question.)

Integrative studies, such as systematic reviews with meta-analyses, are very powerful types of evidence to start with, irrespective of the dental problem in question, as they distil a large body of knowledge from combined primary studies into a readily useable format, thus having the potential to affect oral health care decisions directly. Table 9.2 contains information for choosing the best type of evidence according to the clinical question of interest. To determine whether a given dental intervention (therapeutic or preventive) works for a particular patient population, randomised controlled trials (RCTs) and systematic reviews of several RCTs will be the best type of evidence to look for. To determine the accuracy of a diagnostic test, diagnostic cross sectional studies that systematically compares the results of the test of interest with those of an accepted criterion standard are required. For a question about prognosis or natural history cohort studies of people

assembled at a uniform, early point in the course of their disease are needed.

For harmful exposures/ adverse effects of interventions or aetiology evaluations, other analytical study designs, such as case-control studies, are often needed, as RCTs are not usually available.[3]

Following this guide, as our question is about the comparative effectiveness of two preventive interventions (sealant and fluoride varnish), the first choice of evidence type to look for would be a systematic review/meta-analysis of RCTs (or a large randomised trial, if we can't find a systematic review addressing our topic), because this is considered the highest level of evidence from research into effectiveness.

This is based on the fact that when evaluating the effectiveness of an oral health promotion or preventive intervention, a hierarchy of validity to grade studies based on the rigour of the study design should be followed.[16,17] This hierarchy of decreasing strength of evidence, the best being the highest, reflects how sure one can be that the observed effects are attributable to the intervention and are not the result of other factors (Fig. 9.2). The caveat is that all the research must be of good quality.

Table 9.1 – Structured Clinical question using the PICO format.

Patient/problem (P)	Intervention (I)	Comparison (C)	Outcome (O)
In patients with **P**	Would **I**	When compared with **C**	Result in **O**
In children with	Would fissure sealants	When compared with F varnish	Result in fewer caries
Newly erupted molars			

*A list of all the countries which currently have a scheme in place for free access to The Cochrane Library databases can be found at http://www.thecochranelibrary.com/view/0/FreeAccess.html.

Table 9.2 – The Clinical question and the best type of evidence to search for.

Question	Most appropriate type of evidence
Therapy/prevention	Randomised controlled trials and controlled trials (avoiding non-experimental designs)
Prognosis/natural history	Cohort studies
Harmful exposures/causation	Cohort and case-control studies
Diagnostic tests	Diagnostic cross-sectional studies
All of the above	Systematic reviews

Fig. 9.2 – Hierarchy (of decreasing strength) of evidence of effectiveness.

- Evidence from systematic reviews of randomised controlled trials
- Evidence from at least one randomised controlled trial
- Evidence from controlled trials without randomisation
- Evidence from observational studies such as cohort or case control studies
- Evidence from expert committee reports based on the sources of evidence cited
- Evidence from descriptive studies and opinions of respected authorities based on clinical evidence

Having framed our question appropriately and defined the best type of evidence to search for, where and how do we find the evidence?

Conducting an efficient search in electronic databases and selecting the relevant study

Where to search

Unbiased evidence can be efficiently located by searching high quality, on line databases and resources. Currently, the best resource is provided by the Cochrane Collaboration (http://www.cochrane.org/), an international volunteer organization with some 50 sub-groups, one of which is the Oral Health Group (http://www.ohg.cochrane.org/). The Cochrane Collaboration systematically searches the world's literature for clinical trials and RCTs, and generates systematic reviews of trials that distil and integrate the best evidence to support clinical care. These Cochrane systematic reviews and the randomized controlled trials that are identified (many compiled in these reviews), can be searched in The Cochrane Library CDSR (a database of systematic reviews prepared and maintained within the Cochrane Collaboration) and CENTRAL (the most comprehensive register of RCTs and clinical trials available) respectively, through the Cochrane Library search engine (http://onlinelibrary.wiley.com/o/cochrane/cochrane_clcentral_articles_fs.html). The Cochrane Library search engine can also search additional databases from the Centre for Reviews and Dissemination (CRD). The CRD has 3 databases with distillations of reviews: Database of Abstract of Reviews of Effects (DARE); NHS Economic Evaluation Database (NHS EED); and the Health Technology Assessment Database (HTAD). All three databases can also be simultaneously searched directly from the CRD search page (http://www.crd.york.ac.uk/crdweb/SearchPage.asp).

In Latin America and the Caribbean, access to The Cochrane Library* databases is free via the Brazilian Virtual Health Library BIREME interface (in English, Spanish or Portuguese) at http://cochrane.bireme.br/portal/php/index.php.

Alternatively, general bibliographic databases for biomedical information, such as MEDLINE (largely U.S. English language), EMBASE (largely European), and LILACS (largely Spanish language) can be examined.

MEDLINE is published by the U.S. National Library of Medicine. It is a database of abstracts from some 5,000 health care journals, and provides free internet access to these abstracts through its search engine PubMed (http://www.ncbi.nlm.nih.gov/pubmed/). PubMed also provides linkage to open access journals. EMBASE is a proprietary database owned by Elsevier with access on a subscription or fee basis.

LILACS is the most comprehensive database of scientific-technical literature in health sciences in Latin America and the Caribbean. Free access to LILACS is available via the Virtual Health Library website (http://lilacs.bvsalud.org/). The use of MEDLINE, EMBASE or LILACS is usually reserved for situations where Cochrane or the Centre for Reviews and Dissemination databases cannot provide the information sought.

How to search

Regardless of the database searched, a simple search strategy should be constructed based on the key concepts of the PICO formatted question.

If we elect to use MEDLINE/PubMed in our example, we would create a search strategy based on the "P" problem (caries), the "I" intervention (pit and fissure sealants), the "C" comparison (fluoride varnish). (Table 9.3, steps #1 to #3). These searches are then added together (Table 9.3, step 4). The next step is to limit this search to the highest level of evidence - systematic reviews of trials with meta-analyses (Table 9.3, step 5). (In MEDLINE/PubMed, high levels of evidence (e.g., randomized controlled trials or systematic reviews) can be efficiently located through the use of such methodological filters (limits) based on the type of study design most likely to answer a particular question.)

Once the search has been performed, the titles and abstracts can be scanned to identify those articles that appear to answer the PICO question.

This search strategy identified 7 potentially relevant systematic reviews with meta analysis. An examination of the titles identified a relevant Cochrane systematic review of 4 trials published in 2010 titled: "Pit and fissure sealants versus fluoride varnishes for preventing dental decay in children and adolescents".[18]

(It should be noted that this systematic review (as well as the trial reports) would have also been retrieved if we had searched the information resources included in The Cochrane Library, the CDSR and DARE databases (as well as CENTRAL), which are explicitly geared towards supporting evidence-based approaches to health care.)

Table 9.3 – PubMed Search History (May 2012).

Search	Most Recent Queries	Result
#5	Search #1 AND #2 AND #3 Filters: Systematic Reviews; Meta-Analysis	7
#4	Search #1 AND #2 AND #3	53
#3	Search fluoride varnish	685
#2	Search pit and fissure sealants	2728
#1	Search caries	43019

Critically appraising the evidence - Applying rules of evidence to determine validity and usefulness

Because not all systematic reviews are of high quality, in spite of featuring at the top of the hierarchy of evidence about effectiveness (Fig. 9.2), it is important to critically appraise systematic reviews (and all clinical trials) before acting on their findings.

The three conceptual questions are:
- Is the study valid?
- What are the results?
- Will the results help my patients?

The first question concerns its closeness to the truth – in other words, are the results highly likely to predict what would happen in clinical practice. Validity guides are used to choose the articles most likely to provide a valid answer.

Widely used, self-directed, critical appraisal guides to determine validity were created by the Evidence-Based Medicine Working Group at McMaster University.[14] Two sets of critical appraisal work sheets – one for systematic reviews and one for randomized controlled trials - are provided in Tables 9.4 and 9.5.[19-21] If the answers on the critical appraisal work sheet are positive, usually there is no compelling reason why the study results should not be applied to the patient/population in question.[13]

Table 9.4 – Critical appraisal questions used to evaluate a review article.[19]

	Yes	Can't tell	No
I - Are the results of the study valid, i.e. how close to the truth are they?			
Did it address a focused clinical question? In terms of			
a target population			
intervention(s)			
outcome(s)			
Were the criteria used for selecting studies for inclusion appropriate?			
Is it unlikely that important studies were missed?			
Was the validity of included studies appraised?			
Were assessments of studies reproducible?			
Were data syntheses appropriate and results similar from study to study?			
II - What were the results?			
How large was the treatment effect?			
How precise was the treatment effect?			
III - Will the results help in patient care, can results be applied?			
Where all clinically important outcomes considered?			
Are the likely benefits worth the potential harms and costs?			

Table 9.5 – Critical appraisal questions used to evaluate a therapy article.[20,21]

	Yes	Can't tell	No
I - Are the results of the study valid, i.e. how close to the truth are they?			
Was the assignment of patients to treatment randomised?			
Were all patients who entered the trial properly accounted for and attributed at its conclusion?			
Was follow-up complete?			
Were patients analysed in the groups to which they were randomised?			
Were patients, outcome assessors and care givers "blind" to treatment?			
Were the groups similar at the start of the trial?			
Aside from the experimental intervention, were the groups treated equally?			
II - What were the results?			
How large was the treatment effect?			
How precise was the treatment effect?			
III - Will the results help in patient care, can results be applied?			
Where all clinically important outcomes considered?			
Are the likely benefits worth the potential harms and costs?			

A critical appraisal on the validity of the Cochrane review identified in our search confirmed that it was based on a well defined inclusion criteria (random/quasi-random allocation of sealants versus fluoride varnish for occlusal surfaces of permanent molars of children/adolescents); on a comprehensive search of multiple databases and other sources, without language restrictions; included contacts for unpublished data; and data quality and extraction assessed independently and in duplicate.

The results examined 4 clinical trials, but no meta-analyses were undertaken due to the clinical and methodological diversity between study designs and methods. Two large randomized controlled trials indicated that pit and fissure sealants significantly reduce decay when compared to fluoride varnish. At 23 months, the caries reduction in a split-mouth design trial[22] was 26% (confidence range: 5% to 42%). At 4 years and 9 years the reduction in a cluster RCT[23] was 58% (confidence range: 16% to 79%) and 52% (confidence range: 21% to 71%), respectively. A third small study found no difference.[24] And a fourth trial[25] did not address our comparison of interest. The systematic review concluded that: "Dental sealants reduce more tooth decay in the grooves of back teeth in children than fluoride varnish application, but it was unclear how big the difference in treatment effect is".

Applying the evidence to decision making in practice - Acting on the evidence

Having identified the evidence that is relevant, valid, and important, it will not automatically dictate what to do. It will provide the basis on which decisions can be made after considering other issues related to each particular situation. Some of the issues to take into account in the application of research evidence into practice are highlighted in Box 9.5.

Box 9.5 – Issues in the use of research evidence in decision making.

- There might not be enough high level research to allow us to answer a particular question with any degree of confidence and the best available research evidence may not remove our uncertainties about particular options.
- Research evidence usually describes the average effects of interventions among a group of people in the settings which have been included in trials of effectiveness. It may tell us the chances that a particular outcome will be experienced by an individual who receives a particular intervention/exposure in that particular situation, but sometimes the average effectiveness data will not reflect the range of possible outcomes in different patients (with varying risks) or settings (with other characteristics).
- Most healthcare interventions bring benefits but also risks; clinical decisions thus involve trade-offs between the advantages and disadvantages of different options.
- People may vary in their preferences for particular outcomes (which may or may not have been measured in the studies) and their attitudes to risk. Both affect the way decisions need to be made.

In our example, the evidence from one well conducted systematic review compiling the experimental evidence on the caries preventive effectiveness of sealants versus fluoride varnishes in molar teeth of children is the best currently available evidence answering one particular question. So, how certain do we need to be? Some care providers and decision makers may consider this specific evidence directly comparing the effectiveness of fissure sealants with fluoride varnishes applications in preventing occlusal caries in children very limited, and may be cautious about adopting the findings in clinical care. Others may feel that the evidence for the benefits of sealants is significant enough to warrant the placement of sealants in school-based programs. Still others may want data on the relative costs and benefits. Finally, others may see the benefit of both preventive interventions and implement both. In all of these cases, the central question on whether to move forward is a qualitative one: How much evidence, and what kind of evidence, would convince one to move forward with implementation?

It is worth noting that both sealants and varnishes are relatively simple professionally-applied preventive treatments, both have been available since the 1960s, and widely recommended for clinical, public health, and school-based settings. However, in spite of evidence of effectiveness for both interventions based on Cochrane systematic reviews[18,26-28] and various practice guidelines supporting the use of sealants – two sets of guidelines published by the Scottish Intercollegiate Guidelines Network,[29,30] one guidance document from the British Association for the Study of Community Dentistry,[31] two guidance documents from the American Dental Association[32,33] – the rate of adoption of fissure sealants is slow in both the UK and the US.[34-37]

The reasons for slow adoption of technology for which there is evidence are many. As mentioned earlier, one is the enormity of information and its mis-distribution among clinicians and clinical instructors. Thus, what one learns in school largely determines what one does in practice, and this is unlikely to change. This phenomenon was first documented by Wenberg and Gittleson in 1973.[38] The Dartmouth Atlas of Health care (http://www.dartmouthatlas.org/) now chronicles this phenomenon yearly in the U.S. Guidance from the U.S. Supreme Court in 2012 may now be changing this occurrence and require clinicians to adopt evidence-based methods.[39]

In reality, most clinical and policy decisions are complex and are based on evidence of varying degrees of uncertainty.[40] The evidence-based approach clarifies the level of certainty underlying such complex decisions. Because it starts with the health problems faced by patients and the dental practitioner, rather than with the existing evidence researchers have chosen to generate, this inevitably means that sometimes the evidence available may be far from adequate, but will nevertheless be the best available on which decisions can be based.[41]

Getting EBD into practice

The practice of EBD may seem like a demanding and daunting task for busy clinicians. And yet, this quest for improved health care, based on the current best evidence, is exactly what one normally seeks when considering a new restorative material, implant system, computerized crown preparation, or digital radiographic device. EBD provides a structured way to ask manufacturers a PICO question to assist clinicians in finding answers. And it provides clini-cians a structured way to find answers for themselves.

Some of the factors that contribute to the existence of barriers to implementing EBD and require skills or resources over which dental practitioners have little control are listed in table 9.6. Others are internal factors over which dental practitioners can exert an influence (Table 9.7). Nevertheless, to move the dental profession to a position where routine clinical decisions are evidence-based there is a need to look at ways to:

- ensure existing good quality evidence is available to dental practitioners and presented in useful forms otherwise the potential value of that new knowledge will never be realised.
- assist dental practitioners to make sense of and use up-to-date evidence.
- assist dental practitioners to generate new evidence, mainly from patient-based demand.

Access to on-line search facilities is getting easier day by day in every country or region. The best sources of good quality evidence, such as the databases of systematic reviews in the Cochrane Library, and the journals of secondary publications in Dentistry greatly facilitate the tasks of finding and evaluating the evidence to be used in routine practice. Developments in the use of search filters in electronic databases such as PubMed/MEDLINE and the availability of structured abstracts can make searching and retrieval much more efficient. Postgraduate programmes increasingly include dissemination of information in various formats and via various channels such as more effective continuing education courses, practice guidelines or reminder systems.

Table 9.6 – Factors driving clinical practice requiring external solutions.

Problem	Solutions
Relevant research information not available	
Useful evidence not generated	Promotion of clinicians' and patients' participation in research
not produced	Better research commissioning
not published (publication bias)	Publication of all research findings
not adequately indexed	Better indexing in databases
Research evidence available but not used	
Inaccessible sources/libraries	Extension of open/online access to all clinicians
Poorly reported abstracts in databases	Structured abstracts to facilitate retrieval
Poor quality/biased evidence	Better training of researchers, stringent ethics committees and journal peer review process
Valid studies but too small to produce unequivocal results	Production of systematic reviews
Evidence not presented in forms useful to clinicians	Tougher action and reporting guidelines endorsement by journal editors

Table 9.7 – Factors driving clinical practice over which dental practitioners can have an influence.

Problem	Solutions for the busy dentist
Out-of-date textbooks and biased editorials and reviews	Don't read them for guidance on therapy/prevention
Too much information available (can't keep up)	Read good systematic reviews rather than primary research
Insufficient time	Develop a good scanning strategy
Relevant evidence difficult to find	Improve searching skills in electronic databases
Difficulty in retrieving evidence identified as useful	Go for improved/open access resources
Inability to spot flaws in research	Improve critical appraisal skills
Difficulty in interpreting the data / applying results	Improve statistical and epidemiological skills

Skills training can assist dental practitioners, undergraduates and postgraduates to make sense of and use up-to-date evidence. Relevant training and resources are now available on-line from a number of organisations, not least:

- The Centre for Evidence-based Dentistry (www.cebd.org/)
- The Brazilian Cochrane Center (http://www.centrocochranedobrasil.org.br/)
- EviDentista.org
- The American Dental Association/Forsyth Institute EBD workshop (http://www.ada.org/forsythcourse.aspx)
- There are also short-term intensive EBD courses sponsored by the American Dental Association and the Forsyth Institute in the U.S. (http://www.ada.org/forsythcourse.aspx) and Oxford University in the U.K. (http://www.conted.ox.ac.uk/courses/details.php?id=B900-29)

However, for widespread adoption of the EBD in practice, it must become the basis of training in problem-based curricula for all health education programs.

Evidence Level

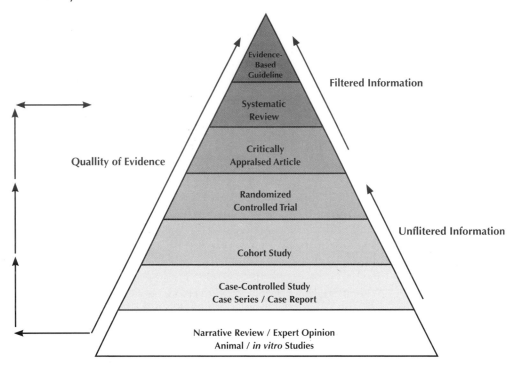

Ability to Demonstrate Cause-Effect

- Evidence-Based Guideline
- Systematic Review
- Critically Appraised Article
- Randomized Controlled Trial
- Cohort Study
- Case-Controlled Study / Case Series / Case Report
- Narrative Review / Expert Opinion / Animal / *in vitro* Studies

Quallity of Evidence

Filtered Information

Unflitered Information

Concluding remarks

Over the last three decades, scientific and software advances supported the development of health care practice and decision making for individual patients or populations. Clinical decision-making can now be based on the current best evidence from clinical trials and systematic reviews of trials. However, there is still a substantial gap between the best clinical evidence and oral health care practice.

Evidence-based Dentistry (EBD) has the potential for bringing oral health care practice into line with research evidence, transforming the practice and teaching of oral health care professionals as they continue to face an exploding volume of literature, rapid introduction of new technologies, deepening concerns about health care costs and increasing attention to the quality and outcomes of oral health care.

By adopting the evidence based practice approach, oral health care professionals will be able to routinely upgrade their knowledge, weigh up the evidence for themselves, and continuously question standard practice. They will also have the opportunity to share the information with patients, and incorporate their values and preferences in the clinical judgements before implementing the scientific findings.

While strategies for inculcating the principles of evidence-based clinical practice will continuously evolve in perpetuity, a number of effective approaches and resources have already been implemented and are available to help the oral health profession to find and translate the best evidence into practice. In this way, the best clinical evidence can be more rapidly disseminated and implemented into practice.

References

1. Richards D. and Lawrence A. Evidence-based dentistry (personal view). British Dental Journal. 1995 Oct 7; 179(7):270-3

2. Evidence-Based Medicine Working Group. Evidence Based Medicine: a new approach to teaching the practice of medicine. JAMA. 1992; 268:2420-2425.

3. Sackett DL, Rosenberg WMC, Gray JAM, Haynes RB, and Richardson WS. Evidence-based medicine: what it is and what it isn't. BMJ.1996; 312:71-72.

4. Cochrane AL (1972). Effectiveness and efficiency: Random Reflections on Health Services (reissued, Royal Society of Medicine Press: London, 1999).

5. Committee on Quality of Health Care in America (1999). Kohn LT, Corrigan JM, Donaldson MS, Editors. To Err Is Human. Building a Safer Health System. Institute of Medicine. National Academy Press, Washington DC.

6. Bastian H, Glasziou P, Chalmers I. Seventy-five trials and eleven systematic reviews a day: how will we ever keep up? PLoS Med. 2010; 7: e1000326.

7. Niederman R, Chen L, Murzyn L, Conway S. Benchmarking the dental randomised controlled literature on MEDLINE. Evidence-Based Dentistry. 2002; 3:5-9.

8. Cochrane AL (1979) 1931–1971: a critical review, with particular reference to the medical profession. In: Medicines for the Year 2000. London: Office of Health Economics. pp.1-11.

9. Sackett DL(1994). On identifying the best therapy. In: Orthodontic treatment: outcome and effectiveness, edited by Trotman, C.A. and McNamara, J.A.Ann Harbor: The University of Michigan, p.7-19.

10. Antman EM, Lau J, Kupelnick B, Mosteler F, and Chalmers TC. A comparison of results of meta-analyses of randomized control trials and recommendations of clinical experts. Treatments for myocardial infarction. JAMA. 1992; 268:240-248.

11. McKibbon KA, Wilczynski N, Hayward RS, Walker-Dilks CJ, Haynes, RB. The medical literature as a resource for health care practice. J Am Soc Inform Sci. 1995; 46:737-42.

12. Sackett DL, Haynes RB, Guyatt GH, and Tugwell P (1991). Clinical epidemiology: a basic science for clinical medicine, Boston: Little, Brown.

13. Sackett, DL, Richardson WS, Rosemberg W, and Haynes RB (1997). Evidence-based Medicine: How to Practice and teach EBM, New York: Churchill Livingstone.

14. Guyatt GH and Rennie D. Users' guides to the medical literature. JAMA. 1993; 270(17):2096-2097.

15. Sackett, DL, Richardson WS, Rosemberg W, and Haynes RB (1997). Evidence-based Medicine: How to Practice and teach EBM, New York: Churchill Livingstone.

16. Deeks J, Glanville J, and Sheldon TA (1996). Assessing the validity of the studies. In: Undertaking Systematic Reviews of Research of Effectiveness. CRD Reports. York: York Publishing Services Ltd. 4:31-39.

17. Gray JAM (1997). Assessing the outcomes found. In: Evidence-based Healthcare. New York: Churchill Livingstone. p.103-154.

18. Hiiri A, Ahovuo-Saloranta A, Nordblad A, Mäkelä M. Pit and fissure sealants versus fluoride varnishes for preventing dental decay in children and adolescents. Cochrane Database Syst Rev. 2010; (3):CD003067.

19. Oxman AD, Cook DJ, and Guyatt GH. Users' guides to the medical literature. VI. How to use an Overview. JAMA. 1994; 272:1367-1371.

20. Guyatt GH, Sackett DL, and Cook DJ. Users' guides to the medical literature. II. How to use an article about therapy or prevention. A. Are the results of the study valid? JAMA. 1993; 270:2598-2601.

21. Guyatt GH, Sackett DL, and Cook DJ. Users' guides to the medical literature. II. How to use an article about therapy or prevention. B. What are the results and will they help me in caring for my patients? JAMA. 1994; 271:59-63.

22. Raadal M, Laegreid O, Laegreid KV, Hveem H, Korsgaard EK, Wangen K. Fissure sealing of permanent first molars in children receiving a high standard of prophylactic care. Community Dentistry and Oral Epidemiology. 1984; 12:65-8.

23. Bravo M, Montero J, Bravo JJ, Baca P, Llodra JC. Sealant and fluoride varnish

in caries: a randomized trial. Journal of Dental Research. 2005; 84:1138-43

24. Florio FM, Pereira AC, Meneghim Mde C, Ramacciato JC. Evaluation of non-invasive treatment applied to occlusal surfaces. ASDC J Dent Child. 2001. Sep-Dec; 68(5-6):326-31, 301.

25. Splieth C, Förster M, Meyer G. Additional caries protection by sealing permanent first molars compared to fluoride varnish applications in children with low caries prevalence: 2-year results. European Journal of Paediatric Dentistry 2001; 2:133-8.

26. Marinho VCC, Higgins JP, Logan S, Sheiham A. Fluoride varnishes for preventing dental caries in children and adolescents. Cochrane Database Syst Rev. 2002; (2):CD002279.

27. Marinho VCC, Higgins JPT, Logan S, Sheiham A. Topical fluoride (toothpastes, mouthrinses, gels or varnishes) for preventing dental caries in children and adolescents. Cochrane Database Syst Rev. 2003; (4):CD002782.

28. Ahovuo-Saloranta A, Hiiri A, Nordblad A, Mäkelä M, Worthington HV. Pit and fissure sealants for preventing dental decay in the permanent teeth of children and adolescents. Cochrane Database Syst Rev. 2008; (4):CD001830.

29. Scottish Intercollegiate Guidelines Network (2005). Prevention and Management of Dental Decay in the Pre-school Child. National Clinical Guideline no. 83, Scottish Intercollegiate Guidelines Network, Edinburgh.

30. Scottish Intercollegiate Guidelines Network (2000). Preventing Dental Caries in Children at High Caries Risk: Targeted Prevention of Dental Caries in the Permanent Teeth of 6–16 Year Olds Presenting for Dental Care. National Clinical Guideline no. 47, Scottish Intercollegiate Guidelines Network, Edinburgh.

31. Department of Health/British Association for the Study of Community Dentistry (2007). Delivering Better Oral Health: an Evidence-based Toolkit for Prevention, Department of Health, London.

32. Beauchamp J, Caufield PW, Crall JJ, Donly K, Feigal R, Gooch B, Ismail A, Kohn W, Siegal M, Simonsen R; American Dental Association Council on Scientific Affairs. Evidence-based clinical recommendations for the use of pit-and-fissure sealants: a report of the American Dental Association Council on Scientific Affairs. J Am Dent Assoc. 2008 Mar; 139(3):257-68.

33. Gooch BF, Griffin SO, Gray SK, Kohn WG, Rozier RG, Siegal M, Fontana M, Brunson D, Carter N, Curtis DK, Donly KJ, Haering H, Hill LF, Hinson HP, Kumar J, Lampiris L, Mallatt M, Meyer DM, Miller WR, Sanzi-Schaedel SM, Simonsen R, Truman BI, Zero DT; Centers for Disease Control and Prevention. Preventing dental caries through school-based sealant programs: updated recommendations and reviews of evidence. J Am Dent Assoc. 2009 Nov; 140(11):1356-65.

34. Solanki GC, Lalloo R, Myburgh NG. Professionally applied topical fluoride and fissure sealants: matching insurance claims with evidence. SADJ. 2007; 62:202-5.

35. Clarkson JE, Turner S, Grimshaw JM, Ramsay CR, Johnston M, et al. Changing clinicians' behavior: a randomized controlled trial of fees and education. J Dent Res. 2008; 87:640-4.

36. Griffin SO, Oong E, Kohn W, Vidakovic B, Gooch BF, et al. The effectiveness of sealants in managing caries lesions. J Dent Res. 2008; 87:169-74.

37. Tellez M, Gray SL, Gray S, Lim S, Ismail AI. Sealants and dental caries: dentist's perspectives on evidence-based recommendations. J Am Dent Assoc. 2011; 142(9):1033-40.

38. Wennberg J, Gittelsohn. Small area variations in health care delivery. Science. 1973 Dec 14; 182(4117):1102-8.

39. Niederman R, Richards D, Brands W. The changing standard of care. J Am Dent Assoc. 2012; May; 143(5):434-7.

40. Logan RL and Scott PG. Uncertainty in clinical practice: implications for quality and costs of health care. Lancet. 1996; 347:595-598.

41. Gilbert R. and Logan S. Future prospects for evidence-based child health. Arch Dis Child. 1996; 75:465-468.

42. Oxman AD, Sackett DL, and Guyatt GH. Users' guides to the medical literature. I. How to get started. JAMA. 1993; 270(17):2093-2095.

Chapter 10

Use of Fluorides in the Control of Dental Caries

Valéria Coelho Catão Marinho
Livia Maria Andaló Tenuta
Jaime Aparecido Cury

Introduction

Epidemiological data have clearly shown that caries levels have decreased substantially in the last 50 years. The decline has been mainly associated with the worldwide use of fluoridated toothpastes.[1] The discovery that fluoride in drinking water lowered rates of caries[2] was the basis for the first theories about the mechanisms of how fluoride acts. That in turn influenced the use of fluoride regimens implemented during the second half of the last century.

However, the belief that fluoride would act pre-eruptively increasing the mineral resistance of the teeth against acid attacks[3] was gradually replaced by evidence of its local post-eruptive action.[4-6] Nevertheless, although it is scientifically recognized that the post-eruptive effect of fluoride (local and nonsystemic effect) is the main factor responsible for the reduced rates of caries observed in modern societies,[7,8] the pre-eruptive paradigm is still present.[9,10] More than a simple matter of knowing the mechanism of action of fluoride, how it works orients how it is used to control caries. The dichotomization of the mode of fluoride use into "systemic" and "topical" shows that an understanding of how caries occurs as a disease (through the accumulation of dental plaque (or biofilm) and frequent exposure to sugars) and of how fluoride is able to reduce the speed of appearance of the clinical signs of this disease, the progression of carious lesions (by interfering with the de-/remineralization of the enamel, when available in the oral fluids),[11] has not yet been incorporated into clinical practice. Hence, for example, when children live in areas where the water is not fluoridated, medications containing fluoride ("nutritional supplements") are still recommended instead of other more rational forms of fluoride use, since the concept that caries can be prevented by fluoride intake (ingestion) is still prevalent, although it is widely acknowledged that the effect of fluoride on the factors responsible for the disease is marginal.[12]

Given that the main mechanism of action of all the methods or forms of fluoride is the same, namely, making fluoride available in the oral fluids, the classification in systemic and topical methods would be better replaced with one that takes into account the scope of fluoride use, such as: community means, for example fluoridated water; individual means, for example, fluoride toothpaste; professional means, for example, application of fluoride in gel, varnishes, or a combination of these.[13,14] Moreover, considering that dental caries results from frequent episodes of demineralization during each exposure of the dental biofilm to sugars,[15] the constant availability of increased fluoride concentrations in the oral fluids is desirable to control caries.[11]

On the other hand, the greater benefits of the availability of fluoride in the mouth has to be weighed up against the risk of developing fluorosis. That may occur by the greater possibility of systemic exposure to fluoride, whether involuntary such as with fluoridated water, or through the inadvertent ingestion of fluoride toothpaste by very young children. In this regard, only the level of fluoride that is ingested and absorbed in the gastrointestinal tract can potentially cause fluorosis when that occurs during the formation and calcification of the teeth. However, when considering the risk of fluorosis, the importance of the bioavailability of fluoride (the fraction of intake that is absorbed and circulates through the bloodstream), has been disguised by numerous studies, showing that children risk developing fluorosis if they ingest fluoride, in their diet and from toothpastes. at levels which are generally higher than the ingested fluoride dose that would provoke fluorosis of lower severity than those causing aesthetic concerns.[16] However, fluoride absorbed and circulating in the bloodstream[17,18] has not been taken into consideration,[19,20] increasing the concern over the use of fluoride by children, causing uncertainty and lack of confidence in the recommendations of use. Therefore, based on overestimated intake doses, recommendations regarding the use of fluoride toothpaste have been made in the absence of good scientific evidence.[21,22] In addition, longitudinal studies have not found any correlation between the dose of fluoride ingested by children during the formation of dental enamel and the degree of resulting fluorosis.[23,24] Accordingly, there is a need to balance the benefits and risks of fluoride use.[7,8] Therefore, considering that all the fluoride maintained constantly in the oral cavity is able to control caries by its local effect,[11] but if ingested

and absorbed daily, the systemic effect can provoke a certain degree of fluorosis in the enamel during the mineralization phase,[25] the choice of the best method(s) of fluoride use to control caries must be based on the best scientific evidence available regarding the balance between benefits and risks of the intervention.

The main focus of this chapter is therefore to present the most recent scientific evidence available on the effectiveness and safety of fluoride use to control dental caries, That is based on the research methods used in pursuit of the best evidence.

Scientific basis for assessing the effects of fluoride

Many studies have attempted to address the uncertainties regarding the effects of the various forms of fluoride-based interventions. This may not come as a surprise, since fluorides has been the subject of basic and clinical research for much more than half a century. A simple and rapid search in PubMed (the free US National Library of Medicine (NLM) electronic database accessing primarily the MEDLINE database of citations on life sciences and biomedical topics), employing the search terms "fluoride" or "fluoride and caries" can be used to indicate the considerable quantity of any kind of research published on the topic in the last six decades. Such a search resulted in 43171 hits for "fluoride" and 8372 hits for "fluoride and caries". These separate search results for the terms "fluoride" and "fluoride and caries" draw attention to the fact that not all studies on the subject are related exclusively to caries, although there have probably been more reports published about the caries-inhibitory properties of fluoride than on any other subject in dentistry. Furthermore, by combining the search terms "fluoride and caries" with specific methodological filters, we can obtain an indication of the amount of research carried out on matters related to the effects of fluoride and of recommendations for its adequate use in controlling dental caries (Fig. 10.1).

Not all these studies, however, will provide reliable information. To be valid, the judgments on the effectiveness and safety of health care interventions based on formal studies should carefully consider the strong and weak points of the methods used by the investigators and the quality of the research produced. Thus, a rational basis can be established for the selection of those studies that will be able to provide more useful and valid evidence. Table 10.1 provides a guide for the different levels of research evidence and their relative strength, where type I is the strongest evidence and type V the weakest. This hierarchy of strength of research evidence reflects the degree to which different methods for evaluating the effects of health care interventions on important outcomes are susceptible to bias or systematic errors, defects, which may render the results less reliable for making inferences. The levels of evidence of research on effectiveness range from simple descriptive studies, for example, case reports, cross-sectional and ecological studies, and go on to include observational studies of individual-based associations, for example, case-control and cohort studies, and end up with formal experiments, for example, randomized clinical trials, and systematic reviews.

While variations of the hierarchy of evidence based on these study designs are still being proposed and employed by health scientists,[26,27] those who proposed them appear to agree that, with regard to the primary study design, randomized clinical trials (RCT) should be considered the most reliable type of design for the assembly of comparison groups on which to base causal inferences about the treatment effects.[28] However, ranked above the experimental studies of adequate size, using proper randomization, are the quantitative scientific summaries of such studies, namely, systematic reviews using meta-analysis of well-designed multiple RCTs. Hence the strongest scientific evidence on effectiveness comes from these quantitative study designs that can provide the best means of minimizing or avoiding systematic errors, or bias,, and at the same time have several observations from a randomized body of evidence which is large enough for the control of random errors, or the effects of chance. This is because in most circumstances, the effect of an intervention will not be clearly evident, and therefore a large amount of randomized evidence is necessary to detect or to refute reliably such moderate, yet potentially important effects.[29]

Epidemiology of different "levels" on a research about fluoride (PubMed search - august 2011)

- Fluoride + Caries = 8372 hits
  - Systematic reviews and meta analysis
  - Reviews = 991
  - Guidelines, recommendation, report of a concensus = 255
  - RCT/trial = 1001

Fig. 10.1 – Number of citations employing the search terms fluoride and caries according to the types of studies (period:1965 to 2011).

The proviso is that all research must be of high quality. The quality of a study is defined as the confidence that its design, conduct and analysis have minimized or avoided bias. The quality or internal validity does not depend on the study design alone, which mostly depends on the question that the study aims to answer; its clinical and epidemiological focus, but also on the way the study was carried out and reported. With this regard, it is important to note that Cochrane reviews, systematic reviews of health care interventions that employ rigorous research methods, have been shown to be of higher methodological quality than other systematic reviews.[30-33] These reviews concentrate mainly, but not exclusively, on synthesizing the evidence from randomized studies, and are published in full in the Cochrane Library (http://www.thecochranelibrary.com) following an editorial process that is common to all the reviews of the Cochrane Collaboration (http://www.cochrane.org/), an international nonprofit organization created in the early 1990s to guarantee that up-to-date information about the effects of health care interventions is readily available all over the world.

Table 10.1 – Levels of evidence of scientific research on the effectiveness of health interventions.[42]

Type	Strength of evidence
I	Strong evidence generated by at least one systematic review of multiple well-designed RCTs
II	Strong evidence generated by at least one well-designed RCT of appropriate size
III	Evidence generated by nonrandomized experimental studies, or observational studies (cohort, multiple time series or case-control studies)
IV	Evidence generated by well-designed non-experimental studies from more than one centre or research group
V	Evidence generated by reports of expert committees based on the sources of evidence cited, descriptive studies (cross-sectional, ecological and case series studies) or opinions of respected authorities based on clinical evidence

Main characteristics of the available evidence on the effects of fluorides on caries control

A variety of study designs have been used to assess the effectiveness of fluorides in controlling caries. While several interventions using fluoride applied topically have been submitted to intensive clinical tests in randomized controlled trials, less conclusive study designs have been used to assess the effectiveness of water fluoridation. Although the aspects that characterize the design and the conduct of studies that assess the effects of therapy with fluoride applied topically are very different from those that assess the effects of water fluoridation, both study types have been traditionally summarized in a similar manner: namely, in narrative literature reviews.

However, traditional narrative methods to compile the evidence available on a topic tend to ignore the levels of evidence and the variable quality of studies, and are therefore unlikely to present an objective view of the evidence. Moreover, such reviews frequently produce very different estimates of effectiveness due to differences in the way the literature to be included was selected, often ignore the uncertainty involved in the estimates of effect, and rarely formally explore the causes of variability in the reported effectiveness. Nevertheless, a large number of these reviews have highlighted important aspects relevant to the evaluation of the effectiveness of fluoride in caries prevention, which were formally taken into account in the systematic reviews/meta-analyses carried out on the topic throughout recent decades[34-58]. Furthermore, the recommendations systematically developed for the appropriate use of fluorides in caries prevention in different contexts and countries are increasingly being made in clinical practice guidelines. Such guidelines are largely based on results of systematic reviews published in the last decade. This is especially noted in relation to the series of Cochrane reviews on the effects of topically-applied fluorides in dentifrices, mouth rinses, gels and varnishes[42-48,57,58] and the systematic review on water fluoridation commissioned by the Centre for Reviews and Dissemination of the National Health Service (NHS CRD) in the United Kingdom, at the University of York.[38]

Considered the most comprehensive and detailed evidence to date, these systematic reviews consistently gather and summarize the large body of knowledge available about the effects of the main modalities of fluorides used nowadays for the prevention of dental caries, and systematically examine the main factors that can influence their effectiveness. In addition, since the York review on the effects of water fluoridation was published,[38] there has been no other high quality systematic review that could change the conclusions of that review, which has been chosen to form the basis of scientific evidence on the

effects of water fluoridation in subsequent overviews on the topic, like in the review produced by the National Health and Medical Research Council in Australia.[59]

Therefore, the evidence originating from the abovementioned York review on the effects of water fluoridation and Cochrane reviews on the effects of fluorides applied topically – in fluoride dentifrices, mouthwashes, gels and varnishes – will be highlighted in the following section. The evidence of the effects of fluoridated milk and of slow-release fluoride devices will be only briefly discussed based on the results of the Cochrane reviews identified on these topics. However, the evidence originating from Cochrane reviews in progress on other fluoride-based interventions, such as on salt fluoridation and on tablets/supplements, is not addressed here, since these are Cochrane reviews under development, and not yet complete when the search was conducted in July 2011.

Evidence from systematic reviews on the effectiveness of fluoride-based interventions in the control of dental caries

The best scientific evidence available on the effects of fluoride in the control of caries was located and selected as reported below:

Relevant Cochrane reviews were sought in the Cochrane Database of Systematic Reviews (CDSR), Edition 7, 2011, of the Cochrane Library, using the terms "Fluoride" and "Caries". All the electronically identified records were scrutinized by title, and all the complete reviews evaluating mainly the effectiveness of a fluoride-based intervention in the prevention of caries in children were selected. Reports of Cochrane reviews in progress in protocol form were not considered. A specific supplementary search to identify the York review on the effects of water fluoridation, using the terms "Fluoridation" and "Caries", was conducted in the Health Technology Assessment (HTA) database, Edition 7, 2011, of the Cochrane Library.

The search in the CDSR yielded 19 reports on Cochrane systematic reviews of controlled trials, produced under the auspices of the Cochrane Oral Health Group (COHG). Four of these reports are outside the scope of this chapter (ozone therapy for caries treatment, chlorhexidine for caries prevention, sealants of pits and fissures vs. fluoride varnish for caries, fluorides for the prevention of white stains in orthodontic patients), and 4 others are reports of relevant reviews still under development in the form of protocols (salt fluoridation to prevent caries, fluoride supplements for caries prevention, fluoride solutions for caries control, and topical fluoride for caries treatments), and for this reason are not covered here. Eleven complete Cochrane systematic reviews on the effects of fluorides in caries prevention were identified and are evaluated below (Table 10.2).

Table 10.2 – Completed Cochrane reviews on fluorides in the CDSR in July 2011 (Cochrane Library, Edition 7, 2011).

Reviews on fluoride dentifrices, mouthwashes, gels and varnishes	
Citation	Title
Marinho et al.[42]	(1st) Fluoride gels for preventing dental caries in children and adolescents
Marinho et al.[43]	(2nd) Fluoride varnishes for preventing dental caries in children and adolescents
Marinho et al.[44]	(3rd) Fluoride dentifrices for preventing dental caries in children and adolescents
Marinho et al.[45]	(4th) Fluoride mouthwashes for preventing dental caries in children and adolescents
Marinho et al.[46]	(5th) Fluorides applied topically (dentifrices, mouthwashes, gels and varnishes) for preventing dental caries in children and adolescents
Marinho et al.[47]	(6th) One topical fluoride (dentifrices, mouthwashes, gels or varnishes) compared to another to prevent dental caries in children and adolescents
Marinho et al.[48]	(7th) Combinations of fluorides (dentifrices + mouthwashes, gels, or varnishes) compared to a single fluoride (dentifrice) to prevent dental caries in children and adolescents
Walsh et al.[57]	(8th) Dentifrices with different concentrations of fluoride to prevent dental caries in children and adolescents
Wong et al.[58]	(9th) Topically appliaed fluoride as a cause of dental fluorosis in children

1.	**Other fluoride reviews**	
2.	Yeung et al. 2005	Fluoridated milk for preventing dental caries
3.	Bonner et al. 2006	Slow-release fluoride devices for the control of dental caries

The search in the HTA produced two reports, of which only the York review on the fluoridation of public water supplies[38] is considered relevant. As mentioned previously, since this was published in October 2000 there has been no other scientifically defensible systematic review capable of changing the results of the York review, hence the continuous recognition of its importance as the main source of evidence for the effects of water fluoridation on caries prevention.[59,60]

A description of the main aspects of the evidence originating from these systematic reviews is presented below in a structured format, to facilitate the understanding and application of the results of the research in practice. The main characteristics of the York review, its results and conclusions are presented first of all. This is followed by a general description of the main methodological features of the Cochrane reviews and a qualitative compilation (summary) of the results of the reviews. This is done mainly in terms of the preventive effectiveness of the various topically-applied fluoride modalities evaluated, and where reported, according to the factors that influence the effectiveness of these interventions, their comparative effectiveness, and that of the combined use of the interventions, as well as in terms of the safety (and acceptability) of these interventions, in an attempt to take into account any assessment of their benefits and undesirable (adverse) effects.

Water Fluoridation

The compiled/reviewed evidence

The NHS CRD review covering all the available evidence on the effectiveness and safety of water fluoridation was published in 2000.[38] The complete report is available on the CRD website (http://www.york.ac.uk/inst/crd/fluorid.htm).

The objectives of the York review

- Which are the effects of fluoridation of drinking water on the incidence of caries?
- If water fluoridation is shown to have positive effects, what is the effect over and above that offered by the use of alternative interventions and strategies?
- Does water fluoridation result in a reduction of caries across social groups and between geographical locations, bringing equity?
- Does water fluoridation have negative effects?
- Are there any differences in the effects of natural and artificial water fluoridation?

Inclusion criteria, search strategy, data collection and analysis

The review specifically analysed the effects of fluoridation of drinking water on dental caries, social inequalities and any harmful effects in the populations that receive fluoridated water. Studies included were classified at levels/hierarchy of evidence (A-C) based on the study design and on adjustment for confounding factors and measurement bias factors. Evidence classified below a moderate level of quality/moderate risk of bias (level B, equivalent to type III in table 10.1) was not considered in the effectiveness assessment. In the safety assessment, all the levels of evidence were considered.

Searches were undertaken in 25 electronic databases, in bibliographies of the studies included, and in other online resources. Published and unpublished studies in any language were sought. Inclusion decisions, quality assessment and data extraction were duplicated by two reviewers and consensus was obtained by discussion or by a third reviewer.

Where the data were in an adequate format, measures of effect and 95% confidence intervals (CI) were plotted. Random effects meta-analysis were carried out where the data could be pooled. Potential sources of heterogeneity were examined in random effects meta-regression analyses (effects of baseline levels of caries, of age, study duration, validity scores and others). Multilevel regression analysis was used to combine studies and to investigate the association of fluoride concentration in water with the prevalence of fluorosis.

Main results of the review

A total of 214 studies were included, with none at level of evidence A (high quality, bias unlikely); In other words, there were no randomized trials of water fluoridation.

The study designs included 102 cross-sectional studies, 47 ecological studies, 45 controlled before-and-after studies, 13 cohort studies, and seven case-control studies. Table 10.3 shows the main characteristics and results of the York review.

Effectiveness of water fluoridation in caries prevention: The best evidence available (level B, moderate quality - 23 controlled before-and-after studies and three cohort studies) from studies on the initiation and discontinuation of water fluoridation suggests that fluoridation effectively reduces the prevalence of caries, both when measured by the proportion of caries-free children and by the mean dmft/DMFT score. The degree of caries reduction, however, is not clear from the available data: The range (median) of the mean difference in the proportion of children without caries

Table 10.3 – Summary of the characteristics of the York Review on the Fluoridation of Public Water Supplies.

Study	Focus	Inclusion criteria	Data gathering/Analysis	Main results/Conclusions
McDonagh et al.[38]	Evaluation of the positive and negative effects of fluoridation of public water supplies to prevent caries	Assessment of efficacy (positive effects - dental caries – studies with level of evidence A and B): Prospective studies comparing at least 2 populations, (F/NF), with at least 2 points in time evaluated. Assessment of safety (adverse effects, including fluorosis) and of social inequalities (SES) – studies with level of evidence A, B or C: Any study design comparing 2 populations (F/NF)	25 electronic databases, other online resources and references (2000) were used to locate published and unpublished studies. Inclusion decisions, quality assessment and extraction of data was duplicated by two reviewers, and consensus obtained by discussion/a third party. Meta-analyses of random effects were carried out in order to group the data, and potential sources of heterogeneity were examined in a meta-regression analysis.	The best evidence available suggests that: Water fluoridation reduces the prevalence of caries. Water fluoridation increases the prevalence of dental fluorosis. There is no conclusive evidence in relation to other adverse effects (the quality of this evidence was methodologically weak). The evidence on the reduction of inequalities in dental health is not clear (also of poor quality). The prevalence of caries increases with the suspension of water fluoridation.

was from -5.0% to 64% (14.6%), the range (median) of mean change in decayed, missing and filled primary/permanent teeth (deft/DMFT) was from 0,5 to 4,4 (2,25) teeth. There was significant heterogeneity among the studies included. Meta-regression showed that the proportion of children without caries at the beginning of the study, the setting (place), and the validity score show a significant association with the difference in risk in the proportion of children without caries. Baseline Decayed, missing and filled primary/permanent teeth (dmf/DMFT), age, setting (place) and study duration show a significant association with the mean difference in DMFT/ dmft.

Effect of the suspension (termination) of water fluoridation on caries levels: Based on 22 analyses (level B, moderate quality), the authors concluded that the prevalence of caries increases after the withdrawal of water fluoridation.

Effect on caries beyond that offered by the use of alternative fluoride-based interventions: An effect of water fluoridation was still evident in studies concluded after 1974 in spite of the assumed exposure to fluoride originating from other sources by the populations studied. However, the small number of studies in this analysis and the poor quality of the studies limited the confidence with which this question could be answered. Moreover, using the study publication date may not have been a sufficiently sensitive factor to identify any change/effect.

Social class effects: The available evidence on social class effects of water fluoridation in reducing caries appears to suggest a benefit in the reduction of the differences in severity of dental caries (measured by dmft/DMFT) between social classes among

five and 12 year-old children, but no effect on the overall measurement of the proportion of caries-free children was detected. The quality of the evidence is low (level C), and is based on a relatively small number of studies.[15] Therefore the association between water fluoridation, caries and social class still needs clarifying.

Negative effects of water fluoridation: These were examined in as comprehensive a manner as possible and the effects on dental fluorosis are the clearest.

There is a dose-response relationship between the level of fluoride in the water and the prevalence of fluorosis (shown in the meta-regression analysis). Fluorosis appears to occur frequently at levels of fluoride typically used in artificial fluoridation schemes (1 ppm F), but the proportion of fluorosis that is aesthetically concerning is lower at these levels: the pooled estimate of the prevalence of fluorosis at a fluoride concentration in water of 1,0 ppm was 48% (95% CI: 40% to 57%) and for fluorosis of aesthetic concern (defined as TF $\geq$ 3, or mild or higher Dean index, or TSIF $\geq$ 2) it was 12,5% (95% CI: 7% to 21,5%). The estimated proportion of the population with any fluorosis at different levels of fluoride in the water ranged from 15% (95% CI: 10% to 22%) at a level of 0,1 ppm F to 72% (95% CI: 62% to 80%) at a level of 4 ppm F. There was, however, considerable heterogeneity between the results of the individual studies. Although 88 fluorosis studies were included, these were of low quality (level C – the majority of the studies were cross-sectional, while only four were controlled before-and-after studies). Additionally, the efforts to reduce observer bias or to control potential confounding factors were not common in the studies included.

The best scientific evidence available on the association of water fluoridation and bone fractures or cancer does not show defined patterns of association.

The various other adverse effects studied did not present enough good quality evidence on any outcome in particular to reach clear conclusions. The outcomes related to infant mortality, congenital defects and IQ indicate the need for further higher quality investigations, using adequate analytical methods to control for confounding factors. While fluorosis can occur within a few years of fluoride exposure during tooth development, other potential adverse effects may require long-term exposure to occur, and this long-term exposure may not have been captured by these studies.

Differences between the effects of natural and artificial water fluoridation: No considerable differences were apparent in this review, where direct comparisons were not possible for most of the outcomes. The available evidence is extremely limited, and was not sufficient to reach a conclusion about this aspect.

Reviewer's (Author's) Conclusions

The review presents a summary of the best and most reliable evidence available on the safety and effectiveness of water fluoridation. The quality of the data on benefits and harms ranges, however, from moderate to low. The evidence of benefit in the reduction of caries should be considered together with the increase in the prevalence of dental fluorosis. The research evidence is of insufficient quality to allow reliable statements about other potential harms, or regarding a possible impact on social inequalities. Any future research on the safety and effectiveness of water fluoridation should be conducted with appropriate methodology.

Fluoride toothpastes, mouthwashes (rinses), gels, varnishes

The compiled/reviewed evidence

The relevant Cochrane reviews on the effects of the main modalitiess of self-applied and professionally-applied fluorides, used separately or in conjunction (with one another), were published from 2003 to 2010[42-48,57,58] and are available in the Cochrane Database of Systematic Reviews CDSR in the Cochrane Library (http://www.thecochranelibrary.com). Cochrane reviews are updated when new evidence appears and in response to comments, and the Cochrane Library should always be consulted for the latest version of these reviews.

Objectives of the Cochrane Reviews

The main issues that were considered in the Cochrane reviews on the effects of the main types/therapies of topical application of fluoride include:

- the potential benefits that can be expected of fluoride therapies in the form of toothpastes, mouthwashes, gels and varnishes, especially in terms of the overall reduction of caries increment;
- how the benefits of these fluoride treatments may vary according to the influence of potentially important effect-modifiers, including the initial level of caries severity, background exposure to other fluoride sources, frequency of application, and more specifically, the fluoride concentration (which has been the focus of a more recent review from the Co-

chrane series, on the relative effectiveness of dentifrices with different fluoride concentrations);

- whether the benefits differ among these fluoride treatments when these are used alone or when used in conjunction;
- the potential adverse effects, especially dental fluorosis, which are, however, rarely investigated or reported in conjunction with the estimates of effectiveness in experimental studies (hence the production of another recent review on the relationship between the use of fluoride applied topically, particularly in toothpaste, and the risk of developing dental fluorosis, which considers the evidence of experimental and observational studies in young children).

Overview of the methodology (inclusion criteria, search strategy, data collection and analysis)

The Cochrane topical fluoride reviews are based on thorough and unprecedented searches of published or unpublished evidence, in the form of randomized clinical trials (RCTs) mainly. These reviews identified and assessed the studies included, using similar methodology and measures of effect for caries. The first four reviews individually investigated the effectiveness of fluoride gel, varnish, mouthwashes and dentifrices in studies using placebo or no treatment control groups, and examined the factors that potentially influence effectiveness (caries reductions). The fifth review was a summary of the first 4, with additional investigations of differences of effectiveness between interventions, based on meta-regression analyses, using the treatments as covariables. The sixth review

collated trials directly compared the 4 treatments; the seventh review also involved direct comparisons between these 4 treatments, but when these were used in combination compared with the use of just one of them (mainly use of fluoride applied topically in combination with fluoride dentifrice versus fluoride dentifrice only). The most recent reviews, eighth and ninth, evaluated the relative effectiveness of fluoride dentifrices of different concentrations (in which a network meta-analysis was employed, using both the direct and indirect comparisons from the RCTs included), and the association between the use of fluoride applied topically in young children and the risk of developing fluorosis (in which the evidence from nonrandomized studies was considered as well).

Overview of the main results and conclusions

The main results and conclusions from the Cochrane topical fluoride reviews are summarized below.

Effect on caries increment in the surfaces of permanent and primary teeth – comparisons with placebo/ untreated groups

The evidence on the beneficial effects of fluoride toothpaste, mouthwash, gel and fluoride varnish is consistent and strong. Research involving more than 65,000 children and adolescents in more than 130 RCTs shows a clear reduction in the increase of caries in both the permanent dentition (for all the forms of topical application of fluoride examined) and the primary dentition (for fluoride gels and varnishes) (Table 10.4).

Table 10.4 – Pooled D(M)FS/d(ef)s estimates of the effects of topical treatment with fluorides, measured as preventive fractions (PF).

Type of Fluoride (**)	Preventive fraction	CI 95%	Type of Fluoride (***)	Preventive fraction	CI 95%
Permanent dentition					
Varnish (7)	46%	30–63%	Varnish (3)	40%	09–72%
Gel (23)	28%	19–37%	Gel (13)	21%	14–28%
Mouthwash (34)	26%	23–30%	Mouthwash (30)	26%	22–29%
Dentifrice (70)*	24%	21–28%	Dentifrice (70)	24%	21–28%
All 4 interventions (133)	26%	24–29%	All 4 interventions (116)	24%	22–27%
Primary dentition					
Varnish (3)	33% PF	19–48%	Varnish (1)	20% PF	2–38%
Gel (2)*	26% PF	-11–63%	Gel (2)	26% PF	-11–63%
Varnish and gel (5)	33% PF	22–44%	Varnish and gel (3)	27% PF	8–48%

CI = Confidence interval; * Comparisons w/Placebo only; ** number of placebo/no treatment comparisons; *** number of placebo comparisons.

Effect of factors that influence the effectiveness of topical application of fluoride in preventing caries

The Cochrane reviews show that topical application of fluoride (compared to placebo/no treatment) can reduce dental caries, regardless of the exposure to water fluoridation. It is also shown that supervising a child in the use of self-applied fluoride (in toothpaste or mouthwash) leads to greater benefits. A significant influence of the initial level of caries, and of the frequency and intensity of fluoride application, was also indicated in the reviews. In particular, the caries-preventive effect fluoride toothpaste can increase with higher initial levels of caries in the population and when a higher concentration of fluoride is used in the dentifrice formulation, even though the benefit is only significant for fluoride concentrations above 1000 ppm F. The effect of fluoride concentration is shown in the results of the Cochrane review on the relative effectiveness of fluoride dentifrices of different concentrations (Table 10.5).

Comparative effect on caries increment among the various topically-applied fluoride modalities

The Cochrane reviews indicate that fluoride toothpaste can protect the teeth against dental caries as much as fluoride mouthwashes or fluoride gels (important comparisons of dentifrices with fluoride varnishes were lacking); the pooled preventive fraction for decayed, missing and filled permanent surfaces, for nine RCTs combined was 1% (95 % CI -13% to 14%). Taking into account these results together with those of a detailed investigation conducted subsequently based on the same data from the Cochrane reviews, on the relative effectiveness of the four main topical fluoride modalities (varnish, gel, mouthwash solution, and dentifrice), in which a simultaneous analysis of direct and indirect comparisons was employed (multiple-treatments or network meta-analysis), no clear evidence was found that any one of the topically- applied fluoride intervention is more effective than another (Salanti et al., 2009).

Table 10.5 – Pooled D(M)FS/d(ef)s estimates of the effects fluoride dentifrices used in different concentrations, measured as preventive fractions (PF) – comparisons with placebo only.

Fluoride concentrations, in ppm F	Direct comparison meta-analysis (Confidence interval of 95%)	Network meta-analysis (Credibility interval of 95%)
Placebo vs. fluoride dentifrices	Preventive fraction	Preventive fraction
250	8,90 [-1,62, 19,42]	9,14 [-3,62, 21,96]
440/500/550	7,91 [-6,11, 21,94]	15,35 [-1,89, 32,53]
1000/1055/1100/1250	22,20 [18,68, 25,72]	22,99 [19,34, 26,58]
1450/1500	22,07 [15,26, 28,88]	29,29 [21,24, 37,46]
1700/2000/2200		33,7 [16,52, 50,77]
2400/2500/2800	36,55 [17,46, 55,64]	35,52 [27,23, 43,62]

Comparative effect on other outcomes

Other outcomes such as acceptability were assessed indirectly in the Cochrane topical fluoride reviews. The acceptability of the various interventions differed. The Cochrane reviews showed that children are more likely to persist with the use of toothpaste than with the use of any other topical fluoride application.

Comparative effect on caries increment between the combined and single fluoride intervention use - direct comparisons

Combining two methods of fluoride treatment, such as fluoride toothpaste with another topically-applied fluoride intervention, produced an additional caries reduction of 10% (95% CI: 2% to 17%) compared to the use of fluoride dentifrice alone. That cannot be considered substantial.

Adverse effects of topically-applied fluoride treatments

The evidence from the relevant Cochrane review on the risk of fluorosis in small children from topical application of fluoride focused mainly on fluoride toothpaste and on the outcome of mild fluorosis. Based mainly on the results of observational studies, there is weak evidence that the use of fluoride toothpaste commenced in children aged under 12 months may be associated with an increased risk of fluorosis. The evidence of an increase in the risk of fluorosis associated with fluoride toothpaste use in the age range between 12 and 24 months is equivocal. Moreover, the use of higher fluoride concentrations in toothpastes of >1000 ppm of F, when evaluated in randomized clinical trials (2 RCTs), was associated with an increase in fluorosis in young children.

Other fluoride-based interventions; fluoridated milk and slow-release fluoride devices

The main features and the results of the two Cochrane reviews published in 2005 and 2006, evaluating other fluoride interventions, are presented in Table 10.6. They assessed the anticaries effect of fluoridated milk[55] and of slow-release fluoride devices.[56] The evidence assessed is considered weak and insufficient to confirm the efficacy of slow-release fluoride devices, because the results of a single trial included participants selected with on the basis of the retention of the device instead of an intention-to-treat analysis. Data from just two trials provided some evidence that fluoridated milk would be beneficial against caries for children of school age.

Tabela 10.6 – Summary of Cochrane reviews on fluoridated milk and slow release fluoride devices.

Study	Inclusion criteria	Methods	Main results
Fluoridated milk for prevention of dental caries[55]	Study design: RCT/ quasi-RCT with an intervention or follow-up of at least 3 years. Intervention: Fluoridated milk vs. non-fluoridated milk. Outcome: changes in the caries experience in the permanent or primary teeth (DMFS or dmfs), Participants: children or adults.	Searches were made in several databases, without language restrictions; authors of the studies contacted for unpublished data; data were extracted and had their quality assessed independently and in duplicate.	2 trials included, involving 353 children. For the permanent teeth, a significant reduction in the DMFT (78.4%, P <0.05) between the test and the control group was shown in one of the trials after 3 years. For the primary teeth, once again, a reduction in the dmf (31.3%, P <0.05) was shown after 3 years in one study, but not in the other. The results could not be pooled owing to the considerable difference in the concentration of fluoride in the milk.
Slow-release fluoride devices for control of dental caries[56]	Study design: RCT/ quasi-RCT. Intervention: The slow-release fluoride devices versus treatment with alternative fluorides, placebo or no intervention. Outcome: changes in the caries experience in the permanent or primary teeth (DMFS and dmfs), and progression of lesions through the enamel and dentine. Participants: children or adults.	Searches were made in several databases, without language restrictions; authors of the studies contacted for unpublished data; data were extracted and had their quality assessed independently and in duplicate.	Only one study included involving 174 children. Although 132 children remained in the study at the point of conclusion (2 years), the examination and the statistical analysis were only carried out on the 63 children who had accumulated the accounts (31 in the intervention group and 32 in the control group). Among them, the caries increment was lower in the intervention group than in the placebo group (mean difference: -0.72 DMFT, CI 95%_ -1.23 to -0.21; and -1.52 DMFS, CI 95%: - 2.68 to -0.36).

Final observations

It can be concluded that the benefit of regular brushing with fluoride dentifrice is firmly established, but there may be continuous scientific controversy concerning the effects of water fluoridation, especially potential adverse effects until better studies are conducted and produce more definitive evidence.

The Cochrane reviews of therapies with fluoride of topical use are being updated, and as the evidence arising from new RCTs is gradually incorporated into existing reviews, the precision of the estimated effects should increase, although no further change is expected in the conclusions. This is the case for fluoride varnishes, with at least seven new additional controlled trials on the effect of fluoride varnishes on the primary teeth being included in the updated review,[61-67] as well as three RCTs assessing the effect of varnishes on permanent teeth.[68-70]

The appropriate use of fluoride has always required an evaluation of its relative risks and benefits. A informed knowledge of the mechanism of action of fluoride and of the rationale and methods used in the evaluation of health care interventions was provided as a basis to understand and to present the scientific evidence available on the effects of the various types of fluoride use in the control of caries. A range of study designs have been used in recent decades to evaluate the various interventions. While the main topically-applied fluoride treatments have been tested intensively in randomized controlled trials, research conducted on the effects of water fluoridation was of inferior methodological quality.

Acknowledgements

The authors would like to thank Professor Aubrey Sheiham for his valuable comments in previous versions of this chapter.

References

1. Petersson GH, Bratthall D. The caries decline: a review of reviews. Eur J Oral Sci. 1996; 104(4(Pt2)):436-43.
2. Dean HT, Arnold FA, Elvove E. Domestic water and dental caries. Pub Health Rep. 1942; 57:1155-79.
3. McKay FS. The study of mottled enamel (dental fluorosis). J Amer Dent Ass. 1952; 44:133-7.
4. Fejerskov O, Thylstrup A, Larsen MJ. Rational use of fluorides in caries prevention. A concept based on possible cariostatic mechanisms. Acta Odontol Scand. 1981; 39(4):241-9.
5. Groeneveld A, Van Eck AA, Backer Dirks O. Fluoride in caries prevention: is the effect pre- or post-eruptive? J Dent Res. 1990; 69 Spec No:751-5.
6. Thylstrup A. Clinical evidence of the role of pre-eruptive fluoride in caries prevention. J Dent Res. 1990; 69 Spec No:742-50.
7. Bratthall D, Hänsel-Petersonn G, Sundberg H. Reasons for the caries decline: what do experts believe? Eur J Oral Sci. 1996; 104:416-22.
8. Tenuta LM, Cury JA. Fluoride: its role in dentistry. Braz Oral Res. 2010; 24 Suppl 1:9-17.
9. Fejerskov O. Changing paradigms in concepts on dental caries: consequences for oral health care. Caries Res. 2004; 38(3):182-91.
10. Buzalaf MA, Pessan JP, Honório HM, ten Cate JM. Mechanisms of action of fluoride for caries control. Monogr Oral Sci. 2011; 22:97-114.
11. Cury JA, Tenuta LM. How to maintain a cariostatic fluoride concentration in the

oral environment. Adv Dent Res. 2008; 20(1):13-6.

12. Dawes C, ten Cate JM: International symposium on fluorides: mechanisms of action and recommendation for use. J Dent Res. 1990; 69.

13. Ellwood RP, Fejerskov O, Cury JA, Clarkson B: Fluoride in caries control. In: Fejerskov O, Kidd E (eds). Dental caries: The disease and its clinical management, 2nd ed. Oxford:Blackwell & Munksgaard. 2008, pp.287-323.

14. Cury JA, Tenuta LM, Ribeiro CC, Paes Leme AF. The importance of fluoride dentifrices to the current dental caries prevalence in Brazil. Braz Dent J. 2004; 15:167-74.

15. Kidd EA, Fejerskov O. What constitutes dental caries? Histopathology of carious enamel and dentin related to the action of cariogenic biofilms. J Dent Res. 2004; 83 Spec No C:C35-8.

16. Burt BA. The changing patterns of systemic fluoride intake. J Dent Res. 1992; 71(Spec. Issue):1228-37.

17. Ekstrand J, Ehrnebo M. Absorption of fluoride from fluoride dentifrices. Caries Res. 1980; 14:96-102.

18. Cury JA, Del Fiol FS, Tenuta LMA, Rosalen PL. Low-fluoride and gastrointestinal fluoride absorption after meals. J Dent Res. 2005; 84:1133-7.

19. Levy SM, Warren JJ, Davis CS, Kirchner HL, Kanellis MJ, Wefel JS. Patterns of fluoride intake from birth to 36 months. J Public Health. 2001; 61:70-77.

20. de Almeida BS, Silva Cardoso VE, Buzalaf MAR. Fluoride ingestion from toothpaste and diet in 1 to 3 year-old Brazilian children. Community Dent Oral Epidemiol. 2007; 35:53-63.

21. European Academy of Paediatric Dentistry. Guidelines on the use of fluoride in children: an EAPD policy document. Eur Arch Paed Dent. 2009; 10(3):129-35.

22. Giacaman RA, Carrera CA, Muñoz-Sandoval C, Fernandez C, Cury JA. Fluoride content in toothpastes commercialized for children in Chile and discussion on professional recommendations of use. Int J Paediatr Dent. 2012 [in press].

23. Martins CC, Paiva SM, Lima YBO, Ramos-Jorge ML, Cury JA. Prospective study of the association between fluoride intake and dental fluorosis in permanent teeth. Caries Res. 2008; 42:125-33.

24. Warren JJ, Levy SM, Broffitt B, Cavanaugh JE, Kanellis MJ, Weber-Gasparoni K. Considerations on optimal fluoride intake using dental fluorosis and dental caries outcomes – a longitudinal study. J Public Health Dent. 2009; 69:111-5.

25. Fejerskov O, Larsen MJ, Richards A, Baelum V. Dental tissue effects of fluoride. Adv Dent Res. 1994; 8(1):15-31.

26. Woolf, S.H., Battista, R.N., Anderson, G.M., Logan, A.G., and Wang, E. Assessing the clinical effectiveness of preventive maneuvers: analytic principles and systematic methods in reviewing evidence and developing clinical practice recommendations. A report by the Canadian Task Force on the Periodic Health Examination. J Clin. Epidemiol. 1990; 43(9):891-905.

27. Guyatt, G.H., Sackett, D.L., Sinclair, J.C., Hayward, R., Cook, D.J., and Cook, R.J. Users' guides to the medical literature. IX. A method for grading health care recommendations. Evidence-Based Medicine Working Group [published erratum appears in JAMA 1996 Apr 24; 275(16):1232]. JAMA. 1995; 274(22):1800-1804.

28. Kleijnen, J., Gotzsche, P., Kunz, R.A., Oxman, A.D., and Chalmers, I. So what's so special about randomisation? In: Non Random Reflections on Health Services Research, edited by Maynard, A. and Chalmers, I.London:BMJ Publishing Group. 1997; p.93-106.

29. Clarke, M.J. and Stewart, L.A. Obtaining data from randomised controlled trials: how much do we need for reliable and informative meta-analyses? BMJ. 1994; 309(6960):1007-1010.

30. Jadad AR, Cook DJ, Jones A, et al. Methodology and reports of systematic reviews and metaanalyses: a comparison of Cochrane reviews with articles published in paper-based journals. JAMA. 1998; 280:278-80.

31. Glenny A M, Esposito M, Coulthard P, Worthington H V. The assessment of sys-

tematic reviews in dentistry. Eur J Oral Sci. 2003; 111:85–92.

32. Jørgensen AW, Maric KL, Tendal B, Faurschou A, Gøtzsche PC. Industry-supported meta-analyses compared with meta-analyses with non-profit or no support: differences in methodological quality and conclusions. BMC Med Res Methodol. 2008 Sep; 9(8):60.

33. Ijaz S, Croucher RE, Marinho VC. Systematic reviews of topical fluorides for dental caries: a review of reporting practice. Caries Res. 2010; 44(6):579-92.

34. Johnson MF: Comparative efficacy of naf and smfp dentifrices in caries prevention: A meta-analytic overview. Caries Research. 1993; 27:328-336.

35. Helfenstein U, Steiner M: Fluoride varnishes (duraphat): A meta-analysis. Community Dentistry & Oral Epidemiology. 1994; 22:1-5.

36. Stamm JW. Clinical studies of neutral sodium fluoride and sodium monofluorophosphate dentifrices. In: Bowen WH, ed. Relative efficacy of sodium fluoride and sodium monofluorophosphate as anti-caries agents in dentifrices. London: The Royal Society of Medicine Press Limited. 1995; 43-58.

37. van Rijkom HM, Truin GJ, van 't Hof MA. A meta-analysis of clinical studies on the caries-inhibiting effect of fluoride gel treatment. Caries Res. 1998; 32:83-92.

38. McDonagh MS, Whiting PF, Wilson PM, et al. Systematic review of water fluoridation. BMJ. 2000; 321:855-859.

39. Bartizek RD, Gerlach RW, Faller RV, et al. Reduction in dental caries with four concentrations of sodium fluoride in a dentifrice: a meta-analysis evaluation. J Clin Dent. 2001; 12:57-62.

40. Strohmenger L, Brambilla E. The use of fluoride varnishes in the prevention of dental caries: a short review. Oral Dis. 2001; 7:71-80.

41. Chaves SC, Vieira-da-Silva LM. Anticaries effectiveness of fluoride toothpaste: a meta-analysis. Rev Saude Publica. 2002 Oct; 36(5):598-606.

42. Marinho VC, Higgins JP, Logan S, Sheiham A. Fluoride gels for preventing dental caries in children and adolescents. Cochrane Database Syst Rev. 2002a; 2:CD002280.

43. Marinho VC, Higgins JP, Logan S, Sheiham A. Fluoride varnishes for preventing dental caries in children and adolescents. Cochrane Database Syst Rev 2002b; 3:CD002279.

44. Marinho VC, Higgins JP, Sheiham A, Logan S. Fluoride toothpastes for preventing dental caries in children and adolescents. Cochrane Database Syst Rev. 2003a; 1:CD002278.

45. Marinho VC, Higgins JP, Logan S, Sheiham A. Fluoride mouthrinses for preventing dental caries in children and adolescents. Cochrane Database Syst Rev. 2003b;3:CD002284.

46. Marinho VC, Higgins JP, Logan S, Sheiham A. Topical fluoride (toothpastes, mouthrinses, gels or varnishes) for preventing dental caries in children and adolescents. Cochrane Database Syst Rev. 2003c; 4:CD002782.

47. Marinho VC, Higgins JP, Sheiham A, Logan S. One topical fluoride (toothpastes, or mouthrinses, or gels, or varnishes)versus another for preventing dental caries in children and adolescents. Cochrane Database Syst Rev. 2004a; 1:CD002780.

48. Marinho VC, Higgins JP, Sheiham A, Logan S. Combinations of topical fluoride (toothpastes, mouthrinses, gels, varnishes) versus single topical fluoride for preventing dental caries in children and adolescents. Cochrane Database Syst Rev. 2004b; 1:CD002781.

49. Ammari AB, Bloch-Zupan A, Ashley PF. Systematic review of studies comparing the anti-caries efficacy of children's toothpaste containing 600 ppm of fluoride or less with high fluoride toothpastes with 1,000 ppm or above. Caries Res. 2003; 37:85-92.

50. Twetman S, Axelsson S, Dahlgren H, et al. Caries-preventive effect of fluoride toothpaste: a systematic review. Acta Odontol Scand. 2003; 61:347-355.

51. Benson PE, Parkin N, Millett DT, et al. Fluorides for the prevention of white spots on teeth during fixed brace treatment. Cochrane Database Syst Rev. 2004; 3:CD003809.

52. Petersson LG, Twetman S, Dahlgren H, et al. Professional fluoride varnish treatment for caries control: a systematic review of clinical trials. Acta Odontol Scand. 2004; 62:170-176.

53. Steiner M, Helfenstein U, Menghini G. Effect of 1000 ppm relative to 250 ppm fluoride toothpaste: a meta-analysis. Am J Dent. 2004; 17:85-88.

54. Twetman S, Petersson LG, Axelsson S, et al. Caries-preventive effect of sodium fluoride mouthrinses: A systematic review of controlled clinical trials", Acta Odontol Scand. 2004; 62(4):223-230.

55. Yeung CA, Hitchings JL, Macfarlane TV, et al Fluoridated milk for preventing dental caries. Cochrane Database Syst Rev. 2005; 3:CD003876.

56. Bonner BC, Clarkson JE, Dobbyn L, Khanna S. Slow-release fluoride devices for the control of dental decay. Cochrane Database Syst Rev. 2006; 4:CD005101.

57. Walsh T, Glenny A, Worthington H, Marinho V, Appelbe P: Fluoride toothpastes of different concentrations for preventing dental caries in children and adolescents. Cochrane Database Syst Rev. 2010 Jan 20; (1):CD007868.

58. Wong MCM, Glenny AM, Tsang BWK, Lo ECM, Worthington HV, and Marinho VCC: Topical fluoride as a cause of dental fluorosis in children. Cochrane Database Syst Rev. 2010 Jan 20; (1):CD007693.

59. NHMRC. A Systematic Review of the Efficacy and Safety of Fluoridation. Australian Government 2007. (http://www.nhmrc.gov.au/guidelines/publications/eh41a) (accessed 14 September 2011)

60. Cheng KK, Chalmers I, Sheldon TA. Adding fluoride to water supplies. BMJ. 2007; 335:699.

61. Autio-Gold JT, Courts F. Assessing the effect of fluoride varnish on early enamel carious lesions in the primary dentition. J Am Dent Assoc. 2001; 132(9):1247-53.

62. Chu CH, Lo EC, Lin HC. Effectiveness of silver diamine fluoride and sodium fluoride varnish in arresting dentin caries in Chinese pre-school children. J Dent Res. 2002; 81(11):767-70.

63. Borutta A, Reuscher G, Hufnagl S, Möbius S. Caries prevention with fluoride varnishes among preschool children. Gesundheitswesen. 2006 Nov; 68(11):731-4.

64. Weintraub JA, Ramos-Gomez F, Jue B, et al. Fluoride varnish efficacy in preventing early childhood caries. J Dent Res. 2006; 85(2):172-6.

65. Hardman MC, Davies GM, Duxbury JT, Davies RM. A cluster randomised controlled trial to evaluate the effectiveness of fluoride varnish as a public health measure to reduce caries in children. Caries Res. 2007; 41(5):371-6.

66. Lawrence HP, Binguis D, Douglas J, et al. A 2-year community-randomized controlled trial of fluoride varnish to prevent early childhood caries in Aboriginal children. Community Dent Oral Epidemiol. 2008; 36(6):503-16.

67. Gugwad SC, Shah P, Lodaya R, Bhat C, Tandon P, Choudhari S, Patil S. Caries prevention effect of intensive application of sodium fluoride varnish in molars in children between age 6 and 7 years. J Contemp Dent Pract. 2011 Nov 1; 12(6):408-13.

68. Moberg Sköld U, Petersson LG, Lith A, Birkhed D. Effect of school-based fluoride varnish programmes on approximal caries in adolescents from different caries risk areas. Caries Res. 2005; 39(4):273-9.

69. Milsom KM, Blinkhorn AS, Walsh T, Worthington HV, Kearney-Mitchell P, Whitehead H, Tickle M. A cluster-randomized controlled trial: fluoride varnish in school children. J Dent Res. 2011 Nov; 90(11):1306-11.

70. Tagliaferro EP, Pardi V, Ambrosano GM, Meneghim Mde C, da Silva SR, Pereira AC. Occlusal caries prevention in high and low risk schoolchildren. A clinical trial. Am J Dent. 2011 Apr; 24(2):109-14.

Chapter 11

Promoting Children's Oral Health – Theory and Practice Toolkits on Guidelines for Prevention: Evidence Based Approaches

John Rogers
Julie Satur

Introduction

There is a considerable literature on oral health promotion and the prevention of oral disease. How can we find what is useful to our situation? What is appropriate for community settings? What is appropriate for cli-nical settings and one-on-one oral health education? This chapter will outline the 'toolkits' that are available to help answer these questions.

A range of recently developed toolkits and how to access them is shown in Table 11.1.

Table 11.1 – Toolkits for the prevention of oral disease.

Resource	Access
Evidence-based oral health promotion resource. Department of Health, Melbourne, Australia, 2011.[1]	http://docs.health.vic.gov.au/docs/doc/evidence_based_oral_health_promotion
Delivering Better Oral Health: An evidence based toolkit for prevention (2nd Ed). National Health Service, London, UK, 2009.[2]	http://www.dh.gov.uk
The Scientific Basis of Oral Health Education, Levine RS and Stillman Lowe CR, 2009.[3]	British Dental Journal Books, London UK, 2009.
Oral Health Promotion Messages for the Australian Public: Findings of a National Consensus Workshop. National Oral Health Promotion Clearinghouse, 2011.[4]	Australian Dental Journal, 2011, vol. 56, pp. 1-5.
The use of Fluorides in Australia. Australian Research Centre for Population Oral Health, 2006.[5]	Australian Dental Journal, 2006, vol. 51(2), pp. 195-199.

The first of these toolkits considers interventions that can be undertaken in the community rather than in the dental clinic. The other publications offer evidence--based advice for individuals. Community approaches will be addressed first and then individual advice.

Community approaches to promoting oral health

The evidence-based oral health promotion resource shown in Table 11.1

was developed to assist health promotion practitioners and policy makers to further promote oral health. By drawing together the evidence and considering implications for practice, the resource is a practical summary for policy development and program implementation. Table 11.2 summarises the methodology used and the contents of the resource.

The strength of the evidence for each intervention was evaluated according to the Haby and Bowen public health criteria shown in Table 11.3.[6]

Table 11.2 – Evidence-based oral health promotion resource, 2011.

Methodology	• Systematic literature review - covering June 1999 to June 2010 • Scope – review of oral health promotion interventions and broader programs (such as nutrition and social marketing) that affect oral health
Results	• 202 articles included encompassing 31 systematic reviews
Content	• Oral disease and determinants • Interventions by seven priority groups and settings • Interventions by Integrated Health Promotion categories • Program planning and evaluation • Gaps in the health promotion literature • Resources

Table 11.3 – Public health strength of evaluation and research evidence for intervention effectiveness

Strength of evaluation and research evidence	Description
1 Strong evidence of effectiveness	One systematic review or meta-analysis of comparative studies; or several good quality randomised controlled trials or comparative studies
2 Sufficient evidence of effectiveness	One randomised controlled trial; one comparative study of high quality; or several comparative studies of lower quality
3 Some evidence of effectiveness	Impact evaluation (internal or external) with pre- and post-testing or indirect, parallel or modelling evidence with sound theoretical rationale and program logic for the intervention
4 Weak evidence of effectiveness	Impact evaluation conducted, but limited by pre- or post-testing only; or only indirect, parallel or modelling evidence of effectiveness
5 Inconclusive evidence of effectiveness	No position could be reached because existing research/evaluations give conflicting results; or available studies were of poor quality
6 No evidence of effectiveness	No position could be reached because no evidence of impact/outcome was available
7 Evidence of ineffectiveness	Good evaluations (high quality comparative studies) show no effect or a negative effect

Oral health promotion interventions found in the literature to have an evidence-base are presented in Table 11.4. The strength of evidence is shown by the font as per the legend at the bottom of the table. Interventions are categorised according to the Integrated Health Promotion (IHP)[7] framework which is

Table 11.4 – Oral health promotion interventions according to the Integrated Health Promotion (IHP) framework.

Individual focus   **Population focus**

Screening, individual risk assessment	Health education and skill development	Social marking and health information	Community action	Settings and supportive environments
Integration of oral health into well persons visits, including, as appropriate, anticipatory guidance, motivational interviewing, Lift the Lip screening and referral for oral health care, by: • *well child nurses* • *general practitioners and nurse practitioners* • *Indigenous health workers* • *school nurses.*			Advocacy for oral health promoting environments: water fluoridation healthy food and drink policies restricted advertising of high sugar content products sugar-free medicine access to preventive oral health care.	**Water fluoridation.** **Targeted use of topical fluoride.** **Sugar-free products - chewing gum and** **Confectionery.** Healthy food and drink policies in key settings, childcare, school, workplace, residential care. Affordable oral health products – toothbrushes and fluoride toothpaste. *Orally healthy policy and practice in residential care settings.* *Restricted advertising of high sugar products.*
	Health and welfare workers as oral health promoters: *aged care workers* *welfare and disability workers, diabetes educators, youth workers* *pharmacists* *midwives* *domiciliary (district) nurses.* *Development and consistent use of evidence-based oral health messages.* *Integration of oral health information with other health information.* *Small groups and peer education.*			
	Smoking cessation, brief intervention by oral health professionals. Use of mouthguards when playing contact sports.	Social marketing via mass media. Use of local media.		
	Community action, multi-strategy programs.			
Legend: Level 1 – **strong evidence;** Level 2 – sufficient evidence; Level 3 – *some evidence.*				

similar to the Ottawa Charter. The IHP model presents interventions on a continuum from more individual 'down stream' to more population 'up stream' approaches.

Relevant studies for interventions for pregnant women, babies and young children are categorised into the eight main approaches that are outlined in Table 11.5. The highest strength of evidence found in studies is shown along with the outcome measure used and the target group.

Studies for children and adolescents are categorised into the six approaches outlined in Table 11.6.

More details about each study plus context for this age group and implementation issues are included in the resource. Studies that were ineffective were also indentified as shown in Table 11.7. These studies had good evaluations and showed no effect.

Table 11.5 – Oral health promotion interventions for pregnant women, babies and young children.

Intervention	Highest strength of evidence*	Outcome measure	Target group
1 Targeted home visits by health workers	2	Behaviour change Prevention of tooth decay	High-risk young children and families
2 Targeted fluoride varnish programs in childhood settings	1	Prevention of tooth decay	
3 Targeted supervised toothbrushing in childhood settings	2	Behaviour change Prevention of tooth decay	
4 Targeted provision of fluoride toothpaste and brushes by mailing, home visit or via clinic	2	Behaviour change Prevention of tooth decay	
5 Healthy food and drink policy in childhood settings	2	Behaviour change Policy change	Young children and families
6 Integration of oral health into well child visits	3	Behaviour change Policy change	
7 Community action, multi-strategy programs	2	Behaviour change Prevention of tooth decay	High-risk communities
8 Community-based preventive programs for expectant and/or new mothers	2	Behaviour change Prevention of tooth decay	Expectant and/or new mothers

* Public Health strength of evidence[6] – see Table 3.

Table 11.6 – Oral health promotion interventions for children and adolescents.

Intervention	Highest strength of evidence*	Outcome measure	Target group
1 Targeted school-based toothbrushing programs	2	Behaviour change Prevention of tooth decay	Primary school children
2 Targeted school-based fluoride mouth rinsing programs	2	Prevention of tooth decay	Primary school children

Table 11.6 – Oral health promotion interventions for children and adolescents. (Continues)

3 School-based oral health education • Link to the home environment • Creative and interactive learning based on students interests • Use of peers	2	Behavioural change Prevention of gum disease Prevention of tooth decay when fluorides and/or dental sealants used	Primary and secondary school children
4 Orally healthy school policies • Integration of oral health into the school curriculum • Increasing fruit and vegetable consumption	2	Behavioural change Prevention of tooth decay Prevention of dental trauma Policy change	
5 Healthy food and drink policy in childhood settings	2	Behavioural change Prevention of gum disease Prevention of tooth decay when fluorides and/or dental sealants used	
6 Targeted chewing gum programs	1	Prevention of tooth decay	

* Public Health strength of evidence[6] – see Table 3.

Table 11.7 – Oral health promotion interventions for children and adolescents shown to be ineffective.

Intervention	Highest strength of evidence*	Outcome measure	Target group
1 Supervised school-based toothbrushing programs; • With low dose fluoride toothpaste in non-fluoridated areas • When not sustained	7	Prevention of tooth decay	Primary school children
2 Annual classroom lessons			
3 Non-integrated health promotion programs to prevent school snacking			

* Public Health strength of evidence[6] – see Table 3.

Principles that can be used to guide the planning of programs include:

• **Address the broader determinants of health.**
The WHO has developed a framework for social determinants entry-points and interventions to address oral health inequalities.[8]

• **Base activities on the best available data and evidence.**

• **Act to reduce social inequities and injustice.**
Effective oral health interventions do not always reduce health inequalities, and may actually increase them. This is probably because the socially

advantaged often have more knowledge, skills and resources to implement orally healthy behaviours.

- **Emphasise active consumer and community participation.**
- **Empower individuals and communities.**

This can occur through information, skill development, support, advocacy and structural change strategies. People need to have an understanding of what promotes health and illness and be able to mobilise resources necessary to take control of their own lives.

- **Explicitly consider difference in gender and culture.**
- **Work in collaboration with key stakeholders.**

Partnerships need to be actively sought across a broad range of sectors.

- **Consider sustainability.**
- **Evaluate appropriately.**
- **Implement an appropriate mix of interventions.**

This often requires a balance of both individual and population-wide interventions, supported by capacity building. Where possible integrate with other health promotion programs while retaining specific oral health promotion elements. Fluoride remains an effective preventive measure against dental caries. The other two specific oral health messages are about oral hygiene and regular oral health checks.

The evidence-based oral health promotion resource provides advice about planning and evaluating oral health promotion programs. It identifies gaps in the literature - such as the paucity of evaluations that consider cost effectiveness. Online resources that are available for oral health promotion are also listed.

Individual approaches to promoting oral health

There are a number of 'toolkits' that offer evidence-based advice regarding oral health practices for individuals. Four recent resources are listed in Table 11.1. The Evidence Based Toolkit developed by the Department of Health and the British Association for the Study of Community Dentistry[2] (the UK Toolkit) plus the Scientific Basis for Oral Health Education compiled by Levine and Stillman Lowe[3] (Scientific Basis), rank the type of evidence which informs their recommendations. The last two documents synthesise evidence on oral health education presented at consensus workshops.[4,5]

The levels of evidence used in the UK Toolkit and the Scientific Basis resources are outlined in Table 11.8.

Table 11.8 – Levels of evidence for individual evidence based advice.

Level	Strength of Evidence
I	Strong evidence from at least one systematic review
II	Strong evidence from at least one well designed, randomised controlled trial
III	Evidence from well designed trails without randomisation such as pre and post intervention, cohort, time series and matched case studies
IV	Evidence from well designed, non experimental studies
V	Opinions of respected authorities based on clinical evidence, descriptive studies or expert committee reports

Source: UK Toolkit[2]

Findings relevant to children and adolescents from the four resources are summarised in Table 11.9. Material from the other three documents has been added to the UK Toolkit template. Generally the advice from each resource is consistent. However there are some differences in recommended toothpaste fluoride concentrations. This is because the UK Toolkit provides advice for non fluoridated communities, whereas the Australian resource was prepared for predominantly fluoridated communities.

Table 11.9 – Evidence-based prevention advice for children and young adults.

Group	Prevention advice to be given	Evidence level	Professional Intervention	Evidence level
Children aged up to 3 years	• Breast feeding provides the best nutrition for babies[1-3]	I	• Children should have an oral assessment by age 3 • Children should have their teeth checked as soon as possible[2]	V V
	• From six months of age infants should be introduced to drinking from a cup,[1-3] and from age one year feeding from a bottle should be discouraged[2,3]	III		
	• Sugar should not be added to weaning foods[1,2]	V		
	• Parents and carers should be warned against the practice of allowing sugar sweetened drinks, juices, cordials and carbonated drinks, especially in bottles and feeder cups.[2,3] Comfort sucking on a bottle should be discouraged[2,3]	III-IV		
	• Normal fluid intake would ideally be water or milk, soy milk can cause caries so care should be taken[2]	V		
	• As soon as teeth erupt in the mouth brush them twice daily[1,2,4]	IV		
	• Parents should brush or help brush their child's teeth[1,2,4]	V		

Table 11.9 – Evidence-based prevention advice for children and young adults. (Continues)

	Where community water supply is not fluoridated: • Use only a smear of toothpaste containing no less than 1,000 ppm fluoride,[1] ensure children do not swallow excessive amounts[2]	I	• Australian guidelines on toothpaste are that variations should be based on professional advice for those at greater risk such as those not drinking fluoridated water. Variations could include more frequent use of fluoridated toothpaste, commencement of toothpaste use at a younger age, or earlier commencement of use of standard toothpaste containing 1,000 ppm fluoride[4]	V
	Where community water supplies are predominantly fluoridated: Australian guidelines[4] are that: • From the time the first teeth erupt to the age of 17 months, children's teeth should be cleaned but not with toothpaste • Children from 18 months-5 years should use a pea-sized amount of lower dose fluoride (eg 400-550 ppm fluoride) toothpaste • Tooth paste s hould always be used under supervision of a responsible adult, and children should spit out, not swallow, and not rinse	V		
	• When starting foods other than milk, try to encourage a variety of foods and savoury tastes[2]	V		
	• The frequency and amount of sugary food and drinks should be reduced and, when consumed, limited to mealtimes.[1,2] • Sugars should not be consumed more than four times per day[1]	III III		
	• Drink plenty of tap water, limit sugary foods and drinks, and choose healthy snacks, e.g. fruits and vegetables[3]	III		
	• Sugar-free medicines should be recommended[1]	III		
	• Children should have an oral assessment by age 23 • Children should have their teeth checked as soon as possible[2]	V V		
All children aged 3–6 years	• Brush twice daily[1-3] • Brush last thing at night and on one other occasion[1,2]	I I	• Apply fluoride varnish to teeth twice yearly (2.2% F–) in non fluoridated areas[1] and for those with an elevated risk of developing caries, including children under the age of 10, in situations where other professionally applied fluoride vehicles may be unavailable or impractical[4]	
	• Brushing should be supervised or helped by an adult[1,2,4]	V		
	Where community water supply is not fluoridated: • Use a pea-sized amount of toothpaste containing 1,350-1,500 ppm fluoride[1,2]	V, I		I

Table 11.9 – Evidence-based prevention advice for children and young adults. (Continues)

	Where community water supplies are predominantly fluoridated: Australian guidelines are that; • Children from 18 months-5 years should use a pea-sized amount of lower dose fluoride (eg 400-550 ppm fluoride) toothpaste • Toothpaste should always be used under supervision of a responsible adult, and children should spit out, not swallow, and not rinse[4]	V	• Australian guidelines on toothpaste use are that variations should be based on professional advice for those at greater risk such as those not drinking fluoridated water. Variations could include more frequent use of fluoridated toothpaste, commencement of toothpaste use at a younger age, or earlier commencement of use of standard toothpaste containing 1,000 ppm fluoride[4]	V
	• Spit out after brushing and do not swallow or rinse[1,4]	IV		
	• The frequency and amount of sugary food and drinks should be reduced and, when consumed, limited to mealtimes[1,2] • Sugars should not be consumed more than four times per day[1]	III III		
	• Limit the frequency of intake of acidic drinks[2] and avoid brushing for one hour after an acidic episode[2]	III-V		
	• Drink plenty of tap water, limit sugary foods and drinks, and choose healthy snacks, e.g. fruits and vegetables[2,3]	III		
	• Sugar-free medicines should be recommended[1]	III		
	• All children need regular dental checks but the frequency depends on individual risk factors[2,3]	V		
	All advice as above, plus: • Use a smear or pea-sized amount of toothpaste containing 1,350-1,500 ppm fluoride[1,2] • Australian Guidelines are that toothpastes use should be varied as needed based on professional advice[4]	I	• Apply fluoride varnish to teeth 3-4 times yearly (2,2% F-)[1,2] • Australian guidelines are to use fluoride varnish for those with an elevated risk of developing caries, including children under the age of 10, in situations where other professionally applied fluoride vehicles may be unavailable or impractical[4]	I
Children giving concern (eg those likely to develop caries, those with special needs)	• Ensure medication is sugar free[1]	V	• Prescribe fluoride supplement and advise re maximising benefit[1]	II

Table 11.9 – Evidence-based prevention advice for children and young adults. (Continues)

	• Give dietary supplements containing sugar and glucose polymers at mealtimes when possible (unless clinically directed otherwise) and not last thing at night. Parents should be made aware of the cariogenicity of supplements and ways of minimising risk[1]	V	• Reduce recall interval[1]	V
			• Investigate diet and assist to adopt good dietary practice[1]	III
			• Ensure medication is sugar free or given to minimise cariogenic effect[1]	III
All children aged from 7-and young adults	• Brush twice daily[1-3] • Brush last thing at night and on one other occasion[1,2]	I V	• Apply fluoride varnish to teeth twice yearly (2,2% F–)[1] for those with an elevated risk of caries[4]	I
	In communities where water supply is not fluoridated use fluoridated toothpaste (1,350 ppm fluoride or above)[1,2]	I	• Australian guidelines are to use fluoride varnish for those with an elevated risk of developing caries, including children under the age of 10, in situations where other professionally applied fluoride vehicles may be unavailable or impractical[4]	
	For those with predominantly fluoridated water supplies use toothpaste containing 1000 ppm[4]	V		V
	• Spit out after brushing and do not rinse[1,4]	IV		
	• Drink plenty of tap water, limit sugary foods and drinks, and choose healthy snacks, e.g. fruits and vegetables[2,3]	III		
	• The frequency and amount of sugary food and drinks should be reduced and, when consumed, limited to mealtimes[2] • Sugars should not be consumed more than four times per day[1]	III III		
	• Limit the frequency of intake of acidic drinks[2] and avoid brushing for one hour after an acidic episode[2]	III-V		
	• Chewing sugar free gum can reduce decay[3]	II		
	• Mouthguards should be worn for all sports where there is a reasonable risk of mouth injury[3]	V		
	• Everyone needs regular dental checks but the frequency depends on individual risk factors[2,3]	V		

Table 11.9 – Evidence-based prevention advice for children and young adults. (Continues)

Those giving concern (eg those likely to develop caries, those undergoing orthodontic treatment, those with special needs)	**All the above, plus:** • Use a fluoride mouthrinse daily (0,05% NaF) at a different time to brushing[1,3,4]		• Fissure seal permanent molars with resin sealant[1]	I
	• Australian guidelines are that for teenagers and adults who are at elevated risk of developing caries, dental professional advice should be sought to determine if they should use toothpaste containing a higher concentration of fluoride (i.e. greater than 1000 ppm fluoride).[4]		• Apply fluoride varnish to teeth 3-4 times yearly (2.2% F–)[1] • Australian guidelines are to use fluoride varnish for those with an elevated risk of developing caries, including children under the age of 10, in situations where other professionally applied fluoride vehicles may be unavailable or impractical[4]	I
			• For those 8+ years with active caries prescribe daily fluoride rinse[1]	I
			• For those 10+ years with active caries prescribe 2,800 ppm toothpaste[1]	I
			• For those 16+ years with active disease consider prescription of 5,000 ppm toothpaste[1]	I
			• Investigate diet and assist adoption of good dietary practice[1]	III

Sources:
1. UK Toolkit (1)
2. The Scientific Basis of Oral Health Education (2)
3. Oral Health Promotion Messages for the Australian Public (3)
4. The Use of Fluorides in Australia (4)

Summary

There are a range of 'toolkits' available that can assist in planning, implementing and evaluating oral health education and promotion.

The Evidence-based oral health promotion resource[1] summarises oral diseases and their determinants and identifies predominantly non-clinical evidence-based interventions. The UK Toolkit[2] presents evidence-based messages and professional interventions for different age groups. These two resources are complemented by the Scientific Basis of Oral Health Education[3] and two resources from consensus workshops.[4,5]

These resources synthesise the vast amount of research and present evidence-based interventions and guidelines for good oral health policy and practice. They provide practical summaries for promoting oral health.

References

1. Rogers J. Evidence-based oral health promotion resource. In: Victorian Department of Health, editor. Melbourne, Victoria: Prevention and Population Health Branch, Government of Victoria, Department of Health. 2011.

2. Department of Health/British Association for Community Dentistry. Delivering Better Oral Health: An evidence based toolkit for prevention. In: Department of Health/British Association for Community Dentistry, editor. Second ed. London. 2009.

3. Levine R. The scientific basis of oral health education. Community Dent Health. 2004 Jun; 21(2):131-3.

4. National Oral Health Promotion Clearing House. Oral health messages for the Australian public. Findings of a national consensus workshop. Aust Dent J. 2011 Sep; 56(3):331-5.

5. Australian Research Centre for Population Oral Health. The use of fluorides in Australia: guidelines. Aust Dent J. 2006; 51(2):195-9.

6. Haby M, Bowen S. Making decisions about interventions. A guide for evidence-informed policy and practice. In: Victorian Department of Health, editor. Melbourne. 2010.

7. Department of Health. Integrated health promotion kit. In: Victorian Department of Human Services, editor. Melbourne. 2003.

8. Kwan S, Petersen P. Oral health: equity and social determinants. Geneva: World Health Organisation. 2010.

Chapter 12

Public Policies for Healthy Eating; Applying the Common Risk Factor Approach

Maria do Carmo Matias Freire
Marcelo Bönecker

Introduction

The types of food eaten has a strong influence current and future health of children (Fig. 12.1). This chapter addresses the effects of nutrition and diet on oral health in early childhood and adolescence, as well as the importance of the public policies for healthy eating in the promotion of oral health, within the context of the common risk factor approach.[1] In this approach, oral diseases and other non-communicablechronic diseases (NCDs) are considered to have a set of risk factors that include diet.

Food and diet: effects on oral health

Both diet and the type of food and nutritional state of the child can affect the teeth during tooth formation (pre--eruptive effect) and after eruption, by a direct local effect (post-eruptive effect). It may result in defects in the tooth structure, dental caries and dental erosion. There is good evidence that nutritional deficiencies have an adverse effect on the periodontal tissues of animals, but in humans the evidence is insufficient.[2] In cases of vitamin C deficiency the periodontal tissues of humans are indeed affected, hindering the inflammatory response.

Epidemiological studies show that the type of diet and the nutritional state protects against oral cancer, mainly through the high consumption of fresh fruit and vegetables.[3,4]

Dietary sugars and dental caries

- There is a wealth of evidence showing that sugars are undoubtedly the most important dietary factor in the development of dental caries.[29]

- There is no good evidence that, with the exception of lactose, the cariogenicity of the different sugars such as sucrose, glucose and fructose varies.
- "Epidemiological studies have shown that starch is of low risk to dental caries. People who consume high-starch/low sugars diets generally have low caries experience whereas people who consume low-starch/high-sugars diets have high levels of caries."[29]
- Starchy staple foods are of little importance in the development of caries.
- Cooked staple starchy foods such as rice, potatoes and bread are of low cariogenicity in humans.[29]
- The cariogenicity of uncooked starch is very low.[29]

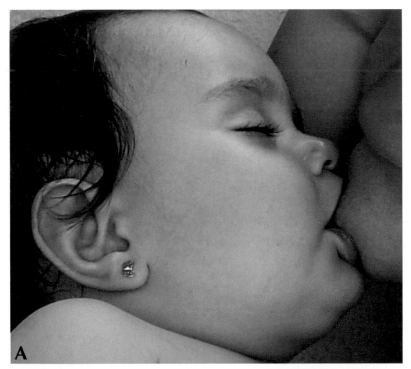

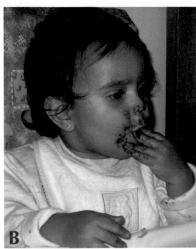

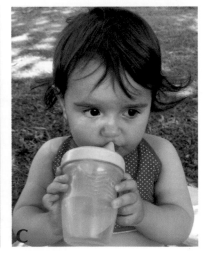

Fig. 12.1A-C – Suitable eating habits are formed in early childhood and influence general and oral health.

Defects in the tooth structure

Nutritional deficiency during tooth formation is one of the causes of defects in tooth structure. The most widely known enamel defect is linear enamel hypoplasia, resulting from hypocalcaemia.[5] Hypoplasia is common in deciduous incisors of children from developing countries where malnutrition is prevalent. Hypoplasia can be associated with the development of caries. Another cause of enamel defect is excessive fluoride intake during tooth formation. That results in fluorosis.

Dental erosion

Although the prevalence of erosion varies widely in the last twenty years[6] and the comparison between studies is difficult owing to the different indices and criteria used to assess the loss of tooth structure, some longitudinal studies have reported an increase in its incidence[7-9] Erosive tooth wear is a condition, which can affect the deciduous and permanent dentitions (Fig. 12.2 and 12.3). This wear is characterised by the progressive loss of tooth structure, due to chronic exposure to acids not of bacterial origin,[10] which is an important differential aspect in relation to dental caries.

The acids involved in the erosive process can be of either extrinsic origin from food, drinks and/or acidic medications, or intrinsic origin, in which organic or psychosomatic alterations (gastroesophageal reflux and bulimia) that causes the acid content of the stomach to come into contact with the oral environment.

Diet is considered the principal factor of the multifactorial etiologyof dental erosion, characterised clinically by tooth substance loss initially on the vestibular and palatine surfaces of the upper incisors (Fig. 12.4) and occlusal surfaces of lower molars (Fig. 12.5), but depending on the intensity and frequency, other teeth and surfaces are equally affected (Fig. 12.6). The frequent consumption of highly acidic solid and liquid food, mainly soft drinks and processed fruit juices, are the main dietary factor.[11] In the deciduous dentition, the risk is higher when these liquids are administered in a baby bottle, which leads to prolonged exposure of the teeth to the acid pH, especially if the bottle is used frequently to calm the child.[12]

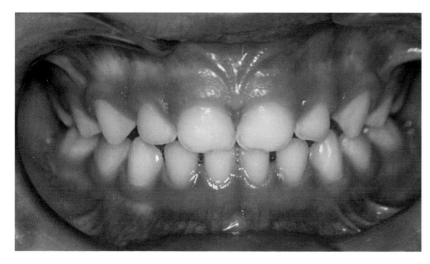

Fig. 12.2 – Dental erosion on deciduous teeth.

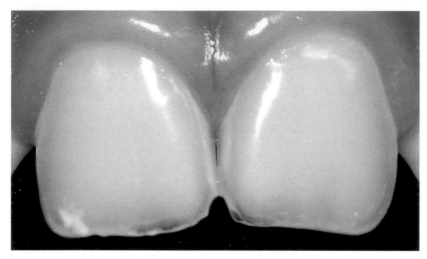

Fig. 12.3 – Dental erosion on permanent teeth.

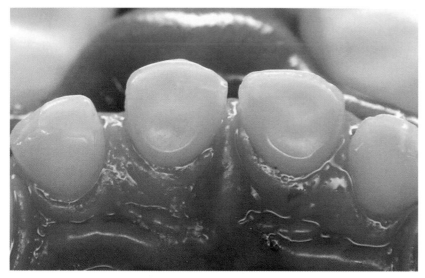

Fig. 12.4 – Dental erosion on palatine surface of deciduous teeth.

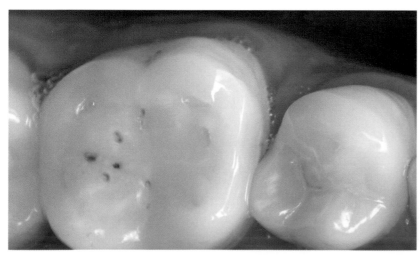

Fig. 12.5 – Dental erosion on occlusal surface of deciduous molars.

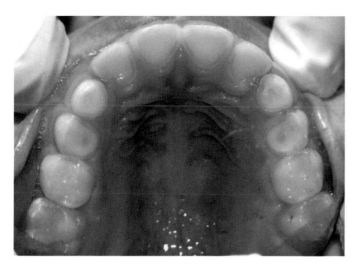

Fig. 12.6 – Dental erosion affecting several surfaces and various teeth.

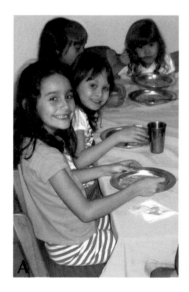

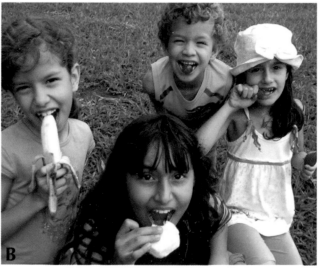

Fig. 12.7 – Schools constitute a pedagogical setting to work with nutritional education.

Although the acidity of food and drinks, represented by the pH value, is an important determinant of erosion,[13] it cannot be considered a unique and exclusive factor. Other chemical parameters inherent to these products, such as concentration of phosphate/calcium/fluoride, presence of chelating agent, type and quantity of acid, buffer capacity, temperature, and adhesion, also present an influence on the erosive potential.[13-16]

The tooth position, the anatomy of the soft tissue, the quality of the dental tissue and the salivary properties may be involved in the erosive process, leading to a greater or lesser risk of erosive lesion.[15,17,18]

Behavioural factors also exhibit a direct influence on the intensity, location and characteristics of erosive lesions. These factors range from frequency, length, form and timing of beverage consumption, to the presence of psychosomatic diseases, such as bulimia.[19,20]

Only one study investigated the association between the prevalence of erosion and nutritional state.[21] Adolescents who were overweight presented a higher incidence of dental erosion, while those at a risk of becoming overweight and underweight presented a lower incidence, yet no statistically significant association was found.

Scientific evidence that serves as a basis for erosion prevention strategies is still limited and/or insufficient and originates from in situ and in vitro studies. The main prevention strategies are related to changes of eating habits, general health treatment, reduction of the mechanical impact of brushing, increased salivary flow, development of less erosive foods and use of fluorides. There are no population studies on dental erosion in the dental literature as there are for dental caries.

Dental caries

Pre-eruptive effect

Malnutrition affects the tooth structure in rodents, delays eruption and results in increased caries, yet this relationship is harder to demonstrate clearly in humans.[22] The best evidence so far comes from a longitudinal study carried out on Peruvian children where the occurrence of anepisode of moderate to severe malnutrition, during the first year of life, was associated with an increase in caries in the deciduous and permanent dentitions many years later.[11]

Three probable mechanisms have been considered to explain the relationship between malnutrition and caries: (a) tooth formation defects[24]; (b) delay in tooth eruption[25]; and (c) alteration in the salivary glands.[26,27]

Malnutrition associated with high sucrose intake constitutes an important risk factor for the development of caries.

Post-eruptive effect

The local post-eruptive effect of the diet has much more influence on caries development than the pre-eruptive effect.[28,29] Sugar is the most cariogenic component of diet, acting as substrate for the production of acids by bacteria from the plaque and subsequent demineralisation of the dental enamel. The frequency, quantity and type of sugar consumed influence its cariogenic potential. Sucrose is the most cariogenic sugar, although glucose, fructose and maltose are also cariogenic. Lactose is the least cariogenic sugar.

Starch can cause caries, but to a much lesser extent than sugars. Basic starchy foods, such as rice, potatoes, bread and pasta are a low risk to the child. When refined, cooked and mixed with sugars, such as crackers or biscuits, and consumed frequently, starch can cause caries. Most caloric sweeteners and all non-caloric sweeteners are non-cariogenic or present very low cariogenicity. Protection elements in the diet include cheese, proteins, fats and casein, but their practical use is uncertain.

Sugars have been classified for dental health purposes by distinguishing between sugars naturally integrated into the cellular structure of the food (intrinsic sugars) and those present in a free form or added to food (extrinsic sugars). Extrinsic sugars are more readily available for metabolism by oral bacteria than intrinsic sugars and are, therefore, potentially more cariogenic. Due to the lower cariogenicity of lactose and the cariostatic nature of milk, sugars naturally present in milk and milk products are classified as 'milk sugars' and are distinguished from other free sugars or 'non-milk extrinsic sugars' (NMES).[30] The sugars that are potentially damaging to dental health are the NMES and include all added sugars, sugars in fresh fruit juices, honey and syrups.[3]

The following classification has been proposed for sugars:[30,31]

Intracellular or intrinsic sugars: those present naturally within the cellular structure of food, such as fruit and vegetables. They present very low cariogenic potential and are important for good nutrition.

Extracellular or non-milk extrinsic sugars: those added to foods, by the actual consumer or by the manufacturer, such as table sugar (generally sucrose) and biscuits, cakes, soft drinks, yoghurts, icecreams and other treats for children and honey. They present high cariogenic potential and deleterious effects on the health when ingested in large quantities.

Milk sugar: the sugar (lactose) present in milk and its by-products. It presents low cariogenic potential and is important for good nutrition.

Sugars, caries and erosion in children

Babies have an innate preference for sweetness because in nature, all sweet foods are safe to eat. So if something is sweet humans are evolved to prefer it to sour foods, which indicates toxicity. The problem of sugar consumption generally starts very early in childhood, with the introduction of sugary foods and drinks in the first months of life. Sugars can have an detrimental effect on their deciduous teeth (Fig. 12.8) and also affect their immediate and future general health, especially through obesity.

We will now address aspects of eating in the main periods of early childhood and adolescence and then the effects of sugars on the oral health of children. Examples of strategies for improving eating habits, emphasising reduction of sugarsin the diet, will also be presented.

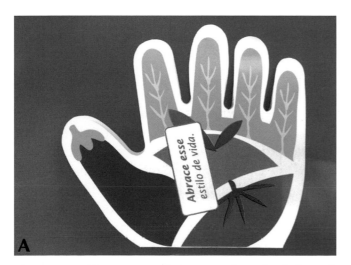
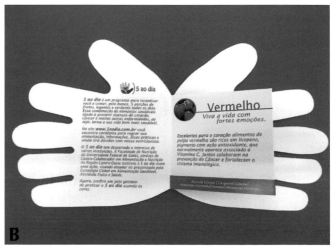

Fig. 12.8 – Diet program known as "5-a-day" diet related program, which emphasises a importance of at least five portions of fruit and vegetables a day.

Breastfeeding

Exclusive breastmilk constitutes the ideal diet at the beginning of a child's life, as it is a complete food, protects against common early childhood infections, is contamination-free and adapts perfectly to the child's metabolism (Figure 12.1-A). During exclusive breastfeeding there is no need to offer other foods or liquids to the child, not even water, since breast milk already contains water. Moreover, breastfeeding is important in the promoting ties between mother and child and is more economic for families.

The World Health Organisation's current recommendation is that children be exclusively breastfed from the first hour after birth up to the age of six months, and that they should continue being breastfed up to two years of age or beyond, with food supplementation from the age of six months.[32] Breastfeeding or bottle feeding with cow's milk without added sugar is not considered cariogenic or erosive. The effects of breastfeeding on oral health also include the good development of the masticatory system.[33]

Human and cow's milk contain 7% and 4,8% of lactose, respectively, but lactose is asugar with the least potential for fermentation toacids by the oral bacteria.[34,35] Milk also contains protective components, such as calcium, phosphorus, antibacterial substances, phosphoproteins(casein) and fats, which help to prevent the dissolution of the enamel and contribute to its remineralisation.

Human milk contains a higher proportion of lactose and a lower proportion of calcium, phosphorus and protein than cow's milk, yet the occurrence of caries in breastfed babies is very rare.[36] Systematic review studies show that there is noscientific evidencethat night-time and on demand breastfeeding is associated with caries.[37,38] Bottle feeding with cow's milk or powdered formula milk (cow's milk processed by the manufacturer), on the other hand, can represent a dental health risk to children. There are few studies on the cariogenicity of formula milk.[39] Several formula milksmarketed in the United States have significant cariogenic potential in animals.[35] Glucose polymers have been added in the processing of formula milks as an energy supplement and there is not enough information on their effect on dental health.[40] Cow's milk without the addition of sugar has cariostatic properties.

Both milk and other liquids with sugar added during their preparation at home or during their industrial processing, frequently result in rampant caries, especially when they are administered before sleeping.[41,42] These liquids are usually teas, chocolate powder mixes, fruit juices,powdered fruit drinks and sugar-sweetened softdrinks. Fruit juices are cariogenic.[42] These liquids also cause dental erosion, which can occur even without the addition of sugar. Some fruit juices are erosive, particularly those with a citric acid base, which have chelating potential.[14]

The effect of breastfeeding or bottlefeeding should not be considered separately. Studies show that low socioeconomic status has an influence on the development of caries in early childhoodand constitutes a stronger determinant ofthe feeding method.[43,44] Moreover, nutritional deficiency in the antenatal period can cause defects in the enamel, predisposing to caries.[44,45]

Feeding from 6 months of age

The complementary feeding period, erroneouslynamed "weaning", should be started from the age of six months, with expansion of the diet, including other solid and liquid foods, besides milk.[46] The eruption of the first teeth generally coincides with or initiates the complementary feeding and its composition is therefore essential for dental health.[47] WHO recommends avoiding drinks with low nutritional value, such as tea, coffee and sugary drinks, as well as limiting the quantity of juices offered.[46]

In Brazil, the Food Guide for Children under Two Years of Age, published by the Ministry of Health in 2002,[48] recommends avoiding sugars, softdrinks, sweets and other delicacies in the first years of life. The recommendations are set out in full are in Table 12.1, which presents the Ten Steps to Healthy Eating.

The nutritional guidance based on the recommendations of the Food Guide for Children was effectivein caries prevention in children.[49] Compared with a control group the group whose mothers received guidance at household visits in the first year of life of the child, there was a reduction of 22% in the incidence of caries and a smaller number of teeth with caries experience at 4 years of age.

Table 12.1 – Recommendations of the Department of Health for the feeding of childrenunder 2 years old.[48]

The "Ten Steps to Healthy Feeding"	
STEP 1	Give only breastmilk until the age of six months, without offering water, teas or any other food.
STEP 2	From the age of six months, slowly and gradually introduce other foods, maintaining breastmilk up to the age of two years or over.
STEP 3	From the age of six months, offer supplemental foods(cereals, tubers, meat, legumes, fruit and vegetables) three times a day if the child receives breast milk and five times a day if they are weaned.
STEP 4	Supplemental food should be offered without strict timetables, always respecting the child's wishes.
STEP 5	Supplemental food should be thick from thestart and offered in a spoon; start with a pasty consistency (mashes/purées), and gradually increase their consistency until the child is eating the same food as the family.
STEP 6	Offer the child different foods every day. A varied diet is a colourful diet.
STEP 7	Encourage the daily consumption of fruit, vegetables and legumes/pulsesduring meals.
STEP 8	Avoid sugar, coffee, canned food, fried food, soft drinks, sweets, savoury snacks and other delicaciesin the early years of life. Use salt with moderation.
STEP 9	Pay attention to hygiene in the preparation and handling of foods; guarantee its appropriate storage and conservation.
STEP 10	Encourage sick and convalescent children to eat, offering their habitual diet and their favourite foods, respecting their acceptance.

Dietary recommendations from the age of two years are generally found in the food guides and other official documents designed for the population in general. There is a consensus about the need to reduce sugar intake levels to improve general health and the prevention of chronic non-communicable diseases. According to WHO's technical report on diet, nutrition and prevention of chronic diseases, non-milk extrinsic sugars should contribute with no more than 10% of the total energy in the diet.[50]

Processed baby food and drinks

Processed baby foods are very common in children's diets and many of them contain sugars, generally sucrose, which can constitute a health risk. Processed sugar-sweetened beverages, such as fruit juices and softdrinks, cause a reduction in the plaque pH,[51] dental caries and erosion,[12,52-55] besides other health problems.[56] The consumption of fruit juices and other acidic drinks has increased in the last 20 years in North America[52] and increased 7 times between the years 1950 and 1990 in the United Kingdom.[52] In Brazil, the soft drink market doubled from 2000 to 2005 and is already the thirdlargest in the world after USA and Mexico.[57]

Some foods without the addition of sucrose contain other extrinsic and cariogenic sugars,such as glucose, fructose, dextrose, honey and glucose polymers or maltodextrins.[31,40] Energy and sports drinks affect oral health.[58] Therefore, it is necessary to provide consumers with clarifications on the various types of sugar and to develop measures to make food labels more informative.[59]

The pH value and calcium, phosphate and fluoride content of erosive agents influence mineral dissolution of the tooth structures.[13,14,60] The food or drink is considered erosive when it is subsaturated in relation to the hydroxyapatite.[60] However, unlike dental caries, there is no specific critical pH value below which erosion occurs.[13,14]

Feeding at childcare facilities – crèches, children's homes and schools

Crèches, schools and other institutions should offer or promote healthy diets for children in their care, as they are appropriate places to develop health promotion measures in the community. There are some studies on the impact of these actions on children's oral health.

Crèches

According to a food guide for children under 5 in child care in England, published by the Caroline Walker Trust,[61] "If children are having sugary foods and drinks, these should be given with meals rather than between meals. Children do not need sugary foods such as sweets, chocolate, softdrinks or honey for energy. Starchy foods - such as potatoes, bread, rice, pasta and yam- are better sources of energy (calories), as these foods contain other important nutrients too." The guide also warns about the risk of dental erosion in this age group.

A study conducted in a Brazilian municipalit showed that low-income children in the care of crèches that have adopted food guidelines, including the reduction of sugar in the diet, had a much lower incidence of caries than that found in children from crèches that did not adopt guidelinee.[62]

Children's homes

At Hopewood House, a home for underprivileged children in southern Australia,the consumption of sugar and refined flour was reduced and the children consuge a lactovegetarian diet and one of starch from potatoes, rice and wholemeal flour. As a consequence, 46% of the 12-year-olds were caries-free, compared with only 1% of those of the same age attending other schools in the same region.[63] A low prevalence of caries was also reported in the Synanon Community, in the USA, where refined sugar was substituted for fruit purees and artificial sweeteners, associated with fluoride tablets and bacterial plaque control.[64]

Schools

Schools constitute a pedagogical setting to work with nutritional education, with actions that range from the inclusion of nutrition contents in the curricula to practical measures for offering healthy diets through the institutional school meal or commercial school canteen programs (Fig. 12.7).

These measures can also benefit other aspects of children's education such as familiarising children with foods that they may not have access to at home; contributing to alter the usual pattern of consumption among children where fruit, for example, is not value; or developing social practices associated with meal schedules. Success in the development and implementation of these measures depends on the collaboration of the local health and education authorities, administrators of school meal programs, head teachers, food handlers and schoolteachers as well as parents or other persons in charge and nutritionists.

Some countries,such as England and Australia,have published technical documents and practical guideline forschool food, including recommendations for reducing the consumption of foods containing sugars.[65,66]

An example of a public measure is the establishment of the guidelines for the Promotion of Healthy Eating at preschool, primary and secondary school private and state-run establishments at a national level in Brazil, by an Interministerial Administrative Ruling (Ministries of Health and of Education).[67] This Ruling establishes the 10 Steps for the Promotion of Healthy Eating at schools, which includes the restriction of the supply and sale of foods with a high content of fat, saturated fat, transfat, free sugar and salt. Before this strategy, some Brazilian locations had already employed similar rulew.[68]

Regarding the impact on oral health, two longitudinal studies conducted at schools in Australia showed that at schools that did not sell sweets in their canteens the children presented a lower incidence of caries over a two-year period, compared with children from schools that did sell sweets.[69,70] At English schools, a link was found between the sale of biscuits and caries experience in incisors.[71]

Action to reduce sugars consumption needs to be a core element of an integrated food policy to improve health. Therefore, guidelines are needed to assist individuals and policy makers, and to provide industry with regulations on the formulation and marketing of their products. Consensus international and national guidelines already exist on the need to reduce sugars consumption.[50] Governments should develop strategies to implement the recommendations of the report of the joint WHO/FAO expert consultation on diet and the prevention of chronic diseases and should support food-based dietary guidelines (Moynihan & Petersen 2004). A prudent upper limit of intake of sugars is no more than 100 calories per day or 15 kgs a year per person.[89]

Sugar in paediatric medications

Liquid medications or syrups for treating chronic diseasesfor long periods of time[72] that containg sugars (sucrose, glucose or fructose) can cause caries when used several times a day, and particularly at night.[72]

Measures to control the use of these medications are necessary and can be integrated into the national medication policy. Several actions have been recommended in developed countries, involving the participation of various segments, from consumers to the manufacturers of these products.[72,73] As a consequence, the pharmaceutical industry is developing alternative formulations, either sugarless or with alternative sweeteners,and lists of sugar-free liquid medicines are made available to the health professionals. In its guide for the prevention of oral problems, the UK Department of Health included a list of sugar-free medications or medications that contain non-cariogenic substitutes.[74]

Oral health and eating in the context of general health

The global and national overview of nutrition and health

Rapid changes in diets and lifestyle are producing a significant impact on the nutritional state of populations, both of developed and of developing countries. Drawing a parallel with malnutrition, obesity is today one of the most visible public health problems, and at the same time the most neglected[75,76]

Obesity is generally caused by excess calories from fats and sugars, and from lack of physical activity. It contributes to the development of several chronic non-communicable diseases, such as diabetes, hypertension, stroke, cardiovascular diseases and some types of cancer. The increase in the prevalence of these diseases lead the World Health Organisation (WHO) to propose a global strategy for their control based on diet and on physical activity.[77]

There is considerable evidence relating diets with highsugar content withchronic diseases other than dental carie; vesical calculi, gastrointestinal problems, deficiency of micronutrients, bone loss and bone fracture.[3,30] The progressive increase in chronic diseases means that attention is also focused on child feeding in the early years of life.[78]

Childhood obesity affects health, increasing the risk of hyperlipidaemia, hypertension and abnormal glucose tolerance, and constitutes an important predictor of adult obesity. Therefore,obesity, the diseases resulting from obesity and dental caries share an important etiological component in eating habits.[79] Therefore, the prevention of these diseases should begin in early childhood, with good eating habits.

Public food policies

The current recommendation for a healthy diet is compatible with that suggested to maintain oral health and includes the reduction of sugar consumption and its substitution by healthy food such as fruit, vegetables and cereals that also are energy sources.[50] In practice, these goals are not easily reached by the population. In the case of sugar, there is strong lobbying pressure on politicians from the industry, which extols the "virtues" of sugars.

It is necessary to develop means of boosting the public's and professionals' awareness of the importance of diet for good health, including oral health. Health education constitutes an important measure in this process. Although individual counselling for each patient is not realistic and generally results in temporary changes,[80] some children may reap particular benefits if their parents receive the necessary information. For changes in the population, broader measures are necessary.

The concept of health promotion includes the development of means of allowing a community or an individual to improve and exercise more control over their health.[81] In this regard, health education should be integrated with a more comprehensive policy able to intervene in the actual determinants of the health-disease process, and enabling the population to have easy access not only to the information required for changes, but also the healthiest options. Making healthy choices the easier choicses and unhealthy choices more difficult. The promotion of oral health should, therefore, be integrated with general health policies and supported by the common risk factor principle, as sugar consumption is an etiological factor both of caries and of other chronic diseases.[1,82] The dietary recommendations for caries prevention coincide with those geared not only towards disease prevention, but also towards the maintenance of general health.

As regards the sugar consumption reduction policy, Sanderson[83,84] proposedthat it should not be based on educational strategies targeting the consumer audience alone, but should also include other strategies, such as regulatios, substitution and pricing strategy, rirected at the various sectors-involver: producers, refiners, manufacturers, intermediaries, distributors, suppliers, consumers, pressure groups, health professionals and public institutions (Table 12.2). In this model, the cooperation between and among the various government institutions and between these and the other sectors is essential. Whatever the kind of strategy chosen it is advisable to make a gradual introduction to avoid confrontation with consumer preferences and to give the industry time to adapt. The increase in fruit consumption by children and adults can be an indirect way of reducing the consumption of sugary food of low nutritional value. Examples of such strategies are the "5-a-day" diet-related program (Fig. 12.8), developed in several countries, which emphasises the importance of at least five portions of fruit and vegetables a day. The message is simple (it does not mention grams or percentages) and positive, suggesting that people eat more and not less. In Brazil, besides this initiative, the Ministry of Health implemented other fruit and vegetable consumption incentive actions in 2009 that involved production policies, family farming, supply, access and education, which constitute a good example of a health promotion measure with an intersectoral approach.[85]

Due to the difficulties in implementing government measures aimed at reducing the consumption soft drinks and other beverages containing sugar, the campaign entitled "Life's Sweeter With Fewer Sugary Drinks" (http://www.fewersugarydrinks.org/tools.html) was launched in the US with the involvement of health workersand civil organisations and other groups.

Table 12.2 – Strategies for a policy to reduce sugar consumption in the population.[84,85]

Strategy	Goals and examples
Education strategy	Persuade people to change their sugar consumption habits through information, counselling and instruction. This strategy has been almost exclusively consumer-oriented. Examples: - Educational programs or activities involving individual or collective diet and nutrition; - Information on labels about the nutritional composition of food.
Substitution strategy	Encourage people to use another product instead of sugar and to find alternatives for the existing sugar production. Examples: - Replacement of processed products with natural products in school meals and meals served by other childcare institutions; - Replacement of sucrose with sweeteners; - Replacement of sugarcane cultivation by another crop, in a rotation system; - Alternative uses for sugar, such as the production of combustible alcohol and of biodegradable plastics.
Pricing strategy	Alter the relative prices of sugar and of alternative products, with nutritional purposes. Example: - Alteration in the farmer incentive system.
Regulatory strategy	Uses legal or quasi-legal instruments to reduce sugar consumption. Examples: - Legislation on the use of alternative sweeteners; - Legislation on the labels of processed foods; - Legislation aiming to reduce the content of sugars in processed food and drinks; - Legislation aiming to control the advertising of processed food products for children.

Food guides and healthy diet

Food guides or guidelines are extremely useful to inform national policies, community initiatives and individual action.[86] These guidelines have been common in European countries and in the United States since the 1960s and include several aspects of nutrition, diet and health, culminating in dietary recommendations with the goal of preventing the health issues resulting from dietary excesses and deviations. They are generally drawn up by government institutions, such as ministries or national health departments, but also by other national agencies and professional associations.

According to these documents, a healthy diet should be rich in fresh fruit and vegetables; include a wide variety of starchy foods, preferably in whole or unprocessed form; and contain modest quantities of meat and dairy products. The lowerthe saturated fats, sugars, salt and alcohol, the better it is for the health.[3,50,77,87]

The vast majority of good guides recommend reducing sugar consumption to prevent several chronic diseases, mainly caries and obesity.[88] However, many of them present vague recommendations, such as "limit", "use with moderation", and "small quantities". In the guides that establish quantitative goals, the maximum recommended consumption level is 10% of the total caloric value of the diet from extrinsic sugars (excluding those that are part of the whole fruit), coinciding with the goal established by the World Health Organisation.[50] This level corresponds to approximately 10-15kg/person/yearconsidered compatible with good dental health.[89] The polysaccharides (starch), in turn, should contribute with 50% to 70% of the energy in the diet.

This recommendation has been adopted in some countries, such as Brazil. The Eating Guide for the Brazilian Population, published by the Ministry of Health in 2006, follows WHO's proposal and adds that people should receive guidance on the maximum consumption of a portion of foods and the acceptable levels of sugars and sweets per day.[90] In Europe, it is recommended that extrinsic sugar consumption should not exceed 60 g/person/day for adolescents and adults and around 30 g/person/day forpreschool ages.[91,92] According to the Department of Health in England, the frequency ofintake of food and drinks containing sugars should not exceed four times a day.[93] Such recommendations should be integrated with the national policies of agriculture, food and health and also influence the conduct of nutritionists and food manufacturers.

Based on the scientific evidence available, and discussed in this chapter, it is possible to identify some important dietary recommendations, which should be considered in the formulation of food and oral health policies (Table 12.3). The main message is to reduce the quantity and frequency of consumption of foods containing extrinsic sugars.

Conclusions

Nutrition and diet have a strong influence on dental health. Malnutrition is related to structural defects of the teeth and to dental caries. The evidence is overwhelming that high levels of consumption of sugars leads to increases in a number of chronic diseases, including dental caries. Therefore, to promote health, food policies should focus on reducing the consumption of sugars. Acid drinks, especially soft drinks and processed juices, can cause dental erosion. In developed countries, several strategies have been implemented seeking the reduction of extrinsic sugars in the diet, and are also necessary in developing countries. Eating habits start in early childhood and are essential for the immediate and future health of children. Hence oral health professionals working with this group of the population have a very important responsibility in promoting healthy eating habits that ensure good general and oral health for the child and future adult. Dental Advocates should integrate their efforts with policy makers from different sectors and develop guidelines for reducing the production and consumption of sugars containing products.

Table 12.3 – Dietary recommendations for oral health.

Recommendations for the population in general
- The consumption of non-milk extracellular sugars, particularly sucrose, should be reduced and replaced with fresh fruit, vegetables and starchy foods (cereals, legumes/pulses, roots and tubers);
- When used, sugary foods should be consumed during meals, and not between meals.
- Non-milk extracellular sugars should contribute no more than 10% ofthe total energy (calories) in the diet.

Specific recommendations for children
- Infants should be exclusively breastfed up to the age of six months;
- If used, the baby bottle should not contain sugary liquids;
- Pacifiers should not be dipped in sugar, honey or sugary drinks and offered to children;
- Food and drinks for children, prepared at home, at institutions for minors, crèchesand schools, do not need extrinsic sugars added;
- Sugary processed products, such as soft drinks, sweetsand other delicacies should not be offered to the child on a routine basis.Foods that contain intrinsic sugars, such as fresh fruit, vegetables and cereals, are healthier sources of energy;
- Sugary syrup-based medications, when used in the long term, should be replaced with medications without sugar or other vehicles.

References

1. Sheiham A, Watt RG. The Common Risk Factor Approach: a rational basis for promoting oral health. Community Dent Oral Epidemiol. 2000; 28:399-406.

2. Enwonwu CO. Interface of malnutrition and periodontal diseases. Am J Clin Nutr. 1995; 61(suppl):430S-6S.

3. World Cancer Research Fund/American Institute for Cancer Research. Food, nutrition, physical activity, and the prevention of cancer: a global perspective. Washington DC: AICR; 2007.

4. Latino-Martel P, Druesne-Pecollo N, Dumond A. Nutritional factors and oral cancers. Rev Stomatol ChirMaxillofac. 2011; 112(3):155-9.

5. Nikiforuk G, Fraser D. The aetiology of enamel hypoplasia: a unifying concept. J Periodontol. 1981; 98:888-93.

6. Jaeggi T, Lussi A: Prevalence, incidence and distribution of erosion. Monogr Oral Sci. 2006; 20:44–65.

7. Dugmore CR, Rock WP. The progression of tooth erosion in a cohort of adolescents of mixed ethnicity. Int J Paediatr Dent. 2003; 13(5):295-303.

8. Ganss C, Klimek J, Giese K. Dental erosion in children and adolescents-a cross-sectional and longitudinal investigation using study models. Community Dent Oral Epidemiol. 2001; 29(4):264-271.

9. El Aidi H, Bronkhorst EM, Huysmans MC, Truin GJ. Dynamics of tooth ero-

sion in adolescents: a 3-year longitudinal study. J Dent. 2010; 38(2):131-137.

10. Imfeld T. Dental erosion. Definition, classification and links. Eur J Oral Sci. 1996; 104 (2(Pt2)):151-155.

11. Asher C, Read MJF. Early enamel erosion in children associated with excessive consumption of citric acid. Br Dent J. 1987; 162:384-7.

12. Smith AJ, Shaw L. Baby fruit juices and tooth erosion. Br Dent J. 1987; 162:65-7.

13. Barbour ME, Lussi A, Shellis RP. Screening and prediction of erosive potential. Caries Res. 2011; 45Suppl 1:24-32.

14. Lussi A, Jaeggi T. Chemical factors. Monogr Oral Sci. 2006; 20:77-87.

15. Magalhães AC, Wiegand A, Rios D, Honório HM, Buzalaf MAR. Insights into preventive measures for dental erosion. J Appl Oral Sci. 2009; 17(2):75-86.

16. Lussi A, Megert B, Peter Shellis R, Wang X. Analysis of the erosive effect of different dietary substances and medications. Br J Nutr. 2011; 30:1-11.

17. Lussi A. Erosive tooth wear - a multifactorial condition of growing concern and increasing knowledge. Monogr Oral Sci. 2006; 20:1-8

18. Hara AT, Lussi A, Zero DT. Biological factors. Monogr Oral Sci. 2006; 20:88-99.

19. Zero DT, Lussi A. Behavioral factors. Monogr Oral Sci. 2006;20:100-105.

20. Lussi A, Jaeggi T, Scharer S. The influence of different factors on in vitro enamel erosion. Caries Res. 1993; 27(5):387-393.

21. McGuire J, Szabo A, Jackson S, Bradley TG, Okunseri C. Erosive tooth wear among children in the United States: relationship to race/ethnicity and obesity. Int J Paediatr Dent. 2009; 19(2):91-8.

22. Alvarez JO, Navia JM. Nutritional status, tooth eruption, and dental caries: a review. Am J ClinNutr. 1989; 49(3):417-26.

23. Alvarez JO, Caceda J, Wooley KW, Baiocchi N, Navia JM. A longitudinal study of dental caries in the primary teeth of children who suffered from infant malnutrition. J Dent Res. 1993; 72(12):1573-6.

24. Mellanby M. The relation of caries to the structure of teeth. Br Dent J. 1923; 44:1-13.

25. Alvarez JO, Lewis CA, Saman C, Caceda J, Montalvo J, Figueroa ML, Izquierdo J, Caravedo L, Navia JM. Chronic malnutrition, dental caries, and tooth exfoliation in Peruvian children aged 3-9 years. Am J Clin Nutr 1988 Aug; 48(2):368-72.

26. Johansson I, Saellstrom A-K, Rajan BP, Parameswaran A. Salivary flow and dental caries in Indian children suffering from chronic malnutrition. Caries Res 1992; 26(1):38-43.

27. Johansson I, Lenander-Lumikari M, Saellström AK. Saliva composition in Indian children with chronic protein-energy malnutrition. J Dent Res. 1994 Jan; 73:11-9.

28. Sheiham A. Dietary effects on dental diseases. Publ Health Nutr. 2001; 4(2B):569-91.

29. Moynihan PJ, Petersen PE. Diet, nutrition and the prevention of dental diseases. Publ Health Nutr. 2004; 7(1A):201-26.

30. Department of Health. Committee on Medical Aspects of Food Policy. Dietary sugars and human disease. London: HMSO; 1989. Report on Health and Social Subjects 37.

31. Moynihan PJ. Update on the nomenclature of carbohydrates and their dental effects. J Dent. 1998; 26(3):209-18.

32. World Health Organization/UNICEF. Global strategy for infant and young child feeding. Geneva: WHO. 2003.

33. Nowak AJ, Warren JJ. Infant oral health and oral habits. Pediatr Clin North Am. 2000; 47(5):1043-66.

34. Rugg-Gunn AJ, Roberts GJ, Wright WG. The effect of human milk on plaque in situ and enamel dissolution in vitro compared with bovine milk, lactose and sucrose. Caries Res. 1985; 19:327-34.

35. Bowen WH, Pearson SK, Rosalen PL, Miguel JC, Shih AY. Assessing the cariogenic potential of some infant formulas, milk and sugar solutions. J Am Dent Assoc. 1997; 128(7):865-71.

36. Hackett AF, Rugg-Gunn AJ, Murray JJ, Roberts GJ. Can breast feeding cause dental caries? Human Nutrition: Applied Nutrition. 1984; 38A:23-8.

37. Erickson PR, Mazhare E. Investigation of the role of human breast milk in ca-

ries development. Pediatr Dent. 1999; 21:86-90.

38. Valaitis R, Hesch R, Passarelli C, Sheehan D, Sinton J. A systematic review of the relationship between breastfeeding and early childhood caries. Can J Public Health. 2000; 91:411-7.

39. Duarte PM, Coppi LC, Rosalen PL. Cariogenicidade e propriedades cariostáticas por diferentes tipos de leite: revisão. Arch Latinoam Nutr. 2000; 50:113-20.

40. Moynihan PJ, Gould MEL, Huntley N, Thorman S. Effect of glucose polymers in water, milk and a milk substitute on plaque pH in vitro. Int J Paediatr Dent. 1996; 6:19-24.

41. Ripa LW. Nursing caries: a comprehensive review. Pediatr Dent. 1988; 10(4): 268-82.

42. Winter GB. Problems involved with the use of comforters. Int Dent J. 1980; 30:28-38.

43. Ismail AI. Prevention of early childhood caries. Community Dent Oral Epidemiol. 1998; 26(suppl 1):49-61.

44. Smith PJ, Moffatt ME. Baby-bottle tooth decay: are we on the right track? Int J Circumpolar Health. 1998; 57(suppl 1):155-62.

45. Davies GN. Early childhood caries: a synopsis. Community Dent Oral Epidemiol. 1998; 26(suppl 1):106-16.

46. Holt RD, Moyhihan PJ. The weaning diet and dental health. Br Dent J. 1996; 181:254-9.

47. World Health Organization. Complementary feeding: report of the global consultation, and summary of guiding principles for complementary feeding of the breastfed child. Geneva: WHO. 2003.

48. Brasil. Ministério da Saúde. Guia alimentar para crianças brasileiras menores de dois anos. Brasília: Ministério da Saúde. 2000.

49. Feldens CA, Giugliani ERJ, Duncan BB, Drachler ML, Vítolo MR. Long-term effectiveness of a nutritional program in reducing early childhood caries: a randomized trial. Community Dent Oral Epidemiol. 2010; 38:324-32.

50. World Health Organization. Diet, nutrition and the prevention of chronic diseases. Geneva: WHO. 2002.

51. Birkhed D. Sugar content, acidity and effect on plaque pH of fruit juices, fruit drinks, carbonated beverages and sport drinks. Caries Res. 1984; 18(2):120-7.

52. Millward A, Shaw L, Smith AJ, Rippin JW, Harrington E. The distribution and severity of tooth wear and the relationship between erosion and dietary constituents in a group of children. Int J Paediatr Dent. 1994; 4(3):151-157.

53. O'Brien M. Children´s dental health in the United Kingdom, 1993. London: OPCS. Her Majesty´s Stationery Office. 1994; 74-76, 113.

54. Watt RG, Dykes J, Sheiham A. Preschool children's consumption of drinks: implications for dental health. Community Dent Health. 2000; 17(1):8-13.

55. Almeida LFD, Abílio GMF, Cavalcante MT, Castro RD, Cavalcanti AL. Cariogenic and erosive potential of industrialized fruit juices available in Brazil. Braz J Oral Sciences. 2010; 9:351-7.

56. Amato D, Maravilla A, García-Contreras F, Paniagua R. Los refrescos y la salud. Rev Invest Clin. 1997; 49:387-95.

57. ABIR. Associação Brasileira das Indústrias de refrigerantes e bebidas não alcoólicas. In. HTTP://www.abir.org.br.

58. American Academy of Pediatrics. Committee on Nutrition and the Council on Sports Medicine and Fitness. Sports Drinks and Energy Drinks for Children and Adolescents: Are They Appropriate?Pediatrics. 2011; 127:1181-90.

59. Celeste RK. Análisecomparativa da legislação sobre rótulo alimentício do Brasil, Mercosul, Reino Unido e União Européia. Rev Saúde Pública. 2001; 35:217-23.

60. Barbour ME, Parker DM, Allen GC, Jandt KD. Human enamel erosion in constant composition citric acid solutions as a function of degree of saturation with respect to hydroxyapatite. J Oral Rehabil. 2005 Jan; 32(1):16-21.

61. The Caroline Walker Trust. Eating well for under-5s in child care: practical and nutritional guidelines, 2nd Edition. Report of an expert working group. London: CWT. 2006.

62. Rodrigues CS, Sheiham A. The relationships between dietary guidelines,

sugar intake and caries in primary teeth in lowincome Brazilian 3-year-olds: a longitudinal study. Int J Paediatr Dent. 2000; 10:47-55.

63. Harris R. Biology of the children of Hopewood House, Bowral, Australia. 4. Observations on dental caries experience extending over 5 years (1957-61). J Dent Res. 1963; 42:1387-99.

64. Silverstein SJ, Knapp JF, Kircos L, Edwards H. Dental caries prevalence in children with a diet free of refined sugar. Am J PublHlth. 1983; 73:1196-9.

65. The Caroline Walker Trust/National Heart Forum. Eating well at school: Nutritional and practical guidelines. London: CWT. 2005.

66. Victorian Government Department of Human Services.Promoting healthy eating for children: A planning guide for practitioners.Australia: DHS. 2005.

67. BRASIL. Portaria Interministerial N° 1.010 de 8 de maio de 2006. Institui as diretrizes para a Promoção da Alimentação Saudável nas escolas de educação infantil, fundamental e nível médio das redes públicas e privadas, em âmbito nacional. Ministério da Saúde/Ministério da Educação, Brasília, 2006. Disponível em: http://dtr2001.saude.gov.br/sas/PORTARIAS/Port2006/GM/GM-1010.htm. [Acessoem: 01 nov.2011]

68. Passos E, Magalhães NP, Gonçalves MEF, Moura VHV, Silva EB. Alimentação saudável nas escolas. Brasília a. 2006; 43:323-8.

69. Fanning EA, Gotjamanos T, Vowles NJ. Dental caries in children related to availability of sweets at school canteens. Med J Austr. 1969; i:1131-2.

70. Roder DM. The association between dental caries and the availability of sweets in South Australian school canteens. Austr Dent J. 1973; 18:174-82.

71. Pengelly JPB, Smith FJA. Incisor caries and primary schools tuckshops. Publ Health London. 1972; 86:183-8.

72. Hobson P. The effects of sugar-based medicines on the dental health of sick children. Br Dent J. 1984; 8:155-6.

73. Dangor CM, Veltman AM. Sugar-free liquid pharmaceuticals. S Afr Med J. 1986 Aug 16; 70(4):199-200.

74. Department of Health/The British Association for the Study of Community Dentistry. Delivering Better Oral Health: An evidence-based toolkit for prevention. London: DH/BASCD. 2007.

75. World Health Organization. Obesity: preventing and managing the global epidemic. Report of a WHO consultation.Tech Rep Ser. 2000.

76. Popkin BM, Gordon-Larsen P. The nutrition transition: worldwide obesity dynamics and their determinants.Int J Obesity. 2004; 28,S2-S9.

77. World Health Organization. Fifty-seven World Health Assembly. Global Strategy on Diet, Physical Activity and Health. Geneva; 2004. Disponível em: http://www.who.int/hpr/NPH/docs/gs_global_strategy_general.pdf. [acessed: 04/11/2011].

78. Flynn MA, McNeil DA, Maloff B, Mutasingwa D, Wu M, Ford C, Tough SC. Reducing obesity and related chronic disease risk in children and youth: a synthesis of evidence with 'best practice' recommendations. Obes Rev. 2006; 7Suppl 1:7-66.

79. Traebert J, Moreira EAM, Bosco VL, Almeida ICS. Transição alimentar: problema comum à obesidade e à cárie dentária. Rev Nutr. 2004; 17:247-53.

80. Croucher R. General dental practice, health education, and health promotion: a critical reappraisal. In: Schou L, Blinkhorn AS, editors. Oral Health Promotion. Oxford: Oxford Medical Publications. 1993; p.153-68.

81. World Health Organization. Otawa Charter for health promotion. Health Promotion. 1987; 1(44): iii-v.

82. Sheiham A. The role of the dental team in promoting dental health and general health through oral health. Int Dent J. 1992; 42:223-8.

83. Sanderson ME. Towards a sugar health policy [dissertation]. Cranfield Institute of Technology. 1984.

84. Sanderson ME. O caminho do futuro: a forçamotriz da política do açúcar. In: ABOPREV. Prática odontológica cen-

trada em prevenção: aspectos básicos. São Paulo, ABOPREV; 1991. Biblioteca Científica, Fascículo 2 - Açúcares: debate atual e ação futura.

85. Brasil. Ministério da Saúde. Coordenação Geral da Política de Alimentação e Nutrição. Ações de incentivo ao consumo de frutas e hortaliças do governo brasileiro. Brasília: Ministério da Saúde. 2009.

86. Martins KA, Freire MCM. Guias alimentares para populações: aspectos históricos e conceituais. Brasília Méd 2008. 45(4):291-302.

87. U.S. Department of Agriculture. Department of Health and Human Services. Dietary Guidelines for Americans 2005.Disponível em: http://www.healthierus.gov/dietaryguidelines. [acessoem: 04/11/2011].

88. Freire MCM, Cannon GJ, Sheiham A. Análise das recomendações internacionais sobre o consumo de açúcares publicadas entre 1961 e 1991. Rev Saúde públ. 1994; 28:228-37.

89. Sheiham A. Why free sugars consumption should be below 15 kg per person per year in industrialised countries: the dental evidence. Br Dent J. 1991; 171:63-5.

90. Brasil. Ministério da Saúde. Secretaria Nacional de Assistência à Saúde. Departamento de Atenção Básica. Coordenação Geral da Política de Alimentação e Nutrição. Guia alimentar para a população brasileira: promovendo a alimentação saudável. Brasília: Ministério da Saúde. 2006.

91. Department of Health. Dietary reference values for food energy and nutrients for the United Kingdom. Report of the panel on dietary reference values of the Committee on Medical Aspects of Food Policy. London: HMSO; 1991. Report on Health and Social Subjects Nº 41.

92. World Health Organization. WHO Regional Office for Europe. CINDI Dietary Guide. Copenhagen: WHO. 2000.

93. Department of Health/The British Association for the Study of Community Dentistry. Delivering Better Oral Health: An evidence-based toolkit for prevention. London: DH/BASCD. 2007.

Chapter 13

The Common Risk Factor Approach: Integrating Oral Cleanliness with General Cleanliness as Demonstrated in the Fit for School Project

Claides Abegg
Bella Monse

This chapter discusses the importance of hygiene habits for health promotion in the perspective of the common risk factor approach. It emphasizes the importance of the integration of oral and general hygiene habits to achieve more effective results. The first section presents a brief review of hygiene and health. This is followed by a discussion about the relationship between general and oral hygiene habits and health. The third section addresses integration of oral and general hygiene habits. In the last section, we describe the Fit for School programme, an example of a health promotion strategy that works with the common risk factor approach.

Hygiene and health: a brief history

Hygiene practices have accompanied humankind throughout history. In ancient times, the main reason for hygiene was concern about contamination. The relationship between human health and the environment began to develop as early as in ancient Greece.[1] Personal or body hygiene was very common in the remote past, but people did not know that invisible organisms are present in the air, on the hands and on the surfaces of objects, and can cause diseases in individuals and populations.[1,2] The idea that microorganisms can cause infectious diseases began to take shape in the 16th and 17th centuries. However, personal hygiene and hygiene of the family environment began to receive more attention from the 19th century onwards.[2]

The benefits obtained from the "modern concept of hygiene" include clean drinking water, basic sanitation, vaccine development and food production and storage. Also in relation to human health, there has been a decline of morbidity and mortality due to infectious diseases in developed countries and in some developing countries such as Brazil. Nowadays, efforts are concentrated more on preservation of environments and cleanliness, aiming to promote health and to preserve human life.[2]

Personal and domestic hygiene has not been extensively studied as it is considered a private topic involving intimate and moral issues.[3] Curtis[3] argues that there is a link between what is considered dirty, repugnant, hygiene and disease. This link has a strong evolutionary basis and is present in all societies.[3]

Ideas about hygiene and its practices are related to the maintenance of order and discipline[4], and is built on cultural foundations and permeates a vast range of societies and religions. At the same time, they are considered intuitive behaviours for avoiding the infection and contagion present since primeval times.[3]

Individuals have different motivations for the adoption of good hygiene practices, such as concern about health, for aesthetic reasons, to cause a good impression among peers and to be socially acceptable, to avoid contamination and protect their children´s health and to , create a pleasant environment to live in.[5,6]

The birth of a child increases the motivation for improved hygiene, with an increase in the frequency of handwashing and of antimicrobial product use.[6]

By caring for the oral and personal hygiene of their children, parents are showing and teaching the child how they should care for their body and mouth[7.]

Thus, during the primary socialization process, children learn hygiene behaviours and habits that are internalized and are not easy to change in adulthood, being integrated into the daily routine of people in an organized and slightly flexible way.[8,9] The routines practised in the morning when waking up and at night before going to sleep, such as tooth brushing and bathing, are considered the least flexible of the daily routines to change.[10] A study with British adults and another with Brazilian adults showed that oral hygiene habits are perceived as routine and are performed in a sequence of activities, time and place.[11,12] These behaviours are part of the "adaptation process to the everyday life of individuals and are integrated into their social relations forming part of a system that adds meaning to their lives".[13]

Hygiene habits and general and oral health

Daily cleaning of the mouth is an important habit in most societies. At the same time, tooth brushing is the most common method for cleaning teeth, and is considered a socially desirable habit. In a first review of literature on the subject, Gift[14] showed that in the United States and Europe brushing frequency was from once to twice a day. In a national study conducted in Finland in the 1970s, 43% of individuals brushed their teeth more than once a day. In a subsequent investigation carried out with schoolchildren from Nordic countries tooth brushing was a daily practice for most of the participants.[15] In a survey about oral hygiene habits in European adolescents reported improvements in tooth brushing lead to reductions in bacterial plaque and gingivitis between the 1970's and 1990's.[16] The United Kingdom National Oral Health Survey[17] showed that two thirds of the individuals said they brushed their teeth twice a day and 6% of the individuals replied that they brushed them less than once a day. Results of the same survey[18] in 2009 evidenced an increase in the percentage of individuals who brushed their teeth twice a day (75%) and a reduction of those who brushed less than once a day; only 2%. In a national study conducted in Chinese 12 and 18 year olds, toothbrushing frequency was mainly once a day.[19] The

brushing standard of once a day was also observed in Iranian adolescents.[5]

Brazilian studies report that the toothbrushing standards tended to be higher than in other countries. Marcenes and Sheiham,[20] in a study carried out with adults from Belo Horizonte, showed that the reported average daily brushing frequency was three times a day. Similarly, while investigating adults from Porto Alegre, Abegg[21] found a brushing frequency with mean and median of three times a day. In a later study conducted with adolescents and adults in southern Brazil, the most commonly reported toothbrushing frequency was three times a day.[22] In another study with adolescents from a satellite town near Porto Alegre, a high brushing frequency was also observed; 77,8% of the adolescents said that they brushed their teeth three or more times a day.[2]

The habit of cleaning the mouth and the teeth starts in early childhood integrating with the learning of other personal hygiene and cleanliness practices such as handwashing and bathing. It is in this period that health-related behaviours and habits are established, and are influenced throughout life by different factors.

Adequate oral hygiene, including brushing the teeth with fluoride toothpaste, is one of the most simple and efficient ways of preventing dental caries and periodontal disease.

Likewise, the practice of washing the hands can reduce the incidence of intestinal infections and of HNI1 flu.[24]

The occurrence of diseases such as type A flu (H1N1), raised the importance of the need for good hygiene habits such as washing the hands with soap on the public health agenda.

Hygiene and Infection

Lack of hygiene, inadequate sanitation and non-drinking water, are important causes of mortality and morbidity. Altogether, these factors are among the most important risk factors for diseases, representing a large portion of the worldwide disease burden. The disease burden due to shortage of drinking water, of sanitation and hygiene was estimated at 1,73 million deaths during the year 2000.[25]

The relationship between the adoption of hygiene measures such as an adequate source of water provision, handwashing before food preparation and early childhood health is imporatant. Epidemiological studies and investigations of diarrhoea have found an association between poor water quality, infectious diarrhoea and gastroenteritis, especially in developing countries. There was an improvement in health conditions, especially of children, after the implementation of adequate sanitation conditions.[26] A study compared the decline of diarrhoea and of malnutrition in children from villages in Bangladesh with and without the intervention of a hygiene education programmes, observing a greater decline in the locations with intervention. The authors also reported that the differences increased over time as a larger number of villages adopted the intervention.[27]

A significant percentage of intestinal infections occur in the family environment.[28] A study carried out in the United Kingdom demonstrated how contamination and transmission with microorganism can occur in the family environment. Of the individuals observed, 20% did not wash their hands with soap after using the toilet and only 43% did so after changing babie's nappies.[6]

In spite of the reduction in mortality caused by infectious and transmissible diseases, intestinal infectious diseases are still common in both developed and developing countries.[2]

A systematic review carried out in 2003 showed that regular handwashing with soap can reduce the rate of diarrhoea by 31% to 47% and that of respiratory diseases by up to 30%[24]

The Relationship between General and Oral Hygiene Habits

There is a relationship between oral hygiene habits and general hygiene habits. In one of the first investigations into the subject, Hodge et al.[29] described the association between the toothbrushing habit and general hygiene habits in English adolescents. The adolescents who brushed their teeth more frequently also bathed and changed their underwear more frequently. Bergler[30] assessed attitudes in relation to hygiene and cleanliness habits in Germany, France and Spain. The author noted a similarity between standards of body hygiene, house cleanliness and hygiene related to changes and washing of clothing. Individuals who brushed their teeth more frequently also cleaned the house and changed their underwear more frequently. A study conducted with Brazilian adults showed that toothbrushing frequency was associated with the use of dental floss. Individuals who brushed their teeth less frequently also used dental floss less often.[12]

Studies with adolescents found that among the youngest ones the group that brushed their teeth and used dental floss most frequently also washed their hands more often after using the toilet.[31,32] In a survey with Kenyan youths between 14 and 17 years of age, an association was observed between toothbrushing, bathing and handwashing after using the toilet.[33]

Dorri, Sheiham and Watts[34] recently proposed an explanatory theoretical model for the association between general and oral hygiene habits (Fig. 13.1).

The model is based on the rationale that general and oral hygiene habits have similar motivations, as well as on the evidence of the association between general and oral hygiene habits. The social and demographic variables are at the distal level, while the Sense of Coherence, which comprehends several psychological factors and has been associated with health-related behaviours, and the social network of peer groups in which quality and quantity are measured, are at the intermediate level.[34]

The model was tested on Iranian adolescents and showed that socio-demographic variables such as sex and education influence general and oral hygiene habits, and the relationship between these, through their impact on the Sense of Coherence and on the networks of peer groups of adolescents. In another study on the same population, the authors found a positive association between oral hygiene habits and general hygiene habits. The adolescents who presented greater brushing frequency also bathed and changed their underwear more frequently.[5]

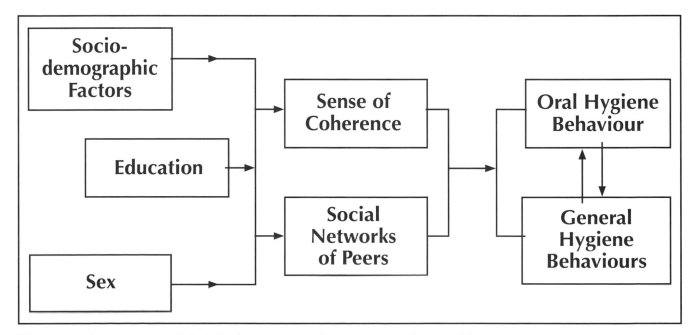

Fig. 13.1 – Theoretical model of the factors that influence oral and general hygiene habits in adolescents.

The reviewed studies provide convincing evidence of the association between general and oral hygiene habits and at the same time suggest that all hygiene habits have similar motivations, emphasizing the importance of the integration of these habits in the planning of health promotion actions. Thus, the incorporation of oral and general health in health promotion activities, for example, at schools, improves the general health conditions of children and adolescents, with a positive impact on their school performance.

> General and oral hygiene habits are associated. Strategies for promoting oral health should be developed together with those of general health.

Health promotion can be performed in different places, the workplace, a university, a nursery or a school. Whichever the place in which the health promotion activities are implemented, their development should cover all the different levels, mobilizing individual and organizational resources with the objective of improving the health of individuals.[35]

The current health promotion proposal is based on the amplified concept of health having appreciation of life, solidarity, completeness, equality and citizenship as a guideline.[36] The different strategies proposed by health promotion emphasize the importance of intersectoral action, encouraging cooperation and partnerships in a conjugated effort with the objective of improving the health of the population as a whole or of specific population groups. Intersectorality can be defined as "the articulation of knowledge and experiences in the participative identification of collective problems, in integrated decisions about policies and investments, aiming to obtain social returns in the perspective of social inclusion"[37] and reduction of inequality. Intersectoral action is not an easy task, considering that it is necessary to respect and understand different views on matters related to health.[36] At the same time, the integrated performance of sectors, both public and private, makes it possible to learn about the functioning of these sectors and to understand the role of each one. In this way it allows planning and development of activities with clearly established goals and adequate knowledge of local needs and resources.[35,36] The need for joint action targeting health promotion by the various sectors of society is widely recognized. The joint efforts and the alliances between government agencies, community organisations, health professionals, urban planners, workers, parents and pupils is considered the most efficient and cost-effective way of developing health promotion programmes.[35]

> The integrated performance of several sectors of society with the participation of different social players is the most efficient and cost-effective strategy for performing health promotion.

Although any social place is suitable for health promotion activities, schools have been one of the main focal points for health promotion activities (See Chapter 18 and 19). In most countries, individuals spend a lengthy period of their lives at school. Thus schools facilitate continuity of health promotion activities, an essential aspect for the success of any programme whose goal is to promote the health of individuals. Moreover, as mentioned previously, it is in childhood and adolescence that health-related behaviours are usually established and integrated in the daily family routine.

Health promotion programmes integrating general hygiene habits with oral hygiene habits are an example of the application of the common risk factor approach bringing benefits both for oral health and for the general health of schoolchildren. Moreover, programmes should be planned taking into account both culture and local practices. As an example, we present below a description of the Fit for School[38] (FFS) health promotion programme for schoolchildren.

Fit for School (FFS)

In 2008, the government of the Philippines launched a nationwide health promotion programme for infants and toddlers (nurseries) and schoolchildren. It is a comprehensive programme developed in partnership by the Ministry of Health, the Ministry of Education and nongovernmental organizations. FFS works on the logic of the involvement of different social players, teachers, carers, parents and pupils, as it considers them jointly responsible for the construction of sustainable health. Although it uses international guidelines and recommendations, the programme is focused on local needs, taking into account the culture and existing knowledge. FFS uses the existing school structure for its implementation, constituting simple interventions, based on scientific evidence, geared towards the most prevalent diseases among children, such as respiratory infections, diarrhoea, worm infections and dental caries.

> Health promotion programmes and strategies should be adapted respecting the local needs, taking into considering the social, cultural and economic differences of countries and regions.

The implemented activities are as follows:
- Supervised daily handwashing with soap
- Supervised tooth brushing with fluoride toothpaste
- Semi-annual de-worming by means of the supervised ingestion of one albendazole pill.

FFS is innovative as it is simple and comprehensive, driven by international guidelines such as the Focusing Resources on Effective School Health model, proposed by UNESCO/WHO and by the actions described in the Ottawa Charter (1986).[39] The Ottawa Charter[39] considers that health cannot be achieved without the coordinated action of different social sectors. To this effect, a decentralized power and leadership were established from the alliance between central and local government, teachers, pupils and the community. The technical and organizational support is offered to the Department for Education and to the local government, by the nongovernmental organization Fit for School Inc. Technical guidelines, informative manuals and practical support are also offered for the programme´s implementation.[40]

FFS managed to overcome the barriers that traditionally exist between the health and education sectors, implementing mutual collaboration aiming to reach a common goal. Furthermore, professionals not belonging to the area of health, such as teachers, schoolchildren, parents and local politicians, are involved and trained to promote health and to prevent disease. At the same time, health professionals play an important role in the training of human resources, in the monitoring and assessment of the programme.[38]

Fit for School is implemented by the education sector. However, the department of health of the local government is responsible for the purchase of the necessary materials (dentifrice, toothpaste, toilet soap and worm medicines), geared towards the development of the programme. The proposal of FFS is to face diseases with a high impact in an all-encompassing manner.

By reaching all children of school and preschool age, using health promotion activities, FFS reduces the disease burden, fostering equity and reducing inequality. In this manner, it stimulates the children's development, facilitating the attainment of proposed targets in relation to health in early childhood, both at a national and international level.[40]

> By means of a set of simple yet effective actions, Fit for School affects part of the population that is in a vulnerable situation in relation to a large number of health problems.[40]

The creation of environments to support health promotion is one of the main actions proposed by the Ottawa Charter, emphasizing the importance of the close relationship between individuals and the environment. In the case of FFS, one of the first initiatives taken to make the school a healthy environment is access to water. When there is no piped water, tippy taps, special pipes made from material that is both recycled (water bottles) and from the actual region (Figs. 13.2 and 13.3), are built. An interesting aspect is the involvement of children, parents and teachers in the preparation of these materials.[38,40] Toothbrushes are also distributed to the schoolchildren, encouraging each pupil to personalize his or her brush, thus allowing its identification (Figs. 13.4 and 13.5). Moreover, special spaces are built to store the brushes (Fig. 13.6). Thus, due to its transformation into a healthy social space, the school favours the assimilation of healthy habits in the first years of life, helping to form a healthy adult. The health education offered to schoolchildren has clear and realistic goals. By proposing the integration of health promotion behaviours in the children's daily routine it favours the lifelong maintenance of these behaviours.

Another important characteristic of the programme is sustainability.[38] The annual cost of materials per child is around 0,50 US dollars, which is relatively low, even for the poorer regions. The planning included the involvement of international development agencies in its initial stage and the gradual reduction of their participation over time, limited to timely intervention in monitoring and evaluation. The responsibilities of all the social players involved are defined in the planning of the programme. Besides being the beneficiaries, the chil-dren are also actively involved in the development in all the programme stages.[40]

The annual assessment is part of the development of FFS. A class is selected at random to be assessed at each school. The schools are also encouraged to perform their own self-assessment. The programme was initially implemented as a community project in one of the provinces of the country. An interesting aspect emphasized in the development of FFS were the gains obtained during the implementation process, such as the increase in access to water and sanitation and the gradual adhesion of the schools. The result was the incorporation of 3,850 in the program by the year 2010.[38]

Children can play the role of educators: older children can educate younger children, obtaining benefits both for the pupil and for the educator.

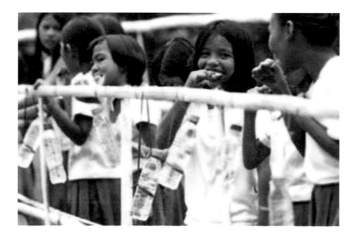

Fig. 13.2 – Water bottles used to supply water for washing hands.

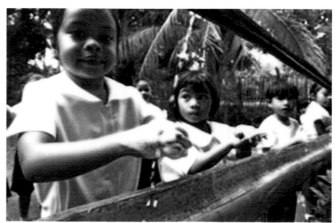

Fig. 13.3 – Tippy taps, special 'pipes' made from localy available natural material.

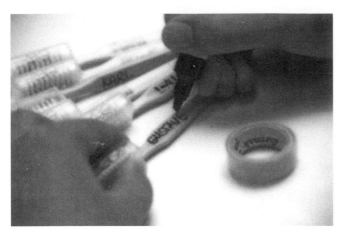

Fig. 13.4 – Toothbrushes with child's name on it.

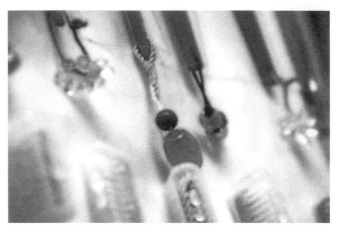

Fig. 13.5 – Toothbrushes with identifiable attachment to personalize them.

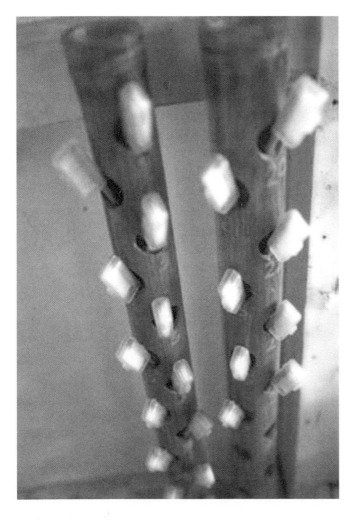

Fig. 13.6 – Special holder madeto store the tooth.

Final considerations

General and oral hygiene habits are learnt by children in their first years of life and become an integral part of the daily routine of families. These routines are generally organized and are not very easy to change. Simple hygiene habits such as brushing the teeth with fluoride toothpaste and washing the hands with soap can assist in the prevention of caries and of periodontal disease, as well as of diseases that are common in early childhood, such as intestinal infection.

There is ample evidence of the association between general and oral hygiene habits. At the same time, the motivations that lead people to develop these habits appear similar, stressing the importance of the simultaneous development importance of general and oral health promotion strategies. The Fit for School programme, developed and implemented at nurseries and schools in the Philippines, is an example of the success of strategies driven by the principles of health promotion and of the common risk factor approach.

References

1. Terpstra PMJ. Hygiene and Disinfection. Int Biodeterior Biodegradation. 1988; 41, 3 e 4: 169-175.
2. Stanwell-Smith R. The infection potential in the home and the role of hygiene: historical and current perspectives. Int J Environ Health Res. 2010; 13, suppl 001.
3. Curtis V. Dirt, disgust and disease: a natural history of hygiene. J Epidemiol Community Health. 2008; 61:660-664.
4. Douglas M. Purity and Danger: an analysis of the concepts of Pollution and Taboo. London: Ark. 1988.
5. Dorri M, Sheiham A, Watt RG. Relationship between general hygiene behaviours and oral hygiene behaviours in Iranian adolescents. Eur J Oral Sci. 2009; 117:407-412.
6. Curtis A, Birana B, Deverel K, Hughes C, Bellamy K, Drasar B. Hygiene in the home: relating bugs and behaviour. Soc Sci Med. In press.
7. Freeman R. The determinants of dental health attitudes and behaviours. British Den J. 1999; 187 1:15-8.
8. Baric, L, Blinkhorn, SA, MacArthur. A health education approach to nutrition and dental health education. Health Educ J. 1974; 33:79-90.
9. Abegg, C, Croucher, R, Marcenes, WS., Sheiham A. How do routines of daily activities and flexibility of daily activi-

ties affect tooth-cleaning behavior? J of Public Health Dent. 2000; 154-158.
10. Cullen IG, Phelps E. Diary techniques and problems of urban life. Joint Unit for Planning Research. University College London. 1975.
11. Croucher R. The performance gap. Health Education Authority Report 23. London: Health Education Authority. 1989.
12. Abegg, C. Factors affecting Tooth Cleaning Pattern, Structure and Performance in Brazilian Adults. Ph.D. Thesis, Department of Epidemiology and Public Health, University College London. 1996.
13. Hunt MS, Macleod M. Health and behavioural change: some lay perspectives. Community Med. 1987; 9 68-76.
14. Gift HC. Current utilization patterns of oral hygiene practices: state-of-the-science review. In Löe, H and Kleinman, DV,(eds.). Dental plaque control measures and oral hygiene practices. Oxford: IRL. 1986; p.39-71.
15. Rise J, Haugejorden O, Wold B, Aarö LE. Distribution of dental health behaviours in Nordic schoolchildren. Community Dent Oral Epidemiol. 1991; 19:9-13.
16. Honkala E, Freeman, R. Oral hygiene behavior and periodontal status in European adolescents: an overview. Community Dent Oral Epidemiol, 1988; 16:194-8.
17. Todd J, Lader D. Adult dental health 1988. United Kingdom. London: HMSO. 1991.

18. Adult Dental Health Survey 2009. Summary Report. [Internet] NHS: The information Centre for Health and Social Care. United Kingdom. [Cited 03/24/2011] Available at: http://www.ic.nhs.uk/pubs/dentalsurveyfullreport09

19. Zhu L, Petersen PE, Wang HY, Bian JY, Zhang BX. Oral health knowledge, attitudes and behaviour of adults in China. Int Dent J. 2005 Aug.; 55(4):231-41.

20. Marcenes WS, Sheiham A. The relationship between work stress and oral health status. Soc Sci Med. 1992; 35:1511-1520.

21. Abegg, C. Hábitos de higiene bucal de adultos porto-alegrenses. Rev Saúde Pública. 1997; 31(6):586-593.

22. Lisboa IC, Abegg C. Hábitos de higiene bucal e uso de serviços odontológicos por adolescentes e adultos do Município de Canoas, Estado do Rio Grande do Sul, Brasil. Epidemiologia e Serviços de Saúde. 2006 out-dez; 15(4):29-39.

23. Freddo SL et al. Hábitos de higiene bucal e utilização de serviços odontológicos em escolares de uma cidade da Região Sul do Brasil. Cad Saúde Pública. Rio de Janeiro, 2008 set; 24(9):1991-2000.

24. Curtis V, Cairncross S. Effect of washing hands with soap on diarrhoea risk in the community: a systematic review. Lancet Infect Dis. 2003; 3:275-281.

25. Prüss A, Kay D, Fewtrell L, Bartram J. Estimating the burden of disease from water, sanitation, and hygiene at a global level. Environ Health Perspect. 2002; 110(5):537-542.

26. Esrey SA. Water, waste, and well-being: a multicountry study. Am J Epidemiol. 1996; 143:608-623.

27. Shahid N, Greenough W, Samadi A, Huq M, Rahaman N. Hand washing with soap reduces diarrhoea and spread of bacterial pathogens in a Bangladesh village. J Diarrhoeal Dis Res. 1996; 14:85-89.

28. Scott EA, Bloomfield SF, Barlow CG. An investigation of microbial contamination in the domestic environment. J Hyg (Lond). 1982; 89:279-293.

29. Hodge, HC, Holloway, PJ, Bell, CR. Factors associated with toothbrushing behaviour in adolescents. Br Dent J. 1982; 152:49-51.

30. Bergler R. Personal hygiene and cleanliness in an international comparison. Zentralbl Bakteriol Mikrobiol Hyg B. 1989; 187:422-507.

31. Macgregor ID, Balding JW. Toothbrushing and smoking behaviour in 14-year-old English schoolchildren. Community Dent Health. 1987; (4):27-34.

32. Macgregor ID, Balding JW, Regis D. Motivation for dental hygiene in adolescents. Int J Paediatr Dent. 1997; (7):235-241.

33. Nzioka BM, Nyaga JK, Wagaiyu EG. The relationship between tooth brushing frequency and personal hygiene habits in adolescents. East Afr Med J. 1993; 70:445-448.

34. Dorri M, Sheiham A, Watt RG. Modelling the factors influencing general and oral hygiene behaviours in adolescence. Int J Paediatr Dent. 2010; 20:261-269.

35. Moyses S, Watt R. Promoção de Saúde Bucal – Definições. In: Buischi, YP, (org.). Promoção de saúde bucal na clínica odontológica. São Paulo: Artes Médicas. 2000; p.1-21.

36. Aerts D, Alves G. G., La Salvia, M. V., Abegg, C. Promoção de saúde: a convergência entre as propostas da vigilância da saúde e da escola cidadã. Cad Saúde Pública. Rio de Janeiro, 2004 jul-ago; 20(4):1020-1028.

37. Junqueira LAP, Inojosa RM. O movimento do setor saúde e o desafio da intersetorialidade. (Cadernos Fundap 21). São Paulo: Fundap. 1996.

38. Monse B, Naliponguit E, Belizário V, Benzian H, W van Palenstein Helderman. Essencial health care package for children – the "Fit for School" programme in the Philippines. Int Dent J. 2010; 60(2):85-93.

39. The Ottawa Charter for Health Promotion 1986. [Internet] WHO. [cited 09/19/2011] Available at: http://who.int/hpr/NPH/docs/ottawa_charter_hp.

40. Monse B et al. Fit for School Inc. Manual for teachers for the implementation of essential health care program in schools. Fit for School Inc., Cagayan de Oro, Philippines. 2010.

Chapter 14

Prevention of Smoking Using the Common Risk Factor Approach: the Roles of Dentists Prevention of Smoking in Adolescents

Mario Vianna Vettore

Introduction

The epidemic of cigarette smoking is a global challenge, as smoking remains the single leading worldwide cause of preventable diseases and deaths. The hazards associated with cigarette smoking have been well documented since the 1950's.[1-3] The World Health Organization estimates that almost 6 million people die each year from direct tobacco use and second-hand smoke.[4] Although the reduction in smoking in recent years, it remains one of the foremost risk factors related to the 63% of all deaths caused by noncommunicable diseases (NCDs).

Cigarette smoking has been directly implicated in numerous oral diseases including oral cancer and precancer, periodontal disease, tooth loss, poor wound healing and implant's failure.[5,6]

In addition to the direct harmful effects of smoking, passive smoking, the so-called secondhand smoke, causes serious respiratory problems in children and adolescents. Exposure to secondhand smoke, where nonsmokers are exposed to environmental tobacco smoke as a result of their proximity to individuals who smoke, is also harmful to health.[7] Older children whose parents smoke get sick more often. Their lungs are less developed than children who do not breathe secondhand smoke, and they get more bronchitis and pneumonia. Children and adolescents with asthma who inhale secondhand smoke have more severe and frequent asthma attacks.[7,8] As will be outlined later, discouraging parents from smoking will not only improve the health of their children but, more importantlt, will decrease the risk of their children smoking.

NCDs and oral diseases are socially determined (see Chapter 7). So are their main proximal determinants: smoking, unhealthy diet, insufficient physical activity and excessive use of alcohol. The greatest effects of these risk factors fall increasingly on low- and middle-income countries, and on poorer people within all countries, mirroring the underlying social determinants.[4]

Different approaches for smoking control have been developed and implemented. They include educational, clinical, regulatory, economic and comprehensive. Notwithstanding, smoking during adolescence remains a paramount public health problem and poses a challenge to reduce tobacco-related diseases.

There are very few reported health promotion activities directed at smoking prevention by oral health services. Dentist's activities have mainly focused on the individual approach of smoking cessation; recording smoking status, providing advice and self-help material.[5] The barriers to dentists implementing cessation counseling are lack of knowledge, time constraints, lack of smoking cessation experts to refer people to, lack of reimbursement, and feeling inadequate.[9] Moreover, the limitations of individual-centred approach in smoking cessation are widely recognized. Therefore a shift is required towards a comprehensive and multidisciplinary approach, such as the common risk factor approach.

In contrast to strategies directed to prevent some specific chronic diseases, the underlying concept of the common risk factor approach is that tackling a few, but relevant number of risk factors, may have a greater impact on a large number of diseases than directing attention to each specific disease caused by that behaviour. Most NCDs are tobacco-related, and are considered important public health problems. They include coronary heart diseases, stroke, cancers, respiratory diseases, metabolic diseases and oral diseases, such as oral cancer, periodontal disease and tooth loss.[10]

Other inadequate health-related behaviours have been implicated in the initiation and progress of different systemic conditions and oral diseases. Poor diet characterized by satured fatty acids and non milk extrinsic sugars is associated with chonic conditions such as cardiovascular diseases, diabetes, obesity and dental caries.[11] High alcohol consumption is related to cardiovascular disease, some cancers, neurological diseases and periodontal disease.[12] The common risk factor approach has positive aspects compared to those directed to specific disease including lower cost, greater efficiency and effectiveness (See Chapter 7).

This chapter highlights the role of dentists in tobacco control in adolescents applying the principles of the Ottawa Charter for health promotion and the common risk factor approach.[13,14] First the prevalence of smoking and current trends among young smokers will be presented. Then, different aspects concerning smoking control in adolescents in a public health perpective are outlined including the clustering of smoking with other health-related behaviours, the social issues related to smoking initiation, the role of tobacco industries on smoking, surveillance and information on smoking, recommendations for implementing smoking cessation policies, role of dentists and other professionals in reducing smoking in adolescents and effectiveness of tobacco control in the dental office.

Prevalence of smoking and current trends among young smokers

Although cigarette smoking in adults declined from the 1960s through to the 1980s, recent reports indicate that smoking prevalence has remained relatively stable through the 1990s. During the last 20 years, a steadly decline in smoking has been reported in most occidental countries.[15]

Table 14.1 shows per capita cigarette consumption in the various regions of the world, according to distribution criteria prepared by WHO.[16] The overall world decrease in consumption between 1970-1972 and 1980-1982 was noteworthy (1.6%). However, cigarette consumption stabilized between 1980–1982 and 1990-1992. The trends varied considerably among the WHO regions and between industrialized and developing countries. While the region of the Americas experienced the highest decline in annual per capital consumption of cigarettes representing -1.5% percentage change, an increase of 3.0% was observed in the Region of the Western Pacific between 1970-1972 and 1990-1992. Both industrialized and developing countries experienced an increase in cigarette consumption between 1970-1972 and 1980-1982. Industrialized and developing countries experienced opposite trends between 1980-1982 and 1990-1992. There was an overall reduction in industrialized countries (-0.5%) and an increase of 2.5% in developing countries.[16]

The current prevalence of daily tobacco smoking in adults aged 15 years and older varied widely among the six WHO regions in 2008 (Fig. 14.1). The highest overall prevalence for smoking is estimated at nearly 29% in the European Region, while the lowest is in the African Region (8%). The highest prevalence of smoking among men was in the Western Pacific Region (46%) and among women in the European Region (20%). In all regions, men smoked more than women, with the largest disparities for daily cigarette smoking being in the Western Pacific Region, where men smoked 15 times more than women, followed by the South-East Asia Region where men smoked 10 times more than women. The smallest disparity between men and women was in the Region of the Americas, where men smoke about 1.5 times more than women. Among men, the highest prevalence of smoking was in lower-middle-income countries. Smoking then declines as country income rises. Among women, relatively high rates (around 15%) are reported in upper-middle and high-income countries, and about five times lower (between 2% and 4%) in low- and lower-middle-income countries.[4]

Table 14.1. Global and Regional estimates and trends in cigarette consumption among adults 15 years and older, 1970–1972 to 1990–1992.

WHO regions and conutries	Average annual per capita consumption		
	1970-1972	1980-1982	1990-1992
Region of Africa	460	570	590
Region of the Americas	2,580	2,510	1,900
Region of the Eastern Mediterranean	700	940	930
Region of Europe	2,360	2,500	2,340
Region of Southeast Asia	850	1,140	1,230
Region of the Western Pacific	1,100	1,610	2,010
Industrialized countries	2,860	2,980	1,590
Developing countries	860	1,220	1,410
World	1,410	1,650	1,660

Source: Pan American Health Organization. Health in the Americas. Washington; 1998.[16]

Fig. 14.1 – Age-standardized prevalence of daily tobacco smoking in adults aged 15 or more years, by WHO Region and World Bank income group, comparable estimates, 2008.

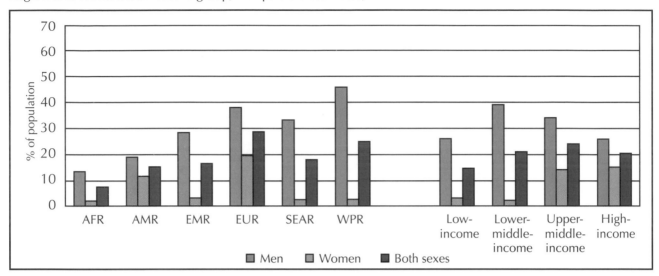

AFR: African countries, AMR: Americas, EMR: Eastern Mediterranean, EUR: Europe, SEAR: South-East Asia Region, WPR: Western Pacific Region
Source: World Health Organization. Global status Report on noncomunicable diseases. Geneva: WHO; 2010.[4]

Data from the last Global Adult Tobacco Survey conducted by the Brazilian Ministry of Health showed 17.2% of people 15 years or older were smokers, representing a total of 26.6 million people. Brazil also experienced a dramatic decline in smoking prevalence. Between 1996 and 2008 there was almost 48% decrease in smoking prevalence among adults aged 18 years or older.[17]

Information on the prevalence of cigarette smoking among adolescents was scarce until the 2000's when the WHO's Tobacco Free Initiative (TFI), and the Centers for Disease Control and Prevention (CDC) Office on Smoking and Health (OSH) have developed the Global Youth Tobacco Survey (GYTS). The GYTS employs a standard methodology completed by a representative school based sample of students primarily between the ages of 13-15 years. In 2002 data representing 43 countries was published. It was estimated that 13.9% of the adolescents are current smokers, defined as having smoked on one or more days in the

30 days preceding the survey. The estimates ranged from 0.5% in Goa, India to 39.6% in Chile. Nearly 25% of students, who smoke, smoked their first cigarette before the age of 10 years.[18]

Figure 14.2 summarizes the 2009 report of the Global Youth Tobacco Survey (GYTS). Overall, 9% of boys and 12% of girls aged 13-15 years old are current smokers. Cigarette smoking prevalence for boys and girls varies between regions, from less than 8% in Eastern Mediterranean to 21% in Europe for the former group, and from 2% in Eastern Mediterranean and South-East Asia to 17% in Europe for the latter 19.

In the last Brazilian school-based national health survey, involving adolescents between 13 to 15 years old from public and private primary schools, the prevalence of those who tried smoking once in a lifetime was 24%. Of them, 49.3% experienced smoking before 12 years old. Frequency of regular smokers less than 13 years old was 3.5%, and increased for 4.8% and 9.7% for those with 14 years and 15 years of age.[20]

Fig. 14.2 – Global cigarette smoking prevalence smoking in adolescents aged 13-15 years.

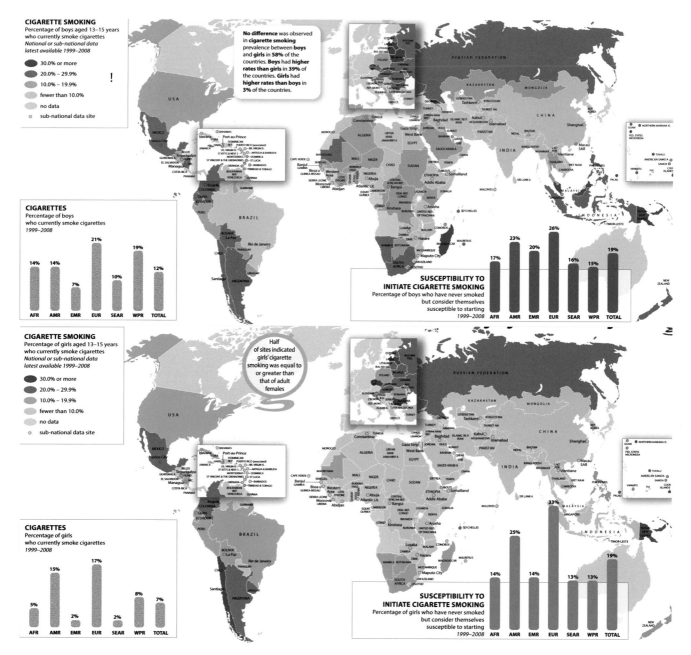

AFR: African countries, AMR: Americas, EMR: Eastern Mediterranean, EUR: Europe, SEAR: South-East Asia Region, WPR: Western Pacific Region

Source: Warren CW, Asma S, Lee J, Lea V, Mackay J. Global Tobacco Surveillance System. The GTSS Atlas. CDC. 2009.[19]

One of the first specific reports focusing on the problem of tobacco use among young people and its trends was published in 1994 by the National Center for Chronic Disease Prevention and Health Promotion, CDC 21. Some successful strategies in reducing adolescent use of tobacco were also proposed by CDC including communitywide efforts that include tobacco tax increases, enforcement of minor's access laws, you-th-oriented mass media campaigns, and school-based tobacco-use prevention programs.[21] The CDC report outlined six key characteristics of the trends among young smokers as presented in Box 14.1.

Box 14.1 – Key characteristics of the trends among young smokers.

1. Nearly all, first use of tobacco occurs before high school graduation; this finding suggests that if adolescents can be kept tobacco-free, most will never start using tobacco.
2. Most adolescent smokers are addicted to nicotine and report that they want to quit but are unable to do so; they experience relapse rates and withdrawal symptoms similar to those reported by adults.
3. Tobacco is often the first drug used by those young people who use alcohol, marijuana, and other drugs.
4. Adolescents with lower levels of school achievement, with fewer skills to resist pervasive influences to use tobacco, with friends who use tobacco, and with lower self-images are more likely than their peers to use tobacco.
5. Cigarette advertising appears to increase young people's risk of smoking by affecting their perceptions of the pervasiveness, image, and function of smoking.
6. Communitywide efforts that include tobacco tax increases, enforcement of minor's access laws, youth-oriented mass media campaigns, and school-based tobacco-use prevention programs are successful in reducing adolescent use of tobacco.

Source: CDC, 1994[21]

Clustering of smoking and other health-compromising behaviour in adolescents

There are a number of key health-compromising behaviours related to numerous chronic and oral diseases. Evidence from health surveys of children and adolescents show that they cluster (See Chapter 4). There are other core features concerning health-compromising behaviours in adolescents. They include the importance of childhood and adolescence as critical periods for initiation of smoking and other unhealthy behaviours. Most importantly, studies show that smoking is a gateway habit for adoption of other health-compromising behaviours and highlight the relationship of social milieu such as peer's influence and family's structure with smoking behaviour and clustering of health-related behaviours.

There are clear temporal developmental stages in the use of licit and illicit drugs from adolescence through to young adulthood. The period of transition from adolescence to adulthood, is critical for establishment of risk factors for chronic diseases that are associated with lifestyle behaviours such as smoking and unbalanced diet, has its roots in this period.[22] The term "youth" refers to a period overlapping with adolescence in which individuals make the transition from the dependency of childhood to the independence of adulthood. It is no longer clear, however, what the boundaries of this stage in the life-course are.[23]

Smoking is usually the first health-compromising behaviour experienced by adolescents and can be considered the gateway behaviour to the initiation and regular use of ilicit drugs and prescribed psychoactive drugs.[24-26] In addition, due to the fact that tobacco is a licit drug and socially acceptable, it usually produces a multiplying effect for the use of other psychostimulant drugs, such as marijuana.[24,25,27] A striking difference is the greater importance of cigarettes among women than among men in the sequence of drug involvement. Cigarettes can precede marijuana and other ilicit drugs in the absence of alcohol use among women, whereas alcohol, even in the absence of cigarettes, consistently precedes marijuana use among men.[25] The identification of developmental sequence in drug involvement does not invariably imply that the use of licit or illicit drugs at a particular stage will lead to the use of other more serious drugs.

Another striking pattern regarding smoking in youth is that once they become weekly smokers, they are unlikely to give up smoking. Furthermore, of the adolescents who are current smokers, an increasing percentage will remain smokers over the forthcoming years since they will be unable or unwilling to quit smoking.[28]

Epidemiological studies show that the distribution of different oral and general health-related behaviours does not occur randomly within populations. In fact, some unhealthy behaviours, which are common risk factors for oral and systemic diseases are concentrated in particular groups of individuals. The clustering phenomenon of behavioural risk factors is also observed in adolescents and smoking is the lifestyle behaviour that presents the strongest associations with a range of other health-compromising behaviours.[20,26,29-35] In addition to poor diet and alcohol, others behaviours, particularly harmful for adolescent's health and their development, have been associated with smoking, including being involved in fights, carrying weapons, engaging in higher-risk sexual behavior and drugs use.[21]

A WHO cross-national study, the 'Health Behaviour in School-aged Children', involved children and adolescents between 11 and 15 years old in 29 European countries and North America. The analysis of health behaviours, health status and social context showed that several risk factors were associated with high smoking prevalences in all countries. There was an increased likelihood of smoking among adolescents in stepfamilies, even after other factors were taken into account.[30]

In Brazil, findings from the last National School-Based Health Survey (PeNSE) showed strong associations between regular smoking and behavioural risk factors in adolescents. Regular smokers were almost 6 times more likely to have consumed alcohol in the last month and almost 7 times more likely to have tried drugs.[20]

There was an association of smoking with alcohol and use of drugs in students from 9 to 19 years of age in the Federal District of Brasília. When stratified by sex, 80% of male students and 73% of female students who smoked also consumed alcoholic beverages. The prevalence of illicit drug use among students who smoked was 24%, and it was greater among boys (32%) than it was among girls

(16%). The association between smoking and alcohol/drug use by adolescent students was greater in public schools than in private schools.[26] Similarly, alcohol use and illicit drug use were linked to smoking in 15 years old adolescents in North-eastern France. The prevalence of alcohol use and illicit drug use were respectively 7 and 10 times higher in smokers than in non-smokers.[29]

A national study in Canada involving 4724 children and adolescents (10-17 years-old) revealed that the prevalence of having three risk factors, and four or five risk factors increased with age while the prevalence of having zero or one risk factor decreased with age, for both males and females. The prevalence of multiple behavioral risk factors did not differ by sex and no association was found between the number of risk factors and socioeconomic status.[33]

Adolescents demonstrating inadequate oral health behaviours also engage in general health-compromising behaviours. Toothbrushing frequency was positively associated with the frequency of taking showers and inversely associated with the frequency of changing underwear.[36] A study of Finnish and Turkish pre-adolescents, 10-12 years old, showed that eating fast foods and drinking fizzy drinks was associated with watching TV for two or more hours per day in school days.[31] Smoking and others behavioural risk factors has been also associated with oral health-related behaviours in adolescents, including frequency of toothbrushing and dental visits.[32,34,35,37,38]

Petersen et al.[32] assessed the interrelationship between general and oral health-related behaviours in Chinese urban adolescents. Adolescents with high levels of preventive oral health practices also demonstrated general health-promoting behaviours. In factor analysis of general and oral health-related behaviours, three factors were isolated: (a) risk behaviours: playing computer games, alcohol habits, tobacco habits, watching TV, physical activity and the consumption of sugary foods/drinks, (b) health-promoting behaviours: oral hygiene practices, healthy dietary habits and general hygiene practices and (c) help-seeking behaviours: visit to the physician and visit to the dentist.

The association between general health-related behaviours, including smoking, and toothbrushing was evaluated in Brazil using the National School-Based Health Survey (PeNSE). Data from almost 50,000 adolescents revealed that sugar intake, smoking, alcohol consumption, drugs use, low levels of physical activity and use of seatbelts were statistically associated with toothbrushing. While toothbrushing frequency was significantly lower among adolescents from low socioeconomic families, smoking and low physical activity were higher among adolescents from socially disadvantage families.[35]

Social causes of smoking in adolescents

Health-related behaviours are associated with social conditions and family structure.[21,26,29-35] Smoking and other licit and illicit drugs are strongly influenced by social and cultural factors, such as social milieu, availability and legislation.

Adolescent's temptations to try smoking, onset of smoke and maintaining smoke are influenced by enabling and prohibition factors of the social environment in which they live. The psychosocial risk factors for initiating tobacco use are presented in Box 14.2.[21]

Box 14.2 – Psychosocial Risk Factors for Initiating Tobacco Use.

1. The initiation and development of tobacco use among children and adolescents progresses in five stages: from forming attitudes and beliefs about tobacco, to trying, experimenting with, and regularly using tobacco, to being addicted. This process generally takes about three years.
2. Sociodemographic factors associated with the onset of tobacco use include being an adolescent from a family with low socioeconomic status.
3. Environmental risk factors for tobacco use include accessibility and availability of tobacco products, perceptions by adolescents that tobacco use is normative, peers' and siblings' use and approval of tobacco use, and lack of parental support and involvement as adolescents face the challenges of growing up.
4. Behavioral risk factors for tobacco use include low levels of academic achievement and school involvement, lack of skills required to resist influences to use tobacco, and experimentation with any tobacco product.
5. Personal risk factors for tobacco use include a lower self-image and lower self-esteem than peers, the belief that tobacco use is functional, and lack of self-efficacy in the ability to refuse offers to use tobacco. For smokeless tobacco use, insufficient knowledge of the health consequences is also a factor.

Source: CDC, 1994[21]

Family members', peers', and best friend's smoking are key factors for smoking in young people.[39,40] The magnitude of the association between peer smoking and current smoking decreases from early adolescence to middle adolescence while the association between smoking at home and current smoking is static across developmental stage, after controlling for gender, race/ethnicity and exposure to tobacco industry and anti-tobacco media.[40]

Positive aspects associated with smoking reported by youths include social situations, such as while talking, relaxing and having a good time when a family member and/or a friend are smokers. Negative effect situations for smoking include severe anxiety and stress, and frustration. Adolescents are more prone to smoke when things are not going their way, when they need something to get through a difficult day, and when they are arguing with their families. Peer situations that favor smoking include when they want to be part of the crowd, with friends at a party, and when they are embarrassed to be a nonsmoker. Curiosity about cigarette smoking is another aspect related to try smoking and include curiosity about how a cigarette tastes and what type of feeling is associated with smoking.[41]

The adoption of smoking during youth is also related to sense of independence as individuals in this age group are beginning to accept responsibility for their own health behaviours and attitudes.[42]

The appeal of early smoking onset is strongly associated with gender norms and social acceptance among their peers and schoolmates.[43] The likelihood of current smoking was significantly associated with peer networks in which at least half of the members smoked and one or two best friends smoked. In addition, there was a significant interaction of popularity and school smoking prevalence. The risk of current smoking was somewhat greater among popular students in schools with high smoking prevalence than among popular students in schools with low smoking prevalence.[39]

Nevertheless, the positive social status related to cigarette smoking is still present within these groups and remains as the main factor that motivates more and more young people to experiment tobacco cigarettes. The abovementioned 'positive functions' are associated with bonding with peers, being independent and mature, and having a positive social image. Therefore, adolescents with lower self-esteem and lower self-images and so emotionally dependents are still the main targets of the tobacco industry.

Smoking rates are declining in most industrialized countries. The worldwide rates of decline of smoking are not similar accross socioeconomic groups. In many countries lower socioeconomic adolescents have been experiencing a slower reduction in smoking prevalence than those who are better off.[44] Hence, there is an increase in social inequality in cigarette smoking in adolescents as well as in other health-related behaviours.[34,35]

The relationship between low family socioeconomic status and smoking prevalence in adolescence is complex. Simplistic analysis report that smoking prevalence and levels of consumption are higher among youths from lower socioeconomic groups whether measured by parental education as in the United States, or parental social class in the United Kingdom.[45,46] In addition, adolescents with more formal years of schooling are significantly less likely to initiate smoking than are individuals with less education.[47] Awareness and literacy are considered important explanations for social class differences concerning smoking. Families and adolescents who are better off economically and with higher educational recognize smoking and exposure to second-hand smoke as risk factors for multiple health problems, and this was often influential in decisions not to smoke. However, although socioeconomic status of adolescents' family is a well-known predictor of smoking in youths, low literacy is not a singular aspect that mediates this relationship. Smoking during adolescence is affected by adolescent's personal income, access to tobacco and tobacco price.[48]

There is a paradox in the link between socioeconomic status backgrounds and smoking in young people. Some report that young people are more prices sensitive than adults, which means that the relation between tobacco price and smoking is important for young people, mainly for higher levels of smoking. In several countries, lower class youths have more personal money compared to their peers from higher social classes. Personal income is much more strongly related to smoking among young people from higher than lower class backgrounds because lower class youths have greater access to cheaper tobacco both from family and friends and from the illicit market. Many studies report that both smoking prevalence and consumption increase directly with the amounts of pocket money or money from other sources such as part-time earnings, which is uncommon in adolescents from wealthy families.[49] The plausible assumption that young people, like adults from higher socioeconomic status backgrounds, have more money and therefore would be more exposed to tobacco is greatly affected by their personal income and access/price of tobacco, which are crucial for tobacco consumption. In fact, individual purchasing power plays an important role in smoking in young people.[48]

For the poor, the increase in tobacco taxation during the last decades produced alternative ways to overcome fiscal policies, and therefore, obtain cheap cigarettes. They purchase smuggled and illicit cigarettes. That might have the unintended consequence of increasing class differentials in youth smoking rather than the reverse.[48]

These socioeconomic determinants of smoking in adolescents should be taken into consideration by dental associations and oral health professionals when they act as advocates and interact with local and national decision- and policy-makers in the development of strategies devoted for tobacco control. They should consider the evidence of clustering of health-related behaviours and the importance of taking into account the complexity of socioeconomic factors related to smoking in young people.

The role of tobacco industries on smoking in adolescents

Young people are a strategically important market for the tobacco industry since adolescents are the chief source of new consumers for the tobacco industry. In addition, young people are the most vulnerable age group to initiate smoking. Apart from the approach directed to health promotion to prevent and control tobacco smoking in adolescents, the 'social image' related to

smoking must be taken into account. This is a useful tool to choose the most appropriate health promotion strategy for each audience.

The boom in tobacco consumption was in the late of the 19th century and especially in the first half of the 20th century, and was strongly influenced by the media and film industry. The link between tobacco smoking and famous actors in Hollywood films, seen as symbols of success, had a strong influence on the onset of smoking spread throughout the world, especially among adolescents and young adults. The major tobacco companies have arisen and expanded using Hollywood actors in their media campaigns creating a false image of smoking as a socially positive behavior. Moreover, American films showing actors smoking referred to stereotypes of beautiful, attractive, strong, healthy and successful people. This strategy was more successful than any advertising campaign since the audience did not associate the product to the manufacturer or sponsor; the tobacco industry.[50,51]

An interesting historical contrast refers to the overlap between the great expansion of smoking and the onset of good scientific evidence about its harmful effects to health from the 1950s. At that time, media and advertising techniques transformed smoking into a social, family and acceptable behaviour. Furthermore, smoking became a desireable addiction because of the false image of success and modernity associated with it. The expansion of smoking occurred in parallel to the first publications of the irrefutable evidence of the harmful effects of smoking on different types of cancer in U.S 1,2 and the UK populations.[3] From the 1970s, when a significant proportion of deaths was attributed to smoking, a sharp overall decline in smoking was reported, but it slowed down from the 1980s. Throughout this period of decline in smoking, the juvenilization of smoking began, namely, an increasingly early onset of smoking, as the main consumer group became adolescents and young adults. The change in smoking onset regarding age group was also accompanied by other changes in the profile of consumers, such as the proportional increase in females, the so-called feminization in smoking, and a shift to socially underprivileged population groups.[22] However, this pattern was not observed in certain populations, like the Middle East.[52]

The changes in age of onset of smoking as well as the shift in smoker's demographic and socioeconomic profile did not occur at random. From the 1980s the scope of marketing of tobacco industry changed. Young adults from medium/high social classes were no longer the target population. Adolescents became a population group strategically important for the tobacco industry. Since most smokers try their first tobacco cigarette before they are 18 years old, young people are the chief source of new consumers for the tobacco industry, which each year must replace the many consumers who quit or die from smoking-related diseases.

The tobacco industry has been focusing on the concept of 'positive functions'. Until recently tobacco industries were allowed to be involved in promotional activities such as sponsorship of sports events to reach new consumers. Furthermore, most of the cigarette advertising used human models to display images of youthful activities, independence, healthfulness and adventure-seeking. In presenting attractive images of smokers, cigarette advertisements appear to stimulate some adolescents who have relatively low self-image to adopt smoking as a way to improve their own self-image. Despite the changes in legislation and other actions against smoking, the exposure to tobacco-related media remains associated with increased current and former smoking in both early and middle adolescence.[40]

Surveillance and information on smoking

Data collection and information availability on tobacco use are relevant components for the establishment of actions and strategies against smoking. Relevant websites concerning information about smoking at both national and international levels are available. They include websites from WHO, CDC US National Library and World Dental Federation (FDI) are presented in Box 14.3. In Brazil, the National Institute of Cancer is the governmental institution responsible for providing information about smoking.

Standardized mechanisms to collect youth tobacco use information on a global basis was established in 1998 by Tobacco Free Initiative (http://www.who.int/tobacco/en/) involving representatives from countries in each of the six WHO regions. The Global Tobacco Surveillance System (GTSS) was developed to "enhance country capacity to design, implement and evaluate tobacco control interventions, monitor key articles of the World Health Organization's (WHO) Framework Convention on Tobacco Control (FCTC) and components of the WHO MPOWER technical package". The GTSS includes the collection of data through four surveys: the Global Youth Tobacco Survey (GYTS); the Global School Personnel Survey (GSPS); the Global Health Professions Student Survey (GHPSS) and the Global Adult Tobacco Survey (GATS). The GYTS focuses on youth aged 13-15 and collects information in schools.

Box 14.3 – Key Website Sources of Information on Tobacco.

WHO Tobacco Free Initiative
    http://www.who.int/tobacco/en/
Global Youth Tobacco Survey (GYTS)
    http://www.who.int/tobacco/surveillance/gyts/en/index.html
Exposure to Secondhand Smoke Among Students Aged 13-15 Years. Worldwide,
    2000-2007
    http://www.cdc.gov/mmwr/preview/mmwrhtml/mm5620a2.htm#tab
WHO Tobacco and Oral Health
    www.who.int/oral_health/publications/ohpd01/en/
WHO Tobacco Control country profiles
    www.whocollab.od.mah.se/expl/tobacco.html
CDC Snmoking and Tobacco Use
    http://www.cdc.gov/tobacco/basic_information/index.htm
MedLine Plus. US National Library of Medicine
    http://www.nlm.nih.gov/medlineplus/smoking.html
Smoking facts
    http://www.smoking-facts.net/
National Institute of Cancer of Brazil
    http://www.inca.gov.br/tabagismo/
FDI World Dental Federation
    http://www.fdiworldental.org:8080/content/tobacco

Smoking cessation policies

Combatting tobacco use has been a public health priority in many countries. The best results are achieved when a comprehensive set of measures to reduce the use of tobacco are implemented together. Tobacco control encompasses a range of supply, demand and harm reduction strategies that aim to improve the health of a population by eliminating, or reducing, consumption of tobacco products and exposure to tobacco smoke.[53,54]

Along with an individual approach (behavioural and/or pharmacological interventions) to smoking cessation and treatment of tobacco dependence, a supportive environment is needed to encourage tobacco consumers in their attempts to quit. Treatment of tobacco dependence should be part of a comprehensive tobacco-control policy along with measures such as taxation and price policies, advertising restrictions, dissemination of information and establishment of smoke-free public places.[54,55] Recommendations to assist countries in implementing smoking cessation strategies were proposed by WHO in 2003 and are summarized in Box 14.4.[55]

Box 14.4 – Key recommendations for implementing smoking cessation strategies.

1. A smoking cessation policy should be part of any comprehensive tobacco--control policy if smoking cessation efforts are to be effective and sustainable;
2. A supportive environment, which includes a decrease in accessibility of tobacco products, a reduction in social acceptance of tobacco consumption and an increase in information, will improve the likelihood of smokers quitting;
3. All tobacco-users should be offered effective treatment for tobacco dependence;
4. Member States should develop evidence-based national policy guidelines for the treatment of tobacco dependence;
5. Awareness should be increased among health-care professionals, administrators, and policy-makers of both the benefits and cost effectiveness of smoking cessation interventions relative to other health-care interventions;
6. Training should be provided to all health-care providers at primary care, community and national level to enable them to deliver smoking cessation interventions effectively;
7. New partnerships are needed to increase commitment and the pool of financial and technical support for implementing evidence-based treatment.

Source: WHO 2003[55]

A public health approach in tobacco control should involve all sectors of society including partnerships between governmental organizations and civil society, and not health sector alone.[14] In this perspective, oral health professionals can contribute significantly to reduce smoking rates amongst young people. Dentists can work through academic and governmental instituitions as well as recognized professional associations in advocacy and providing guidelines and policy support. Advocacy involves influencing decision- and policy-makers to ensure that tobacco control is placed upon their agendas. Creating and strengthening partnerships with other sectors of the society is a key element for success.[56] Dental education is predominantly individual and patient-centred and therefore working across professional boudaries is a challenging task for dentists. Contemporary dental education should be expanded and dental professionals must develop appropriate skills in comunication and team working.

Tobacco control should be on the agenda of policy makers in all sectors and at all levels. The results will be as stronger as they are more planned and implemented using intersectoral approaches. The WHO Framework Convention on Tobacco Control was the first globally binding public health treaty. Box 14.5 provides an overview of the key elements of the WHO FCTC.[53]

In 2008 WHO introduced the MPOWER measures, which are intended to assist the WHO FCTC implementation at country-level of effective interventions to reduce the demand for tobacco.[54] The package encourages policy-

-makers along with the rest of society, including civil society, health-care providers and others, to envision a world free of tobacco use by promoting a legal and socio-economic context that favours tobacco-free living. Policies and interventions of the MPOWER package are displayed in Box 14.6.[54]

Box 14.5 – Key elements of the WHO FCTC.

1. Monitor tobacco use and prevention policies
   - Country specific comparable data
   - Sign up to WHO FCTC
   - Ratify WHO FCTC
   - National tobacco control policies
2. Protect people from tobacco smoke
Core demand reduction provisions are:
   - Price and tax measures to reduce the demand for tobacco, and
   - Non-price measures to reduce the demand for tobacco, namely:
      Protection from exposure to tobacco smoke;
      Regulation of the contents of tobacco products;
      Regulation of tobacco product disclosures;
      Packaging and labelling of tobacco products;
      Education, communication, training and public awareness;
      Tobacco advertising, promotion and sponsorship; and
      Demand reduction measures concerning tobacco dependence and cessation.
Core supply reduction provisions are:
   - Illicit trade in tobacco products;
   - Sales to and by minors; and,
   - Provision of support for economically viable alternative activities.
3. Offer help to quit tobacco use
   - quitlines (toll-free)
   - treatment services, including brief advices, behavioural support and NRT
   - training of educators in tobacco control and smoking cessation
4. Warn about the dangers of tobacco
   - education, information and public awareness most countries provide information and education on the harm caused by tobacco through school programmes and/or public awareness campaigns
   - consumer information, packaging, warnings, etc
5. Enforce bans on tobacco advertising, promotion and sponsorship
   - direct and indirect advertising
   - promotion of tobacco products on non-tobacco products
   - sponsorship of events, etc
6. Raise taxes on tobacco
   - price and taxation policy

Source: WHO FCTC 2003[53]

Box 14.6 – MPOWER - Policies and interventions.

M. Monitor Tobacco Use: obtain nationally- representative and population- based periodic data on key indicators of tobacco use for youth and adults.

P. Protect people from tobacco smoke: Enact and enforce completely smoke-free environments in health-care and educational facilities and in all indoor public places including workplaces, restaurants and bars.

O. Offer help to quit tobacco use: Strengthen health systems so they can make tobacco cessation advice available as part of primary health care. Support quit lines and other community initiatives in conjunction with easily accessible, low- cost pharmacological treatment where appropriate.

W. Warn about the dangers of tobacco: (i) Require effective package warning labels, (ii) Implement counter-tobacco advertising and (iii) Obtain free media coverage of anti-tobacco activities.

E. Enforce bans of tobacco, advertising, promotion: (i) Enact and enforce effective legislation that comprehensively bans any form of direct tobacco advertising, promotion and sponsorship; (ii) Enact and enforce effective legislation to ban indirect tobacco advertising, promotion and sponsorship.

R. Raise taxes on tobacoo products: (i) Increase tax rates for tobacco products and ensure that they are adjusted periodically to keep pace with inflation and rise faster than consumer purchasing power; (ii) Strengthen tax administration to reduce the illicit trade in tobacco products.

Source: WHO 2008[54]

In 2003, the release of the World Bank report offered relevant useful evidence to combat cigarette smoking.[57] One of the foremost actions related to such decrease in cigarette consunption was the introduction of the comprehensive smoke-free legislation.[58] Taxation on the price of tobacco has been pointed out a promising strategy to fight against cigarette smoking in young people. According to the World Bank, a price rise of 10% promotes an 8% decrease of tobacco use in low and middle-income countries.

While for adults a 10% increase in the price of cigarettes would decrease adult consumption by 3-5%, it was expected that youths would be up to three times as responsive to price as adults. However, because of the multifactorial aspects related to smoking in youth and young adults they are at least as responsive to price as adults are. Cigarette price showed a larger impact on adolescent's decisions to smoke rather than on average amount smoked by smoker. Data from nationally representative longitudinal surveys in the US between 1991 and 1993 revealed that had a 10% increase in the federal excise tax been enacted during the time of study, and had that tax been fully passed on to consumers, the probability of daily smoking initiation among youth would have declined by approximately 10%. Individual social characteristics including education and personal higher income from employment were significantly associated with cigarette smoking initiation.[47]

Tobacco taxation, advertising, sponsorship and production regulation were covered by a groundbreaking World Health Organization public health treaty to control tobacco supply and consumption in the Assembly in 2003.[59] The main estimated consequence of fiscal policies on smoking control in young people was the decrease in social inequalities since young people with less income are more price sensitive than their better-off peers, and as a result fiscal policies would reduce social differentials in smoking.[48] However, governmental actions must include not only the increase on cigarette excise tax because the initiation and regular use of cigarettes by adolescents from the low social class are highly influenced by the difficuly or ease of access to cigarettes. The frequency of current smokers adolescents between 13-15 years old who purchased cigarettes in a store was significantly higher in developing countries compared to industrialized ones. For example, in Chile and Buenos Aires the rates were 60.4% and 59.6%, while it was 9.6% in USA.[18]

Price increases are the most effective, and cost-effective, deterrent to tobacco use, especially for young people and low-income people.[57] Nevertheless, it is recognized that price is not the single aspect of affordability. Higher taxes will generate additional government revenue though few countries earmark tobacco tax revenues for tobacco prevention. Poor smokers who decide to quit or cut back smoking will gain health and in-

come. The challenge is posed for those who do not reduce smoking in the face of price increases as they will pay more. Compensanting tax and price cuts on healthy foods must be considered as well as target cessation programs.

Ineffective or partially effective measures to reduce smoking include improvements in consumer information about the harms of smoking, mass media campaign against tobacco and health warnings on cigarette boxes such as large and unappealing tobacco products packaging. Restricting access by youth and prohibition of smoking as well as crop substitution efforts and trade restrictions has little impact on early onset of smoking. Moreover, most measures to reduce supply are ineffective, control of smuggling is the exception, and is the key supply-side measure to pursue. Even though the real benefits of comprehensive bans on all advertising and promotional products of tobacco on smoking reduction are inconclusive, countries that have implemented such actions have reduced tobacco use much more quickly and to lower levels than other countries.

People from different countries and even from different areas within the same city may face a wide variety of cultural, social and political scenarios. Therefore, actions and efforts devoted to reduce and preventing tobacco smoking should be adapted to local needs and available resources. Since adolescents are a group of the population at greater risk of starting smoking compared to the whole population, the targeted-population approach would be an initial and reasonable approach. Nevertheless, the core strategy to obtain better results for prevention of tobacco in adolescents is the adoption of the whole-population approach.[60] The effectiveness of the whole-population approach, namely, smoke-free envirnoments, and flaws of the higher risk approach, ie, smoking cessation program, in tobacco control will be discussed next.

Tobacco control through legislation has been effective in reducing smoking prevalence in many countries as they have succeeded in reducing the incidence of cancers, heart disease and respiratory diseases. Smoking free places is central to creating supportive environments regarding tobacco cessation. The developement of supportive environments banning tobacco should occur at local national and local levels. Smoke-free places such as restaurants, health facilities, public transports, cinemas shops and workplaces are becoming increasingly common. Partial bans are not effective and if full bans are politically unfeasible, strong restrictions, and significant counter-advertising should be pursued.[57]

Since 1986 several actions to reduce cigarette smoking in Brazil have been developed and implemented. They include bans and restrictions on advertising of tobacco products, creation of specific tax for tobacco-derived products, insertion of varied text-warning messages on the packages and on the marketing material of tobacco products, prohibition of the use of cigarettes in public or private collective facilities, prohibition of the sale of tobacco products to children and adolescents and on the internet.[61] In 2011, the Brazilian government introduced a law banning smoking in all enclosed public spaces in Brazil. It amends a 1996 law, which allowed smoking in specially designated, ventilated areas. The new law will make Brazil the largest country

in the world to go smoke-free, adding momentum to a movement sweeping across Latin America to protect citizens from the deadly toll of tobacco use and secondhand smoke. The smoking ban in enclosed spaces was already implemented in states like Sao Paulo, Rio de Janeiro and Parana, in line with laws passed by local legislatures. The new federal law requires all enclosed workplaces and public places to be smoke-free, bans tobacco advertising at point of sale, increases tobacco taxes and requires large health warnings on both sides of cigarette packs.

Children and adolescents can greatly benefit from smoking free schools. The risk of current smoking was higher in schools with high smoking prevalence.[39] Health Promoting Schools (HPS) is a broad strategy, which encompasses a range of envirnomental and educational changes to promote oral and general health in schools[62,63] (See Chapter HPS). HPS is a successful comprehensive health promotion strategy based on the guiding principles of the Ottawa Charter for Health Promotion that encompasses the whole-population approach combined with the common risk factor approach. HPS provides an effective setting for health promoting not only for students but also for the school staff, families and community members.[64,65] Health-related HPS policies include ban on smoking in all school premises, prevention of early onset tobacco smoking, smoking cessation services and counseling.[63] The impact of HPS on children's oral health was evaluated in 33 schools in deprived areas in Curitiba. Smoking policy composed one of the components of the school's levels of support for health promotion, which was positively correlated with percentage of caries-free children. In addition, supportive schools had higher levels of caries-free and less dental trauma than non-supportive schools.[62]

Role of dentists and other professionals in reducing smoking in adolescents

Initiation of tobacco use begins primarily during childhood and adolescence, and physicians and dentists can play a major role in preventing the onset of tobacco use through advising youths not to start using tobacco. Physicians are therefore recommended to incorporate the four A's in their practices that promote smoking prevention and cessation: Ask, Advise, Assist, and Arrange follow--up.[15] Those who care for children and adolescents should also include a fifth A, Anticipatory guidance, which is the practice of providing counsel regarding potential problems derived from tobacco smoking. According to four A's model of intervention, providing messages that are appropriate to the patient's age and developmental stage, physicians can intervene in early stages of tobacco use. It was believed that doctors and dentists are role models and leaders, and as such they could also influence attitudes in the schools and community.[66]

Quit rates among adolescents are less dramatic than in adults.[67] Therefore, prevention of smoking at early ages is crucial to reduce smoking prevalence. The development of the personality during adolescence is usually accompanied by the maturation of personal beliefs, development of skills and coping strategies in response to social pressures and other psychosocial factors that affect personality and therefore their lifetime habits. Individual lifestyle approach in preventing tobacco use ne-

glects social circumstances where adolescents are embedded.[13,56]

The evidence of the effectiveness of programs to prevent initiation of tobacco use by adolescents conducted by dentists is very limited.[68,69] In fact, health promotion activities involving dentists are restricted to dental health education, which has been traditionally focused on dietary changes, knowledge and attitudes.[70]

According to the WHO, health promotion involves "any process that enables individuals or commuitites to increase control over the determinants of their health".[14] Therefore, the role of dentists in the prevention of smoking in adolescents should go beyond the dental office were they do individual counseling concerning the risks of smoking for health. They should be encouraged to engage in tobacco control advocacy through taking part in governmental and non-governmental instituitions against tobacco. The provision of scientific evidence and relevant information related to harmful effects of smoking to oral tissues and oral diseases would strengthen the global movement against tobacco. Also, the benefits to oral health obtained from tobacco reduction should also be disseminated.

Although the involvement of dental professionals in health promotion activities against tobacco is low, many initiatives have encouraged dentists to get involved in tobacco cessation activities. The First National Dental Symposium on Smoking Cessation was held at the American Dental Association (ADA) in 1989.

In 2003, the World Oral Health Report emphasized the ethical, moral and practical reasons why oral health professionals should strengthen their contributions to tobacco-cessation programmes. The reasons are presented in Box 14.7.[59]

Box 14.7 – Reasons for the involvement of oral health professionals in tobacco-cessation programmes.

1. They are especially concerned about the adverse effects in the oropharyngeal area of the body that are caused by tobacco practices.
2. They typically have access to children, youths and their caregivers, thus providing opportunities to influence individuals to avoid all together, postpone initiation or quit using tobacco before they become strongly dependent.
3. They often have more time with patients than many other clinicians, providing opportunities to integrate education and intervention methods into practice.
4. They often treat women of childbearing age, thus are able to inform such patients about the potential harm to their babies from tobacco use.
5. They are as effective as other clinicians in helping tobacco users quit and results are improved when more than one discipline assists individuals during the quitting process.
6. They can build their patient's interest in discontinuing tobacco use by showing actual tobacco effects in the mouth.
7. Oral health professionals and dental associations worldwide should consider this platform for their future work and design national project(s) jointly with health authorities. Tobacco prevention activities can be translated through existing oral health services or new community programmes targeted at different population groups.

Source: Petersen/WHO 2003[59]

The majority of tobacco control studies performed in dental settings focused on smoking cessation or smokeless tobacco use in adults. They were predominantly conducted in the USA and in the UK in different seetings such as university clinics, private dentists and hospital clinics. Different methods for assisting smoking cessation were tested including the use of nicotine gum (2 and 4 mg), regular reminder and advice to quit smoking and oral health education. Smoking quit rates varied considerably among methods reaching 12% for nicotine gum and 2 to 8% for advice and dental health education. Test groups consistently showed better but modest results. Critical aspects of tobacco control trials in dental settings are the follow-up period since they were no longer than one year and few of them were randomized trials.[71-76]

A recent systematic review assessed the effectiveness of tobacco use cessation in dental settings.[77] Most studies were in dental office settings, involving smokeless tobacco patients seeking assistance with tobacco use. The predominant intervention was counseling 5A's and in 7 of the 8 studies the follow-up period was 6 months. It was demonstrated that interventions for tobacco users in the dental setting increase the odds of quitting tobacco. However, the evidence is derived largely from patients using smokeless tobacco. Pharmacotherapy, such as nicotine replacements, bupropion and varenicline is recommended for tobacoo use cessation in medical settings but has received little assessment in dental applications. Whether the dental setting or referral to specialist tobacco use cessation services is the most effective strategy to help people to quit tobacco use remains unclear.[77] The meta-analysis showed statistically significant increase in the odds of tobacco abstinence (OR=1.60 CI95%=1.09-2.35). However, subgroup analysis showed statistically significant greater odds for quitting in studies with smokeless tobacco users (OR=1.86 CI95%=1.10-3.14) but not for cigarette smoking (OR=1.09 CI95%=0.71-1.69).[77]

There are several reasons for the modest tobacco cessation rates in adolescents and adults regardless of the method, and the ineffectiveness of tobacco initiation prevention programs in dental settings. The first weakness is the adoption of the lifestyle and behaviour change approach. In lifestyle approach, dentists have focused on changing behaviours of their patients as the main meaning of promoting health. Harmful behaviours, such as smoking, are considered a conciously chosen personal behaviour and smoking understood as a personal decision the individual make. In this approach, psychosocial factors and features of social context are not taken into account when planning and developing smoking prevention techniques.

The future of tobacco cessation in dental setting is highly dependent on the education of dentists. Victoroff et al.[78] assessed the incoming dental student's attitudes toward tobacco cessation promotion in dental setting. Nearly all incoming students agreed that it is the dental professional's responsibility to educate patients about the risks of tobacco use. Most agreed that it is part of the dental professional's role to ask patients if they use tobacco, to discuss the benefits of stopping, and to advise tobacco users to quit. Moreover, dental students may have reservations about the extent to which tobacco cessation services fit within the scope of dental practice. That is, some students are not certain that all activities within each of the five A's categories fall within the scope of dental practice. Finally, some students may be skeptical about the extent to which tobacco cessation promotion is effective in helping patients to quit.[78] The implementation of effective tobacco use prevention and cessation in a dental school setting requires a multidisciplinary approach involving the school's entire teaching personnel and external experts. In general, a knowledge base attained through lecture, Problem-Based Learning (PBL), or E-Learning, and clinical skills attained through clinical instructions and practices is required. It is suggested that curriculum content should include the biological effects of tobacco use, the history of tobacco culture and psychosocial aspects of tobacco use, prevention and treatment of tobacco use and dependence, and development of clinical skills for tobacco use prevention and cessation.[79]

Evidence-based clinical treatment methods that substantially increase quit rates are available in the Public Health Service clinical practice guideline, which recommendations are as useful to dental clinicians. In 2008, the U.S. Department of Health and Human Services published a guideline named "Treating Tobacco Use and Dependence: 2008 Update" in which effective clinical treatments and recommendations for tobacco dependence were elaborated by a panel.[80] The Panel employed an explicit, science--based methodology and expert clinical judgment to develop recommendations on the treatment of tobacco use and dependence. The recommendations regarding tobacco dependence counseling and medication treatments are presented in Box 14.8.[80] The first point was the recognition that tobacco dependence is a disease and not a social behaviour or a life style without harmful consequences to health. Treating tobacco dependence by a physician is effective through different approaches including counseling and motivational treatments and medications.

Box 14.8 – Recommendations regarding tobacco dependence counseling and medication.

1. Tobacco dependence is a chronic disease that often requires repeated intervention and multiple attempts to quit. Effective treatments exist, however, that can significantly increase rates of long-term abstinence.
2. It is essential that clinicians and health care delivery systems consistently identify and document tobacco use status and treat every tobacco user seen in a health care setting.
3. Tobacco dependence treatments are effective across a broad range of populations. Clinicians should encourage every patient willing to make a quit attempt to use the counseling treatments and medications.
4. Brief tobacco dependence treatment is effective. Clinicians should offer every patient who uses tobacco at least the brief treatments shown to be effective.
5. Individual, group, and telephone counseling are effective, and their effectiveness increases with treatment intensity. Two components of counseling are especially effective, and clinicians should use these when counseling patients making a quit attempt:
   - Practical counseling (problemsolving/skills training)
   - Social support delivered as part of treatment
6. Numerous effective medications are available for tobacco dependence, and clinicians should encourage their use by all patients attempting to quit smoking — except when medically contraindicated or with specific populations for which there is insufficient evidence of effectiveness (i.e., pregnant women, smokeless tobacco users, light smokers, and adolescents).
   - Seven first-line medications (5 nicotine and 2 non-nicotine) reliably increase long-term smoking abstinence rates:
   – Bupropion SR – Nicotine gum – Nicotine inhaler – Nicotine lozenge – Nicotine nasal spray – Nicotine patch – Varenicline
   - Clinicians also should consider the use of certain combinations of medications identified as effective.
7. Counseling and medication are effective when used by themselves for treating tobacco dependence. The combination of counseling and medication, however, is more effective than either alone. Thus, clinicians should encourage all individuals making a quit attempt to use both counseling and medication.

8. Telephone quitline counseling is effective with diverse populations and has broad reach. Therefore, both clinicians and health care delivery systems should ensure patient access to quitlines and promote quitline use.

9. If a tobacco user currently is unwilling to make a quit attempt, clinicians should use the motivational treatments shown to be effective in increasing future quit attempts.

10. Tobacco dependence treatments are both clinically effective and highly cost-effective relative to interventions for other clinical disorders. Providing coverage for these treatments increases quit rates. Insurers and purchasers should ensure that all insurance plans include the counseling and medication identified as effective as covered benefits.

Source: Treating Tobacco Use and Dependence: 2008 Update[80]

Conclusions

Relevant changes have been observed in the last few decades regarding the prevalence and age of onset of cigarette smoking. While until the 1970s male adults were the predominant consumers of cigarette smoking, the lowering of the age of onset of cigarette consumption is noteworthy since then. Young people are a strategically important market for the tobacco industry since adolescents are the chief source of new cigarette consumers for the tobacco industry. The main policy affecting the decline in youth cigarette smoking prevalence over the past decade has been the adoption of policies restricting youth access to tobacco products. Prevention of smoking in adolescents is still a challenge for oral health professionals. The effectiveness of individual approach programmes of tobacco prevention performed by oral health professionals is unclear. Further investigations with longer follow-up periods to assess their effectiveness are needed. There are few population based approaches used by oral health professionals, and there is no good evidence of the effectiveness of focusing only on individual and using a high risk approach in tobacco smoking control.

Oral health professionals can contribute to preventing the early uptake of tobacco smoking by supporting other groups involved in anti-smoking policies and using whole-population approaches, advocating for smoke-free legislation that includes smoking-free places initiatives and taxation on the price of tobacco. Dentists must recognize the importance of partnerships with other health sectors as the best approach to fight against adolescent's tobacco initiation and addiction. However, current dental curricula needs changing to an urgent shift towards population and community approaches to change dental students into oral health professionals committed to effective oral health promotion.

References

1. Levin ML, Goldstein H, Gerhardt PR. Cancer and tobacco smoking: a preliminar report. JAMA. 1950; 143:336-8.
2. Wynder EL, Graham EA. Tobacco smoking as a possible etiological factor in bronchogenic carcinoma: a study of 684 proved cases. JAMA. 1950; 143:329-36.
3. Doll R, Hill AB. A study of the aetiology of carcinoma of the lung. Br Med J. 1952; 13:1271-86.
4. World Health Organization. Global status Report on noncomunicable diseases. World Health Organization 2010. Available at http://whqlibdoc.who.int/publications/2011/9789240686458_eng.pdf
5. Warnakulasuriya S, Dietrich T, Bornstein MM, Casals Peidró E, Preshaw PM, Walter C, Wennström JL, Bergström J. Oral health risks of tobacco use and effects of cessation. Int Dent J. 2010; 60:7-30.
6. Hanioka T, Ojima M, Tanaka K, Matsuo K, Sato F, Tanaka H. Causal assessment of smoking and tooth loss: a systematic review of observational studies. BMC Public Health. 2011 8; 11:221.
7. Centers for Disease Control and Prevention. Smoking & Tobacco Use. Health Effects of Scondhand Smoke. March 21, 2011. Available at: http://www.cdc.gov/tobacco/data_statistics/fact_sheets/secondhand_smoke/health_effects/
8. U.S. Department of Health and Human Services. The Health Consequences of Involuntary Exposure to Tobacco Smoke: A Report of the Surgeon General. Atlanta: U.S. Department of Health and Human Services, Centers for Disease Control and Prevention, Coordinating Center for Health Promotion, National Center for Chronic Disease Prevention and Health Promotion, Office on Smoking and Health. 2006 [accessed 2011 Nov 10].
9. Helgason AR, Lund KE, Adolfsson J, Axelsson S. Tobacco prevention in Swedish dental care. Community Dent Oral Epidemiol. 2003; 31(5):378-85.
10. Vellappally S, Fiala Z, Smejkalová J, Jacob V, Somanathan R. Smoking related systemic and oral diseases. Acta Medica. 2007; 50(3):161-6.
11. Burt BA, Kolker JL, Sandretto AM, Yuan Y, Sohn W, Ismail AI. Dietary patterns related to caries in a low-income adult population. Caries Res. 2006; 40(6):473-80.
12. Amaral Cda S, Vettore MV, Leão A. The relationship of alcohol dependence and alcohol consumption with periodontitis: a systematic review. J Dent. 2009; 37(9):643-51.
13. Sheiham A, Watt RG. The common risk factor approach: a rational basis for promoting oral health. Community Dent Oral Epidemiol. 2000; 28:399-406.
14. World Health Organization. Ottawa Charter. Ottawa: World Health Organization. 1986.
15. Gordon JS, Severson HH. Tobacco cessation through dental office settings. J Dent Educ. 2001; 65:354-63.
16. Pan American Health Organization. Health in the Americas. Vol 1, 1998 edition. Washington, D.C.: PAHO.
17. Almeida LM, Szklo AS, Souza MC, Sampaio MMA, Mendonça AL, Martins LFL (orgs.). Global Addult Tobacco Survey – Brazil Report. Rio de Janeiro: INCA. 2010.
18. The Global Youth Tobacco Survey Collaborative Group. Tobacco use among youth: a cross country comparison. Tobacco Control. 2002; 11:252-270.
19. Warren CW, Asma S, Lee J, Lea V, Mackay J. Global Tobacco Surveillance System. The GTSS Atlas. CDC. 2009.
20. Barreto SM, Giatti L, Casado L, Moura L, Crespo C, Malta DC. Smoking exposure among school children in Brazil. Cien Saude Colet. 2010; 15 Suppl 2:3027-34.
21. U.S. Department of Health and Human Services. Preventing Tobacco Use Among Young People: A Report ofthe Surge & General. Atlanta, Georgia: U.S. Department of Health and Human Services, Public Health Service, Centers for Disease Control and Prevention, National Center for Chronic Disease Prevention and Health Promotion, Office on Smoking and Health. 1994.
22. Ferreira I, Twisk JW, van Mechelen W, Kemper HC, Stehouwer CD. Develop-

ment of fatness, fitness, and lifestyle from adolescence to the age of 36 years: determinants of the metabolic syndrome in young adults: the amsterdam growth and health longitudinal study. Arch Intern Med. 2005 10; 165(1):42-8.

23. West P. Health inequalities in the early years: is there equalisation in youth? Soc Sci Med. 1997; 44(6):833-58.

24. Kandel D. Stages in Adolescent Involvement in Drug Use. Science. 1975; 190(4217):912-4.

25. Yamaguchi K, Kandel DB. Patterns of drug use from adolescence to young adulthood: II. Sequences of progression. Am J Public Health. 1984; 74(7):668–72.

26. Rodrigues MC, Viegas CA, Gomes EL, Morais JP, Zakir JC. Prevalence of smoking and its association with the use of other drugs among students in the Federal District of Brasília, Brazil. J Bras Pneumol. 2009; 35(10):986-91.

27. Iglesias V, Cavada G, Silva C, Cáceres D. Early tobacco and alcohol consumption as modifying risk factors on marijuana use. Rev Saude Publica. 2007; 41(4):517-22.

28. Kelder SH, Perry CL, Klepp KI, Lytle LL. Longitudinal tracking of adolescent smoking, physical activity, and food choice behaviors. Am J Public Health. 1994; 84(7):1121-6.

29. Challier B, Chau N, Prédine R, Choquet M, Legras B. Associations of family environment and individual factors with tobacco, alcohol, and illicit drug use in adolescents. Eur J Epidemiol. 2000; 16(1):33-42.

30. Griesbach D, Amos A, Currie C. Adolescent smoking and family structure in Europe. Soc Sci Med. 2003; 56(1):41-52.

31. Cinar B, Murtomaa H. Clustering of obesity and dental health with lifestyle factors among Turkish and Finnish pre-adolescents. Obes Facts. 2008;1(4):196-202.

32. Petersen PE, Jiang H, Peng B, Tai BJ, Bian Z. Oral and general health behaviours among Chinese urban adolescents. Community Dent Oral Epidemiol. 2008; 36(1):76-84.

33. Alamian A, Paradis G. Clustering of chronic disease behavioral risk factors in Canadian children and adolescents. Preventive Medicine. 2009; 48:493-9.

34. Jung SH, Tsakos G, Sheiham A, Ryu JI, Watt RG. Socio-economic status and oral health-related behaviours in Korean adolescents. Soc Sci Med. 2010; 70:1780-8.

35. Vettore MV, Moysés SJ, Sardinha LMV, Iser BPM. Condição socioconômica, frequência de escovação dentária e comportamentos em saúde em adolescentes brasileiros: uma análise a partir da PeNSE. Cad Saúde Pública. In Press.

36. Dorri M, Sheiham A, Watt RG. Relationship between general hygiene behaviours and oral hygiene behaviours in Iranian adolescents. Eur J Oral Sci. 2009; 117(4):407-12.

37. Sanders AE, Spencer AJ, Stewart JF. Clustering of risk behaviours for oral and general health. Community Dent Health. 2005; 22(3):133-40.

38. Park YD, Patton LL, Kim HY. Clustering of oral and general health risk behaviors in Korean adolescents: a national representative sample. J Adolesc Health. 2010; 47(3):277-81.

39. Alexander C, Piazza M, Mekos D, Valente T. Peers, schools, and adolescent cigarette smoking. J Adolesc Health. 2001; 29(1):22-30.

40. Villanti A, Boulay M, Juon HS. Peer, parent and media influences on adolescent smoking by developmental stage. Addict Behav. 2011; 36(1-2):133-6.

41. Pallonen UE, Prochaska JO, Velicer WF, Prokhorov AV, Smith NF. Stages of acquisition and cessation for adolescent smoking: an empirical integration. Addict Behav. 1998; 23(3):303-24.

42. Coates, T. J., Peterson, A. C. and Perry, C. (eds) Promoting Adolescent Health. A Dialog on Research and Practice. AcademicPress, NewYork. 1982.

43. McCleary-Sills JD, Villanti A, Rosario E, Bone L, Stillman F. Influences on tobacco use among urban Hispanic young adults in Baltimore: findings from a qualitative study. Prog Community Health Partnersh. 2010; 4(4):289-97.

44. Rasmussen M, Due P, Damsgaard MT, Holstein BE. Social inequality in ado-

lescent daily smoking: has it changed over time? Scand J Public Health. 2009; 37:287-94.

45. Green G, Macintyre S, West P, et al. Like parent, like child? Associations between drinking and smoking behaviour of parents and their children. Br J Addict. 1991; 86:745–58.

46. Powell L, Tauras J, Ross H. The importance of peer effects, cigarette prices and tobacco control policies for youth smoking behavior. J Health Econ. 2005; 24:950-68.

47. Tauras JA, O'Malley PM, Johnstin LD. Effects of price and access las on teenage smoking initiation: a national longitudinal study. NBER Working paper No. 8331, JEL No. 11, June 2001. Available at: http://www.nber.org/papers/w8331.

48. West P, Sweeting H, Young R. Smoking in Scottish youths: personal income, parental social class and the cost of smoking. Tob Control. 2007; 16(5):329-35.

49. Ross H, Chaloupka F, Wakefield M. Youth smoking uptake progress: price and policy effects. Eastern Econ J. 2006; 32:355-67.

50. Casitas R, García-García R, Barrueco M. The cinema as a vector of expansion of the smoking epidemic. Gac Sanit. 2009; 23:238-43.

51. Sargent JD. Smoking in film and impact on adolescent smoking: with special reference to European adolescents. Minerva Pediatr. 2006; 58:27-45.

52. Shafey O. Global epidemiology and health hazards of tobacco use: Arab world patters. Ethn Dis. 2007; 17(Sup 3):S3-13-S3-15.

53. World Health Organization. Framework Convention on Tobacco Control [FCTC]. Geneva: World Health Organization. 2003.

54. World Health Organization. MPOWER. A policy pachage to reverse the tobacco epidemic. Geneva: World Health Organization. 2008.

55. World Health Organization. Policy recommendations for smoking cessation and treatment of tobacco dependence Tools for public health. Geneva: World Health Organization. 2003.

56. Daly B, Watt R, Batchelor P, Treasure E. Principles of oral health promotion. In: Essential Dental Public Health. Oxford University Press. 2002.

57. World Bank. Tobacco control at a glance. Washinton DC: Word Bank. 2003.

58. Gallagher JE, Alajbeg I, Büchler S, Carrassi A, Hovius M, Jacobs A, Jenner M, Kinnunen T, Ulbricht S, Zoitopoulos L. Public health aspects of tobacco control revisited. Int Dent J. 2010; 60:31-49.

59. Petersen PE. The World Oral Health Report 2003. Continuous improvement of oral health in the 21st century and the approach of the World Health Organization Global Oral Health Programme. Geneva, World Health Organization. 2003.

60. Rose G. The strategy of preventive medicine. Oxford. Oxford University Press. 1992.

61. Szklo AS, de Almeida LM, Figueiredo VC, Autran M, Malta D, Caixeta R, Szklo M. A snapshot of the striking decrease in cigarette smoking prevalence in Brazil between 1989 and 2008. Prev Med. 2011. [Epub ahead of print].

62. Moysés ST, Moysés SJ, Watt RG, Sheiham A. Associations between health promoting schools' policies and indicators of oral health in Brazil. Health Promot Int. 2003; 18(3):209-18.

63. Kwan SY, Petersen PE, Pine CM, Borutta A. Health-promoting schools: an opportunity for oral health promotion. Bull World Health Organ. 2005; 83:677-85.

64. World Health Organization. WHO's Global School Health Initiative: Health Promoting Schools; a Healthy Setting for Living, Learning and Working (WHO/HPR/HEP/98.4). WHO, Geneva. 1998.

65. World Health Organization. WHO Information Series on School Health. Oral Health Promotion through Schools. Document 11. Geneva: WHO. 2003.

66. Epps RP, Manley MW. The clinician's role in preventing smoking initiation. Med Clin North Am. 1992; 76:439-49.

67. Warnakulasuriya S. Effectiveness of tobacco counselling in the dental office. Journal of Dental Education. 2002; 66:1079-87.

68. Hovell MF, Slymen DJ, Jones JA, Hofstetter CR, Burkham-Kreitner S, Conway

TL, Rubin B, Noel D. An adolescent to-bacco-use prevention trial in orthodon-tic offices. Am J Public Health. 1996; 86:1760-6.

69. Russos S, Keating K, Hovell MF, Jones JA, Slymen DJ, Hofstetter CR, Rubin B, Morrison T. Counseling youth in to-bacco-use prevention: determinants of clinician compliance. Prev Med. 1999; 29:13-21.

70. Kay EJ. Locker D. Is dental health edu-cation effective? A systematic review of current evidence. Comm Dent Oral Epi-demiol. 1996; 24:231-5.

71. Christen AG, McDonald JL, Olson BL, Drook CA, Stookey GK. Efficacy of nico-tine chewing gum in facilitating smok-ing cessation. J Am Dent Assoc. 1984; 108:595- 7.

72. Cohen SJ, Stookey GK, Katz BP, Drook CA, Christen AG. Helping smokers quit: a randomized controlled trial with pri-vate practice dentists. J Am Dent Assoc. 1989; 118:41-5.

73. Cooper TM, Clayton RR. Stop-smok-ing program using nicotine reduction therapy and behavior modification for heavy smokers. J Am Dent Assoc. 1989; 118:47-51.

74. Severson HH, Andrews JA, Lichtenstein E, Gordon JS, Barckley MF. Using the hygiene visit to deliver a tobacco ces-sation program: results of a randomized clinical trial. J Am Dent Assoc. 1998; 129:993-9.

75. Macgregor IDM. Efficacy of dental health advice as an aid to reducing cigarette smoking. Br Dent J. 1996; 180:292-6.

76. Smith SE, Warnakulasuriya KAAS, Feyer-abend C, Belcher M, Cooper DJ, Johnson NW. A smoking cessation programme conducted through dental practices in the UK. Br Dent J. 1998; 185:299-303.

77. Needleman IG, Binnie VI, Ainamo A, Carr AB, Fundak A, Koerber A, Ohrn K, Rosseel J. Improving the effectiveness of tobacco use cessation (TUC). Int Dent J. 2010; 60(1):50-9.

78. Victoroff KZ, Dankulich-Huryn T, Haque S. Attitudes of incoming dental students toward tobacco cessation promotion in the dental setting. J Dent Educ. 2004; 68:563-8.

79. Ramseier CA, Christen A, McGowan J, McCartan B, Minenna L, Ohrn K, Walter C. Tobacco use prevention and cessa-tion in dental and dental hygiene under-graduate education. Oral Health Prev Dent. 2006; 4(1):49-60.

80. Treating Tobacco Use and Dependence: 2008 Update. Clinical Practice Guide-line. U.S. Department of Health and Hu-man Services, Public Health Service May 2008. http://www.surgeongeneral.gov/tobacco/treating_tobacco_use08.pdf

15

The Prevention of Traumatic Dental Injuries Using a Common Risk Factor Strategy

Jefferson Traebert
Maria Ilma Cortes
Marcelo Bönecker
Wagner Marcenes

Introduction

Injuries are among the most under--recognized and neglected public health problems of the 21st century. Unintentional injuries are one of the leading causes of morbidity, death, hospitalization and disability across the world. Two-thirds of the global burden of injury is classified as unintentional and are mainly caused by road traffic injuries and falls. The burden of all injuries is expected to be equal to that of all communicable diseases worldwide by 2020. Of the total burden of global disease, just over 12% is attributable to injuries. Despite being a worldwide major public health problem, limited attention has been paid to the prevention of injuries. The injury burden caused by exposure to major risk factors is an important guide to policies and priorities for prevention.

Traumatic dental injuries (TDI) have aroused considerable interest in the scientific community in recent years. TDI affect the mineralized tissues of the tooth, the pulp, as well as its supporting dental tissues. The outcome of these injuries depends not only on the individual repair potential of the cells involved, but also on the interaction of the various tissues.[1] In dental trauma, unlike other parts of the body, the healing and repair processes do not occur soon after the incident. The repair of a traumatized tooth can take years to consolidate.

The increase in the levels of violence and in the number of traffic accidents and the greater participation of children in sporting activities has transformed dental trauma into an emerging public health issue.[2] Dental trauma affects a large portion of the population of children and adolescents. The prevalence of dental trauma is high throughout the world, ranging from 3,9% to 58%.[3-5] Most epidemiological studies are cross--sectional, only a few are on incidence.[6]

The major variation among the results of the different epidemiological studies conducted is due to the socioeconomic, behavioural and cultural differences among the populations of countries, and also to the fact that we do not yet have a methodological criterion considered standard for such studies.

Dental trauma can have a considerable impact on the quality of life of children and adolescents. Damage to the teeth and face of children and youths is traumatic, not only in the physical sense, but also in the emotional and psychological sense, leading to the anxiety and anguish of the child, adolescent and parents.[7-9] The psychosocial impact on the quality of life of people affected by TDI is important as the aesthetic impairment of fractured upper central incisors affect facial appearance.[7,10,11] Children and adolescents with TDI expressed dissatisfaction with the appearance of the traumatised teeth,[7] as did those who had their teeth restored after a TDI.[11] A fractured anterior tooth can lead to physical disability, such as difficulty in chewing, phonation, and other oral functions. It can also produce social and psychological embarrassment, such as avoidance of smiling, affecting the social relationship. A population--based case-control study carried out in Brazil[12] showed that adolescents with dental trauma, either untreated or with unsatisfactory treatment according to normative standards, had 2.1 times more chances of presenting a negative impact in comparison with the group of individuals without dental trauma. Among the adolescents with dental trauma treated satisfactory, the negative impact was not statistically significant. Another study[9] showed that children with a previous history of dental trauma were 1.9 times more likely to suffer an impact on quality of life than children without dental trauma, and two times more in children with treated dental trauma than in children without a history of dental trauma. By contrast, dental trauma did not appear to be associated with lower quality-of-life indices in preschool children.[13]

Despite these results, due to its high prevalence, dental trauma is responsible for a high percentage of demand in dental emergency services.[14] Although there are established methods of treating TDI, most TDI are untreated.[2,15,16]

The extensive prevention and control strategies[6,7,10,11,17-22] and the high cost, which results in direct expenses with treatment,[18] or indirect expenses such as loss of days of work and school absenteeism[17] contributes to the importance of TDI as a dental public health issue. In Denmark, TDI account for most of the dental resources.[19]

Traumatic dental injuries can result in a small fracture of the enamel or to the loss of the permanent tooth. Loss of tooth structure, sensitivity, pain, tooth mobility, radicular resorption and pulp necrosis can be observed in individuals who have sustained dental trauma. In the deciduous dentition the most common injuries mainly affect the periodontal tissue due to the greater plasticity of the alveolar bone in very young children. So, trauma more frequently results in dislocations and displacements. In the permanent dentition the most common injuries mainly affect the coronal portion of the upper anterior teeth, resulting more frequently in fractures of different degrees of complexity. Similar to what occurs in deciduous dentition, the upper central incisors are the most strongly affected teeth (Fig. 15.1).

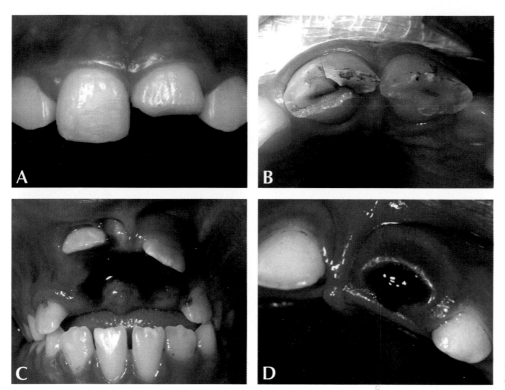

Fig. 15.1A-D – (A) Fracture in the permanent central incisor. (B) Dental trauma involving enamel, dentin, pulp and periodontal tissue. (C) Fracture in the maxillary anterior region. (D) Avulsion of deciduous tooth.

Multiple traumas, injuring two or more teeth, can occur. Moreover, children and adolescents can have repeated episodes of trauma.[20] This recurrent pattern may lead to an inadequate response to treatment, leading to an unfavourable prognosis. Studies have demonstrated that radical endodontic treatment in teeth with roots not completely formed presents an unfavourable long-term prognosis, even when the apexification is successful.[21,22]

Distribution of TDI by age and sex

Most dental trauma occurs in childhood and adolescence. A cohort study in 16-year-olds conducted in Sweden[23] showed that in permanent dentition, the peak age is between 8 and 11 years for males and 9 years for females. It is estimated that 71% to 92% of all dental trauma sustained over a lifetime occurs under 19 years of age.[24-27] The prevalence of dental trauma increases with age. The greater prevalence of dental trauma in individuals in higher age groups does not necessarily reflect a greater risk of occurrence, since dental trauma is cumulative. When using an index that allows the collection of data on treatment provided and presence of trauma sequelae it is possible to observe a greater prevalence in children and adolescents from higher age groups. The prevalence and the incidence of dental trauma according to age and sex in a group of children from Copenhagen, monitored continuously from the age of 2 to 14 years, showed that the peak appears for the first time between 2 and 4 years of age. At age 7, 28% of the girls and 32% of the boys sustained dental trauma in the deciduous dentition. In the permanent dentition, a sharp increase in the incidence of dental trauma was observed in boys between 8 and 10 years of age, while the incidence was very stable among girls.[28-31] This peak of incidence in boys is probably related to the fact that they habitually engage with more vigour in games and horseplay in this age group in comparison with girls.[29-32]

Studies show that male children sustain more traumatic injuries to the teeth than females.[33-35] The ratio of occurrence of dental trauma between boys and girls varies significantly. The fact that boys sustain almost double the dental trauma than girls in the permanent dentition appears to be related to their more active participation in contact sports.[24-27,36] However, other evidence[22,36] indicates that there is no difference with regard to the occurrence of dental trauma between the sexes in the deciduous dentition. Similarly, some studies involving permanent dentition also demonstrated that there is no statistically significant difference of sex-related prevalence.[11,37,38] A cohort study conducted in Brazil[39] also reached the same conclusion. One of the possible explanations for this phenomenon may lie in the fact that girls also take part in sporting and leisure activities, and are exposed to violence in a manner similar to boys,[14,39,40] a striking feature of modern-day society.

Social and environmental determinants

The home is the main site of risk for the occurrence of unintentional traumatic injuries of every sort, in children.[41] As far as TDI is concerned, the main sites of occurrence are the home, school and streets.[2,14,37,42-51] In a study conducted in Sweden,[52] the home was the leading site of occurrence in children in the age groups of 0 to 6 years and of adults from 16 to 30 years; and the school for the age group from 7 to 15 years. Studies carried out in developed and developing countries, such as Iraq, India, Australia, Norway and England, showed that the majority of injuries occurred outside the school environment.[30,44,53,54] In addition, a larger number of severe injuries occurred after classes had ended.[55] It is significant that in most studies, a high percentage of children said they were unable to remember where the event had occurred.

One of the main environmental determinants of dental trauma is socioeconomic vulnerability. Data from the United Kingdom show a greater prevalence in poor areas (43% in Newham[15] and 34% in Bury and Salford[56]) in comparison with the overall prevalence of 17% and 15% recorded in the United Kingdom and in England, respectively.[57] Moreover, even inside a deprived area, the more underprivileged children have more dental trauma than the others. Overcrowding was the main environmental factor related to its occurrence.[58] Deprived areas have fewer playgrounds, sports facilities, and more streets, schools and houses that are less safe. This unsafe environment facilitates falls and collisions, leading to TDI.

A study conducted in Curitiba, Brazil showed that components related to the environment and to the development of public policies were significantly associated with dental trauma. Deprivation, in its broadest sense, was associated with the greater risk of dental trauma. The spatial analysis of dental trauma pointed to the fact that geographical space had an effect on this outcome variable, with significant concentration in the western region of Curitiba. Many of the cases occurred in places of residence outside the potential coverage area of Health Centers.[59]

Many studies show that low socioeconomic status is associated with a greater risk of unintentional injuries. General accidents are more common in groups with lower socioeconomic status than in groups with higher socioeconomic status.[58] Since accidents are the main cause of traumatic injuries, a similar association can be expected between TDI and low socioeconomic status. Rivara and Barber,[60] Nersesian et al.[61] and Pless et al.[62] showed that in poverty-stricken environments there is an increased risk of injuries involving pedestrians, especially children. However, most of these data were collected based exclusively on traffic accidents in industrialized countries.

In relation to TDI, there is no clear association with the socioeconomic status. Few studies have included this variable, and those that include it show conflicting results, as some have indicated significant associations between prevalence and variables that indicate better socioeconomic status,[63] others have shown that there is no association,[2,16,33] while some have shown greater prevalence among children of lower socioeconomic status.[9,64,65] Cortes et al.[7] demonstrated that children with a high socioeconomic level were 1,4 times more likely to present TDI than children with a low socioeconomic status. The greater risk of occurrence of TDI among children and adolescents of higher socioeconomic status may be related to the fact that these have more access to swimming pools, bicycles, skateboards, ice skates, rollerblades, water skiing, riding and others.[66] Moreover, individuals from poorer families may practice sports and games in unsafe environments, without the necessary safety equipment. The differences between results of the few studies that included socioeconomic variables suggests that more surveys should be conducted to better understand the effect of the socioeconomic status on the occurrence of TDI.[67]

Effects of human behaviour on occurrence of injuries

Human behaviour plays an important role in the occurrence of injuries and TDI. Children with a high-risk behaviour tend to have more TDI than those with less risky behaviour. Children suffering from relationship problems with schoolmates, such as victims of mockery or bullying, have TDI much more frequently than other children.[68] The same study reported a tendency for children with more social behaviour to have fewer dental injuries than the others. Lalloo[69] reported that hyperactive children have significantly more TDI than non-hyperactive children. On the other hand, Odoi et al.[68] did not demonstrate a significant relationship between these variables. These conflicting results are easy to understand and suggest that the environment plays a stronger role in the determination of TDI than human behaviour. A child can be hyperactive without risk of accident if they are in a safe environment.

Few studies have concentrated on investigating the role of the family in the etiology of trauma. The family as an interrelated system represents a significant context for the health of each one of its members. A study reported that the psychosocial factors related to the occurrence of unintentional general traumatic injuries were related to family conflicts. The greater the family conflicts, the greater the occurrence of the injuries, regardless of other study variables. Families with a high degree of conflicts tended to be more disorganized and less cohesive, and less able to protect their children against the occurrence of injuries, than families with a low degree of conflicts.[41] With reference to TDI, a case-control study concluded that there is no association between TDI and the occurrence of adverse vital events involving the family.[70]

Studies on stressful emotional states measured by biological markers or questionnaires also reported the presence of an association with TDI.[34,71,72] Nicolau et al.[73] used the life course approach to elucidate its causes and concluded that adolescents experiencing adverse psychosocial environments over the course of their lives had more TDI than others who experienced more favourable environments. This included living in a nonnuclear family and experiencing high levels of paternal punishment.

Predisposing biological factors

An increase in incisal overjet and inadequate lip coverage are predisposing factors for TDI.[2,35,74-82] A systematic review addressed the relationship between size of incisal overjet and TDI and concluded that children with an incisal overjet over 3 mm have approximately twice the chance of sustaining traumatic injuries to the anterior teeth than children with an overjet up to 3 mm. The effect of overjet on the risk of TDI is weaker in boys than in girls, in the same overjet size group.[78] Children with inadequate lip coverage have a greater chance of sustaining TDI. It is not the lip posture alone that is an important predisposing factor for TDI, nor does oral respiration constitute a risk factor. The degree of TDI risk is better evaluated by the overjet measurement (Fig. 15.2).[78] This fact has important implications for the dentist and for the public service, to the effect that it is necessary to provide dental treatment for the more severe malocclusions, including increased overjet.[20]

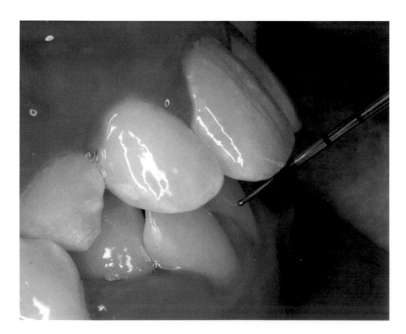

Fig. 15.2 – Measurement of overjet.

TDI is approximately twice as frequent in children with protruding incisor teeth than in children with normal occlusion,[79,80] and that the greater number of injured teeth in the individual patient is associated with protrusive occlusion.[81] Inadequate lip coverage demonstrated a three times higher risk of occurrence of TDI in the superior incisors, in comparison to adequate lip coverage,[38,83] while other studies do not show any significant relationship between inadequate lip coverage and TDI.[33,39] The study that showed a significant association did not take other risk factors into account. The study conducted by Marcenes et al.[33] took the environment into account, and showed a significant association between lip coverage and TDI before considering other factors in the data analysis, but not after adjusting the results to the levels of deprivation experienced. Therefore, the conflicting results may be due to the interaction between the predisposing factors (e.g., overjet size and lip coverage) and environmental factors (e.g., type of playground,) and/or behavioural factors (e.g., risk assumption). Unfortunately, few studies took all these factors together into account.

Little is known about other morphological characteristics related to TDI. A study showed a greater prevalence of TDI in children with greater space deficiency in the superior arch, greater anterior posterior intermaxillary discrepancy and greater inclination of the incisors in relation to the palatal plane.[79]

Many studies[14,40,84,85] have mentioned falls and collisions as the main causes of TDI. However, few have focused on studying the anthropometric measurements of children as a possible contributory factor in such falls and collisions. A study[86] showed that the chance of obese children sustaining TDI was significantly greater than in non-obese children. Studies conducted in Brazil arrived at conflicting results. While in one study[34] the overweight children had 1.93 more chance of sustaining TDI when compared with the children with adequate weight/height ratio. In another study[14] no statistically significant association was observed.

Etiology and prevention strategies

Contact sports, practiced without the proper protection by children and adolescents; overcrowded recreation settings equipped with apparatus that has a sharp-edges; neglecting to use seatbelts and special car seats for children and the increasing violence in cities are directly related to the occurrence of TDI.

TDI can be classified based on its etiology, taking into account the event itself or the intention, as proposed by the Consumer Safety Institute of the European Commission in the Data Dictionary for Minimum Data Sets on Injuries.[87] The event related to the TDI is defined as the activity in the incident. It includes falls, collisions, leisure-time physical activities, traffic accidents, games of intense physical contact, violence, inappropriate use of the teeth and biting very hard objects. The latter two events are relatively common, but not applicable to general injuries. The intention represents human involvement in the occurrence of the TDI. It can be unintentional, intentional and iatrogenic (Table 15.1).

Table 15.1 – Events related to TDI.

Events related to occurrence of TDI	
Unintentional	Intentional
Falls and collisions	Violence
Leisure-time physical activities	Iatrogenic procedures
Traffic accidents	
Inappropriate use of the teeth	
Biting very hard objects	
Presence of disease, physical limitations or learning difficulties	

Intentional and unintentional external causes should be the subject of public policies and of attention from professionals, as they are among the true causes of TDI. Traebert et al.[88] demonstrated the high burden of disease due to external causes in the state of Santa Catarina, Brazil. A total sum of 1247.7 Disability Adjusted Life Years (DALY) per 100 thousand inhabitants was estimated in the state in 2005. The highest rate was due to "traffic accidents" (39.6%) followed by "violence" (21.5%).

Urban and domestic violence, fights, traffic accidents, violence resulting from excessive consumption of alcoholic beverages, and unsuitable environments for the pursuit of leisure activities and failure to use safety equipment are among the main causes of TDI. In addition, such conditions are responsible for a series of situations of risk involving safety and general health.

The causes of TDI are common to those of injuries to other parts of the body. Therefore it is appropriate to use a Common Risk Factor Approach to preventing TDI.

Preventive Strategies

Adequately planned and executed measures for the promotion of public and domestic safety, promotion of health and prevention, educational, legislative and punitive measures can reduce situations that result in injuries, also reducing the occurrence of TDI. The adaptation of public environments and schools to pose less risk of incidents involving children, in addition to better supervision of physical activities and playtime by qualified adults, can help prevent trauma in general. For example, the surveillance of TDI can constitute an opportunity for preventive measures for more severe musculoskeletal injuries.[89]

Depending on the etiological aspects related to the events, the strategies for prevention of TDI assume importance beyond the dental sphere. For this reason, the Common Risk Factor Strategy conforms to the prevention of TDI.

The basis of this approach is to focus attention changing the factors that determine the disease or event. The underlying fundamental concept is based on the idea that by controlling a small number of risk factors, it is possible to achieve a major impact on a number of diseases and health events at a lower cost, with greater efficiency and efficacy than specific approaches.[90] Figure 15.4 presents a broad array of injury prevention actions and policies through Health Promoting Schools.

1. Personal and social growth to develop essential skills for conflict resolution, relationship problem solving, and to avoid improper use of alcohol and drugs.
2. School policy on bullying and violence among the students to create an environment of social support inside the school.
3. Physical environment – leisure areas, pitches conceived and built in compliance with strict safety standards.
4. School health policy for the training of teams in first aid procedures.
5. School policy to curb the consumption of alcoholic beverages on the school premises.
6. Provision of mouthguards for sports.
7. Ties with the health services – establishment of emergency procedures, training of the team in triage programs and support in health-related matters.

Fig. 15.4 – Actions and policies to reduce injuries.[90]

Etiological events of TDI and prevention in the light of the Common Risk Factor Strategy

Objectively, TDI is caused by a collision that can generate sufficient mechanical energy to produce the injury. Any animate or inanimate object in motion has energy that depends on its mass and speed. The increase in mass and/or energy increases the speed. Thus it is important to understand the vehicles and the circumstances that generate mechanical energy which, in turn, cause TDI. Furthermore, it is important to know the "causes of the causes" of the TDI. What causes people to fall or to experience a collision? What causes them to sustain an injury while driving, riding a bicycle or walking along the street? What causes them to sustain an injury while practicing sports? What causes them to fight? The answers to these questions lead us to the environmental and behavioural causes of TDI.

The matrices developed by Haddon[91] can be applied to prevention strategies for TDI.

Haddon's injury prevention matrix

The lack of full understanding of the possibility of controlling so-called accidental injuries may be responsible for the pessimistic view that injuries cannot be prevented and controlled.

Haddon[91] developed a matrix to assess the injury and to identify the prevention methods. The first dimension spans elements of the epidemiological triad, the host (the injured person), the agent (that caused the injury) and the environment (the physical and social context in which the injury occurred). These aspects are arranged in four columns in the Haddon matrix and are examined in terms of time, which presents three intervals: pre-event, event and post-event, arranged in three rows, constituting the second dimension. Haddon[91] defines injury or damage as predictable and avoidable. His matrix comprises the basic concepts of development of the disease (host, agent, physical environment and social environment) with the circumstances before, during and after the injury. It is a suggestive picture for assessing damage and identifying prevention methods. By using this picture, we are able to evaluate the relative importance of the different factors and to plan interventions. After identifying the interventions that fit inside each cell of the matrix, we can generate a list of strategies to treat a variety of injuries.[91,92]

The prevention of injuries is provided for during the various phases and covers:

Pre-event – prevents the existence of the agent, prevents the release of the agent, separates the agent from the host, and provides protection for the host.

Event – minimizes the quantity of agents present, controls the pattern of release of the agent to minimize the damage, controls the interaction between agent and host to minimize the damage, increases the host's resistance.

Post-event – provides a quick treatment response for the host, provides treatment and rehabilitation for the host.

Figure 15.5 exemplifies the use of the Haddon matrix for the prevention of injuries in children (child restraints for use in cars). Figure 15.6 presents an example applied to the prevention of falls based on the study of McClure et al.[93]

Phase	Host	Vehicle	Physical environment	Social environment
Pre-event	Driver ability; driver training.	Maintenance of brakes; vehicle inspection programs; installation of child restraint; child restraint checking programs.	Adequate roadway markings; correct installation of child restraint; format of the seats: suitable for height and weight.	Context in relation to alcohol consumption and driving; speed.
Event	Human tolerance in thinking that the accident will not happen to oneself; wearing of seatbelt; having child in a correctly fitting child restraint	Crash worthiness of the vehicle; format of the child restraint (for example, avoid head extrusion).	Presence of fixed objects adjacent to the road; presence of unsecured objects inside the vehicle.	Application and monitoring of the compulsory use of the seatbelt and of child restraints.
Post-event	General state of health of crash victims.	Fuel tanks designed to minimize the likelihood of post-accident fire.	Availability timely and effective response to emergencies.	Public service prepared to handle trauma and rehabilitation.

Fig. 15.5 – Haddon Matrix for the prevention of injuries to children.[94]

	Host	**Vehicle**	**Physical environment**	**Social environment**
Pre-fall	Bone density; flexibility; balance and strength	Appropriateness of type of shoe (such as slippers, for example)	Nonslip flooring, handrails on all stairs; use of medications that can alter balance.	A perception of the inevitability of older people falling over and having accidents discouraging physical activity in older people.
Event (fall)	Human tolerance to the thought that the fall will not happen to oneself; use of hip protectors.	Proper use of hip protectors; quality and durability of the hip protector.	Height of the fall and surface fallen onto; contact with other objects.	Anti-slip flooring requirements in public spaces, hospitals and homes of elderly people.
Post-fall	General state of health of victims of falls, fractures and other wounds.	Alarm systems in case of falls.	Availability of timely and effective response to emergencies	Public service prepared to handle trauma and rehabilitation.

Fig. 15.6 – Haddon Matrix for prevention of falls by elderly people.[95]

Unintentional TDI

Falls and collisions

Falls are common among children and older adults. Falls and collisions are the main events related to the high incidence of TDI in small children, under school age,[24,28,96,97] with the child's first efforts to move around. Due to their lack of experience and coordination, the frequency of falls increases as the child starts to walk and tries to run (Fig. 15.7). Therefore, prevention strategies should always take into account the causes of falls and collisions. As regards children in the initial stages of independent locomotion, the competent supervisory role is an important determinant. As small children lack the natural protective reflexes movement with the hands in cases of falls, children often literally fall on their faces, considerably increasing the risk of dental subluxations and avulsions. At the same time as children should be given freedom to create confidence and autonomy to learn to walk, a carer should always be nearby to protect them from natural falls during this learning process. Such care should be taken both at home and at nurseries and school.

Old adults experience the same challenges as small children. Falls and collisions are responsible for a large proportion of their TDI. However, the event that caused the fall or collision is the most important element for prevention. They are the real cause that results in TDI.

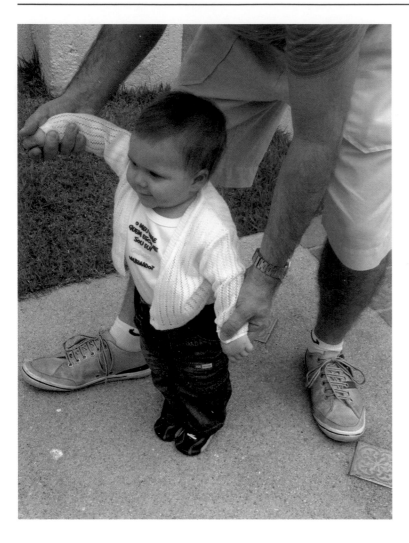

Fig. 15.7 – First steps – situation of risk for TDI. Have competent adult supervision.

Victims of abuse tend to give a vague account when asked about the cause of the wound. The fall is a perfect example of these vague reports. Moreover, falls among children are related mainly to negligent care by those responsible and can often be avoided through better parent or guardian supervision and by houses built with more safety devices.

In the study of the etiology of TDI, a fall or collision due to a push, for example, should not be classified just as a simple fall or collision. This is an undesirable risk behaviour, which greatly increases the likelihood of occurrence of the event, and can represent a minor case of violence or bullying. A study evaluated the human intention at the time of occurrence of TDI. 7.4% of causes of TDI were due to collisions and 2.5% to falls, which occurred with the intentional participation of other people. In addition, 16.5% of the TDI cases occurred due to leisure activities involving other people, 1.6% due to horseplay, such as fights between children and 1.2% due to violent incidents, such as robbery. Thus, 29.2% of the total TDI incidents was a result of the action of other people (Fig. 15.8).[20]

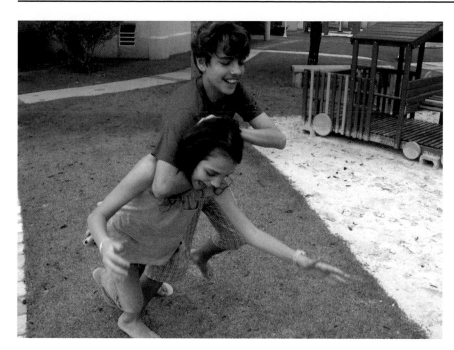

Fig. 15.8 – Two brothers in simulation of high-risk games for TDI, although the natural grass surface absorbs the shock from the fall.

Both at home and at school, in addition to competent supervision, the environment should be adequately prepared for this phase of life. Stairs should be properly blocked with gates or small fences to prevent the child from falling, when crawling or taking their first steps. Tables, counters and other household or school furniture, especially those with heights close to that of the child's head, should be in rounded shapes, reducing the risk of collisions that result in injury to the child. Slippery mats and toys spread around the floor also increase the risk of falls.

As it is almost inevitable that the child will walk freely among their toys spread around the floor, their favourite play place should be well prepared. This includes a spacious environment, without furniture with risk potential and with flooring that attenuates the results of possible falls. Rubber or ethylene vinyl acetate (EVA) mats, used extensively nowadays, can be an alternative for these places.

Clearly, many of these household precautions also apply to elderly people. Mats and an excess of furniture in the home hinder unimpeded walking, especially when vision or locomotion problems are present. The elderly person who has their autonomy reduced also needs competent supervision to avoid falls that result in injures and fractures of every kind, including TDI.

Guidance given to the parents or carers by the paediatric dentist, geriatric dental specialist or by the general practitioner is essential. However, the strategy should include guidelines within a broader context to avoid events that result in any type of injury or damage to children or to the elderly. This dramatically expands the role of the dentist, demonstrating an all-encompassing concern for the health of children or the elderly, and not with the TDI itself. Guidance on the risk factors common to any type of damage or injury includes the dentist in the role of professional involved in these types of incident and brings the guidance messages to the patient or to the population.

In the school environment, adequate supervision increases in importance. Moments of concentration of many children, such as during break times, for example, require the presence of an appropriate number of properly qualified adults to avoid the occurrence of events that increase the risk of any type of wound and injury. Special importance is attributed to the adequacy of the environment in which these children and adolescents concentrate.

Firstly, it is appropriate for children of very different ages to have differentiated break or recreation times or to play in different environments, since the nature of the games is also different. Collisions involving smaller children, in games with older children or adolescents, will thus be avoided.

The type of flooring in leisure areas made available to the children and adolescents in houses, gated communities or in schools is extremely important. A fall occurring on a concrete floor, for instance, can produce very different results if compared with a fall in an area with soft sand or natural grass (Fig. 15.9).

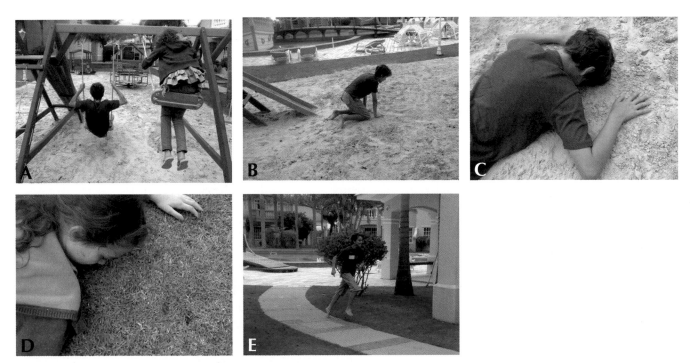

Figs. 15.9A-E – (A) Appropriate flooring for a playground – soft sand. (B) Falls are common in children's games (simulation). (C) In case of falls, the soft fall absorbs the shock of impact, reducing the risk of TDI (simulation). (D) In case of falls, natural grass also absorbs the shock of impact, reducing the risk of TDI (simulation). (E) Sides of swimming pools and leisure areas with stone or concrete floors increase the risk of TDI.

Physical education lessons are times that require special attention. They should always be delivered by qualified instructors, which is not always the case, especially in developing countries. Moreover, preventive measures should be adopted for sports involving physical contact, including the compulsory use of a mouthguard as safety equipment (Fig. 15.10). The school health policy should also focus on the training of personnel in first aid procedures.[91]

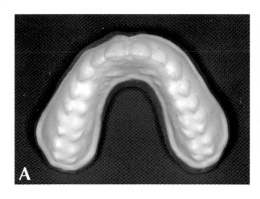

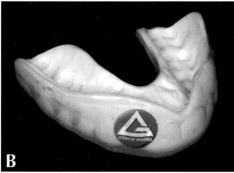

Figs. 15.10A,B – (A) Mouthguard. External view. (B) Mouthguard. Side view.

Leisure-time physical activities

Injuries during adolescence are often due to sports.[98-110] The World Dental Federation divided sports into two categories according to the risk of TDI: high-risk sports that include American football, hockey, ice hockey, lacrosse, martial arts, rugby and skating; and medium-risk sports, which include basketball, diving, squash, gymnastics, parachuting and water polo (Fig. 15.11).[111]

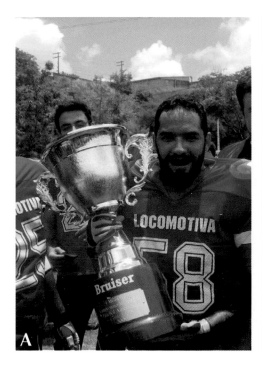

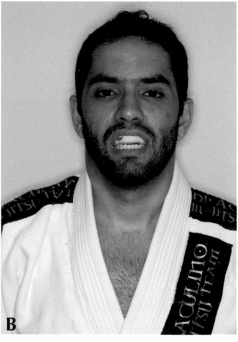

Figs. 15.11A,B – (A) American football – high-risk sport for TDI. Athletes use a mouthguard. (B) Martial arts – high-risk sport for TDI. Athletes use a mouthguard.

Studies confirm that contact sports, such as ice hockey, football, baseball, American football, basketball, rugby, wrestling and handball[112-122] are the main events that cause TDI. The severity of this problem was addressed in a series of studies, which report that 1.5% to 3.5% of the children who take part in contact sports are victims of TDI every year,[114,115,123,124] and at least one third of all the TFDI and up to 19% of injuries to the head and face are related to the sport.[125-130] There is little doubt that special precautions, such as the use of resistant helmets[131] and a well-fitting mouthguard, can reduce the occurrence of TDI (Figs. 15.12 and 15.13).

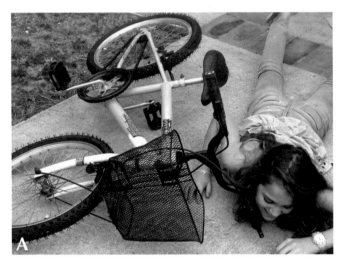
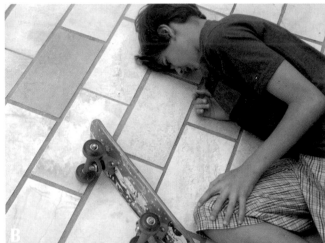

Figs. 15.12A,B – (A) Falls from bicycles are common events in cases of TDI (simulation). Note failure to use safety equipment. (B) Child riding a skateboard without adequate protection (simulation).

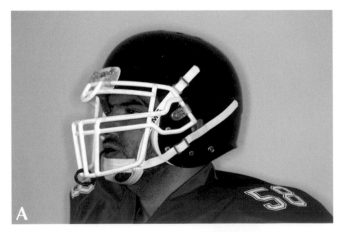
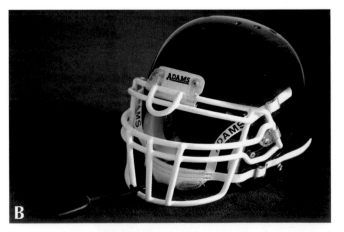

Figs. 15.13A,B – (A) Use of appropriate helmet. (B) American football helmet with mouthguard.

As a prevention strategy, dental professionals should provide children and adolescents with well-fitting mouthguards for use when participating in sports. Dental professionals should also press for the use of protective devices in risky physical activities to be made compulsory by law. Health education should concentrate on increasing awareness of the risk of engaging in physical activities without suitable protection; for example, when using skates or skateboards without protective devices. Health education should also emphasize the benefits of formal training and of the improvement of fitness levels before getting involved in leisure-time physical activities that involve risks.[14] Health workers and public managers should create incentives for the use of mouthguards during the practice of sporting activities, especially those that involve physical contact between the participants. Moreover, the use of safety equipment in leisure activities that include the use of bicycles, skates and ice skates, and the creation of safe environments, both for the practice of sports and for other leisure activities, is essential.[39]

However, there is not yet enough evidence that planned intervention is effective in reducing the prevalence or incidence of sports injuries that affect the mouth and face.[132] TDI due to leisure-time physical activities can also be drastically reduced through environmental changes. This includes a better design for playgrounds and buildings and using appropriate surfacing in recreation settings. Ground surfaces of soft sand and natural grass can be considered a lower risk for the occurrence of TDI, when compared with concrete floors.

Traffic accidents

Traffic accidents can involve pedestrians, producing wounds, often caused by bicycles and cars. Facial and dental injuries resulting from car accidents are seen more frequently among older adolescents.[133,134] The front seat passenger is particularly prone to facial injuries. This pattern of injury is seen when the front passenger or driver hits the steering wheel or dashboard.[135-137]

Wounds related to bicycles have been widely disseminated, resulting in severe TDI, due to the elevated force of impact caused by the vehicle's speed.[24,106,138] Mouth injuries related to bicycles appear to be more common up to the age of 14, in comparison with non-oral wounds (Fig. 15.12).[139]

Prevention strategies include a series of measures such as the establishment and the observation of speed limits for cars, use of seatbelt, airbags and special restraint seats for smaller children in motor vehicles. However, new types of facial trauma have been reported and are attributable to airbag deployment defects.[140,141]

The use of a helmet when riding a bicycle can reduce the risk of severe facial injury in the middle and upper regions of the face. But there is no protection for the lower jaw and cervical spine.[142] To reduce TDI it is necessary to enlarge the area of coverage of the helmet.[138,143] The use of a mouthguard connected to the helmet is also recommended (Fig. 15.13).

Inappropriate use of the teeth

Few studies have assessed this event, the inappropriate use of the teeth. However, many individuals traumatize their teeth when using the teeth as a tool to open bottles, for example. Inappropriate use of the teeth leading to TDI was reported in between 3,3% and 8,5% of children.[14,34,144,145] The most common inappropriate uses of teeth are biting pens, opening hair clips, bags of savoury snacks and key rings, attempting to repair electronic equipment or to change batteries, cutting or securing objects, opening bottle caps, adjusting watches and others. The prevention strategies should include guidance from the dentist on the appropriate use of the teeth, mainly directed at adolescents, since the occurrence of the abovementioned events can be greater among them.

Biting hard (stiff) objects

Another event related to the occurrence of TDI is the act of biting very hard objects. A high percentage (20.5%) of TDI related to eating was reported by Huang et al.[145] The Taiwanese food culture could be the reason for this: people often grind bones and open crab's claws with their teeth. Al-Majed et al.[146] suggested a similar scenario in Saudi Arabia in relation to the custom of eating raw nuts and dried melon seeds. In Brazil, Traebert et al.[14] reported that less than 3% of TDI results from eating hard foods, while others did not mention any relationship between foods and TDI.

TDI were observed among patients who have piercing. Patients and health professionals should be informed about the procedures and risks associated with the use of tongue and oral piercings.[147-149] Levin et al.[150] found that of the 400 patients aged between 18 and 24 who had a dental consultation at a military base, 20% had some kind of oral piercing. More than half of these patients were not aware of the dangers of using this ornament. Partial information shows that piercings can cause chips, fractures and wear and tear of teeth and fillings and pulp damage.[147,151,152] Information about systemic complications resulting from tongue piercings was presented as case reports. Campbell et al.[149] showed a prevalence of chipped teeth of 19.2% among individuals who used tongue piercing, especially of the molars and premolars.

Diseases, physical limitations or learning difficulties

The onset of diseases is a rare cause of TDI in the general population, but is more common in individuals suffering from epilepsy, cerebral paralysis, anaemia and dizziness. Epileptic patients present special risks and problems with TDI.[153-157]

The prevalence of 57% of TDI in a group of individuals with cerebral paralysis was considered much higher than that of the healthy population groups, despite the fact that the individuals with the disease did not take part in violent sporting activities as did the healthy children. This should serve as a warning to the health authorities for them to conduct an in-depth investigation of the events that result in dental injuries in individuals with disabilities and to suggest methods to reduce this type of morbidity.[158]

Similarly, a very high frequency of TDI was found among the patients with learning difficulties,[159] probably related to various factors such as lack of motor coordination, conditions of large gatherings of people at institutions or concomitant epilepsy. O'Donnell[160] reported that completely blind children and young adults in Hong Kong were at a greater risk of injury to the anterior teeth than people with full or partial vision. Children had a greater risk of injury to the anterior teeth than people with full or partial vision. Children with auditory or visual disorders had a greater incidence of TDI than children without these problems.[161] Many drug addicts sustain fractures of molars and premolars, apparently resulting from violent clenching of the teeth 3 to 4 hours after intake of drugs.[162,163]

Intentional TDI

Violence

The role of violence due to the intentional action of another person was also identified as an important cause of TDI. This can be related to physical abuse, including bullying. Attitudes such as hitting a schoolmate on the head when they are using a drinking fountain, for example, or sticking a foot out in front of a mate, who is running to get them to fall down, cannot be considered "horseplay". Other violent attitudes on the part of adolescents involving head butting, thumping, slapping, or throwing of objects against the body and face of other adolescents cannot be considered simple horseplay either. These are violent and undesirable attitudes that increase the risk of a traumatic event.

The prevention strategies in these cases include the school's policy against bullying and violence among the students to create an environment of social support inside the school, as pointed out by Sheiham and Watt.[90]

Oral health professionals should be able to identify violence and act against it. It is important for dentists to start recognizing the signs and symptoms of physical abuse, developing practice policies and procedures to document and report suspected cases, and to collaborate with other members of the community to help prevent violence.[14]

The tragic cause of oral injuries in small children manifests in children who suffer severe physical abuse or beatings.[164-180] Many children are exposed to physical abuse and are referred to hospital with wounds on the head, face, mouth or neck.[181] Child abuse occurs in approximately 0.6% of children[164,175] and 10% of all injuries to such abused children involve the teeth.[175] The official data on the number of child abuse cases generally reflect the reported cases and not the actual number of incidents.[182] From 16% to 29% of dentists declared they have already seen a case or suspected case of child abuse, but only 6% to 14% declared that they communicated the case to the relevant authorities.[183,184] Physical abuse takes place mainly at home[181] and the dentist has the obligation to notify the competent authorities of incidents of child neglect and abuse.[185,186]

Physical attacks, together with traffic accidents, were responsible for 71% of the maxillofacial injuries in a study conducted in the United Kingdom.[186] In this context, it should be mentioned that recent data showed that domestic violence is a universal problem.[187-194] These attacks generally result in wounds in the facial region. Characterizing the victim as a beaten person is complicated as they rarely want to press charges. Social entities for the provision of care and counselling to these victims exist in many countries and should be called upon.[191]

A type of harmful injury that is apparently becoming more and more frequent is that of wounds in the oral and facial region of tortured people.

Most of these victims, in addition to other atrocities that were inflicted on them, suffered torture involving the oral region.[195-197] A study described the results of examinations of 34 former prisoners from 6 countries, who had been submitted to torture involving the facial region.[195] The most common type of torture was beating, which resulted in avulsion, loosening or fracturing of teeth and laceration of soft tissues. Deliberate fracturing of teeth with pliers was also observed. In addition, they reported the occurrence of electrical torture in which the electrodes were placed on the teeth, lips, tongue and soft tissues in the temporomandibular joint. In the latter case, the muscle spasm caused a very strong occlusion. The result was the loosening and fracturing of teeth, as well as intense pain in the muscles and in the temporomandibular joint.

Under the auspices of Amnesty International, workgroups of dentists and physicians were formed in several countries with the objective of collecting proof to document the torture of prisoners.

Iatrogenic procedures

The incidence of perianaesthetic TDI ranges from 0.04% to 12.1%[198] and is considered the most frequent cause of lawsuits against dentists, related to anaesthesia in the United Kingdom. That represents approximately one third of all the confirmed lawsuits.[198] A retrospective study in France showed an average incidence of 9.5 accidents/100 applications of anaesthesia/year,[199] while other studies have shown an annual incidence ranging from 1:150 to 1:1000 cases.[200,201] The risk of injuries to the teeth can be re-duced by a pre-surgical inspection of the oral cavity and assessment of the individual anatomical conditions in the region of the head and neck, which can interfere in endotracheal intubation.[202,203] Using a mouthguard is a simple way of preventing TDI during general anaesthesia and has little effect on the intubation difficulty.[204] Nevertheless, such recommendations should be subject to cost/benefit analysis before their generalized application,[198] especially after Skeie and Schwartz[205] pointed out that 0.062% of patients under general anaesthesia sustained TDI even though they were using a mouthguard, in comparison with 0.063% of those not using a mouthguard. Nowadays, the use of a mouthguard for each intubation does not appear reasonable, but the teeth should be considered in this situation.[206]

Conclusions

As the etiology of TDI is focused on sociobehavioural events, its prevention requires actions that surpass the dental sphere and even the health sector. Hence the Common Risk Factor Strategy is appropriate for dealing with this increasing health problem, since it includes the problem in the agenda of prevention of several other health conditions.

Aspects related to violence, traffic accidents, falls and collisions, inappropriate household and school environments and failure to use safety equipment while practicing sports transcends the role of the dentist, but do not exclude them from the preventive strategy. On the contrary, they increase the dentist's responsibility as a member of the team of healthcare professionals that deals with intentional and unintentional external causes.

REFERENCES

1. Andreasen JO, Andreasen FM, Andersson L. Textbook and color atlas of traumatic injuries to teeth. 4.ed. Oxford: Blackwell Publishing. 2007; 897p.
2. Traebert J, Almeida IC, Garghetti C, Marcenes W. [Prevalence, treatment needs, and predisposing factors for traumatic injuries to permanent dentition in 11-13-year-old schoolchildren]. Cad Saude Publica. 2004 Mar-Apr; 20(2):403-10.
3. Côrtes, MIS, Bastos, JV. Epidemiologia do traumatismo dentário. Pro-odonto. Prevenção. 2011; 5:113-49.
4. Glendor U. Epidemiology of traumatic dental injuries - a 12 year review of the literature. Dent Traumatol. 2008; 24(6):603-11.
5. Glendor U, Marcenes W, Andreasen JO. Classification, epidemiology and etiology. In: Andreasen JO, Andreasen FM, Andersson L. Textbook and color atlas of traumatic injuries to teeth. 4.ed. Oxford: Blackwell Publishing. 2007; p.217-254.
6. Bastone EB, Freer TJ, Mcnamara JR. Epidemiology of dental trauma: A review of the literature. Aust Dent J. 2000; 5(1):2-9.
7. Côrtes M, Marcenes W, Sheiham A. Impact of traumatic injuries to the permanent teeth on the oral health-related quality of life in 12-14-year-old children. Community Dent Oral Epidemiol. 2002; 30(3):193-8.
8. Fakhruddin KS, Lawrence HP, Kenny DJ, Locker D. Impact of treated and untreated dental injuries on the quality of life of Ontario schoolchildren. Dent Traumatol. 2008; 24:309-13.
9. Bendo CB, Paiva SM, Torres CS, Oliveira AC, Goursand D, Pordeus IA et al. Association between treated/untreated traumatic dental injuries and impact on quality of life of Brazilian schoolchildren. Health Qual Life Outcomes. 2010; 8:114.
10. Robertson A, Noren JG. Subjective aspects of patients with traumatized teeth. A 15-year follow-up study. Acta Odont Scand. 1997; 55:142-7.
11. Ramos-Jorge M, Bosco V, Peres M, Nunes A. The impact of treatment of dental trauma on the quality of life of adolescents - a case-control study in southern Brazil. Dent Traumatol. 2007; 23(2):114-9.
12. Souza ML, Jorge MLR, Traebert J, Peres MA, Ghisi CZ, Bosco VL. Impacto do traumatismo dental sobre a qualidade de vida relacionada à saúde bucal. [Abstract 062]. Braz Oral Res. 2004; 18:95.
13. Abanto J, Carvalho TS, Mendes FM, Wanderley MT, Bonecker M, Raggio DP. Impact of oral diseases and disorders on oral health-related quality of life of preschool children. Community Dent Oral Epidemiol. 2011; 39(2):105-14.
14. Traebert J, Almeida IC, Marcenes W. Etiology of traumatic dental injuries in 11 to 13-year-old schoolchildren. Oral Health Prev Dent. 2003; 1(4):317-23.
15. Marcenes W, Murray S. Social deprivation and traumatic dental injuries among 14-year-old schoolchildren in Newham, London. Endod Dent Traumatol. 2001; 17(1):17-21.
16. Oliveira LB, Marcenes W, Ardenghi TM, Sheiham A, Bonecker M. Traumatic dental injuries and associated factors among Brazilian preschool children. Dent Traumatol. 2007; 23(2):76-81.
17. Wong F, Kolokotsa K. The cost of treating children and adolescents with injuries to their permanent incisors at a dental hospital in the United Kingdom. Dent Traumatol. 2004; 20(6):327-33.
18. Glendor U, Jonsson D, Halling A, Lindqvist K. Direct and indirect costs of dental trauma in Sweden: a 2-year prospective study of children and adolescents. Community Dent Oral Epidemiol. 2001; 29(2):150-60.
19. Borum M, Andreasen J. Therapeutic and economic implications of traumatic dental injuries in Denmark: an estimate based on 7549 patients treated at a major trauma centre. Int J Paediatr Dent. 2001; 11(4):249-58.
20. Ramos-Jorge ML, Peres MA, Traebert J, Ghisi CZ, de Paiva SM, Pordeus IA, et al. Incidence of dental trauma among adolescents: a prospective cohort study. Dent Traumatol. 2008 Apr; 24(2):159-63.

21. Cvek M. Prognosis of luxated non-vital maxillary incisors treated with calcium hydroxide and filled with gutta-percha. A retrospective clinical study. Endod Dent Traumatol. 1992; 8:45-55.

22. Cvek M. Endodontic management and the use of calcium hydroxide in traumatized permanent teeth. In: Andreasen JO, Andreasen FM, Andersson L, (eds) Textbook and Color Atlas of Traumatic Injuries to the Teeth (4th ed). Oxford: Blackwell/Munksgaard. 2007; p.598-657.

23. Borssén E, Holm AK. Traumatic dental injuries in a cohort of 16 years-old in northern Sweden. Endod Dent Traumatol. 1997; 13(6):276-80.

24. Andreasen JO. Etiology and pathogenesis of traumatic dental injuries. A clinical study of 1298 cases. Scand J Dent Res. 1970; 78:339-42.

25. Gutz DP. Fractured permanent incisors in a clinic population. ASDC J Dent Child. 1971; 38:94-121.

26. Oluwole TO, Leverett DH. Clinical and epidemiological survey of adolescents with crown fractures of permanent anterior teeth. Pediatr Dent. 1986; 8:221-3.

27. Skaare AB, Jacobsen I. Dental injuries in Norwegians aged 7-18 years. Dent Traumatol. 2003; 19(2):67-71.

28. Andreasen JO, Ravn JJ. Epidemiology of traumatic dental injuries to primary and permanent teeth in a Danish population sample. Int J Oral Surg. 1972; 1:235-9.

29. Ravn JJ. Dental injuries in Copenhagen schoolchildren, school years 1967-1972. Community Dent Oral Epidemiol. 1974; 2:231-45.

30. Hansen M, Lothe T. Tanntraumer hos skolebarn og ungdom i alderen 7-18 år i Oslo. Norske Tannlægeforenings Tidende. 1982; 92:269-73.

31. Ravn JJ, Rossen I. Hyppighed og fordeling of traumatiske beskadigelser of tænderne hos københavnske skolebørn 1967/68. Tandlægebladet. 1969; 73:1-9.

32. Magnusson B, Holm AK. Traumatised permanent teeth in children - a follow-up. I. Pulpal complications and root resorp. In: Nygaard J, Ostby B, Osvald O, eds. Nordisk Klinisk Odontologi. Copenhagen: A/S Forlaget for Faglitteratur 1964: Chapter 11, 111, 1-40.

33. Marcenes W, Alessi ON, Traebert J. Causes and prevalence of traumatic injuries to the permanent incisors of school children aged 12 years in Jaragua do Sul, Brazil. Int Dent J. 2000 Apr; 50(2):87-92.

34. Nicolau B, Marcenes W, Sheiham A. Prevalence, causes and correlates of traumatic dental injuries among 13-year-olds in Brazil. Dent Traumatol. 2001; 17(5):213-7.

35. Côrtes MI, Marcenes W, Sheiham A. Prevalence and correlates of traumatic injuries to the permanent teeth of schoolchildren aged 9-14 years in Belo Horizonte, Brazil. Dent Traumatol. 2001; 17(1):22-6.

36. Bonini GAVC, Marcenes W, Oliveira LB, Sheiham A, Bonecker M. Trends in the prevalence of traumatic dental injuries in Brazilian preschoolchildren. Dent Traumatol. 2009; 25(6):594-8.

37. Chen YL, Tsai TP, See LC. Survey of incisor trauma in second grade students of Central Taiwan. Chan Gung Med J. 1999; 22:212-9.

38. Marcenes W, al Beiruti N, Tayfour D, Issa S. Epidemiology of traumatic injuries to the permanent incisors of 9-12-year-old schoolchildren in Damascus, Syria. Endod Dent Traumatol. 1999; 15(3):117-23.

39. Cecconello R, Traebert J. Traumatic dental injuries in adolescents from a town in southern Brazil: a cohort study. Oral Health Prev Dent. 2007; 5(4):321-6.

40. Rocha MJ, Cardoso M. Traumatized permanent teeth in Brazilian children assisted at the Federal University of Santa Catarina, Brazil. Dent Traumatol. 2001 Dec; 17(6):245-9.

41. Harris MJ, Kotch, JB. Unintentional infant injuries: sociodemographic and psychosocial factors. Public Health Nurs. 1994; 11(2):90-7.

42. Traebert J, Bittencourt DD, Peres KG, Peres MA, de Lacerda JT, Marcenes W. Aetiology and rates of treatment of traumatic dental injuries among 12-year-old school children in a town in southern Brazil. Dent Traumatol. 2006 Aug; 22(4):173-8.

43. Eilert-Petersson E, Andersson L, Sörensen S. Traumatic oral vs non-oral injuries. An epidemiological study during one year in a Swedish county. Swed Dent J. 1997; 21:55-68.

44. Blinkhorn FA. The etiology of dentoalveolar injuries and factors influencing attendance for emergency care of adolescents in the north west of England. Endod Dent Traumatol. 2000; 16(4):162-5.

45. Amorim LF, Costa LR, Estrela C. Retrospective study of traumatic dental injuries in primary teeth in a Brazilian specialized pediatric practice. Dent Traumatol. 2011; 27(5):368-73.

46. Chan YM, Williams S, Davidson LE, Drummond BK. Orofacial and dental trauma of young children in Dunedin, New Zealand. Dent Traumatol. 2011; 27(3):199-202.

47. Hasan AA, Qudeimat MA, Andersson L. Prevalence of traumatic dental injuries in preschool children in Kuwait - a screening study. Dent Traumatol. 2010; 26(4):346-50.

48. Granville-Garcia AF, Vieira IT, Siqueira MJ, de Menezes VA, Cavalcanti AL. Traumatic dental injuries and associated factors among Brazilian preschool children aged 1-5 years. Acta Odontol Latinoam. 2010; 23(1):47-52.

49. Wendt FP, Torriani DD, Assunção MC, Romano AR, Bonow ML, da Costa CT, Goettems ML, Hallal PC. Traumatic dental injuries in primary dentition: epidemiological study among preschool children in South Brazil. Dent Traumatol. 2010; 26(2):168-73.

50. Noori AJ, Al-Obaidi WA. Traumatic dental injuries among primary school children in Sulaimani city, Iraq. Dent Traumatol. 2009; 25(4):442-6.

51. Malikaew P, Watt RG, Sheiham A. Prevalence and factors associated with traumatic dental injuries (TDI) to anterior teeth of 11-13 year old Thai children. Community Dent Health. 2006; 23(4):222-7.

52. Petersson E, Andersson L Sörensen S. Traumatic oral vs non-oral injuries. Swed Dent J. 1997; 21(1/2):55-68.

53. Davis GT, Knott SC. Dental trauma in Australia. Aust Dent J. 1984; 29:217-21.

54. Baghdady VS, Ghose LJ, Alwash R. Traumatized anterior teeth as related to their cause and place. Community Dent Oral Epidemiol. 1981; 9:91-3.

55. Liew VP, Daly CG. Anterior dental trauma treated afterhours in Newcastle, Australia. Community Dent Oral Epidemiol. 1986; 14:362-6.

56. Hamilton FA, Hill FJ, Holloway PJ. An investigation of dento-alveolar trauma and its treatment in an adolescent population. Part 1: The prevalence and incidence of injuries and the extent and adequacy of treatment received. Br Dent J. 1997; 182(3):91-5.

57. O'Brien M. Children's dental health in the United Kingdom 1993. London: Her Majesty's Stationary Office. 1994.

58. Marcenes W. Murray S. Changes in prevalence and treatment need for traumatic dental injuries among 14-year-old children in Newham, London: a deprived area. Community Dent Health 2002; 19(2):104-8.

59. Moysés SJ, Moysés ST, McCarthy M, Sheiham A. Intra-urban differentials in child dental trauma in relation to healthy cities policies in Curitiba, Brazil. Health Place. 2006; 12(1):48-64.

60. Rivara FP, Barber M. Demographic analysis of childhood pedestrian injuries. Pediatrics. 1985; 76:375-81.

61. Nersesian WS, Petit MR, Shaper R, Lemieux D, Naor E. Childhood death and poverty: a study of all childhood deaths in Maine, 1976 to 1980. Pediatrics. 1985; 75:41-50.

62. Pless IB, Verreault R, Arsenault L, Frappier JY, Stulginskas J. The epidemiology of road accidents in childhood. Am J Public Health. 1987; 77:358-60.

63. Marcenes W, Zabot NE, Traebert J. Socio-economic correlates of traumatic injuries to the permanent incisors in schoolchildren aged 12 years in Blumenau, Brazil. Dent Traumatol. 2001 Oct; 17(5):222-6.

64. Soriano EP, Caldas AF, Diniz De Carvalho MV, Amorim Filho HA. Prevalence and risk factors related to traumatic den-

tal injuries in Brazilian schoolchildren. Dent Traumatol. 2007; 23(4):232-40.

65. Robson F, Ramos-Jorge ML, Bendo CB, Vale MP, Paiva SM, Pordeus IA. Prevalence and determining factors of traumatic injuries to primary teeth in preschool children. Dent Traumatol. 2009; 25(1):118-22.

66. Kemp A, Sibert J. Childhood accidents: epidemiology, trends, and prevention. J Accid Emerg Med. 1997; 14(5):316-20.

67. Traebert J. Accidents, sports, and physical leisure activities are the most frequent causes of traumatic dental injury and the rate of pulp necrosis is high following its occurrence in Pilsen, The Czech Republic. J Evid Based Dent Pract. 2011 Jun; 11(2):102-4.

68. Odoi R. Croucher R. Wong F. Marcenes W. The relationship between problem behaviour and traumatic dental injury amongst children aged 7-15 years old. Community Dent Oral Epidemiol. 2002; 30(5):392-6.

69. Lalloo R. Risk factors for major injuries to the face and teeth. Dent Traumatol. 2003; 19:12-14.

70. Traebert J. Traumatismo dentário: um estudo de caso controle com escolares de 11 a 13 anos de idade e suas famílias. Florianópolis, SC: Tese de Doutorado. Universidade Federal de Santa Catarina. 2002.

71. Vanderas AP, Papagiannoulis AP. Urinary catecholamine levels and incidence of dento-facial injuries in children: 2-year prospective study. Endod Dent Traumatol. 2000; 16:222-8.

72. Perheentupa U, Laukkanen P, Veijola J, Joukamaa M, Jarvelin MR, Laitinen J, Oikarinen K. Increased lifetime prevalence of dental trauma is associated with previous non-dental injuries, mental distress and high alcohol consumption. Dent Traumatol. 2001; 17(1):10-6.

73. Nicolau B. Marcenes W. Sheiham A. The relationship between traumatic dental injuries and adolescents' development along the life course. Community Dent Oral Epidemiol. 2003; 31(4):306-13.

74. Forsberg CM, Tedestam G. Etiological and predisposing factors related to traumatic injuries to permanent teeth. Swed Dent J. 1993;17(5):183-190.

75. Bauss O, Rohling J, Schwestka-Polly R. Prevalence of traumatic injuries to the permanent incisors in candidates for orthodontic treatment. Dent Traumatol. 2004; 20(2):61-6.

76. Shulman JD, Peterson J. The association between incisor trauma and occlusal characteristics in individuals 8-50 years of age. Dent Traumatol. 2004; 20:67-74.

77. Soriano EP, Caldas Jr AF, Góes PSA. Risk factors related to traumatic dental injuries in Brazilian schoolchildren. Dent Traumatol. 2004; 20:246-250.

78. Nguyen QV, Bezemer PD, Habets L, Prahl-Andersen B. A systematic review of the relationship between overjet size and traumatic dental injuries. Eur J Orthod. 1999; 21:503-15.

79. Lewis TE. Incidence of fractured anterior teeth as related to their protrusion. Angle Orthod. 1959; 29:128-31.

80. McEwen JD, McHugh WD, Hitchin AD. Fractured maxillary central incisors and incisal relationships. J Dent Res. 1967; 46:1290.

81. Eichenbaum IW. A correlation of traumatized anterior teeth to occlusion. ASDC J Dent Child. 1963; 30:229-36.

82. Baccetti T, Antonini A. Dentofacial characteristics associated with trauma to maxillary incisors in the mixed dentition. J Clin Pediatr Dent. 1998; 22(4):281-84.

83. Burden DJ. An investigation of the association between overjet size, lip coverage, and traumatic injury to maxillary incisors. Eur J Orthod. 1995; 17(6):513-7.

84. Caldas AF, Burgos M. A retrospective study of traumatic dental injuries in a Brazilian dental trauma clinic. Dent Traumatol. 2001; 17(6):250-3.

85. Gulinelli JL, Saito CT, Garcia-Junior IR, Panzarini SR, Poi WR, Sonoda CK et al. Occurrence of tooth injuries in patients treated in hospital environment in the region of Araçatuba, Brazil during a 6-year period. Dent Traumatol. 2008; 24(6):640-4.

86. Petti, Cairella G, Tarsitani G. Childhood obesity: a risk factor for traumatic injuries to anterior teeth. Endod Dental Traumatol. 1997; 13(6):285-8.

87. European Commission DGfHaCP. Implementation of the Minimum Data Sets on Injuries (MDS-Is). http://ec.europa.eu/health/ph_projects/2001/injury/fp_injury_2001_frep_01_en.pdf. Acesso em 10/10/2011.

88. Traebert J, Calvo MCM, Lacerda JT. Relatório final do Projeto Estimativa da Carga de Doença de Santa Catarina. Florianópolis, SC: FAPESC/SES/MS2009.

89. Traebert J, Marcon KB, Lacerda JT. [Prevalence of traumatic dental injuries and associated factors in schoolchildren of Palhoca, Santa Catarina State]. Cien Saude Colet. 2010 Jun; 15 (Suppl 1):1849-55.

90. Sheiham A, Watt R. The common risk factor approach: a rational basis for promoting oral health. Community Dent Oral Epidemiol. 2000 Dec; 28(6):399-406.

91. Haddon Jr W. The changing approach to the epidemiology, prevention, and amelioration of trauma: the transition to approaches etiologically rather than descriptively based. Am J Public Health. 1968; 58:1431-8.

92. Haddon Jr W. Advances in the epidemiology of injuries as a basis for public health policy. Public Health Rep. 1980; 95:411-21.

93. McClure R, Stevenson M, McEvoy. The scientific basis of injury prevention and control. IP Communications: Melbourne. 2004.

94. Queensland Government, http://www.health.qld.gov.au/chipp/what_is/matrix.asp. Acesso em 08/10/2011.

95. Queensland Government, http://www.health.qld.gov.au/stayonyourfeet/injury_prevention/matrix.asp. Acesso em 10/10/2011.

96. Schützmannsky G. Unfallverletzungen an jugendlichen Zähnen. Dtsch Stomatol. 1963; 13:919-27.

97. Johnson JE. Causes of accidental injuries to the teeth and jaws. J Public Health Dent. 1975; 35:123-31.

98. Hedegård B, Stålhane I. A study of traumatized permanent teeth in children aged 7-15 years. Part I. Swed Dent J. 1973; 66:431-50.

99. O'Mullane DM. Some factors predisposing to injuries of permanent incisors in school children. Br Dent J. 1973; 134:328-32.

100. Knychalska-Karwan Z. Trauma to the anterior teeth in sportsmen in the light of statistics. Czas Stomatol. 1975; 28:479-84.

101. Haavikko K, Rantanen L. A follow-up study of injuries to permanent and primary teeth in children. Proc Finn Dent Soc. 1976; 72:152-62.

102. O'Mullane DM. Injured permanent incisor teeth. An epidemiological study. J Irish Dent Assoc. 1972; 18:160-73.

103. Lees GH, Gaskell PH. Injuries to the mouth and teeth in an undergraduate population. Br Dent J. 1976;1 40:107-8.

104. Szymanska-Jachimczak EI, Szpringernodzak M. Statistical analysis of traumatic damage to permanent teeth in children and adolescents treated at the outpatient clinic of the department of pediatric stomatology institute of the medical academy in Warsaw in the years 1960-1975. Czas Stomatol. 1977; 30:689-93.

105. Nysether S. Dental injuries among Norwegian soccer players. Community Dent Oral Epidemiol. 1987; 15:141-3.

106. Järvinen S. On the causes of traumatic dental injuries with special reference to sports accidents in a sample of Finnish children. A study of a clinical patient material. Acto Odontol Scand. 1980; 38:151-4.

107. Häyrinen-Immonen R, Sane J, Perkki K, Malmström M. A six-year follow-up study of sports-related dental injuries in children and adolescents. Endod Dent Traumatol. 1990; 6:208-12.

108. Brat M, Li SH. Consumer product-related tooth injuries treated in hospital emergency rooms: United States, 1979-87. Community Dent Oral Epidemiol. 1990; 18:133-8.

109. Sandham A, Dewar I, Craig J. Injuries to incisors during sporting activities at school. Tandlægebladet. 1986; 90:661-3.

110. Rodd HD, Chesham DJ. Sports-related oral injury and mouthguard use among Sheffield school children. Community Dent Health. 1997; 14(1):25-30.

111. Federation Dentaire International (FDI). Commission on dental products, Working Party No. 7:1990.

112. Edward S, Nord CE. Dental injuries of school-children. Sver Tandlakarforb Tidn. 1968; 61:511-6.

113. Hawke JE. Dental injuries in rugby football. N Z Dent J. 1969; 65:173-5.

114. Kremer LR. Accidents occurring in high school athletics with special reference to dental injuries. J Am Dent Assoc. 1941; 28:1351-2.

115. Roberts JE. Wisconsin Interscholastic Athletic Association 1970. Benefit plan summary. Supplement to the 47th Official Handbook of the Wisconsin Interscholastic Athletic Association. 1970:1-77.

116. Lees GH, Gaskell PH. Injuries to the mouth and teeth in an undergraduate population. Br Dent J. 1976; 140:107-8.

117. Hill CM, Crocher RF, Mason DA. Dental and facial injuries following sports accidents: a study of 130 patients. Br J Oral Maxillofac Surg. 1985; 23:268-74.

118. Linn EW, Vrijhoef MMA, Wijn Jr DE, Coops RPHM, Cliteur BF, Meerloo R. Facial injuries sustained during sports and games. J Maxillofac Surg. 1986; 14:83-8.

119. Seguin P, Beziat Jl, Breton P, Freidel M, Nicod C. Sports et traumatologie maxillo-faciale. Aspects étiologiqes et cliniqes à propos de 46 cas. Mesures de prévention. Rev Stomatol Chir Maxillofac. 1986; 87:372-5.

120. Stockwell AJ. Incidence of dental trauma in the Western Australian School Dental Service. Community Dent Oral Epidemioll. 1988; 16:294-8.

121. Chapman PJ, Nasser BP. Prevalence of orofacial injuries and use of mouthguards in high school Rugby Union. Aust Dent J. 1996; 41(4):252-5.

122. Lang B, Pohl Y, Filippi A. Knowledge and prevention of dental trauma in team handball in Switzerland and Germany. Dent Traumatol. 2002; 18(6):329-34.

123. Roberts JE. Dental guard questionaire summary. Wisconsin Interscholastic Athletic Association report to the National Alliance Football Rules Committee. 1962.

124. Cohen A, Borish AL. Mouth protector project for football players in Philadelphia high schools. J Am Dent Assoc. 1958; 56:863-4.

125. Meadow D, Lindner G, Needleman H. Oral trauma in children. Pediatr Dent. 1984; 6:248-51.

126. Lephart SM, Fu FH. Emergency of athletic injuries. Dent Clin North Am. 1991; 35:707-17.

127. Understanding and Improving Health and Objectives for Improving Health. 2nd ed. Washington, DC: US Department of Health and Human Services, Healthy People 2010; 2000.

128. Oral Health in America: a report of the surgeon general. Rockville, MD: US Department of Health and Human services. National Institutes of Health, National Institute of Dental and Craniofacial Research. 2000.

129. Burt CWW, Overpeck MD. Emergency visits for sports-related injuries. Ann Emerg Med. 2001; 37:301-8.

130. Billings RJ, Berkowitz RJ, Watson G. Teeth. Pediatrics. 2004; 113(4 Suppl):1120-7.

131. Lucht U, Lie HR. Ridesportsulykker. II. Ulykkerne belyst gennem en prospektiv sygehusundersøgelse. Ugeskr Læger. 1977; 139:1689-92.

132. Nowjack-Raymer Re, Gift HC. Use of mouthguards and headgear in organized sports by school-aged children. Public Health Rep. 1996; 111:82-6.

133. Kulowski J. Facial injuries: a common denominator of automobile casualties. J Am Dent Assoc. 1956; 53:32-7.

134. Kulowski J. Crash injuries. Springfield, Illinois: CT Thomas, 1960. p.306-22.

135. Schultz RC. Facial injuries from automobile accidents: a study of 400 consecutive cases. Plast Reconstr Surg. 1967; 40:415-25.

136. Huelke DF, Sherman HW. Automobile injuries - the forgotten area of public health dentistry. J Am Dent Assoc. 1973; 86:384-93.

137. Worrall SF. Mechanisms, pattern and treatment costs of maxillofacial injuries. Injury. 1991; 22(1):25-8.

138. Gassner RJ, Hackl W, Tuli T, Fink C, Waldhart E. Differential profile of facial injuries among mountainbikers compared with bicyclists. J Trauma. 1999; 47(1):50-4.

139. Eilert-Petersson E, Schelp L. An epidemiological study of bicycle-related injuries. Accid Anal Prev. 1997; 29(3):363-72.

140. Roccia F, Servadio F, Gerbino G. Maxillofacial fractures following airbag deployment. J CranioMaxillofac Surg. 1999; 27:335-8.

141. Mouzakes J. Koltai PJ, Kuhar S, Bernstein DS, Wing P, Salsberg E. The impact of airbags and seat belts on the incidence and severity of maxillofacial injuries in automobile accidents in New York State. Arch Otolaryngol Head Neck Surg. 2001; 127:1189-1193.

142. Thompson DC, Rivara FP, Thompson R. Helmets for preventing head and facial injuries in bicyclists (Cochrane Review). In: The Cochrane Library, Issue 1, 2003. Oxford: Update Software.

143. Acton CH, Nixon JW, Clark RC. Bicycle riding and oral/maxillofacial trauma in young children. Med J Aust. 1996; 165(5):249-51.

144. Tapias MA. Prevalence of traumatic crown fractures to permanent incisors in a childhood population: Mostoles, Spain. Dent Traumatol. 2003; 19(3):119-22.

145. Huang B, Marcenes W, Croucher R, Hector M. Activities related to the occurrence of traumatic dental injuries in 15- to 18-year-olds. Dent Traumatol. 2009; 25(1):64-8.

146. Al-Majed I, Murray JJ, Maguire A. Prevalence of dental trauma in 5-6- and 12-14-year-old boys in Riyadh, Saudi Arabia. Dent Traumatol. 2001; 17:153-8.

147. Botchway C, Kuc I. Tongue piercing and associated tooth fracture. J Can Dent Assoc. 1998; 64(11):803-5.

148. Fehrenbach MJ. Tongue piercing and potential oral complications. J Dent Hyg. 1998; 72(1):23-5.

149. Campbell A, Moore A, Williams E, Stephens J, Tatakis DN. Tongue piercing: impact of time and barbell stem length on lingual gingival recession and tooth chipping. J Periodontol. 2002; 73(3):289-97.

150. Levin L, Zadik Y, Becker T. Oral and dental complications of intra-oral piercing. Dent Traumatol. 2005; 21(6):341-3.

151. Reichl RB, Dailey JC. Intraoral body piercing: a case report. Gent Dent. 1996; 44:346-7.

152. De Moore RIG, De Witte AMJC, De Bruyne MAA. Tongue piercing and associated oral and dental complications. Endod Dent Traumatol. 2000; 16:232-237.

153. Bessermann K. Frequency of maxillofacial injuries in a hospital population of patients with epilepsy. Bull Nord Soc Dent Handicap. 1978; 5:12-26.

154. Buck D, Baker GA, Jacoby A, Smith DF, Chadwick DW. Patients' experiences of injury as a result of epilepsy. Epilepsia. 1997; 38(4):439-44.

155. Ogunbodede EO, Adamolekun B, Akintomide AO. Oral health and dental treatment needs in Nigerian patients with epilepsy. Epilepsia. 1998; 39(6):590-4.

156. Pick L, Bauer J. Zahnmedicin und Epilepsi. Nervenarzt. 2001; 72 (12):946-9.

157. Chapman PJ. Medical emergencies in dental practice and choice of emergency drugs and and equipment: a survey of Australian dentists. Aust Dent J. 1997; 42(2):103-8.

158. Holan G, Peretz B, Efrat J, Shapira Y. Traumatic injuries to the teeth in young individuals with cerebral palsy. Dent Traumatol. 2005; 21(2):65-9.

159. Snyder JR, Knoops JJ, Jordan WA. Dental problems of non-institutionalized mentally retarded children. North-West Dent. 1960; 39:123-33.

160. O'Donnell D. The prevalence of non-repaired fractured incisors in visually impaired Chinese children and young adults in Hong Kong. Quintessence Int. 1992; 23(5):363-5.

161. Alsarheed M, Bedi R, Hunt NP. Traumatised permanent teeth in 11-16-year-old Saudi Arabian children with a sensory

impairment attending special schools. Dent Traumatol. 2003; 19:123-5.

162. Wikström L. Narkotika och tänder. Sver Tandlakarforb Tidn. 1970; 62:1152-5.

163. von Gerlach D, Wolters HD. Zahn and Mundschleimhautbefunde bei Rauschmittelkonsumenten. Dtsch Zahnärtztl. 1977; 32:400-4.

164. Tate RJ. Facial injuries associated with the battered child syndrome. Br J Oral Surg. 1971; 9:41-5.

165. Laskin DM. The battered-child syndrome. J Oral Surg. 1973; 31:903.

166. Schwartz S, Woolridge E, Stege D. Oral manifestations and legal aspects of child abuse. J Am Dent Assoc. 1977; 95:586-91.

167. Laskin DM. The recognition of child abuse. J Oral Surg. 1978; 36:349.

168. Becker DB, Needleman HL, Kotelchuck M. Child abuse and dentistry; orofacial trauma and its recognition by dentist. J Am Dent Assoc. 1978; 97:24-8.

169. Hazlewood AI. Child abuse. The dentist's role. N Y Dent J. 1970; 36:289-91.

170. Malecz RE. Child abuse, its relationship to pedodontics: a survey. ASDC J Dent Child. 1979; 46:193-4.

171. Davis GR, Domoto PK, Levy RL. The dentists role in child abuse and neglect. ASDC J Dent Child. 1979; 46:185-92.

172. Kittle PE, Richardson DS, Parker JW. Two child abuse/child neglect examinations for the dentist. ASDC J Dent Child. 1981; 48:175-80.

173. Schmitt BD. Types of child abuse and neglect: an overview for dentists. Pediatr Dent. 1986; 8:67-71.

174. Schmitt BD. Physical abuse: specifics of clinical diagnosis. Pediatr Dent. 1986; 8:83-7.

175. Needleman HL. Orofacial trauma in child abuse: types, prevalence, management, and the dental professions involvement. Pediatr Dent. 1986; 8:71-80.

176. Kittle PE, Richardson DS, Parker JW. Examining for child abuse and child neglect. Pediatr Dent. 1986 ;8:80-2.

177. Dubowitz H. Sequelae of reporting child abuse. Pediatr Dent. 1986; 8:88-92.

178. Wagner GN. Bitemark identification in child abuse cases. Pediatric Dent. 1986; 8:96-100.

179. Casamassimo PS. Child sexual abuse and the pediatric dentist. Pediatr Dent. 1986; 8:102-6.

180. Haug RH, Foss J. Maxillofacial injuries in the pediatric patient. Oral Surg Oral Med Oral Pathol Oral Radiol Endod. 2000; 90(2):126-34.

181. Fonseca MA, Feigal RJ, ten Bensel RW. Dental aspects of 1248 cases of child maltreatment on file at a major county hospital. Pediatr Dent. 1992; 14(3):152-7.

182. Miller CA, Fine A, Adams-Taylor S: Monitoring Children´s Health: Key Indicators. 2nd ed. Washington. DC: American Public Health Association. 1989. pp.144-52.

183. McDowell JD, Kassebaum DK, Fryer GE Jr. Recognizing and reporting dental violence: a survey of dental practitioners. Spec Care Dentist. 1994; 14(2): 49-53

184. Ramos Gomez F, Rothman D, Blain S. Knowledge and attitudes among California dental care providers regarding child abuse and neglect. J Am Dent Assoc. 1998; 129(3):340-8.

185. Welbury Rr, Murphy JM. The dental practitioner's role in protecting children from abuse. 2. The orofacial signs of abuse. Br Dent J. 1998; 184(2):61-5.

186. Dimitroulis G, Eyre J. A 7-year review of maxillofacial trauma in a central London hospital. Br Dent J. 1991; 170(8):300-2.

187. Gayford JJ. Wife battering: a preliminary survey of 100 cases. Br Med J. 1975;194-7.

188. Parker B, Schumacher DN. The battered wife syndrome and violence in the nuclear family of origin. A controlled pilot study. Am J Public Health. 1977; 67:760-1.

189. Scott PD. Battered wives. Br J Psychiatry. 1974; 125:433-41.

190. Rounsaville B, Weissmann MM. Battered women; A medical problem requiring detection. Int J Psychiatry. 1977-78; 8:191-202.

191. Rounsaville BJ. Battered wives. Barriers to identification and treatment. Am J Orthopsychiatry. 1978; 48:487-94.

192. Petro JA, Quann PL, Graham WP. Wife abuse. The diagnosis and its implications. J Am Dent Assoc. 1978; 240:240-1

193. Laskin DM. Looking out for the battered woman. J Oral Surg. 1981; 39:405.

194. Young GH, Gerson S. New psychoanalytic perspectives on masochism and spouse abuse. Psychotherapy. 1991; 28:30-8.

195. Bolling P. Tandtortur. Tandlægebladet. 1978; 82:571-4.

196. Diem CR, Richling M. Dental problems in Navy and Marine Corps repatriated prisoners of war before and after captivity. Milit Med. 1978; 143:532-7.

197. Diem CR, Richling M. Improvisational dental first aid used by American prisoners of war in Southeast Asia. J Am Dent Assoc. 1979; 98:535-7.

198. Chadwick RG, Lindsay SM. Dental injuries during general anaesthesia. Br Dent J. 1996; 180(7):255-8.

199. Chadwick RG, Lindsay SM. Dental injuries during general anaesthesia: can the dentist help the anaesthetist? Dent Update. 1998; 25(2):76-8.

200. Lockhart PB, Feldbau EV, Gabel RA, Connoly SF, Silversin JB. Dental complications during and after tracheal intubation. J Am Dent Assoc. 1986; 112:480-3.

201. Hyodo M, Kurimoto KM. Statistical observation about the injury to the teeth caused by endotracheal intubation. Masui. 1991; 20:1064-7.

202. Folwaczny M, Hickel R. Oro-dental injuries during intubation anesthesia. Anaesthesist. 1998; 47(9):707-31.

203. Mebius C, Soras A, Raf L. Tooth injuries in connection with intubation anesthesia: severity of the disease and dental status. Lakartidningen. 1998; 95 (24):2848-9.

204. Brosnan C. Radford P. The effect of a toothguard on the difficulty of intubation. Anaesthesia. 1997; 52:1011-4.

205. Skeie A, Schwartz O. Traumatic injuries of the teeth in connection with general anaesthesia and the effect of use of mouthguards. Endod Dent Traumatol. 1999; 15:33-6.

206. Lacau Saint Guily J, Boisson-Bertrand D, Monnier P. Lesions to lips, oral and nasal cavities, pharynx, larynx, trachea and esophagus due to endotracheal intubation and its alternatives. Ann Fr Anesth Reanim. 200; 22(1):81-96.

Chapter 16

Effectiveness of Oral Health Education

Simone Tetu Moysés
Julie Satur
Jonathon Timothy Newton

Introduction

This chapter addresses aspects of the effectiveness of methods of oral health education. First there is a brief conceptual discussion about health education practices, pointing out the limitations of education centred approaches in the transmission of knowledge and the importance of social and environmental influences in the determination of health related behaviours. As it is vitally important for planners of programs to be aware of evidence of the available evidence on the effectiveness of oral health education practices, the effectiveness is reviewed next. Then we discuss theories about behaviour changes and how they should be the motivational approaches should be incorporated. The chapter ends with the presentation of a brief outline of health education practices in Brazil, exploring opportunities for the incorporation of effective actions in the context of Primary Health Care in Brazil.

The effectiveness of oral health education

There is an obvious and recognized need to transmit oral health information to people to enable them to maintain their own oral health. An understanding of biomedical models of disease has been considered essential to achieving protective behaviours. Dental and other health professionals have engaged in transmitting information and advice to target causes of illnesses through preventive and educational approaches. The underlying theory behind these approaches is that once individuals acquire the relevant knowledge and skills, they will then alter their behaviour to maintain optimal oral health.[1] These bio-medical models of individual oral health education based on giving information have been shown to be largely ineffective.[2-5]

Traditional notions of health education have relied upon teaching and learning approaches - providing information in ways that people can absorb and use it. Green defined health education in 1980 as '...*any combination of learning experiences designed to facilitate voluntary adaptations of behaviour conducive to health...*'.[6] Green's emphasis was not on what information was used, but on how it impacted on behaviour change that was *voluntary*. The emphasis here is on voluntary - the way in which people perceive their own problems and choose to act on them. The evidence shows that many people also choose not to act on information.[2-4]

While there is evidence that behaviour change does sometimes occur through motivating, sustained change has been difficult to achieve. There is also evidence to show that health education based on information giving approaches can actually increase inequalities because of unequal capacity to act on the information provided; that health education may be actively disempowering.[2,3,5] Health education activity must not overlook the broader context determining human behaviours, including factors such as the social, economic, political and environmental circumstances, known as the social determinants of health.[7] Oral diseases are not only affected by the social determinants of health, and the cultural and social circumstances in which people live, they interact with them.

Oral health behaviours are inextricably connected to the other behaviours people apply to cope with and manage their lives. For children, the oral health behaviours of their parents are influential, but the social and living conditions of their parents and families that place pressures on their lives and ability to cope are of far greater influence

(See Chapter 8). Added to this are the behaviours arising out of the developmental stage of a child that creates an interactive social learning environment that may reward habits and behaviours that are not always directly related to oral health. These behaviours and habits and the interaction between parent and child establish the context in which oral health behaviours are established. The ability of a parent, and also a child, to apply information and knowledge in the context of their lives is far more complex than simply 'know and do'.

More recently, health literacy has emerged as an important concept to explain a person's ability to obtain, process and communicate and use information about health. People with poor health literacy are less likely to respond to health education and to use preventive approaches. Health literacy encompasses task-based abilities (reading, writing, cognition - the ability to understand clinical and health related information) and skills-based abilities (the ability to use and act on information, analyse and apply it to changing circumstances and exert greater control over life). Improving health literacy involves more than translation of health information into culturally appropriate language although that is an elementary task. There is also a requirement for enabling and empowering activity to improve a person's confidence in dealing with the health system, their ability to act on the knowledge and work with the support of others.[8,9]

So, while oral ill health conditions are almost completely preventable, data on the prevalence of disease indicates that approaches based on providing mainly information for prevention are often ineffective. This raises the question of what is effective health education.

Importance of evidence-base for planning and actions on health education

"Blind faith and unquestioning belief that we are doing good are weak substitutes for sound evidence".[10]

If we want to make our health education effective we need to understand how and why people behave as they do, how they use information and what features in their social setting affect the way they act. This will naturally differ from person to person so the ability to 'educate' either an individual, or a group of people will depend on their individual levels of health literacy, their learning styles, their perceptions of the disease and its risk factors, the context in which the behaviours are taking place and their ability to change their coping behaviours and be empowered to take control of their own health within that context.

The importance of self-efficacy, a person's belief in their own ability to complete a task or action, must be recognised to identify which activities a person will undertake or avoid.[8] Identifying a person's specific needs and concerns when attempting to initiate behaviour change is important, as is the recognition that change is a process and that new skills and knowledge must be integrated into their everyday life. As a person integrates new skills into their daily life, self efficacy and confidence in their ability to effect and maintain the change is built.

It is also important to identify context and culture. If we only ever provide people with information we never create the opportunity to find out what conditions, influences and coping mechanisms people use to manage their lives, we are likely to be ineffective.

There is an important need for counselling type approaches using active listening to gather information to enable tailored approaches to working with people rather than the traditional paternalistic and normative approaches that many clinical encounters produce. There is a critical need to respect people's expertise and ability to cope and flourish in the context of their own lives.

A number of research based models exist to inform health education interventions which draw on theories of self efficacy, motivation, counselling and behaviour change. These models offer frameworks to consider the processes of behaviour change and the influences of social circumstances. They are important instruments in the planning of effective interventions to address oral health behaviours.

Reviews/evidence of effectiveness of dental health

Evidence based reviews provide a method of identifying the most effective and efficacious interventions. Their limitations are that they rely on the availability and quality of published evidence and as a result there are gaps in the evidence which necessitate the need for local and practitioner experience in the use of evidence to inform intervention planning. The early reviews of the evidence of effectiveness for oral health promotion interventions was conducted by Sprod et al.[3] by Kay and Locker.[2] Kay and Locker reported that a meta-analysis of 37 studies which met quality criteria, concluded that small positive, but temporary effects on plaque levels (10% change) could be achieved through dental health education activities. There was no evidence from this review that oral health education activities reduce dental caries, even if changes in behaviour were achieved. Kay and Locker concluded that the most effective interventions were expensive in time and resources and that more rigourous approaches to evaluation were required.

Sprod, Anderson and Treasure acknowledged the limitations inherent in evaluating oral health promotion effectiveness and used methods that identified reliable studies and also recognised the findings of weaker study designs in order to present accumulated findings and to capture as much learning as possible from the review process. They concluded that there was evidence that oral health education can be effective in improving people's knowledge and oral health at all ages but that '...*longer term health gains are possible if the social environments of the very young are targeted...*'. They found that modifying personal oral hygiene skills can be demonstrated relatively easily in the short term but that one-off interventions are likely to be insufficient. Innovative interventions based on behaviour models for education and behaviour change were shown to be effective and participative approaches acknowledging the full range of social, cultural and personal norms were valuable, particularly in achieving longer term change. They noted that '...*although they should not be relied upon to give evidence of effectiveness on their own, community based interventions may still be very well-designed studies...*' and able to provide insights into the effectiveness of programs at community level. Although causality may be difficult to establish, such programs are also useful for highlighting potential areas or approaches worthy of further attention.[3]

Wright, Satur and Morgan.[4] used the data of the two previous studies and the addition of systematically reviewed papers published from 1994 to 1998. In relation to health education interventions, this study reinforced the findings of earlier studies and additionally concluded that clinical preventive approaches (advice, fluorides, fissure sealants) were effective in reducing dental caries but often did not reach those in greatest need. Interventions that improve knowledge were useful but there were acknowledged limitations related to motivation, readiness to change, learning styles, and the need for repetitive sessions. Many media (instruction materials, videos, pamphlets) were supportive when used in tailored ways; appropriate language and simple messages are important. Individual persuasive approaches were effective where individuals had sought information and were ready to change. Short term change was easier to achieve and dietary change more difficult. Advice from dental professionals about smoking cessation was also shown to be effective in motivated individuals. Group health education interventions had similar levels of effectiveness with most useful being those using peer educators and participative approaches, engaging with cultural approaches and addressing barriers to change. Increasing knowledge among primary health carers was also shown to be effective particularly in settings with regular contact with parents and those involved early socialisation in childhood learning settings.[4]

In 2006 Satur, Gussy, Morgan Calache and Wright reviewed 243 studies from 1998 to 2005, 98 of which met inclusion criteria to add to the previous work in this area.[4] Strong and moderate evidence of effectiveness of interventions found in this study were summarised. Interventions addressing vertical transmission of streptococcus mutans in mothers were found to be of limited effectiveness unless clinical therapeutic interventions were included or good oral hygiene practices were established. Interventions in dental settings for smoking cessation showed promise particularly where individuals were counselled using methods built on the Stages of Change model, although evaluations were mostly process and impact rather than long term. There was evidence from a number of 'information giving' approaches in schools and clinical settings, which produced changes in knowledge, but with little or no effect on plaque scores and dental caries levels. The authors accepted that knowledge is important for oral health literacy but their findings reinforced the concept that information giving alone is not an effective approach to improving oral health status. Activities that increased knowledge (capacity to promote oral health) among primary carers and health workers was effective as did the incorporation of oral health education in training settings and undergraduate programs for health workers. There was also support for the notion that the profile raising and observational activity that accompanies an oral health promotion programme may in itself stimulate increased attention to oral health in these settings, suggesting support for approaches that incorporate accreditation standards, advocacy and networking. There was also promising evidence emerging from community based participatory programs with flexible educational delivery mechanisms meeting local needs. The authors acknowledged difficulty with isolating cause and effect but supported the notion of the role of the oral health practitioner as an expert resource (rather than driver) to support the delivery of culturally located oral health promotion programs in community settings.[11]

In 2010, the Victorian Health Department again commissioned a review of evidence to inform the development of an oral health promotion resource to inform policy development and program implementation. Building on previous work, the search included studies published between 1999 and 2010 and locally available evaluations published outside the peer reviewed literature. Findings of this review are summarised in Chapter 11 and those relevant to oral health education are reported here.[12]

Rogers found that the provision of oral health education and risk assessment by non dental personal has shown effectiveness in a number of programs, particularly with high risk children and their families. Education for oral health of gatekeepers such as primary health care support personnel including maternal and child health nurses, paediatricians, nutrition fieldworkers, home health visitors, teachers and childcare workers thus, continues to be effective. The value lies in increasing their oral health knowledge and capacity for health education and risk assessment and referral in settings where children and their parents are participants. It also adds to their ability to develop common risk approaches to improving oral health and for advocacy to raise and maintain the profile of oral health in general health settings. Mailing or gifting health education information and oral hygiene aids (toothpaste and toothbrushes) to families of young children was also effective in reducing dental caries among children in non fluoridated communities.

Providing information through Health Fairs has also had some limited effectiveness.[12]

The use of peer educators has also shown effectiveness by providing information in culturally relevant ways in both community settings with parents and school settings with children. Oral health education in schools through annual classroom lessons was found to be ineffective because of the isolated or 'stand alone' nature of the intervention; more embedded approaches have shown improvements in children´s oral hygiene practices over the short term but not sustainability. Innovative approaches using educational theory and teachers expertise was more effective in improving children´s knowledge and motivation. Embedding oral health education in school curricula and in health promoting schools approaches is supported by evidence of effectiveness particularly where participative approaches are utilised. There is also evidence that generic educational outcomes can be met by using oral health content in school curricula. Actively involving parents and generating community ownership of interventions around child oral health, particularly in pre and primary school settings, makes interventions more likely to be successful.[12] Rogers also found evidence to support the use of health behaviour theory as a basis for more effective interventions with adolescents.[12] This finding was supported by a review of the evidence for oral health education interventions with individuals conducted by Yevlahova and Satur.[13] They reviewed 89 studies and included 32 which met the selection criteria and found that the strongest evidence for effectiveness was in shown where counselling approaches and motivational interviewing were used, followed by

models based interventions and lastly clinical prevention and health education models.[13] There was strong evidence to suggest that clinical prevention, treatment and educational interventions can lack effectiveness because of a range of practitioner and client based barriers. Educational interventions assessed here were those that used information giving in the form of advice in a standardised way with a passive patient. Practitioners' workloads often limit the time required in a clinical encounter to deliver preventive advice in effective ways and they were found to lack insight into patient risk factors and operate with values differences between patients and clinicians. Oral health education provided in a clinical encounter with adolescents was found to be generally positively, but vaguely remembered and not always applied into practice. This study showed that even people who displayed knowledge of oral health topics did not always succeed in practising healthy habits. Additionally, for many people the stress of the clinical encounter acts as a barrier to absorbing information. These approaches that used standardised messages were described as palliative in nature and were considered to be ineffective. Counselling approaches using more interactive information giving approaches that address individual behaviour, were found to be relatively ineffective in general health environments but effective in oral health settings in combination with clinical preventive interventions. The inclusion of clinical prevention interventions meant that the effect of the counselling could not be isolated to allow an explanation of the reduction in need for care.[13]

Interventions based on models of health behaviour were effective in reducing disease and risk behaviours among adolescents and adults. The Health Belief Model, Theory of Planned Behaviour, Theory of Reasoned Action, Locus of Control and Protection Motivation Theories have all underpinned effective interventions to improve oral hygiene among adults with periodontal disease. Intervention's such as smoking cessation, improving adherence to oral hygiene instructions and reductions in consumption of carbonated drinks were also found to be effective when built on behaviour models. Tobacco cessation programs delivered by dental practitioners, built on behaviour models which included counselling were found to be effective in two systematic reviews. The Trans-Theoretical Model (TTM, or Stages of Change) was effective in initiating behaviour change in 45% of adolescents included in an intervention to reduce carbonated drink consumption. The study supported the TTM's predictions about the balance between the 'pros and cons' of change, which varied depending on which stage of change the individual was in. The influence of self-efficacy, family, friends and social circumstances were important to the health decision making process in these studies. Observational studies evaluating the Ecological Principles of Behaviour Change model showed that the comprehensive inclusion of intra-personal influences, policies and physical environmental influences was useful for planning behaviour change interventions and that this approach was feasible in primary health care settings.[13]

Motivational Interviewing (MI), a counselling approach that uses the Stages Of Change model as the basis for interactive interviewing to motivate behaviour change, was effective across a range of health based interventions.[13]

The focus of this approach is to prepare people for change by developing salience, exploring and resolving ambivalence and the impediments to change and enabling them to make their own decisions about why and how to proceed.[14] A meta-analysis of MI based interventions found that 51% of people who received MI treatment improved behaviour at follow up compared with 37% receiving no treatment or treatment as usual.[15] Another systematic review of 29 studies found that 60% of participants demonstrated at least one significant behaviour change.[16] Clients were mostly prepared for change over a small number of sessions with additional sessions to help them initiate and maintain the changes. The studies showed that the time invested in MI was useful in actively engaging people in an evaluation of their behaviour. There was evidence to show that the intervention effects did not appear to fade completely over time and that even single sessions were beneficial. MI impacted on clients in broad and relevant ways; they felt 'listened to' and understood by their health practitioners. Health practitioners were able to recognise a client's readiness to change and the steps toward it rather than seeing the outcome as the only goal. This approach seems to be consistent with several models of health behaviour. It shares elements such as recognition of the consequences of change, the influence of self efficacy and personal control, the influence of the settings and social contexts over behaviour, and the placing of the client/patient at the centre as the expert in their own lives. MI allows people to integrate information into their own social context in a supported way. The authors of this review endorsed the effectiveness and explanatory powers of the Trans-Theoretical Model and Motivational Interviewing as a technique to use it with individuals for behaviour change.[13]

The evidence presented above makes it clear that traditional bio-medical approaches to health education based on normative, information giving strategies are largely ineffective. It is also clear that a range of models based interventions can be effective and that their value lies in understanding and addressing the complexity of behaviour change. Client centred approaches to health education have been useful where people have stable lives and social supports, economic resources and a good sense of control over the determinants of their health. These approaches use 'active listening', respect the autonomy and expertise of the individual in their own lives, seek active participation and problem solving and draw on theories of behaviour change that allow for planning and practice. People must have identified the need to change themselves and be ready to change. Using motivational interviewing approaches that incorporate behaviour change models have been shown to be effective in working with people to prepare for change where their resources for change are good. Where people are marginalised by disability, social inequality or poverty, their ability to alter their circumstances or have any power over their lives is limited and approaches to health education must move to empowerment models.[5]

Models of Health Related Behaviour

There is a wide range of psychological models and theories that provide an important framework for increasing our understanding of the determinants of adherence to recommendations concerning health behaviours. Therefore they underpin the provision of effective dental health education. Social cognition models (SCMs) in particular have been repeatedly applied to predict and explain behaviour changes such as screening attendance, dieting, and oral hygiene behaviour.[17] 'Social cognitions' are beliefs, thoughts and attitudes concerning behaviours, which are believed to relate to whether or not a person undertakes a particular behaviour. All these models share the common assumption that an individual's behaviour is best understood by examining their attitudes and beliefs. The following models will be reviewed in relation to oral health related behaviours:

- Health Belief Model
- Protection Motivation Theory
- Locus of Control
- Social Learning Theory
- Theory of Planned Behaviour
- Implementation intentions
- Stages of Change model or Transtheoretical model

We shall focus only on three of the models which have particular relevance for oral health: the Theory of Planned Behaviour; Implementation intentions; and the Stages of Change model. For each model an outline of the constructs involved and their relationships will be given. This will be followed by a review of research exploring the relationship between the theory and health-related behaviours, including where possible oral health-related behaviours. Finally, intervention studies based on targeting the cognitions in each model will be discussed. Overall, the application of social cognition models to behaviour change interventions is still in its infancy and so there are relatively few published intervention studies.

Theory of Planned Behaviour

The theory of planned behaviour[18] builds upon the theory of reasoned action.[19] The latter was originally formulated in an attempt to explain the mediating processes between attitudes and behaviour, which according to this theory is the intention to act. This assumes intentions are a product of careful deliberation of available information. Ajzen and Fishbein further thought to incorporate evidence from previous studies by developing the 'principle of compatibility', which states that the relationship between attitudes and behaviour is greatest if both are measured to the same degree of specificity, especially along the following four dimensions: action, target, context and time. According to this principle, the relationship between attitudes and behaviour is greatest if the behavioural statement corresponds with the target behaviour along those dimensions. Thus, specific behaviours are best predicted by specific attitudes and general behaviours are best predicted by general attitudes. For instance, specific repeated single behaviours, such as flossing, require the targeting of specific attitudes, rather than more general attitudes that may predict general behaviours such as healthy eating. Originally, this theory was formulated to explain purely volitional behaviour. Behaviours that require resources which are not freely available, such as skills, time, costs or opportunities, were not originally within the remit of this model. In order to account for behaviours that are not under complete volitional control, Ajzen[18] added the perceived behavioural control construct. This extension of the Theory of Reasoned Action was named the theory of planned behaviour.

The theory of planned behaviour states that intention to perform an action is the most immediate predictor of behaviour (Fig. 16.1). This intention, in turn, is determined by attitudes towards the behaviour, perceptions of personal control over the behaviour and beliefs about social norms. The concept of 'attitudes' in this theory refers to a general evaluation of the positive and negative aspects of the behaviour. For instance, a given behaviour might be evaluated as unpleasant-pleasant, unwise-wise, bad-good, unnecessary-necessary, and uncomfortable-comfortable. In general, positive attitudes are thought to predict positive intentions to perform the behaviour. Subjective norm refers to the perceived social pressure to perform or not perform the behaviour and is usually assessed through two items. Normative beliefs are measured with items such as 'Those important to me think I should do x' whereas motivation to comply is assessed through a further item, such as 'It's important to me to do what others think I should do'. According to this theory, an individual is more likely to engage in a given behaviour if he or she perceives that significant others endorse the behaviour and they wish to conform to this pressure. Both attitudes and subjective norm are thought to be direct antecedents of intention. Therefore, intention is the mediating variable between attitudes and subjective norm and behaviour. Perceived behavioural control describes the constraints as perceived by the individual. The general tenet holds that individuals are more disposed to engage in behaviours they feel are achievable and under their personal control. The direct relationship between perceived behavioural control and behaviour is thought to reflect the extent to which measures match actual control.

Armitage and Conner[20] conducted a meta-analysis of studies that had used the Theory of Planned Behaviour. Across all behaviours, intention and perceived behavioural control (PBC) accounted for 27% of the variance in behaviour. Overall, PBC adds a further 2% to the prediction of behaviour, over and above intention. Assessing the predictive power of the subjective norm, attitudes and perceived behavioural control variables, the authors found that 39% of the variance in intention was accounted for by these three variables. Assessed individually, the subjective norm variable was the weakest predictor of intention, compared to attitudes and PBC.

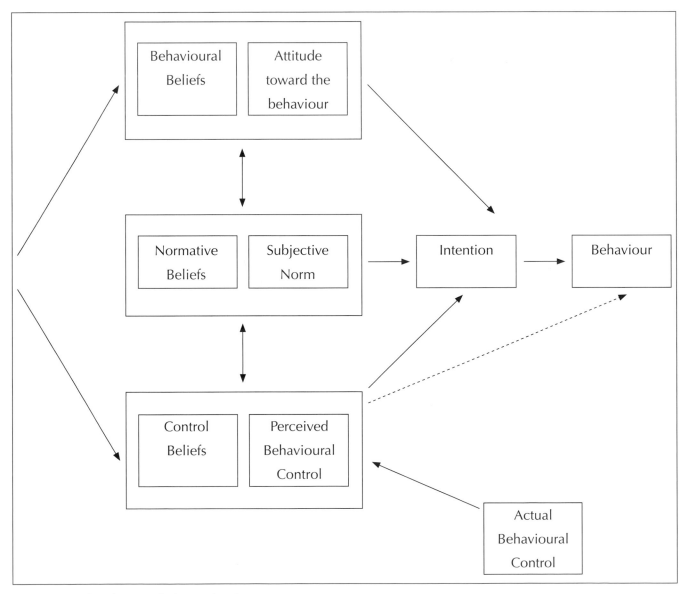

Fig. 16.1 – The Theory of Planned Behaviour.

Source: Ajzen[60]

Exploring studies that examine the relationship between oral hygiene behaviour and the theory of planned behaviour in more detail, McCaul et al.[21] assessed self-efficacy in conjunction with the theory of reasoned action variables as applied to oral hygiene behaviour. They found that self-efficacy beliefs further predicted brushing and flossing intention, but failed to increase the amount of variance explained in self-reported behaviour. A similar study assessed self-efficacy and TRA in combination to predict oral hygiene behaviour in a sample of periodontal patients and found that self-efficacy added to the variance explained by the TRA constructs.[22] While the combined constructs of the TRA explained 46% of variance for self-reported brushing and 38% for flossing behaviours, adding self-efficacy raised the amount of variance explained to 51% and 66% respectively. These findings were supported in later studies[22] in periodontal patients and in diabetic patients.[23]

Lavin and Groarke[24] recruited 199 university students to a study exploring the relationship between TPB constructs and self-reported use of dental floss. The Theory of Planned Behaviour variables predicted 46% of the variance in intention and 29% of the variance in behaviour. Similarly McCaul et al.[25] found that the theory of planned behaviour predicted oral hygiene behaviour in undergraduate students.

In summary, the theory of planned behaviour has been tested in a large variety of settings and populations, and a further number of studies have tested the application of this model to the design of behaviour change interventions. The model explained around 20-30% of the variance in behaviour and around 30-50% of the variance in intention. Whi-le the subjective norm variable is often found to be the weakest predictor of intention and behaviour, when applied to the study of oral hygiene behaviour this variable seemed to produce more promising correlations. However, this is a difficult construct to target for interventions. Studies combining the theory of reasoned action with self-efficacy confirm the strong relationship between self-efficacy beliefs and oral hygiene related behaviours.

Implementation intentions

The Theory of Planned Behaviour includes the notion of 'intention' as the key motivation to engage in a behaviour. Research using this model has focused on factors that determine or strengthen intentions, assuming that intention strength is a good predictor of behaviour. Correspondingly, much of the adherence literature assumes that a patient's lack of adherence is an indication of their lack of willingness or motivation to engage in the recommended behaviour. However, since the mid 1990s a growing body of research has addressed the apparent gap between intention and behaviour, indicating that this relationship may not always be as straightforward as formerly assumed. Motivation may be a necessary prerequisite for behaviour but not sufficient in itself to induce behavioural change. Gollwitzer[26] distinguishes between goal intentions and implementation intentions. Whereas goal intentions are formed in the motivational phase, implementation intentions are important in the post-motivational (or volitional) phase to ensure translation of intentions into action by linking the behaviour to an anticipated situational context. More specifically, goal intentions are commitments to engage in a certain behaviour (i.e. 'I intend to do x'), whereas implementation intentions are plans committing the individual as to when, where and how the behaviour is to be implemented (i.e. 'I intend to do x whenever the situational conditions y are met'). Implementation intentions promote the initiation and effective execution of a goal-directed activity by stating a specific plan of where, when and how this activity should occur. In order to form an implementation intention, the individual must first identify a goal-directed behaviour and anticipate a suitable situational context to initiate it. For example, the individual might specify "flossing" as the behaviour and a suitable situation as "in the bathroom in the evening after brushing my teeth".

Gollwitzer[26] summarises research conducted into implementation intentions. Studies were included in this review if the implementation intentions formed by participants were assessed in relation to a goal-directed behaviour, and if a statistical association between the formation of an implementation intention and behavioural outcome variable was reported or could be obtained. A meta-analysis of the findings from the studies provides evidence that forming implementation intentions makes an important difference in whether or not people successfully translate their intentions into actions. This finding was robust across a variety of behavioural domains, study designs and outcome measures.

Two studies applied implementation intentions to oral hygiene-related behaviour. Schüz et al.[27] found that planning was the only significant predictor of adherence to a daily regime of flossing in university dental students. Sniehotta et al.[28] developed a brief intervention to enhance intention implementations in a group of university students. By asking participants to plan where and when they would floss their teeth, Sniehotta and colleagues were able to demonstrate an improvement in the proportion of participants who were flossing three times a week or more.

Stages of Change model

The Transtheoretical Model of behaviour change, commonly referred to as the 'stages of change model',[29] describes how people modify their behaviour over time. The five *'stages of change'* summarised in figure 16.2 are:

- *Precontemplation* (the individual has no intention to take action in the foreseeable future Many individuals in this stage are unaware or unaware of their problems).
- *Contemplation* (they are aware that a problem exists and intend to take action within the next six months).
- *Preparation* (they intend to take action within the next 30 days and/or have unsuccessfully taken action in the past year).
- *Action* (they have changed a behaviour for less than six months).
- *Maintenance* (the stage in which people work to prevent relapse and consolidate the gains attained during action. For addictive behaviors like smoking this last stage extends from six months to an indeterminate period past the initial action).

Individuals are seen to progress through each stage to achieve successful maintenance of a new behaviour. These stages, however, do not always occur in a linear pattern and an individual may cycle from stage to stage and then back again i.e. relapse before achieving a long term behaviour change.

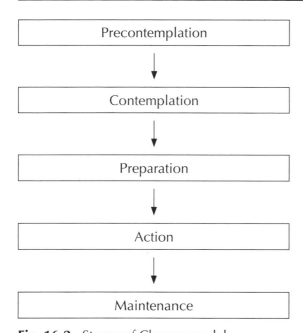

Fig. 16.2 –Stages of Change model

Source: Prochaska, DiClemente, and Norcross.[30]

Transitions between the 'stages of change' are effected by a set of independent variables known as the *'processes of change'* which are the activities and experiences that individuals engage in to progress through the stages. The ten 'processes of change' are divided into two broad categories; *'experimental (cognitive-affective) processes'* which include activities that could be related to thinking about changing behaviour, and *'behavioural processes'* that are categorized as behaviours which are helpful in behaviour change.[30]

The Transtheoretical model has been used extensively in research on smoking and smoking cessation. Cross-sectional studies have used the 'stages of change' to identify the distribution of current smokers within each stage.[31,32] The extent to which the variables in the Transtheoretical model predict an individual's movements between sta-ges is equivocal. It predicts that different types of interventions should be targeted at individuals within different stages of change; however, a systematic review of 23 studies found that there was limited evidence for the effectiveness of stage-matched interventions in changing smoking behaviour.[33]

Only one published study has used the Stages of Change framework in an attempt to improve oral hygiene in patients with periodontitis. Stewart et al. (1996)[34] found that a group of patients who received a psychological intervention based on the stages of change model demonstrated significantly higher change in self-efficacy scores for flossing at post--intervention compared to the other two groups. However, the magnitude of differences between groups was small.

In summary there is clear evidence for the existence of the 'stages of change', particularly in individuals who smoke, and that the processes of change identified within each stage are also prevalent. However, there is less convincing evidence that asking people to engage in the processes of change is related to behaviour change or move through the stages. What seems most probable is that the processes of stages of change are effective targets for behaviour change irrespective of the 'stage' which an individual is in.

Psychological models of behaviour change have identified a great many thought processes that are related to oral hygiene behaviour. There has been much less research addressing whether change in these thought processes can effect change in behaviour. There are several promising targets for interventions. The distinction between motivational and volitional stages appears to be important. Clinicians should distinguish between individuals who lack the motivation to change their oral hygiene behaviour, and those who are motivated but require support in planning and maintaining behaviour change. Targets for motivational interventions that appear to be important are placing an emphasis on the benefits of behaviour change and enhancing self-efficacy beliefs about oral hygiene behaviours. (For specific interventions which could target self-efficacy see Abraham & Michie;[35] British Psychological Society Division of Health Psychology Team 2008). For volitional interventions planning where, when and how the individual will engage in the oral hygiene behaviour, appears to be a highly effective brief intervention.

Oral health education realities and practices in Primary Health Care in Brazil

"No-one educates anyone; no-one educates himself alone, people educate each other, mediated by the world". Paulo Freire

Health education in Brazil reflects political and ideological contexts of health intervention and the dominant conceptions of health and education at different times in recent history.[36] Three main approaches that guide health education coexist in the health care system:

- prescriptive and coercive educational practices, centred on the conception of health based on medicalization and hygiene used in the early 20th century;
- individualistic approach focused on risk factors and the need for changes of individual behaviours dominant since the preventivist perspective of the second half of the 20th century;

- health promoting education based on the contemporary recognition of the importance of empowerment and of autonomy for the democratization and construction of health, dominant in public health policies from the Brazilian Health Reform Movement and implementation of the Unified Health System (SUS), in 1988.

Traditionally, health education, including the field of oral health, has been used to control disease from the perspective of accountability of individuals for the reduction of health risks.[37] Despite the evidence on the limitations of clinical and educational interventions focused exclusively on individuals bringing about sustainable improvements in oral health,[3,38-41] strategies of this nature are still very common in Brazilian health services. Based on a pedagogic approach of transmission of knowledge (Fig. 16.3), this sort of educational practice ignores determining factors of oral health/disease, and can induce "victim blaming",[42] as individual changes of behaviour are often beyond the control of individuals. As a result, people living in social and materially deprived conditions are frequently blamed for not making the appropriate changes, even after having received information and having been "trained" in self care in health, disregarding the fact that personal changes of behaviour can be much more difficult for them.[43]

The impacts of these approaches at an individual and social level reinforce individualism, dependence and detachment from reality.[44] They may also increase inequalities in health[45] as their response is conditioned by individual capacities related to differentiated contexts of life in an unequal society.

The transmission...

Ideas and knowledge about health are the most important points of communication. "Banking education" leads the student to receive knowledge passively, making him or her a deposit of information provided by the educator,[54,61] and seldom provoking individual behaviour changes.

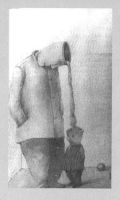

Individual impact

- passivity
- distancing between theory and practice
- Social impact
- conformism, individualism, lack of participation and cooperation
- lack of recognition of own reality

The conditioning...

Emphasis on behavioural results, attitudes and skills, through stimuli and rewards capable of "conditioning" the student to emit responses desired by the educator. Reproduction of predefined and uncontextualized behaviours.

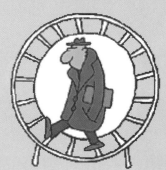

Individual impact

- efficiency in the learning of predetermined processes
- tendency toward individualism, competitiveness

Social impact

- emphasis on productivity and efficiency
- limited creativity and originality
- dependence
- lack of critical consciousness and of cooperation

The problematization...

Health problems/determinants of health and disease are identified and understood with a basis on the critical analysis of the reality observed, reaching a level of consciousness of this reality, in order to act on it, enabling social transformation.

Fig. 16.3 – Educational approaches in health.

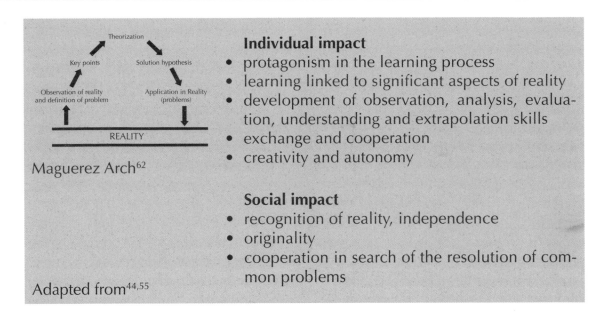

Individual impact
- protagonism in the learning process
- learning linked to significant aspects of reality
- development of observation, analysis, evaluation, understanding and extrapolation skills
- exchange and cooperation
- creativity and autonomy

Social impact
- recognition of reality, independence
- originality
- cooperation in search of the resolution of common problems

Maguerez Arch[62]

Adapted from[44,55]

Important conceptual changes are needed that focus on the determinats of health and the search for evidence on the effectiveness of actions for disease prevention and health promotion for the reduction of inequalities. That has criticized the health care models focused on biomedical/behavioural approaches geared towards the transmission of information. A radical reorientation of these models towards effective health promotion strategies is needed as the main means of promoting health and reducing inequality.[46]

In the 1980s, health promotion was recognized as "the process of enabling people to increase control over their health and its determinants, and thereby improve their health".[47] A parallel movement in Brazil, during the 8th National Health Conference, aimed to guarantee equal opportunities and the right to health, and reaffirmed the need to train people, by means of popular health education, to achieve their health potential. The enabling elements that were highlighted were:
- environments favourable to health,
- access to contextualized information,
- the development of skills for better living, and
- the creation of opportunities to make healthier choices.[48]

Health promotion concerns the "lifestyle structure", namely, the complex forms of interaction between patterns of individual behaviour, collective behaviour, organizational behaviour and available resources.[49] From this perspective, the search for the development of autonomy and individual empowerment through access to information, communication and popular health education, has become recognized as an essential strategy for health-oriented behaviour change, action on the social determinants, besides favouring the strengthening of social participation in tackling health inequities. Effective health education focused on autonomy as part of the actions proposed by the current National Health Promotion,[50] Basic/Primary Health Care,[51] and Oral Health Policies in Brazil.[52]

Popular health education emphasizes the enlargement of spaces for cultural interaction and negotiation among those involved in the social determination of health for the shared construction of knowledge and cooperation for action on these determinants and not the knowledge transmission process.[53] It therefore relates to a liberating and reality transforming action.[54] Individuals and groups that understand the factors that influence their health, know how to act on the factors and seek help when they need it. This is only possible by means of a reality problematizing pedagogic approach (Fig. 16.3). According to Pereira,[55] this approach, besides promoting valuing people´s learning and instrumentalization for the transformation of their reality and of themselves, enables the effectuation of citizens´ right to information so as to establish their active participation in health actions.

Opportunities for effective practices of education for the oral health of families and children in Primary Health Care scenarios in Brazil

As discussed previously, health education can enhance abilities of families and children to apply information and knowledge. Applying information and knowledge can be favoured by living in interactive social environments that consider the relational, political and environmental influences on the behaviours adopted to care for their health. Hence it is important to identify environments favourable to health education practices, focused on oral health, which favour positive and autonomous behaviours of these groups in the context of Primary Health Care. The main challenges are the involvement of different players, both inside and outside the Health Sector, training for mobilization and development of effective practices in different environments, besides the effectuation of liberating educational practices that build the autonomy of families and children for self-care.

Intersectoral scenario

Different living spaces of families and children can favour the development of general and oral health education actions. The city, the neighbourhood, the workplace of the parents, besides crèches and schools, are spaces for actions spearheaded by other sectors besides the Health Sector (Figs. 16.4 and 16.5). Collective spaces in the city frequented by families and children can provide an opportunity for interactive and contextualized collective educational practices, addressing the importance of care for life and for the environment where we live.

Crèches and schools take on a prominent role in the development of educational strategies with an impact on oral health, either in the pursuit of the problematization of health care and of people's relationship with their environment, or in the development of skills for life (See Chapter 18).

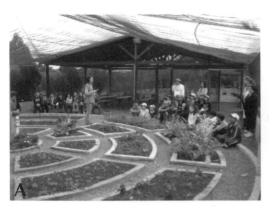
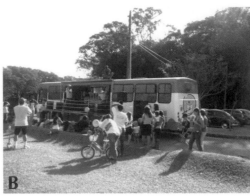

Fig. 16.4 – Oral health education in the city.

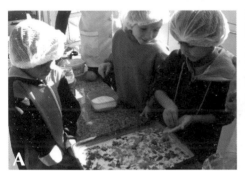
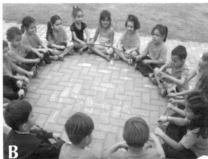
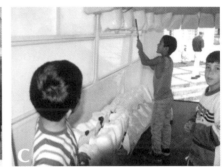

Fig. 16.5 – Oral health education at school.

Community scenario

In the community scenario of health education practices in Primary Health Care in Brazil, the performance of the Community Health Agent is prominent. Incorporated in the health team, especially in those working according to the principles of the Family Health Strategy, in defined territories, the Community Health Agent is, at the same time, a member of the local community and part of the professional team responsible for the health care of its community. Their specific duties include establishing a link between people and health teams, permanent contact with families, recognizing their needs and developing individual and collective educational actions in homes and in the community, targeting health care and promotion.[51] In the everyday routine of the services, their principal actions in the community have been providing families with guidance on disease prevention, child care and hygiene of people and environments.[56]

The educational practices performed by Community Health Agents could be linked to their greater ability to recognize the macro determinants that influence individual decisions relating to the health of communities, since they are part of them and live there. Paradoxically, their inclusion in health teams has brought about a tendency to reproduce prescriptive practices and those of adaptation to the norms of behaviour dictated by biomedical knowledge. The main challenge lies in recognizing the importance of their learning, different from technical knowledge, and in the qualification for their work as an educator capable of identifying problems and local needs and realities.[56]

The role of Community Health Agents in the promotion of oral health in the local communities is important in Primary Health Care. However, addressing topics related to oral health, oral hygiene and healthy eating, and even guidance for seeking clinical care, can be considered difficult by the Agents because of the awkwardness that these topics can cause people.[56]

Scenario of the clinic

The approach to common risk factors, which bridges the gap between oral health/disease conditions and other chronic conditions, such as diabetes, hypertension and cardiovascular diseases, can support health education practices in the primary health care clinic. Dental caries and gingivitis in children are chronic conditions, dependent on risk factors related to diet, hygiene and stress.

New approaches to the management of chronic conditions have reinforced the need for multidisciplinary care in an expanded clinic perspective that recognizes the personal and collective context which determines individual behaviours. Supportive self care is one of the strategies to be used in the clinic, and is defined as the systematic provision of health education and supportive actions to boost the confidence and increase the skills of people in managing their problems.[57] The principal objectives of supported self care are to generate knowledge and skills in individuals with chronic diseases to know their problem; to decide on and choose their treatment; to adopt, change and maintain behaviours that contribute to their health; to use the necessary resources to support

changes and to overcome the barriers against the improvement of their health.[58]

Based on human behaviour theories, especially the Theory of Planned Behaviour, of Implementation Intentions, and the Stages of Change Model, the construction of supported self care requires a set of strategies that vary according to the level of knowledge, the beliefs about health conditions, the attitudes towards changes, the level of confidence, the robustness of social support networks and the level of motivation.[57] The motivational interview (MI) has been considered an important strategy to support the construction of a self care plan, besides being recognized as the most effective method for providing support to behaviour changes in health within the sphere of the clinic, with important potential to be incorporated by oral health professionals.[59]

According to Mendes[57a] the joint preparation of a self care plan by the health team and the person responsible for the child, besides the involvement of the child him/herself, should utilize a methodology that includes assessment, counselling, concordance, assistance and monitoring. The assessment consists of an understanding of the disease, self-care capacity, knowledge, beliefs and behaviours of the person and their guardian. The Stages of Change models and the motivational interview are tools that have been used here. Counselling should be based on a problematizing approach that considers the disease recognition process, identification of significant information and of possible care strategies, to support the formulation of an action plan. Concordance consists of the preparation of the action plan based on the priorities, convictions and confidence to change of people. Assistance is the identification of the personal barriers, of the strategies, of the problem solving technologies and of the social and environmental supports for self care. Finally, a regular and systematic action monitoring plan is defined jointly and can include strategies such as regular visits to the health unit, telephone, electronic mail, and peer groups.[57]

The record of a self care plan, built by means of a motivational interview (MI), is considered an important strategy for the monitoring of what is decided. An example of a supported self care plan built by the mother of a 3-year-old child with early childhood caries, together with health professionals, is presented in figure 16.6.

Fig. 16.6 – Supported self care plan.

Name of child: Ana Alice Name of the mother/guardian: Maria da Graça Date: 20 April, 2011
1.Target: What? Where? How Much? When? How frequently? This week I will reduce my daughter´s nighttimes consumption of bottle-fed milk, decreasing the number of times I offer the milk day by day.
2.The main barriers to achieving this goal are: • my daughter will wake up at night crying and ask for the bottle • my husband will get mad at me, as he needs to sleep at night to work during the day • my daughter will be hungry at night
3.The actions that I can undertake to overcome these barriers are: • I can feed my daughter well before her bedtime, so that she does not miss the bottle as much during the night • I can ask my husband to be patient for a while, as I know that our daughter will soon no longer need the bottle at night • I can ask my friend for help, as she has already experienced this situation with her son, and can give me some advice
4.My degree of confidence in attaining the goal is (from 0, totally unconfident, to 10, totally confident)[8]

5. Monitoring

Day	Checklist	Remarks
Monday		
Tuesday		
Wednesday		
Thursday		
Friday		
Saturday		
Sunday		

Adapted from Mendes.[57]

The routine incorporation of the strategy of the supported self care plan for the management of chronic diseases is still not common in Brazil, although there is evidence of its effectiveness in other countries.[57] Its adoption, especially in oral health care, will lead to improvements in the quality of health education practices and of care offered by the Health System.

The need to refine oral health education practices is a current challenge of dentistry. It is necessary to strengthen education as a tool to increase social and political consciousness, in the search for sustainable improvements in oral health. The chronic nature of the main oral diseases and the profile of inequities in oral health, demand educational actions that support self care, an indispensable factor for instrumentalization individuals and groups to act to enhance health in an equitable manner. The involvement of different people and institutions qualified to develop effective educational practices can shift away from the over reliance of information, through the inclusion of essential knowledge for understanding and action on the determinants of health. Finally, the incorporation of theoretical benchmarks that support behaviour changes and evidence of their impact in different contexts can sustain the redefinition of health education practices.

References

1. Watt RG. Strategies and approaches in oral disease prevention and health promotion. Bulletin of the World Health Organization. 2005; 83(9):711-8.
2. Kay EJ, Locker D. Effectiveness of Oral Health Promotion: A Review. London: Health Education Authority. 1997.
3. Sprod A, Anderson R, Treasure E. Effective oral health promotion: literature review. Cardiff: Health Promotion Wales. 1996.
4. Wright FAC, Satur J, Morgan MV. Evidence Based Health Promotion; Resources for Planning. Victoria. 2000.
5. Keleher H, MacDougall C, Murphy B. Understanding Health Promotion. South Melbourne: Oxford University Press. 2007.
6. Green LW, Kreuter MW. Health promotion planning: an educational and environmental approach. 2nd ed. Mountain View, Toronto, London: Mayfield Publishing Company. 1991.
7. Marmot M, Wilkinson RG, editors. Social determinants of health. 1st ed. Oxford, New York: Oxford University Press. 1999.
8. Glanz K, Rimer B, Viswanath K. Health behavior and health education. Theory, research and practice. San Francisco: Jossey-Bass. 2008.
9. Nutbeam D, Harris E, Wise M. Theory in a Nutshell; a practical guide to health promotion theories. Australia: McGraw Hill Medical. 2010.
10. Glanz K. Achieving best practice in health promotion:Future directions. Health Promot J. 1996; 6:25.
11. Satur JG, Gussy MG, Morgan MV, Calache H, Wright FAC. Review of the evidence for oral health promotion effectiveness. Health Education Journal. 2010; 69(3):257-66.
12. Rogers J. Evidence-based Oral Health Promotion Resource. Melbourne: Prevention and Population Health Branch Victorian Department of Health. 2011.
13. Yevlahova D, Satur J. Models for individual oral health promotion and their effectiveness: a systematic review. Australian Dental Journal. 2009 Sep; 54(3):190-7.
14. Miller WR, Rollnick S. Motivational interviewing: Preparing People for Change. 2nd ed. New York: Guilford Press. 2002.

15. Burke BL, Arkowitz H, Menchola M. The efficacy of motivational interviewing: a meta-analysis of controlled clinical trials. J Consult Clin Psychol. 2003; 71:843-61.

16. Dunn C, Deroo L, Rivara FP. The use of brief intervention adapted from MI across behavioural domains: a systematic review. Addiction. 2001; 96:1725-42.

17. Conner M, Norman P. Predicting health behaviour: A social cognition approach. In: Conner M, Norman P, editors. Predicting health behaviour. Maidenhead: Open University Press. 2005; p.1-27.

18. Ajzen I. The theory of planned behaviour. Organizational Behaviour and Human Decision Making Processes. 1991; 50:179-211.

19. Fishbein M, Ajzen I. Belief, attitude, intention, and behaviour. Reading MA: Addison-Wesley. 1975.

20. Armitage CJ, Conner M. Efficacy of the Theory of Planned Behaviour: a meta-analytic review. Brit J Soc Psychol. 2001; 40:471-99.

21. McCaul KD, O'Neill K, Glasgow RE. Predicting the performance of dental hygiene behaviors: An examination of the Fishbein and Ajzen model and self-efficacy expectations. J App Soc Psych. 1988; 18:114-28.

22. Tedesco LA, Keffer MA, Fleck-Kandath C. Self-efficacy, reasoned action, and oral health behaviour reports: A social cognitive approach to compliance. Journal of Behavioural Medicine. 1991; 14(4):341-55.

23. Syrjälä AM, Ylostalo PV, Mirka CN, Knuuttila ML. Relation of different measures of psychological characteristics to oral health habits, diabetes adherence and related clinical variables among diabetic patients. Eur J Oral Sci. 2004; 112:109-14.

24. Lavin D, Groarke A. Dental floss behavior: A test of the predictive validity of the theory of planned behavior and the effects of implementation intentions. Psychology Health and Medicine. 2005; 10:243-52.

25. McCaul KD, Glasgow RE, O'Neill HK. The problem of creating habits: establishing health-protective dental behaviour. Health Psychol. 1993; 11:101-10.

26. Gollwitzer PM, Sheeran P. Implementation intentions and goal achievement: A meta-analysis of effects and processes. Adv Exp Soc Psych. 2006; 38:69-119.

27. Schüz B, Sniehotta FF, Wiedemann A, Seemann R. Adherence to a daily flossing regimen in university students: effects of planning when, where, how and what to do in the face of barriers. J Clin Periodontol. 2006; 33:612-9.

28. Sniehotta FF, Soares VA, Dombrowski SU. Randomized controlled trial of a one-minute intervention changing oral self-care behavior. J Dent Res. 2007; 86:641-5.

29. Prochaska JO, DiClemente CC. The transtheoretical approach. Homewood IL: J Irwin. 1984.

30. Prochaska JO, DiClemente CC, Norcross JC. In search of how people change. Applications to addictive behaviors. Am Psych. 1992; 47:1102-14.

31. Turner Y, Ashley FP, Wilson RF. Effectiveness of oral hygiene with and without root planing in treating subjects with chronic periodontitis. Brit Dent J. 1994; 177:367-71.

32. Velicer WF, Fava JL, Prochaska JO, Abrams DB, Emmons KM, Pierce JP. Distribution of smokers by stage in three representative samples. Prev Med. 1995; 24(4):401-11.

33. Riemsma RP, Pattenden J, Bridle C, Sowden AJ, Mather L, Watt IS, et al. Systematic review of the effectiveness of stage based interventions to promote smoking cessation. BMJ. 2003; 326:1175-7.

34. Stewart JE, Wolfe GR, Maeder L, Hartz GH. Changes in dental knowledge and self-efficacy scores following interventions to change oral hygiene behaviour. Pt Educ and Couns. 1996; 27:269-77.

35. Abraham C, Kelly MP, West R, Michie S. The UK National Institute for Health and Clinical Excellence public health guidance on behaviour change: a brief introduction. Psychol Health Med. 2009 Jan; 14(1):1-8.

36. Silva CMdC, Meneghim MdC, Pereira AC, Mialhe FL. Educação em saúde: uma reflexão histórica de suas práticas. Health education: a historical reflection of its practices. Ciência & Saúde Coletiva. 2010; 15(5):2539-50.

37. Albuquerque PC, Stotz EN. A educação popular na atenção básica no município: em busca da integralidade. Interface- Comunic, Saúde, Educ. 2004; 8(15):259-74.

38. Brown LF. Research in dental health education and health promotion: a review of the literature. Health Education Quarterly. 1994; 21(1):83-102.

39. Schou L, Locker D. A review of the effectiveness of health education and health promotion. Utrecht: Landelijk Centrum GVO 1994. Report No.: 4.

40. Kay L, Locker D. Is dental health education effective? A systematic review of current evidence. Community Dentistry and Oral Epidemiology. 1996; 24:231-5.

41. Kay E, Locker D. A systematic review of the effectiveness of health promotion aimed at improving oral health. Community Dentistry and Oral Epidemiology. 1998; 15(3):132-44.

42. Raymond JS. Behavioral epidemiology: the science of health promotion. Health Promotion. 1989; 4(4):281-6.

43. Tones K, Tilford S. Health education: effectiveness, efficiency and equity. 2nd ed. London, Weinheim, New York, Tokyo, Melbourne, Madras: Chapman & Hall. 1994.

44. Bordenave JED. Alguns fatores pedagógicos. In: L. JPSJ, Castro, editors. Capacitação em Desenvolvimento de Recursos Humanos CADRHU. Natal: Ministério da Saúde Organização Pan-Americana da Saúde Editora da UFRN. 1999; p.261-8.

45. Schou L, Wight C. Does dental health education affect inequalities in dental health? Community Dent Health. 1994 Jun; 11(2):97-100.

46. Watt RG. From victim blaming to upstream action: tackling the social determinants of oral health inequalities. Community Dentistry and Oral Epidemiology. 2007 Feb; 35(1):1-11.

47. WHO - World Health Organization. Ottawa Charter for Health Promotion. Health Promotion. 1987; 1(4):iii-v.

48. Buss PM, Carvalho AI. Development of health promotion in Brazil in the last twenty years (1988-2008). Ciencia & Saude Coletiva. 2009 Nov-Dec; 14(6):2305-16.

49. Rutten A. The implementation of health promotion: a new structural perspective. Social Science and Medicine. 1995; 41(12):1627-37.

50. Brasil, Ministério da Saúde. Política Nacional de Promoção da Saúde. Brasília: Ministério da Saúde, Série Pactos pela Saúde. 2006.

51. Brasil, Ministério da Saúde. Política Nacional de Atenção Básica. Brasília: Ministério da Saúde, Série Pactos pela Saúde. 2006.

52. Brasil, Ministério da Saúde, Coordenação Nacional de Saúde Bucal. Diretrizes da Política Nacional de Saúde Bucal. Brasília: Ministério da Saúde. 2004.

53. Vasconcelos EM. O Paulo da Educação Popular. In: BRASIL, Saúde Md, Participativa SdGEe, Participativa DdAàG, editors. Caderno de Educação Popular e Saúde. Brasília: Ministério da Saúde. 2007; p.31.

54. Freire P. Educação e Mudança. 24ª ed. Rio de Janeiro: Editora Paz e Terra. 2001.

55. Pereira ALdF. As tendências pedagógicas e a prática educativa nas ciências da saúde.Pedagogical approaches and educational practices in health sciences. Cadernos de Saúde Pública. 2003; 19(5):1527-34.

56. Mialhe FL, David HMSL. Os discursos dos agentes comunitarios de saúde sobre suas práticas educativas. In: Mialhe FL, editor. O Agente Comunitario de Saúde. Campinas: Unicamp. 2011; p.83-120.

57. Mendes EV. As Redes de Atenção à Saúde. Belo Horizonte: ESP-MG. 2009.

58. Morrison S. Self management support: helping clients set goals to improve their health. Nashville: National Health Care for the Homeless Council. 2007.

59. Watt RG. Motivational interviewing may be effective in dental setting. Evid Based Dent. 2010; 11(1):13.

60. Ajzen I. Perceived behavioural control, self-efficacy, locus of control, and the theory of planned behaviour. Journal of Applied Social Psychology. 2002; 32(4):665-82.

61. Freire P. Pedagogy of the Oppressed. Harmondsworth: Penguin. 1972.

62. Bordenave JD, Pereira AM. Estratégias de ensino-aprendizagem. 14ª ed. Petrópolis: Vozes. 1994.

Chapter 17

Primary Care as a Setting for Promoting Health

Sabrina Susan Fuller
Paulo Goes

Introduction

Primary care is the first point of contact with the health service and, in countries with well-developed primary care services, is the setting in which most care is provided. Because good oral health is an integral part of good general health, the primary care team have great potential as advocates, enablers and mediators for oral health. Attempts to support behaviour change can be categorised into four areas: education, communication, technologies, and resources. Primary care has a key role in each of these.

This chapter outlines the characteristics of primary care and how its organisation varies between countries. It demonstrates the place of oral health in primary care through the context of good general health and sets out the contribu-tion that oral health makes to the physical and mental health and wellbeing of children. Conversely it shows that oral health is one integral component of children and families' health, well-being and life experience. Given the close links between the range of health indicators and other indicators such as family income and educational attainment of child and parents, a whole systems approach to improving oral health in the context of general health is required.[1]

This chapter offers a model for strategic planning for oral health in the context of primary care, based on an analysis of need which includes the views of children and their families and offers holistic support to the family. Some of the principles which must underpin action are set out – including tailoring the response to the level of health need, building on community assets and strengthening family competence to self-manage health; an emphasis on early years and early intervention; a family focus, and a personalised approach to delivering services.

To support this evidence-based approach practical advice is offered on how to implement the promotion of oral health successfully through primary care. Finally a series of case-studies are provided which illustrate how such an approach can be delivered in a variety of settings in Brazil and in the United Kingdom.

Primary care as a setting for promoting health

The characteristics of primary care

The World Health Organisation has identified primary care as a key force in promoting the health of the population.[2] Starfield defines primary care is

the provision of first contact, person--focussed on-going care over time that meets the health-related needs of people.[3]

Continuity of care means that primary care workers can be effective in promoting health, as advice can be tailored to need and reinforced over time. Primary care's role as co-ordinators of care and its person-focus supports the integration of their oral health needs in the context of overall health, wellbeing and other needs.

Organisation of primary care in different settings

The system of organisation of primary health care varies between countries, and there is also considerable variation within countries in the way that individual practices are organised. Both of these will influence the potential of primary care to improve health as shown in Table 17.2.

Table 17.1 – Characteristics of primary care as defined by WHO[2] and by Starfield.[3]

WHO	Starfield
First level of contact of individuals, family and the community with health system	
Brings health care as close as possible to where people live and work	Person focussed meeting health needs
First element of a continuing process	Continuity of care
Central function and main focus of health system	Refers only what is too uncommon to maintain competence
Provides essential health care based on practical, acceptable and evidence-based methods	Co-ordinates care
Cheap and accessible technologies	Better health outcomes
	Lower cost
	Greater equity in outcomes (evidenced by inter and intra-national comparisons)

Table 17.2 – Factors influencing the potential of primary care to improve health.

Health system characteristics	Practice characteristics
Type of system	Content and featurs of first contact
System of finance	Development of relationship between professional and patient
Level of specialism within primary care	Comprehensive system
How costs are apportioned	Co-ordination of care
Whether practices have lists of patients	Focus on needs of families
Whether out-of-hours service provided	Focus on needs of communities
Academic support	

The extent to which primary dental care is part of general primary care will also vary between systems, for example in parts of Brazil prevention and treatment of oral disease is delivered as an integrated part of the Family Health Strategy. This model is described as a case study later in the chapter.

Oral health supporting the aims of primary care

Contribution of oral health to physical and mental health and wellbeing

Chapter 1 on a life course approach to health sets out how healthy children can form the basis for a healthy society, and how good oral health contributes to the health of children. It is, therefore, not difficult to interest primary care professionals in promoting oral health within the context of good overall health and wellbeing.

Linking oral health into primary care priorities

General health

- Affecting the ability to eat a healthy diet
- Chronic abcesses as a source of sepsis
- Acute infections, cellulitis
- Avoidable general anaesthetics for dental treatment as a potential risk to life

Mental health and wellbeing

- Pain and distress from toothache
- Lost nights' sleep

- Taste or odour from chronic abcesses
- Effect of decayed teeth on appearance, self esteem and self confidence
- Phobia or fear of dental treatment

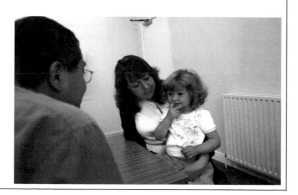

They can be motivated to prevent dental disease through understanding that it is a preventable disease, and no child, especially a child who already has multiple needs, need suffer from its consequences. The effects of poor oral health on the child population can be described through a rigorous needs assessment process.

Not only does oral health make an important contribution to the physical health of a child but, equally, it contributes to good self-esteem and emotional wellbeing which in turn supports healthy lifestyles and general health. Children – and adults – are extremely self-conscious about the appearance of their teeth. Decayed or missing teeth affect a child's appearance and also their self-confidence.

Oral health in the context of general health

Poor oral health is closely associated with child poverty and multiple deprivation. The survey of child dental health in the United Kingdom found marked differences in the proportion of children with decay into dentine and obvious decay experience according to whether the school they attended was situated in an area of socio-economic deprivation or not. The relationship holds for primary and permanent teeth.

These differences should be seen in the context of overall health as described by Tsakos and Alzahrani in chapter 4. Children and young peoples' health indicators published for the North West of England show that low birth weight, measles, whooping cough, road traffic accident casualties, dental health, teenage conceptions, childhood obesity and reported health status are all related to levels of socio-economic deprivation. Children and young people in poorer areas of the North West England have worse health status than those in the more affluent areas. Other risk factors and determinants of health – low income, education, numbers of children dependent on state benefits, lone parents, and children at risk from abuse or neglect are also significantly worse in the most socio-economically deprived areas.

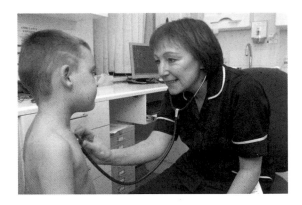

Oral health in the context of general health and wellbeing:
Oral health is associated with socio-economic status which also links to families':
- Income
- Attainment
- Employment
- Housing
- Risk from accidents
- Physical health
- Mental health

Primary health care professionals have to tackle families' needs – for example supporting healthy family diet – in the context of the family's environment and experience. The environment that children are born into and grow up in is a complex mix of influences on health – physiological, familial, domestic, social and physical. Addressing these determinants of health and wellbeing for children and adolescents will improve population health and wellbeing overall and reduce inequalities. This requires coordinated interventions by all agencies.

This underlines the need to integrate initiatives to improve oral health into more general intervention to support good physical and mental health. Oral health cannot be tackled in isolation, hence the importance of involving a range of primary care professionals to advocate for, enable and mediate to achieve population oral health.

Fair Society: Healthy Lives[4]

Professor Marmot found that there is an unequal distribution of resources across families in terms of wealth, living conditions, levels of education, supportive family and community networks, social capital and parenting skills. Abundant evidence suggests that socioeconomic status is associated with a range of developmental outcomes for children. Furthermore, the literature suggests strongly that socioeconomic gradients in early childhood replicate themselves throughout the life course.

He set out principles of effective action to tackle inequalities including:
- Give every child the best start in life
- Enable children, young people and adults to maximise their capabilities and have control over their lives
- Ensure a healthy living standard of living for all
- Create and develop healthy and sustainable places and communities
- Strengthen the role and impact of ill health prevention.

Subsequent sections of this chapter will demonstrate how these principles can be woven into the primary health care role in improving the oral health of children and young people.

Integrating oral health into strategic primary care service planning

At whatever level dental professionals are operating – whether at a local operational or regional or national strategic level - they should work to ensure that oral health is integrated into service planning.

The first step is needs assessment – a structured process which offers a basis for shared action. It identifies oral health as a priority to be addressed and sets out the needs of the different sections of the population and how they can be addressed effectively. It involves all stakeholders including service users in consultation on the findings and conclusions of the needs assessment and in the development of its recommendations. The process gives all those involved a stake in implementation of the resulting strategy and delivery plan.

Needs assessment[5-7]

A structured approach to needs assessment can include the following:

- Reasons that this is a public health issue – national prevalence and trends, contribution to mortality, morbidity and chronic illness.
- Local prevalence and trends, benchmarked against the national and regional data.
- Vulnerable groups and how they are represented locally – segmenting the needs of different sub-groups of the population
- Evidence for effective intervention – for whole population and for particular sub-groups, based on literature reviews or policy guidance.
- Relevant results of local and national consultations with communities, patients and staff.
- Overview of services currently in place and identification of gaps in service
- Draft conclusions based on the findings of each section.
- Review findings and conclusions with a wide range of stakeholders including service users and formulate recommendations in partnership.

Oral health needs assessment supports partnership working as it offers a sound basis for:

- A shared understanding of local needs and how to meet them effectively-enabling primary care and other partners to agree on what constitutes effective action.
- Existing services, policies, pathways, environment and provision are reviewed against this. Gaps are identified as well as the potential for disinvestment in ineffective or non-priority interventions.
- Partners identify the total resource available.
- Partners agree a costed delivery plan to meet need and consult on the plans. These may include advocacy, enabling and mediating oral health initiatives integrated into the work of a range of professionals.
- Projected improvements in outcome from the different components of the programme can be modelled.

- Accountabilities for delivery are agreed.
- Monitoring and evaluation of delivery, impact and outcomes will form an integral part of the plan.

Because all stakeholders – communities, families, young people, and the relevant professional groups – have developed a shared understanding of local need is and how to meet it effectively; and have together formulated a delivery plan outlining the contribution of each group, then comprehensive initiatives to improve oral health are delivered in an integrated fashion to meet the needs of the population, community or family, without duplication of effort.

Underlying principles for planning for effectively improving oral health

Some principles for effective action are set out below. These principles are closely interlinked and interdependent.

Proportional universalism

Focusing solely on the most disadvantaged will not reduce health inequalities sufficiently. To reduce the steepness of the social gradient in health, actions must be universal, but with a scale and intensity that is proportionate to the level of disadvantage. This is called proportionate universalism. Greater intensity of action is likely to be needed for those with greater social and economic disadvantage, but focusing solely on the most disadvantaged will not reduce the health gradient, and will only tackle a small part of the problem.

Increasing the strengths, assets and resilience of communities, families and young people

Resilient communities, families and young people will be much more likely to value and care for their own health and well-being, including their oral health. Conversely good oral health is an asset which builds self-esteem – itself underpinning healthy lifestyle and physical and mental health. Promoting strengths, assets and resilience should be a key role of all primary health care professionals working with communities, families and young people.

Every Child Matters[8]

The factors underpinning childhood resilience were set out in the UK's Every Child Matters framework which recognised the interdependency on the range of factors which bear on a child's life:

- Being healthy - having good physical and emotional health; leading a healthy lifestyle; not consuming illegal drugs; being sexually healthy and safe.
- Staying safe - from neglect, maltreatment, violence and sexual exploitation; being safeguarded from accidental death and injury; not bullied or discriminated against; not affected by anti-social behaviour; feeling secure and cared for, with stability at home. -Enjoying and achieving - attending, enjoying and achieving at school.
- Making a positive contribution through being involved in decision making and supporting the community and engaging in positive, law-abiding behaviour; learning to deal with the significant transition periods, changes and challenges.
- Achieving economic independence by being involved in further education, employment and training, living in sustainable communities and homes, and having access to material goods and transport.

Children who are challenged in one aspect of the factors listed above are likely to face multiple and related challenges. While these factors may not seem immediately related to oral health they all underpin good health and wellbeing including oral health. Primary care is often concerned with a holistic approach to a child's health and wellbeing, for example safeguar-

ding. Poor oral health may be an indicator of wider neglect of a child and breakdown in parenting skills leading to abuse.

The general principles of respect and support for young people implicit in the different components of Every Chid Matters should underpin the provision of all primary care services including those promoting oral health.

Focus on early formative years to achieve maximum health gain in later years – intervene early

There is strong evidence that early intervention - pre-conception and during pregnancy - involving both parents, is important. By identifying those families at higher risk and with lower protective factors early in the pregnancy, it is possible to build resilience and achieve healthier outcomes.

Easily accessible and tailored approaches for preparation for parenting and parenting support have been shown to improve outcomes for the child and family, especially for those more at risk. The Marmot Review identifies the need for high quality maternity services across the social gradient that support positive outcomes of pregnancy and infancy to give children the best start in life.[4]

Advice on good oral health and dental attendance for parent and child should be a part of preparation for parenting and parenting support and this can be achieved through training midwives, and those staff or volunteers who support a parent in the early years of a child's life – examples include health visitors in the United Kingdom.

Family focus, building parenting skills, links with family mental health and wellbeing - many oral health behaviours are closely linked to parenting

- Breast-feeding promotes bonding between mother and child and makes it less likely that the child will be given sweet drinks in bottles.
- Weaning on to healthy family foods is closely linked to parenting skills. Sweets are commonly used to manage a child's behaviour – as bribes, pacifiers and expressions of love.

- A parent who is confident in their parenting skills and who has the information that they need on starting toothbrushing early, healthy infant feeding, weaning diet and family food has the basis for bringing up a child with a healthy mouth and teeth.
- Success in infant feeding and tooth brushing routines will strengthen a parent's feeling of competence promote mental health and wellbeing.

Personalisation

Partnership with families, children and young people to build family/ young people friendly services: children, young people and their families are at the core of providing quality services. Promoting the participation of children and young people in decision making and policy development – and as active contributors to everyday family and community life – is a central part of policy and programme initiatives. It is also an international priority through the UN Convention of the Rights of the Child.[9]

It is important to consider children and young peoples' views and experiences when developing services. If not, it is likely that services will not meet local needs and consequently not offer value for money. Children and young people can participate in many different ways to improve services, including actually commissioning services, recruiting and selecting staff, ensuring the governance of health services and in developing health care research.

The Marmot Review includes a policy objective to enable all children, young people and adults to maximise their capabilities and to have control over their lives. Building confidence and aspirations in young people is key to their involvement and engagement in civil society, which helps them increase responsibility and to articulate how and what they want from services. This includes disabled children, those from black and minority ethnic groups, those living in rural areas, disaffected children and young people and those who do not access education, training or employment in order to develop services which will meet their needs. The voice of young people not attending or using services also needs to be heard. These groups need to be identified and supported to make use of services. This may require working with community groups or employing different communication tools to reach them and would especially apply to independent teenagers or to vulnerable minority groups. Greater understanding is needed about why services may not reaching those most in need.[4]

Case study: an integrated, primary care-based approach to tackling inequalities in oral health in Brazil

The Brazilian model of integrated dental prevention and care within the national Family Health Strategy was developed in order to tackle inequalities in oral health and access to dental care, especially related to socio-economic deprivation.

The model illustrates many of the themes of this chapter: integration of oral health into primary care and working closely with non-dental health professionals, involvement of communities, tackling inequalities, a strong preventive emphasis, and integrated strategic planning, based on an assessment of need, involving professionals, managers and community representatives.

The major challenge for the unified health system in Brazil has been to increase access to dental services and overcome the tendency for dentists to work within the biomedical model of care and instead, to adopt an oral health promotion model based in population-oriented common risk factor approach .

The Brazilian Constitution of 1988 established the National Health System (SUS) based on universal coverage and care. The system was implemented in 1990 and emphasises equal opportunity of access to health services for equal needs, decentralization of actions and integrating delivery of care.

Defined responsibilities for ensuring access to health care and its effectiveness have been delegated to local governing bodies and local people. There is strong emphasis on primary care which manages the most part of population health and ensures that only complex cases – respresenting reach secondary care.

The programme has developed Community Health Agents and adopted a Healthy Family Strategy. Communities are closely involved in the design and delivery of health services. Programme delivery is monitored and outcomes evaluated.

Although not initially a part of the programme, dental services were included in response to the stark inequalities in access to care. Barros and Bertoldi (2002) reported a low level of use dental services; about 77% of children aged 0-6 years and 4% of adults ages 20-49 years had never attended a dentist. Among adults, comparing the 20% poorest to the 20% richest, the proportion of those not receiving care was 16 times higher among the former. In 0-6 year old children those in the 20% richest families had received five times more care than the 20% poorest in the previous year.

In the light of these findings the Ministry of Health decided in 2000 to include oral health teams in the Family Health Strategy supported by investment in both treatment and prevention. The aims of the oral health services were defined as improving oral health and improving access to care, and in order to do this oral health workers had a remit to work closely with other health workers, identifying families at risk and working with communities to promote oral health. This led to a restructuring of dental services, with a shift in emphasis from clinical intervention to prevention; incremental improvements in families' access to preventive and restorative dental services; monitoring of quality and evaluation of improvements in health – all supported by continuing professional development of dental personnel. The challenge now is to maintain and extend access to dental care – reflecting the high priority placed upon oral health by the Brazilian population.

Successful implementation has resulted in an increase in oral health workers from just over four thousand in 2002 to nearly 21 thousand in 2011. The scheme has grown in coverage from just over two thousand municipalities in 2002 to more than five thousand in 2011. Most importantly there appears to have been major improvements in the oral health of 12 year olds, up to 25% reductions in average numbers of Decayed, Missing and Filled Teeth over a seven year period between 2003-10.

In Pernambuco State an oral health information management programme uses clinical epidimological data collected by standardised examiners and non-clinical data as a basis for joint strategic planning by community representatives, dental professionals, managers and the Health Board working together.

Engaging primary care workers in improving oral health

Increasing the profile of oral health in general health

Working across primary care is fundamental to improving oral health through a common risk factor approach. A range of different professional groups, support workers and volunteers can influence the determinants of oral health. Multi-disciplinary work requires a shared agenda and negotiation of priorities. The first step to involving different primary care professionals in promoting oral health is to convince them that good oral health makes an important contribution to the health and well-being of their clients or patients.

Needs assessment – especially if it includes good quality local data - forms a robust basis for this as described. Primary care professionals will be influenced by benchmarking data which demonstrates which if they have outlier status: trend data can highlight changes in incidence and prevalence, and needs assessments also provide information about particularly vulnerable groups. On a personal level primary care workers may themselves have witnessed the infection, pain, loss of function, loss of aesthetics or anxiety that dental disease or its treatment can bring.

As set out by Sheiham and Watt in Chapter 7, a common risk factor approach focuses not on specific illnesses but on shared risk factors and their reduction. Risk factors such as nutrition, poor hygiene and smoking will affect levels of dental caries, periodontal disease and oral cancer as well as other cancers, coronary heart disease and stroke, and many other infectious and non-infectious diseases.

The common risk factor approach fits well into a primary care setting, where the interventions that are most likely to be implemented are those which are simple and appropriate. Risk factors are often linked, and someone who succeeds in making changes in one aspect of lifestyle may then be ready to improve other health-related behaviours.

By working closely with all members of the primary health care team the prevention of oral disease can take its place in a common risk factor approach. All information the public receive from health professionals should be consistent and correct, thereby maximising the credibility of the message with the target group.

Those with the potential to include oral health in the advice they give, or to influence oral health through developing policy or creating a supportive environment include doctors, nurses, midwives, dentists and their teams, pharmacists, dietitians or nutritionists and community health workers. If all primary health care professionals work as a team giving scientifically based, consistent advice, and if they reinforce their message through the features of the environment that they provide for their patients and clients, then together they present a formidable alliance in the fight against preventable disease.

Roles of primary care professionals in improving oral health

As set out in the introduction and by Baelum and Watt on the principles of health promotion, primary health care professionals have a range of roles in promoting health – including advocacy, enabling and mediation. Advocacy acknowledges the influence that political, social, cultural, environmental, behavioural and biological factors can have on the health of individuals or communities and aims to make those conditions favourable to health. To support oral health primary care professionals may argue for healthy eating policies in schools and pre-school settings, or for tobacco control policies or for fluoridation of water supplies.

Enabling recognises that people cannot fulfil their fullest potential unless they are able to take control of the factors which determine their health. Enabling includes providing a supportive environment, access to information, life skills and opportunities for making healthy choices. Advice on health is one part of this – supported by increasing opportunities for families to follow the advice giving. Giving advice effectively is dealt with in the next section.

Mediation recognises that improvements in health can only be achieved through co-ordinated action by governments, health and other social and economic sectors, by non-governmental and voluntary organisations, by local authorities, by industry and the media. Improvements in health involve individuals, families and communities. Health personnel have a responsibility to mediate between the different interests in society for the pursuit of health.

Giving oral health advice effectively

Behaviour change interventions are grounded in behaviour change theory– either explicitly or implicitly – and seek to encourage people to cease or adopt singular or multiple behaviours. Primary care has been identified as a suitable setting in which to deliver behaviour change interventions. Large numbers of people use primary care services and many of them – including some of the most vulnerable - use them frequently. Interventions can be delivered at individual, household, community or population levels using various techniques. A number of models of health behaviour change exist.

Models of behaviour change[10,11]

Brief advice usually involves giving information about the importance of behaviour change and simple advice to change behaviour. Brief advice usually takes only a few minutes. It raises awareness and assesses a person – or parent's - willingness to engage in further discussion about healthy lifestyle issues. Brief advice is usually given opportunistically and linked to an individual's reason for seeking help or using a service. Brief advice has been shown to be effective in increasing smoking quitters, increasing physical activity and decreasing alcohol use. The percentages of those advised who change behaviour are relatively small, but the potential for change on a population level - if brief advice is systematically integrated into health care interventions - is considerable.

Brief interventions, like brief advice, involve opportunistic advice, discussion, negotiation or encouragement. They are used quite frequently in a range of areas in health promotion and can be performed by a variety of health and community care professionals. A brief intervention usually contains an assessment of a person's commitment to behaviour change, advice and sign-posting or referral to support services. They offer a structured way to give advice and may include giving follow-up support or linking people in to other services. They differ from brief advice in that they equip people with tools to change attitudes and handle underlying problems.

Motivational interviewing can be an effective technique to use in a brief intervention. It involves the use of listening skills to explore and evoke a person's motivation through helping them identify the arguments for change. This is a technique that facilitates change based on the expressed aspirations of service users and it supports self efficacy which is, as already discussed, a fundamental principle of improving oral health effectively. This is especially true where oral health related behaviours are closely linked to more fundamental issues such as parenting skills.

Engaging primary healthcare workers in improving oral health

Promoting oral health through a partnership approach across primary care starts with an analysis of which professions, groups, disciplines or sectors can affect the determinants of oral health through their advice, advocacy or enabling. Some will build oral health into policies, others can create supportive environments or made healthy choices easier choices for the target groups. Some will build individuals' knowledge and skills, while others will be involved in supporting the development of communities.[12]

Methods to raise the profile of oral health with primary care professionals and with others who can influence the determinants of oral health:
-Meetings with key individuals, speaking at meetings and participatory training
-The media including national or local newspapers, local or national radio or television, the web, social networking sites, Twitter, professional journals, magazines or newsletters.
A constant feed of information through these channels builds and maintains awareness. Locally relevant information is particularly interesting to primary health care professionals.

Training is the most effective way of engaging primary health care professionals in promoting oral health. To be effective training needs to address the barriers primary care professionals may perceive or encounter in improving oral health.

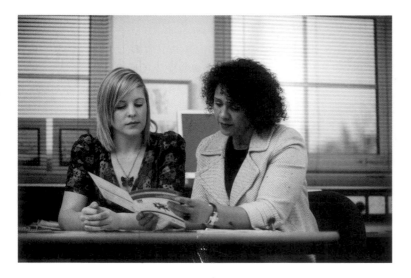

- Among staff with an established relationship with service users there is some concern that delivery of behaviour change conflicts with maintenance of rapport with their client group, or that approaching sensitive issues – and the close link of oral health with parenting can make it a potentially sensitive issue – will stigmatise the patient or client. There is a need to disseminate information about the efficacy of interventions to improve oral health in order to increase confidence in the methods, as lack of confidence will deter staff from attempting to deliver interventions.

- Organisational support is vital to successfully delivery of interventions so it is important to engage management as well as front-line staff in understanding the importance and efficacy of interventions to improve oral health. Lack of time to conduct interventions is a frequently cited problem. Training therefore needs to consider the environment in which staff are working and provide realistic targets for implementing

interventions. Management should be targeted before front-line staff in order to ensure managerial support for interventions and their incorporation into standard practice.

- A perceived lack of knowledge can deter staff from undertaking interventions- whether this relates to areas of behaviour, referral processes or available sources of support. Training for health care professionals should be carried out by credible experts - that is by those with a good knowledge and background in oral health who can support them in developing the level of knowledge they require and need.

- Not only can primary care workers be put off by a lack of confidence in their knowledge on oral health, but also their perceived lack of skills in supporting behaviour change. This can include not knowing which patients to target for such advice, not knowing how to best give advice, not knowing how to deal with those who reject their advice and reluctance to raise sensitive subjects.

- Trainers need to ensure that they capture their audience's attention and help staff to prioritise training in improving oral health. Training should be tailored to fit into staff work schedules and other barriers – such as childcare – which they may face to attending training. Where time is limited training may be delivered through self directed training packages, especially on-line training, through the appointment of an oral health specialist to advise other staff, through using existing professional development networks or other training programmes.

- Training should be made relevant to the target audience and tailored to participants' level of knowledge in order to make best use of professional time and to enhance learning effectiveness. It must be applicable to trainees' professional roles and to the type of relationship they have with service users. Trainers should therefore explore the occupational remit of their training group prior to the delivery of any training session to ensure that the training content relates to the everyday practice of participants. It is useful to draw on participants' everyday clinical experience in order to shape the training.

- For those who may need particular support in understanding how to support behaviour change – for example clinical primary dental care staff – training may include the evidence for the efficacy of interventions, theories of behaviour change, topic specific training, skills for assessing readiness to change, skills for building rapport and facilitating discussion and learning how to deal with different client groups.

Promoting the oral health of children through primary care – practical examples using a life-course approach

A life course approach

Chapter 1 sets out a life course approach; with healthy children forming the sound basis of a healthy society. Applying a life course approach to the health and wellbeing of children and young people takes into account the impact of disadvantage, which starts before birth and accumulates throughout life. Previous sections of this chapter have emphasised how circumstances through the formative years influence health and life chance later on in life, and the complex interaction between social, behavioural, biological and genetic factors across the life course. Taking a life course approach to the promotion of oral health supports consideration of these relationship in the design of strategy and effective interventions.

Some practical examples of how oral health can be built into such an approach are set out below.

Preconception and pregnancy
Early support for a healthy pregnancypreparing for parenthood

Birth and infancy
Working with families to protect the new born child

Early years
Laying the foundations to give the child the best start in life

Children 6-10 years
Bulding health behaviours

Young people 11-18 years
Enjoying adolescence safely

Fig. 17.1 – a life course approach to the health and wellbeing of children.

Pregnancy

It is recognised that women should be at optimal health at the time of conception, and also the importance of establishing maternal healthy lifestyles for the health and lifestyle of the child. This includes the use of healthcare support workers; building on what works to improve services – including dental services – for the most vulnerable women and their families, listening to what women say works, and developing antenatal care which supports healthy lifestyles.

Birth and infancy

It is recognised that optimal infant nutrition, especially breastfeeding, is a protective factor for the health of babies and mothers. It increases the child's chances of leading a future healthy life. It reduces the risk of dental caries and childhood and adult obesity. There is a positive association between breast-feeding and parenting capability particularly among lone or low-income parents.

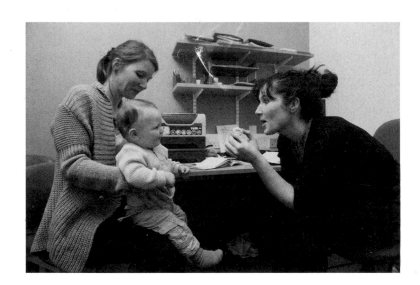

CASE STUDY: distribution of fluoride toothpaste at 12 month developmental check in Tameside (Greater Manchester, England)

Health visitors are trained nurses or midwives with training in promoting community and child health. They and their teams are offered annual training/ update sessions by the oral health team. This training enables health visitors and teams to provide evidenced and informed advice and information to parents and carers. Health visitors state that they feel more confident when delivering advice after the training and it enables oral health advice to be delivered to parents of young children using a common risk factor approach.

The 12 month developmental check offers an ideal opportunity for health visitors to discuss a child's oral health. This is also an excellent opportunity to discuss the whole family's dental needs. Health visiting teams can advise the parents and carers of young children to support the uptake of early tooth brushing, family nutrition and infant feeding in line with local guidance.

The Health Visiting Team are provided with toothpaste, tooth brush, a leaflet and an advice sheet to disseminate which gives information on accessing local publicly funded dental services and how to obtain affordable brushes and paste from their local Children's Centres. The Health Visitor gives the parent or carer one to one advice and information around the safe and effective use of fluoride toothpaste.

This initiative builds on the existing successful relationship between the oral health team and the health visiting team. Health Visitors are well placed to offer support and advice to parents at age appropriate intervals until five years old. Health Visitors feel able to contact the oral health team to ask for more specific information regarding oral health, and for specific oral health advice for children with additional social/physical needs. The initiative is evaluated through asking parents their views and feedback has been very positive.

Early years

The period of primary socialisation, in the first years of life, is when habits and routines, many of them health related, are established. The routines learnt through primary socialisation are based on those of the family members, especially the parents, with whom the child has a strong affective relationship. Such behaviours are learnt unquestioningly as a taken-for granted reality. Habits and routines are particularly important in health related behaviour, because they are dependable. They require no thought or intention so are more reliable than decision based behaviours which readily break down under stress.

Primary care professionals who have a health education role with the parents of young children have unrivalled opportunities for encouraging the early adoption of routines and behaviours to support good dental health for life. Twice daily toothbrushing with fluoride toothpaste and a liking for unsweetened foods and drinks are behaviours that, if learnt in the first years of life, will continue into adulthood.

CASE STUDY: practice nurses in primary care teams in Tameside, Greater Manchester, UK

As members of the primary care team practice nurses provide vaccination and immunisation programmes to young children. This initiative aims to embed oral health into generic health advice given at an immunisation visit.

Practice nurses are offered an oral health update session before they start the scheme. Practice nurses give out a toothbrush, fluoride toothpaste and information around how to start bushing. Information is also included around accessing publicly funded dental services. The general practice is provided with promotional material to inform parents about the oral health scheme.

This initiative ensures that oral health advice to be offered to the parents and carers of young children at an age appropriate time – just before their first teeth come through. It ensures continuity, and reinforces oral health messages that parents and carers have received from the other health professionals.

Children and adolescents

Oral health is important to general health and wellbeing, to overall quality of life, to self-esteem and social confidence – particularly important as children move into adolescence and young adulthood.

The importance of engaging children and adolescents in the design of services to meet their needs has already been described in this chapter, emphasising the importance of building their self esteem and supporting them in feeling valued.

Children and young people are part of families and so all efforts to improve to reduce sugar in the diet – in the context of a healthy diet and the prevention of obesity - and introduce other oral health related behaviours should take a family focus.

Primary prevention of smoking – that is discouraging children from starting smoking as well as supporting them to quit – is part of promoting long-term oral health because tobacco consumption can predispose to periodontal disease and – with harmful levels of alcohol consumption – to oral cancer, as well as being the main preventable cause of reduced life expectancy.

Many young people suffer from trauma to their front teeth while taking part in sport. This can be reduced by efforts to make the environment safer as well as by promoting the use of gum shields in contact sports.

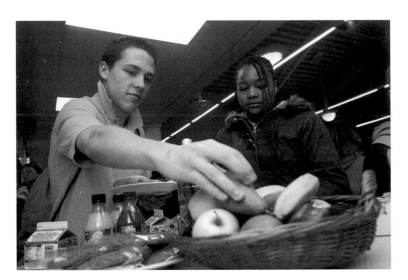

CASE STUDY: School Nurses (including School Nurse Assistants) in Tameside, Greater Manchester, UK

School Nurses deliver health programmes in schools including health and sex education; developmental screening; health interviews, and immunisation programmes.

School nurses and their teams are offered annual training and update sessions on oral health. School nurse teams approached the oral health team to request a teaching resource that they could use to engage with young children and their families. They wanted a resource that was child friendly, and would enable the named school nurse to begin to build a relationship with the children. It was hoped that this would introduce the children to the nurse, and therefore facilitate the other screening initiatives that the school nurse would carry out later in the year such as developmental checks.

The resource offered an opportunity to inform the parents and carers of new starters at school about the benefits of brushing children's teeth with fluoride toothpaste. A fun pack was developed by the oral health team in collaboration with the school nurse assistants. The pack was designed to involve parents and carers. This was achieved by sending pre- evaluation questionnaires home to parents asking about their existing oral behaviours, and followed by letters home to inform them of what their child had learnt in school that day. Post evaluation questionnaires were then sent home at the end of the topic.

The pack is used by school nurses in the context of the school nurse's role in promoting general health. It facilitated contact between the school nurse team and parents and helped parents understand the role of the school nurse. It builds on the oral health advice that parents and carers have received through early years settings in the area.

Vulnerable groups or those with special needs.

Evidence indicates that most people with disabilities have poorer health than the rest of the population. Their access to health services is often characterised by problems that undermine their own dignity and safety and their ability to make decisions. They are often systematically disengaged from mainstream primary health care services. Early intervention and a community approach can prevent deterioration of disabled young people's health. Disabled young people – especially those who display challenging behaviour – have more difficulty accessing assessment and treatment for general health problems unrelated to their disability such as dental care.

Summary

This chapter has shown how oral health forms an integral part of good general health, and how primary care forms a natural setting for improving oral health. It demonstrates the key role that oral health has in contributing to good physical, mental and social well-being and how, conversely, poor oral health often represents just one aspect of multiple deprivation. It therefore proposes that oral health staff should work closely with other health professionals who are working to reduce risk factors and support families to health and wellbeing. It explains how needs assessment can underpin joint strategic working in partnership with service users themselves and with primary care professionals. It sets out how to support the non-specialist workforce in improving the oral health of the population. These principles are illustrated through case studies describing national and local initiatives to improve oral health through integrated working with primary care.

Acknowledgement: thanks are due to Carole Hill for providing the UK case studies.

References

1. North West Children and Young People's Health Indicators. North West Public Health Obervatory; 2008. Available from www.nwph.net.
2. World Health Organisation. Declaration of Alma Ata. International conference on primary care. WHO Geneva. 1978.
3. Starfield B, Shi L, Macinko J. Contribution of Primary Care to Health Systems and Health. Millbank Quarterly. 2005; 83(3):457-502.
4. Fair society: healthy lives. The Marmot Review. Published by the Marmot Review; 2010. Available from www.marmotreview.org.
5. Health needs assessment a practical guide: National Institute of Clincal Excellence. London. 2005.
6. Stevens A, Raferty J, Health Care Needs Assessment. Radcliffe. 2004.
7. Pencheon D, Oxford Book of Public Health Practice. Oxford University Press. 2003.
8. Every child matters. Department for Education; 2003. Available from www.education.gov.uk.
9. Unicef: convention of the rights of the child.;1989. Available from www.unicef.org/crc/index_30160.html.
10. National Institute for Clinical Excellence. Behaviour change at a population, community and individual level. London; 2007. Available from www.nice.org.uku.
11. Powell K and Thurston M. Commissioning training for behaviour change interventions: evidence and best practice in delivery. University of Chester. 2008.
12. A guide for commissioners of children's, young people's and maternal health and wellbeing services: NHS North West 2010. Available from: www.northwest.nhs.uk/.

Chapter 18

Promotion of Oral Health in Nurseries and Preschool Settings: the importance of a good start

Cecile Soriano Rodrigues

Introduction

The growing recognition of the social determination of health, associated with the expansion of human and social rights in contemporary societies has stimulated the implementation of public policies geared towards the improvement of quality of life, focusing on strategies for health promotion in collective environments. Nursery and preschool environments are potentially important for the promotion of oral health of preschool children. The global perspective of expansion of this educational level over the next few years,[1] the development of oral epidemiological technologies[2-4] and especially the evidence of the effectiveness of health promotion interventions in this population group,[5-7] are factors that favour this approach.

The aim of this chapter is to discuss some aspects that are essential for the understanding of oral health promotion strategies in nursery and preschool environments. Therefore we will initially present conceptual elements referring to the creation of healthy environments in nurseries and preschools. This is followed by a brief presentation of the early childhood, or preschool education environments in Brazil. We will also discuss epidemiological findings relating to the oral health of under five year old children. The last section involves a critical evaluation of oral health promotion strategies/interventions in nurseries and preschools.

Creation of Healthy Environments in Nurseries and Preschools

Numerous international conferences and documents recommend the creation of healthy environments as one of the priority fields of action for health promotion.[8-10] The recommendations address multiple influences in the determination of health. The interventions focus on environmental changes to reduce health inequities.[11-13] In these approaches, the physical and social environment are important mediators whereby socioeconomic stratification influences the health situation. The adoption of health promotion measures, in collective environments, should make healthy choices the easiest to adopt. Good air quality, universal availability of treated water, improvement of main roads and fluoridated public water supplies are some examples of health promoting environmental measures.

Studies on chronic diseases have also incorporated specific factors such as the environment and health in early childhood as an important determinant of adult health.[12,14] The scientific evidence indicates that the development of effective strategies for the promotion of equity in health includes a specific focus on early childhood. The model underlying these studies, the Life Course Approach, suggests that diseases originating in early childhood and lifetime cumulative risks (biological and social) influence chronic diseases,[15] including oral conditions[16,17] in later stages of life. Considering that nurseries and preschools represent the

first level of basic education in many countries, concepts and strategies of the Global School Health Initiative (GSHI) of the World Health Organization9,10 and International Union for Health Promotion[18] are applicable in this context (Fig. 18.1).

The GSHI emphasizes the importance of changes in the traditional approach of health programs focused on the individual and specific health problems, to an approach that supports the full development of children and youths and improvement of quality of life and well-being of the school community.[19] The creation of a healthy environment in preschool settings is able to produce positive effects on the lives of children under five years of age.[20,21] However, some evidence indicates that GHSI programs, especially in nurseries and preschool settings, should include more contact with parents and the support of home visits to increase parental

STRATEGIES	DEFINITIONS
Healthy School Policies	Regulations and practices that promote health and well-being in school.
Physical Environment of the School	Physical structure, architecture, equipment, surroundings, location that facilitates learning, physical activity and healthy eating.
Social Environment of the School	It is considered positive when there is a combination of quality of relationships between and among employees and students.
Individual Skills and Competencies for Action	Activities in which the student gains knowledge and experience to act for the purpose of improving their health and that of their community. Refers both to the formal and informal curriculum.
Ties with the community	Relations between school, family, students and community leaders.
Health Services	Can be local or regional based on the school or linked to the school, and are responsible for the health care of children and youths, including those with special needs.

Fig. 18.1 – Essential strategies for promotion of health in schools.[18]

involvement with the child's development.[22,23] Intensive home visits and support from basic health units appear to be effective at increasing the resilience and competence of children and parents, helping to prevent health problems.[22] In that study, the term competence involves ideas of empowerment and autonomy, necessary to help people think for themselves and develop long-lasting attitudes and values to guide consistent and ethically healthy behaviours.[25]

In Brazil, a clear perspective of adopting heath promotion policies in schools was assumed by the Federal Government from 2006, with the establishment of the National Health Promotion Policy[26] and in 2007 with the School Health Program (SHP).[27,28] The latter undertakes to establish strategies for integration and permanent coordination between health and education policies and actions, with the participation of the school community, involving the family health and basic education teams.[27] Basic education in Brazil encompasses nurseries and preschools.[28] However, in spite of the richness of some Brazilian[29] and Latin American experiences,[19] a comprehensive

assessment of the initiative in Latin America identified that the diffusion of GSHIs occurs unequally between and within countries from the region.[19]

An evaluation of the impact on health of the GHSI/SHP approach was not in the scope of this chapter. However it is important to emphasize that few evaluative studies were carried out focusing on GSHI/SHP in nurseries and preschool settings.

The Context of Nurseries and Preschools

Historically, the Brazilian nursery system was structured in social welfare policies resulting from demands of social movements linked to the rights of working women, from the 1970s up to the present time (Fig. 18.2).[30] At the end of the 1980s, influenced by groups connected to the university and educational specialists, nurseries began to be seen as a children´s right and were recognized as constituents of the early education system.[30] The nursery sector is currently undergoing a transition and is being gradually incorporated into the municipal educational system.

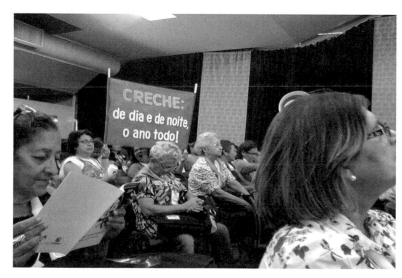

Fig. 18.2 – Plenary Sitting of the III State Conference on Politics for Women 2011. Recife, 24 October, 2011.

Preschools, on the other hand, have always been linked to the education system.[30] As of 2007, a new change in the Brazilian legislation established that early childhood education would extend until the age of 5 years, with nursery for children aged from 0 to 3 years and preschool for those aged between 4 and 5 years.[31] Early childhood education in nurseries and preschools is not compulsory. Education becomes compulsory at the age of 6 years when the child enters elementary school.[32] Nowadays in Brazil, basic education encompasses early childhood education (nurseries and preschool), primary education (9 years) and secondary school (3 years).

Despite the regulatory effort, access of Brazilian children to nurseries is still very limited. In 1995, nurseries catered for 7% of children up to the age of three,[33] while in 2010 the percentage was only 20%.[34] Major inequalities in access to nursery still persist. The greatest inequalities are when children are compared in relation to the location of their homes. In the urban areas 19,6% attended nurseries in 2007 compared to 6.6% in rural areas.[35] Differences in relation to race, income, and region of the country also exist.

Access to preschool is better. In 2007, 77.6% Brazilian children attended preschool.[36] In spite of improvements, inequalities in access to preschool persist. For children situated in the highest income quintile, preschool attendance is 92% while for the poorest quintile access was 71%.[35,36] On the other hand, less developed regions such as the northeast have a higher preschool attendance (82%), while in the South and Midwest attendance was 67% and 66% respectively.[35,36] This may reflect compensatory federal policies and programs.

From the perspective of improvement in the Brazilian educational system the National Education Plan (NEP) 2010/2020, under discussion in the Brazilian Congress[37] included a target for early education, (Box 18.1).

Box 18.1 – Brazilian target for early education of NEP 2010-2020.[37]

Target 1
Achieve universal access to school for the population between four and five year of age by 2016, and expand the supply of early childhood education by 2020, in order to respond to the needs of fifty percent of the population aged three years or under.

The concern about expansion of education in early childhood is international. The Education for All Framework of Action (EFA) undertaken by the governments in Dakar, Senegal, in 20001, established six main goals and specific targets to be reached by 2015. The Dakar goals are shown in figure 18.3. Target 1 specifically addresses the expansion of nurseries and preschools.

Education for All
1. Expand and improve early childhood care and education, specifically in the case of more vulnerable children in a situation of greater need.
2. Guarantee that all children, particularly girls, living in difficult circumstances and those belonging to ethnic minority groups, have access to free, compulsory and high quality primary education by 2015.
3. Guarantee that the learning needs of all youths and adults are met through equitable access to appropriate learning and life training programs.
4. Achieve, by 2010, a 50% improvement in adult literacy levels, especially as refers to women, as well as equitable access to basic and continued education for all adults.
5. Eliminate gender disparities in primary and secondary education by 2015, achieving gender equality in education in 2015, mainly aiming to ensure that girls have full and equal access, as well as good performance, in good quality primary education.
6. Improve all the aspects of education quality and guarantee the excellence of all, so that recognized and measurable learning results are achieved by everyone, especially in linguistic competence and mathematical literacy and in essential training for life.

Fig. 18.3 – The six goals approved during the Dakar Conference of 2000 to be attained in 2015.[1]

It is also important to emphasize that armed conflict is one of the greatest obstacles faced for the expansion of early education and effectuation of the EFA goals, especially in poorer countries. A report published by UNESCO[38] indicates that during the decade, until 2008,[35] countries had armed conflicts, of which 30 were low-income and lower-middle-income nations. The report also indicates that children in poor countries affected by conflicts have twice as much chance of dying before the age of 5 years than children from other poor countries. The report acknowledges that education has a vital role to play in the construction of resistance against violent conflicts.

Understanding about modern social standards, their economic, political and social environments and their repercussions on early education are essential for the development of global health promotion strategies involving children under 5 years old.

Oral Health of Children Under 5 Years of Age

In Brazil, oral epidemiological national surveys are part of the main strategy of the health surveillance, which guides decisions on the national oral health policy.[39] Thus far four national oral health epidemiological surveys have been conducted. The data gathering years of the surveys were 1986, 1996, 2003 and 2010. Of these only the last two gathered information about dental caries in children under the age of five. The survey carried out in 2003 included, besides oral clinical exams, data relating to socioeconomic situation, oral self--assessment and access to dental services.[40] The prevalence of caries at the age of 5 years was approximately 60% and dmf was 2.8. The caries component was 82% of the dmf. The main criticism made against this survey was the sampling procedures.[41] In relation to the survey conducted in 2010, the only data to be published so far is preliminary.[42] There has been a decline of 17% in the average number of teeth affected at the age of 5 years, between the surveys of 2003 (dmft = 2,8) and 2010 (dmft = 2,4).[42] It was also identified that, at this age, 80% of carious teeth have not yet been treated, indicating a strong need for improvements in the system of access to dental care for young children within the scope of basic care.

Some local oral epidemiological studies were also carried out in nursery environments. In the 1990s, studies conducted with 3-year-old children in Goiânia[43] and Recife[6] found that 49.5% and 53% respectively were caries-free. In 2007, a study conducted at state nurseries in Canoas, Rio Grande do Sul, found that 46.1% were caries-free.[44] The studies clearly indicate that, in Brazil, oral health policies need to focus more on oral health promotion strategies targeting children under five years of age.

Health Promotion Interventions in Nurseries and Preschools

Some oral health promotion interventions in nursery and preschool environments have proven effective at maintaining good oral health in early childhood, although the topic still represents a considerable challenge to governments and society. We illustrate here some interventions with potential impact in this area, such as the use of nutrition guides, use of fluoride dentifrices, tobacco-free nurseries and schools and training of carers/teachers.

Dietary guidelines

Adequate food and nutrition are essential requirements for good physical development at all ages, especially among children under the age of five.

Excessive sugar consumption is an important determinant of dental caries.[45-47] After an analysis of the available evidence on the role of diet in the prevalence of dental caries, WHO/FAO[48] recommended that the maximum sugar consumption level be limited to 10% of the total daily calorie intake or between 15-20 kg person/year. In Brazil the guidelines for decreasing sugar consumption in early childhood were included in the Dietary Guide for Children under 2 Years of Age, an initiative of the Ministry of Health and Health Promotion and Protection Program of the Pan American Health Organization (PAHO/Brazil).[49] The guide was prepared with the intention of training professionals who work in the field of infant/early childhood feeding, especially nutritionists and family health teams, and contains ten steps recommended for improving the early childhood feeding of children in Brazil (Fig. 18.4).

The impact of the application of the Ten Steps to Healthy Eating was evaluated in low-income families.[50] The results showed that the intervention was associated with a higher proportion of exclusive breastfeeding at the age of 4 months (RR = 1,58; CI95%: 1,21-2,06) and 6 months (RR = 2,34; CI95%: 1,37-3,99) and infants breastfed at 12 months (RR = 1,26; CI95%: 1,02-1,55) and the lower proportion of children who presented diarrhoea (RR = 0,68; CI95%: 0,51-0.90), respiratory problems (RR = 0,63; CI95%: 0,46-0,85), use of medications (RR = 0,56; CI95%: 0,34-0.91) and dental caries (RR = 0,56; CI95%: 0,32-0,96) in the age bracket 12 to 16 months. As regards caries, the intervention decreased the occurrence of cariogenic feeding practices suggesting that guidelines for delaying the introduction of sugar and avoiding sweet foods are potentially effective on the feeding pattern in the first year of life.

STEP 1	Give only breast milk for the first six months, without offering water, teas or any other food.
STEP 2	From the age of six months, slowly and gradually offer other foods, continuing to breastfeed up to the age of two years or over.
STEP 3	From the age of six months, give supplementary foods three times a day if the child receives breast milk and five times a day if the child has been weaned.
STEP 4	Supplementary food should be offered without having set times, always respecting the child´s wishes.
STEP 5	Supplementary food should be thick right from the start and offered in a spoon; begin with a pasty consistency (mushy/pureed food), and gradually increase their consistency until you are offering what the family eats.
STEP 6	Offer the child different food every day. A varied diet is a colourful meal.
STEP 7	Encourage the daily consumption of fruit and vegetables in meals.
STEP 8	**Avoid sugar, coffee, canned and fried foods, soft drinks, sweets, savoury snacks and other delicacies in the first years of life. Use salt in moderation.**
STEP 9	Be mindful of hygiene when preparing and handling food; ensure its appropriate storage and conservation.
STEP 10	Encourage sick and convalescent children to eat, offering their habitual diet and their favourite foods, respecting their acceptance.

Fig. 18.4 – Ten steps of healthy eating.[49]

The effects of guidelines to reduce sugar consumption on caries rates were evaluated in a longitudinal epidemiological study conducted with 3-year-olds enrolled in state nurseries of Recife.[5] The study adopted the recommendation of WHO[51] for the definition of a sugar consumption pattern considered appropriate in relation to the prevention and reduction of the impact of chronic diseases. Children enrolled in nurseries that adopted the WHO recommendation, developed four times less caries than children enrolled at nurseries which did not adopt the recommendation. The results of this study reinforce the evidence that highlights sugar consumption as an important determinant of dental caries.

Use of fluoride dentifrices

Recommending fluoride dentifrice use has been emphasized.[46,52,53] Brushing with fluoride dentifrice is a simple and economical method that involves self-care and supervision actions in smaller children, besides the regulation and monitoring of the dentifrice manufacturing industry. The effectiveness of fluoride dentifrices for dental caries prevention has been well documented, but few studies have been done on the primary dentition. In 2003, a systematic review examined 70 clinical trials, using caries measurements for permanent dentition in children and youths, and concluded that the preventive fraction of fluoride dentifrices was 24% (CI 95%, 21% to 28%; p<0.0001).[54] In that study, the effect of the use of fluoride dentifrice increased with higher initial levels of caries, higher concentration of fluoride, greater frequency of use and supervised brushing and was not influenced by exposure to fluoridated water.

A recent systematic review included primary dentition studies and confirmed the benefits of fluoride dentifrices when used in fluoride concentrations above 1000 ppm.[7] However, it is important to consider that the use of dentifrices by smaller children is associated with some inadvertent ingestion of some paste,[55] which gives rise to concern about adverse effects of excessive fluoride intake, namely, development of dental fluorosis. Although the mechanism through which dental fluorosis develops has not been fully elucidated, there is some evidence of that excessive levels of fluorides is involved.[56]

Considering the issues raised above, another systematic review described the relationship between topical use of fluorides dentifrices and dental fluorosis.[57] There is evidence that dentifrices containing more than 1000 ppm, between 12-24 months of age was associated with the risk of dental fluorosis. They recommend that the fluoride concentration in children´s dentifrices be lower than 1000 ppm. The authors also emphasized that for populations of children with a high risk of caries, the benefit of caries prevention should be weighed against the risk of fluorosis.

In summary, the daily use of fluoride dentifrice through supervised tooth brushing is recommended in nurseries and pre-schools as a strategy to promote oral health in early childhood, and it is important to assess the ideal concentration of fluorides in dentifrices, according to the exposure to fluoride already existing in the region.

Tobacco-Free Nurseries

Although chronic diseases such as mouth cancer commonly manifest in adulthood, tobacco use and exposure, determining factors of the disease, start in early childhood and adolescence.[58] WHO already considers tobacco use a paediatric disease.[60] In early childhood, passive smoking is associated particularly with diseases of the respiratory system, sudden death syndrome and adverse effects on neuropsychological development and on growth.[58] In Brazil some surveys have recorded the early start of tobacco use. In Rio Grande do Sul, a study involving 4980 adolescents from primary and secondary school identified the prevalence of cigarette experimentation in around 36% with start age ranging between 5 and 22 years.[61] In Belém do Pará the occurrence of cigarette experimentation was 44%, with 52% in state schools and 36% in private schools.[62] In 2009, the National Schoolchildren Health Survey (PENSE)[63] identified that 24% of year 10 state and private school students had already experimented with cigarettes at least once in their lives.

In 1993 WHO included tobacco use in the Tenth Revision of the International Classification of Diseases (ICD10) in the group of mental and behavioral disorders resulting from the use of psychoactive substances (nicotine)[59]

The protection of children and youths against the effects of tobacco use is a concern that is on the international agenda of tobacco control policies whose coordination produced the first global public health treaty, the Framework Convention on Tobacco Control (FCTC), negotiated under the auspices of WHO and in force since 2005. Brazil ratified the FCTC in the same year, 2005, making the commitment of implementing the treaty at the domestic level, especially through the National Tobacco Control Policy. Today 192 countries have ratified the FCTC whose goal is "to protect present and future generations from the devastating health, social, economic and environmental consequences of tobacco consumption and exposure to tobacco smoke by providing a framework for tobacco control measures, to be implemented by the Parties at the national, regional and international levels in order to reduce continually and substantially the prevalence of tobacco use and exposure to tobacco smoke.[58]

Generally speaking the core measures proposed by the FCTC are related to the reduction of the supply and demand of tobacco products. The implementation of the FCTC in the Americas was evaluated through an analysis of the World Reports on the Tobacco Epidemic of 2008 and 2009.[64] The study concluded that a small group of countries implemented effective policies relative to specific aspects of the control of tobacco use analyzed. However, most countries already have specific legislations in the area.

In 2008, WHO[65] adopted six strategies, known as MPOWER, which help countries to apply effective measures to reduce the tobacco epidemic in accordance with the FCTC (Fig. 18.5). Some of the MPOWER strategies can be put into practice in nursery environments, such as the implementation of tobacco-free environments. There is evidence that smoke-free environment policies protect workers against tobacco smoke, decrease the chances of youths becoming tobacco-dependent and increases tobacco use cessation.[66] Many countries have specific legislation that makes the effect of smoke-free environments a compulsory policy and not a case of voluntary action. In Brazil, the prevailing legislation is under discussion with regards to aspects such as the ban on smoking areas in closed environment. Since 2006, in Recife, all the municipal nurseries have adopted the proposal of 100% tobacco-free environments, based on guidance of the local tobacco control policy[67] (Fig. 18.6). The experience was documented by PAHO, as an example of good practice and successful implementation.

MPOWER Strategy	Definition
Monitor	Surveillance of tobacco use and prevention policies.
Protect	Protect the population from tobacco smoke and products.
Offer	Offer help to quit tobacco use.
Warn	Warn about the dangers of tobacco use.
Enforce	Enforce bans on tobacco advertising, promotion and sponsorship.
Raise	Raise taxes on tobacco

Fig. 18.5 – MPOWER Strategy[65]

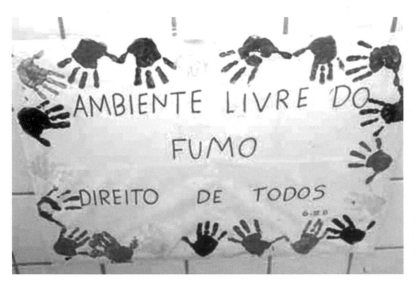

Fig. 18.6 – Recreational activity performed during the implementation of Smoke-Free Environments at a nursery from the municipal early education network. Recife in 2006. Photo: Maristela Menezes

Training carers/teachers in early childhood health promotion

The qualification of carers and teachers to work at nurseries and preschools still admittedly represents a major challenge for the quality of education in nurseries and preschools in Brazil. Numerous evaluative surveys reviewed by Campos[30] indicate that the low level of qualification of carers and teachers is one of the serious problems of early childhood education. Strong discrepancies were also pointed out between the education of professionals who work at nurseries and preschools (the deficiency is more severe at nurseries) and a lack of adaptation of the existing vocational training courses to early childhood education needs.

The National Council of Women´s Rights[68] also identified problems in the education of the team of early childhood education workers. The document assembled reports on experiences of nursery teachers and carers, who were emphatic in emphasizing the urgency of training for professionals from the area, since the carers were seen to adopt attitudes that demonstrated education based on rigid and authoritarian values and a perception that the nursery work merely consisted of "watching over the child". Thus, the provision of technical and pedagogic support to the teams of carers and teachers of nurseries and preschools is crucial for the development of sustainable strategies of promotion of oral health of children. In the United Kingdom, a document produced by the Health Education Authority,[69] entitled "Smiling for Life", was prepared to support teams of carers in the promotion of healthy nutritional and oral practices in preschools. The document highlights reasons why carers are important:

- Many children spend a significant length of time being cared for by the nursery team.
- They have access to the child when the first teeth erupt, especially those from low-income families.
- Carers can help parents make the family environment healthier for their children

The document emphasizes topics such as healthy eating for children under 5 years of age, consumption of sugar, sweeteners, snacks, food labels, tooth brushing, use of fluoride, visits to the dentist, accidents, use of pacifiers and bottles, among others. The guide also covers the partnership with parents, emphasizes the importance of offering options to the child and helping them assume responsibilities when making decisions as well as other broader topics such as the issue of self-esteem.

The account of some Brazilian health promotion experiences in nurseries 0,71 reinforces the need to execute a systemic education project with teams of carers/teachers and with health professionals who work in the field of early children education.

Conclusion

This chapter presented an overview of health promotion at nurseries and preschools, indicating a dynamic situation, with important changes introduced in the last decade and with the advance of a new global awareness of the importance of early childhood education. The environment of nurseries and preschools can favour the promotion of oral health, providing adequate strategies are adopted. Scientific evidence and good practices were highlighted. The chapter mainly explored specific strategies within the scope of healthy eating, use of fluoride, tobacco smoke-free environments and carer/teacher training, which can contribute to the development of the necessary competencies to improve the oral health of children enrolled in nurseries and preschools.

References

1. UNESCO (2008). Relatório de monitoramento de educação para todos Brasil 2008: educação para todos em 2015; alcançaremos a meta? – Brasília: Organização das Nações Unidas para a Educação, a Ciência e a Cultura - UNESCO, 2008.

2. Sheiham A, Cushing A, Maizls, JMA. The Social Impact of Dental Disease In: G D. Slade (editor). Measuring Oral Health and Quality of Life. Proceedings of a conference held June 13-14, 1996, at the University of North Carolina-Chapel Hill, North Carolina(US). p. 47-55. Disponível em: http://arcpoh.adelaide.edu.au/publications/report/ miscellaneous/pdf_files/MeasuringOralHealthAndQualityOfLife.pdf Acessado em: 01/09/2011.

3. McGrath C, Broder H, Wilson-Genderson M. Assessing the impact of oral health on the life quality of children: implications for research and practice.

4. Community dent. oral epidemiol. 2004 April; 32(2):81-85.

5. Gherunpong S, Sheiham A, Tsakos G. A sociodental approach to assessing children´s oral health needs: integrating an oral health-related quality of life (OHRQoL) measure into oral health service planning. Bull. World Health Organ. 2006; 84:36-42.

6. Rodrigues CS, Watt RG, Sheiham A. Effects of dietary guidelines on sugar intake and dental caries in 3-year-old nursery children in Brazil. Health promot. internation. 1999; 14(4):329-35.

7. Rodrigues CS, Sheiham A. The relationships between dietary guidelines, sugar intake and caries in primary teeth in low income Brazilian 3-year-olds: a longitudinal study. Int J Paediatr Dent. 2000 Mar; 10(1):47-55.

8. Walsh T, Worthington HV, Glenny A-M, Appelbe P, Marinho Valeria CC, Shi X. Fluoride toothpastes of different concentrations for preventing dental caries in children and adolescents.

Cochrane Database of Systematic Reviews. In: The Cochrane Library, Issue 08, 2011. Art. No. CD007868. DOI: 10.1002/14651858.CD007868.pub1

9. WHO. Ottawa Charter for Health Promotion. First International Conference on Health Promotion. Ottawa, 21 November 1986 - WHO/HPR/HEP/95.1. 1986. Disponível em: http://www.who.int/hpr/NPH/docs/ottawa_charter_hp.pdf.

10. WHO. WHO's Global School Initiative: health promoting schools. World Health Organization. Geneva, Switzerland. 1998.

11. WHO. Creating an Environment for Emotional and Social Well-Being: An important Responsibility of a Health-Promoting and Child-Friendly School. WHO.

12. Information Series on School Health; Document 10; Geneva, Switzerland. 2003.

13. Whitehead M. Tackling inequalities: a review of policy initiatives. In: Tackling Inequalities in Health – An agenda for action. Ed. Michaela Benzeval, Ken Judge, Margareth Whihead. King´s Fund. London; 1995.

14. Mackenbach JP, van de Mheen H, Stronks K. A prospective cohort study investigating the explanation of socio-economic inequalities in health in The Netherlands. Social Science Medicine. 1994 Jan; 38(2):299-308.

15. Frieden TR. A Framework for Public Health Action: The Health Impact Pyramid. Am J Public Health. 2010; 100(4):590-595.

16. Wadsworth M and Butterworth S. Early life. In: Michael Marmot and Richard G. Wilkinson (editors). Social Determinants of Health. 2ª ed. Oxford: Oxford University Press. 2006; p.31-53.

17. Blane D. The life course, the social gradient, and health. In: Michael Marmot and Richard G. Wilkinson (editors). Social Determinants of Health. 2ª ed.Oxford: Oxford University Press. 2006; p.54-77.

18. Peres MA et al. The Influence of Family Income Trajectories Form Birth to Adulthood on Adult Oral Health: Findings From the 1982 Pelotas Birth Cohort. Am J Public Health. 2011 April; 101(4):730-6.

19. Nicolau, B, Marcenes, W, Bartley, M., Sheiham, A. (2003). A Life Course Approach to Assessing Cause of Dental caries Experience: The Relationship between Biological, Behavioural, Socio-Economic and Psychological Conditions and Caries in Adolescents. Caries Res. 37:319-26.

20. UIPES. União Internacional para Promoção da Saúde. Construindo Escolas Promotoras de Saúde: directrizes para promover a saúde em meio escolar. Versão 2 do documento anterior denominado "Protocolos e Directrizes para as Escolas Promotoras de Saúde" 2009. Disponível em: http://www.iuhpe.org/uploaded/Publications/Books_Reports/HPS_GuidelinesII_2009_Portuguese.pdf.

21. OPAS. Escuelas Promotoras de la Salud. Fortalecimiento de la Iniciativa Regional Escuelas Promotoras de la Salud. Estrategias y Líneas de Acción 2003-2013. Serie Promoción de la Salud N°4. Organización Panamericana de la Salud. Oficina Regional de la Organización Mundial de la Salud. Washington DC. 2003.

22. Anderson, L.M., Shinn, C., Fullilove, M.T., Scrimshaw, S.C., Fielding, J.E. Normand, J, Carande-Kulis, V.G. & the Task Force on Community Preventive Services. (2003). The effectiveness of early childhood development programs: A systematic review. Am.j. prev. med. 24(3S):32-46.

23. Sylva, K, Melhuish, E, Sammons, P, Siraj-Blatchford, I and Taggart, B.

24. Effective pre-school and primary education 3-11 project (EPPE 3-11) a longitudinal study funded by the DfES (2003-2008) Promoting Equality in the Early Years: Report to the Equalities Review. London: Institute of Education. 2007. Disponível em: http://archive.cabinetoffice.gov.uk/equalitiesreview/upload/assets/www.theequalitiesreview.org.uk/promoting_equality_in_the_early_years.pdf.

25. Jané-Llopis E, Barry M, Hosman C, Patel V. Mental health promotion works: a review. Promot. educ. 2005; 2:9-25.

26. Barry MM et al. Review of Evidence-based Mental Health Promotion and Primary/Secondary Prevention. Report prepared for the Department of Health. London. 2009; p.257.

27. Antunes, C. Resiliência – A construção de uma pedagogia para uma escola pública de qualidade. 6ª. edição. Petrópolis, RJ. Ed. Vozes. 2009.

28. Weare, K. Promoting mental, emotional and social health: a whole school approach. London: Routledge. 2000

29. Brasil, 2006. Política Nacional de Promoção da Saúde. Portaria nº 687 MS/GM, de 30 de março de 2006. Ministério da Saúde. Brasília. 2006.

30. Brasil a 2007. Decreto 6286. Presidência da República.

31. Casa Civil Subchefia para Assuntos Jurídicos. Brasília 05 de dezembro de 2007.

32. BRASIL 2008. Portaria 1861. Presidência da República.

33. Casa Civil Subchefia para Assuntos Jurídicos. Brasília 04 de setembro de 2008.

34. Brasil. Ministério da Saúde. Escolas Promotoras de Saúde : experiências do Brasil / Ministério da Saúde, Organização Pan-Americana da Saúde – Brasília: Ministério da Saúde, 2006. 272 p. – (Série Promoção da Saúde; nº 6)

35. Campos MM, Füllgraf J, Wiggers V. A Qualidade da educação Infantil Brasileira: Alguns Resultados de Pesquisa. Cadernos de Pesquisa; 36(127):87-128; 2006.

36. Brasil. Lei de Diretrizes e Bases da Educação Nacional. Lei no. 9.394/1996. Brasília, 1996.

37. Brasil b (2006). Lei Federal 11.274. Presidência da República.

38. Casa Civil Subchefia para Assuntos Jurídicos. Brasília 06 de fevereiro de 2006.

39. Instituto Brasileiro de Geografia e Estatística (IBGE). Pesquisa Nacional por Amostra de Domicílios – 1995. (Microdados).

40. Ministério da Educação. MEC Financia Construção de Creches no País. Disponível em: http://www.brasil.gov.br/noticias/arquivos/2011/01/06/mec-financia-construcao-de-creches-no-pais.

41. Castro JA. Evolução e desigualdade na educação brasileira. Educ. Soc., Campinas, vol. 30, n. 108, p. 673-697, out. 2009.

42. Instituto Brasileiro de Geografia e Estatística (IBGE). Pesquisa Nacional por Amostra de Domicílios – 2007. (Microdados).

43. Brasil. Câmara dos Deputados. Projeto de Lei No.8035.2010. Disponível em: http://www.camara.gov.br/proposicoesWeb/fichadetramitacao?idProposicao =490116.

44. Unesco. Relatório de Monitoramento Global de EPT. Relatório Conciso. A crise oculta: conflitos armados e educação. Edições UNESCO. 2011.

45. Roncalli AG. Projeto SB Brasil 2010: elemento estratégico na construção de um modelo de vigilância em saúde bucal. Cad. Saúde Pública, 26(3):428-429, mar, 2010.

46. BRASIL. Departamento de Atenção Básica, Secretaria de Atenção à Saúde, Ministério da Saúde. Projeto SB Brasil 2003. Condições de saúde bucal da população brasileira, 2002-2003: resultados principais. Brasília: Ministério da Saúde. 2004.

47. Queiroz RCS, Portela MC, Vasconcellos MTL. Pesquisa sobre as Condições de Saúde Bucal da População Brasileira (SB Brasil 2003): seus dados não produzem estimativas populacionais, mas há possibilidade de correção. Cad. Saúde Pública, 25(1):47-58, jan, 2009.

48. Brasil 2010. SBBrasil 2010. Pesquisa Nacional de Saúde Bucal. Disponível em: http://portal.saude.gov.br/portal/arquivos/pdf/apresentacaonova_28210.pdf

49. Freire MC, de Melo RB, Almeida, Silva S. Dental caries prevalence in relation to socioeconomic status of nursery school children in Goiânia-GO, Brazil. Community Dent Oral Epidemiol.;24(5):357-61. Oct 1996.

50. Ferreira SF, Béria JU, Kramer PF, Feldens EG, Feldens CA. Dental caries in 0- to 5-year-old Brazilian children: prevalence, severity, and associated factors. International Journal of Paediatric Dentistry. 2007; 17:289-296.

51. Sheiham A, Watt RG: The Common Risk Factor Approach: a rational basis for promoting oral health. Community Dent Oral Epidemiol. 2000; 28: 399-406.

52. Petersen (2003). The World Oral Health Report 2003: continuous improvement of oral health in the 21st century - the approach of the WHO Global Oral Health Programme. Community Dent and Oral Epidemiol 2003;31 Suppl 1:3-23(ou 24?).

53. Harris R, Nicoll AD, Adair PM, Pine CM. Risk factors for dental caries in young children: a systematic review of the literature. Community Dental Health (2004) 21 (Supplement), 71-85

54. WHO/FAO. Diet, Nutrition and the Prevention of Chronic Diseases: report of a joint WHO/FAO expert consultation, Geneva, 28 January - 1 February 2002. WHO Technical Report Series; 916.

55. Brasil. Ministério da Saúde. Secretaria de Política de Saúde. Organização Pan Americana da Saúde.Guia alimentar para crianças menores de dois anos / Secretaria de Políticas de Saúde, Organização Pan Americana da Saúde. – Brasília: Ministério da Saúde. 2002.

56. Vitolo MR, Bortolini GA, Feldens CA, Drachler M de L. Impactos da implementação dos dez STEPs da alimentação saudável para crianças: ensaio de campo randomizado. Cad. Saúde Pública, 21(5):1448-1457, set-out. 2005.

57. WHO. Diet, Nutrition and the Prevention of Chronic Diseases. Technical Report No.797. World Health Organization. Geneva. 1990.

58. Pertersen (2004). Effective use of fluorides for the prevention of dental caries in the 21st century: the WHO approach. Community Dent Oral Epidemiol. 2004; 32: 319-21

59. WHOb (2003). The World Oral Health report 2003. Geneva: World Health Organization ; 2003. Disponível em: http://www.who.int/oral_health.

60. Marinho VCC, Higgins JPT, Sheiham A, Logan S. Fluoride toothpastes for preventing dental caries in children and adolescents. (Cochrane Review). In: The Cochrane Library, Issue 1, 2003. Chichester: JOhn Wiley & Sons Ltd.

61. Martins CC, Pinheiro NR, Paiva SM. Perfil de crianças portadoras de fluorose dentária quanto às diversas formas de acesso ao flúor. JBP. 2002; 27(5):396-402.

62. Kubota K, Lee DH, Tsuchiya M, Young CS, Everett ET, Martinez-Mier EA, et al.Fluoride induces endoplasmic reticulum stress in ameloblasts responsible for dental enamel formation. Journal of Biological Chemistry. 2005; 280(24):23194-202.

63. Wong MCM, Glenny AM, Tsang BWK, Lo ECM, Worthington HV, Marinho VCC. Topical fluoride as a cause of dental fluorosis in children. Cochrane Database of Systematic Reviews, 2010, issue 1, article no. CD007693, p.1-49

64. Instituto Nacional do Câncer (Brasil). Organização Pan-Americana da Saúde. Pesquisa especial de tabagismo. PETab: relatório Brasil. Rio de Janeiro. INCA. 2011.

65. Ministério da Saúde. Instituto Nacional do Câncer. Programa Nacional de Controle do Tabagismo e Outros Fatores de Risco de Câncer. Modelo Lógico e Avaliação. 2ª ed. Brasília. 2003.

66. Shafey O, Eriksen E, Ross H, Mackay J. El Atlas del Tabaco. 3ª Ed. American Cancer Society. World Lung Foundation. p.128.

67. Pasqualotti, A., Migott A.M. B., Maciel E. N., Branco M. M. N., Carvalho R. M. A. de, Pizzol, T. da S. D., Gehlen C. T., Solda D. A., Gressler M. Experimentação de Fumo em Estudantes do Ensino Fundamental e Médio de Área Urbana na Região Sul do Brasil. Revista Interamericana de Psicología/Interamerican Journal of Psychology. 2006; 40(2):213-218.

68. Pinto D da S, Ribeiro AS. Variáveis relacionadas à iniciação do tabagismo entre estudantes do ensino médio de escola pública e particular na cidade de Belém – PA. J Bras Pneumol. 2007; 33(5):558-564.

69. Instituto Brasileiro de Geografia e Estatístico/IBGE. Ministério da Saúde. Ministério do Planejamento Orçamento e Gestão. Pesquisa de Saúde do Escolar. Rio de Janeiro. 2009.

70. Sandoval RC, Blanco, A. Estado de la implementación del Convenio Marco para el Control de Tabaco en Región de

las Américas. Salud Publica de México vol.52, suplemento. 2010; 2:270-276.

71. Organización Mundial de la Salud. Informe OMS sobre la epidemia mundial de tabaquismo, 2009: consecución de ambientes libres de humo de tabaco. Geneva. Organización Mundial de la Salud. 2010

72. WHO. Protection from exposure to second-hand tobacco smoke. Policy recommendations. Geneva. World Health Organization. 2007; p.50.

73. Organização Pan-Americana da Saúde. Recife Respira Melhor: a implantação de ambientes livres de fumo. Estudo de Caso. Brasília: Organização Pan-Americana da Saúde. 2010; p.68.

74. Conselho Nacional dos Direitos das Mulheres. Creche Urgente: relatos de experiência. Brasília; Série de Manuais sobre Creche.1988.

75. Health Education Authority. Nutrition & Oral Health: Guidelines for pre-schools. London. 1999.

76. Gonçalves, FD et al. Health promotion in primary school. Interface - Comunic., Saúde, Educ. 2008 jan/mar; 12(24):181-92.

77. Oliveira M de N, Brasil ALD, Taddei JAde-AC. Avaliação das condições higiênico-sanitárias das cozinhas de creches públicas e filantrópicas. Ciência & Saúde Coletiva. 2008; 13(3):1051-1060.

Chapter 19

The Approach to Common Risk Factors and Health Promotion in Schools

Simone Tetu Moysés
Bella Elisabeth Monse

Introduction

Care, and the creation of opportunities for the development of people's potential for quality of life commences in early childhood. That has been recognized as an essential strategy for tackling inequities in health.[1] Experiences during the first years of life, including access to health and education, are considered crucial for a person's later development.[2] Social advantages and disadvantages accumulated or grouped at critical periods of human development, particularly in early childhood and adolescence, are possible determinants of inequities of health, including oral health.[3,4] Therefore, to have opportunities to maintain their health children need to live in safe, healthy, caring and responsible environments. The physical and the relational environments can prevent problems and promote well--being, influence views, perceptions and actions.[6]

Schools are social environments that contribute to the development of academic skills and capabilities and knowledge as well as social and individual skills. Those skills assist affect the lives of children and adolescents and the lives of others with whom they come into contact.[7] To this end, they should favour the developmeny of autonomy and individuality to prepare people to live in society, strengthening their critical consciousness and expanding their liberty and resilience in vulnerable situations.[8,9] The influence on health, is therefore manifested not only in the attitudes and behaviours of children and teenagers in relation to health, but also in their actions as citizens in the community when they are adults.[10,11]

This chapter addresses the role of the school as a favourable environment for health promotion and reducing inequities. We shall explore the movements that incorporate integration approaches based on the wider concept of health and its determinants. The effectiveness of health promotion practices at schools with an impact on oral health are discussed, and examples of successful school health programs that incorporate the principles and values of health promotion and the approach to common risk factors of chronic conditions, such as those linked to oral health and disease, are presented.

The role of the school in health promotion

The school is a privileged setting for promoting the health of its students, employees and local communities.[12,13] A school that assumes its responsibility for actions related to health and tackling of inequities values the expansion of knowledge, and develops capabilities of its teachers, employees, parents and of the community to act on the health and determinants of quality of life. It establishes partnerships for the development of intersectoral actions that provide support to the health of its community. It prioritizes investments of resources geared towards health promotion actions of proven effectiveness. It favours collective participation and empowerment, acknowledging and valuing diversities and supporting collective actions within the scope of health and education.[14] Practices developed in the school environment can favour the building of citizenship or the repression, the protection or the expansion of vulnerabilities, care or violence.[14] However, schools can sometimes become a conflictive environment, especially in the urban contexts where there are social, economic, health and education inequities.

Actions relating to health in schools have reproduced these conflicts throughout history. Beattie[15] described how schools have been used as a testing space for public health interventions since 1900. Medical counselling, as part of sanitary principles, established by hygiene control actions by means of the inspection of the children, physical examinations and the introduction of the school meal, were strategies introduced during the first half of the 20 century to build "health consciousness" and to establish personal health and hygiene. From 1950 to 1990, the actions were geared towards changes of student lifestyle and the recognition of the psychosocial origins of risk behaviours, such as tobacco or drug use, and sexuality.

When approaches changed from social control to control over personal health, health education was introduced in schools all over the world. For many years, traditional health education programs were implemented as part of the school curriculum. Teachers were supposed to present packages of information about risky health behaviours in the expectation of providing the children with the necessary knowledge to influence their behaviour. These practices were based on a prescriptive and coercive education model, focused on the reproduction of values and behaviours, instead of a participative process that generates opportunities for well-being and personal and collective growth, paving the way for control over one's own health.[16]

Although some school programs during the 1980s incorporated innovative methods for the development of skills and attitudes to support the students to make healthy lifestyle choices, health education actions proved to have short-term minimal effects.[17] Evidence of systematic reviews of the literature about oral health education programs using traditional methods reinforce that conclusion.[18-23]

An important element for making the school an environment for positive learning and construction of life is the creation of a space that explicitly supports the physical, emotional and social well-being of its students, besides their academic achievement. The recognition of the fact that health behaviours are also defined by the characteristics of living environments (See Chapter 8), reaffirms the need to act on the school environment. The "Healthy School" described by Young and Williams,[24] goes beyond the limits of the formal curriculum. It considers the school´s ethos, its environment and social context to furnish the children with the necessary knowledge, confidence and skills to make choices that promote health.

New school health intervention approaches have been introduced in recent years, linked to the movements of the education sector, from the perspective of valuing the school´s role as a hub of social development of the community by means of the principles of inclusive education, of participation and of democratization of knowledge.[25] This new view of the school enlarges the perspective for health actions in this environment by means of the extension of health care services for students and employees, the creation of physical and social environments of support to health and the expansion of the curriculum beyond classroom activities.[14] The expanded curriculum now incorporates a variety of health-related topics, including healthy diet, physical activity, prevention of violence, safety and accident prevention, substance use and abuse, healthy growth and development, mental health, grounded in the qualification of teaching and of programs, in the assurance of a healthy physical environment and a supporting social environment, as well as in the valuing of partnerships with the school community (Fig. 19.1).[26]

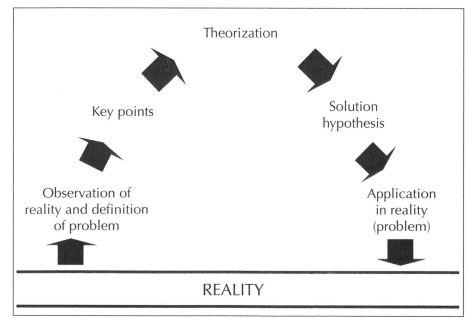

Fig. 19.1 – Educational approach in health.

Integrated School health Promotion Approaches

International movements, including initiatives of organizations such as WHO (World Health Organization), UNI-CEF (United Nations Children´s Fund), UNESCO (United Nations Educational, Science and Cultural Organization) and the World Bank, the international commitment to Focusing Resources on Effective School Health (FRESH) and the networks of Health Promoting Schools, besides worldwide national movements and policies, such as the School Health Program in Brazil, have favoured the enlargement of perspectives for the development of integrated health promotion practices at schools.

The concept of Health Promoting Schools (HPS) emerged during the 1980s, with the support of WHO, as a mechanism for integration of different elements that combined health and education.[24,27,28] These elements would include the curriculum, the school environment, the health services offered by the school, partnerships with the community and the school policies of support to health. Therefore, a Health Promoting School can be defined as "a school that constantly strengthens its capacity as a healthy setting for living, learning and working".[29] Its principles and values are based on the Ottawa Letter,[30] and on the Convention on the Rights of the Child[31] and include participation, equity, local empowerment, partnerships and the sustainability of practices.[32] Its goals for strengthening autonomy over health and structural / environmental performance manifest in action programs that:

- Endeavour to improve the health of school employees, families and members of the community, besides that of the students;
- Reinforce health and learning with all the available measures;
- Involve health and education employees, teachers and their representative organizations, students, parents and community leaders in efforts to make the school a healthy environment;
- Seek to provide a healthy environment, school health education and health services in partnership with community projects, health promotion programs for employees, eating and nutrition programs, opportunities for physical activity and recreation practices and counselling, social support and mental health promotion programs;
- Implement policies and practices that respect the self-esteem of individuals, promote multiple opportunities for success and recognize efforts and positive intentions, as well as personal accomplishments.

This concept of HPS has spread around many parts of the world as an important strategy that provides opportunities to decrease health iniquities. Evaluations of the impact of this approach have emphasized that the available evidence is limited, but promising.[10,17,33-35] Health promotion actions based on HPS values and principles have been implemented, leading to changes in school policies and in curriculums, favouring the participation of parents and of local communities.[35] In a systematic review of the literature to assess the effectiveness of Health Promoting Schools, Lister-Sharp and collaborators[17] emphasize evidence of impact on the social and physical environment of the school in terms of development of employees, provision of school meals, physical exercise programs and social relations, besides improving aspects of health-related behaviours. There is some evidence that this approach can produce a positive impact on aspects of mental and social health, such as self--esteem and control of violence.

From the perspective of education, an integration strategy, launched by the World Education Forum in 2000, with the support of WHO, UNESCO, UNICEF and the World Bank, proposed the focalization of resources for the development of effective school health strategies, aiming to improve quality and equity in basic education. This strategy, known as FRESH (Focusing Resources on Effective School Health),[36] recognized that children's ability to reach their full potential is directly related to the synergistic effect of good health, good nutrition and appropriate education. Hence to reach the proposed goal of "Education for All", it was considered essential to create safe, healthy, inclusive and equitable educational environments that provide an opportunity for excellence in learning. This movement recommends four cost-effective components as a starting point for all schools:

- the development of school health policies;
- the provision of safe water and sanitation;
- health education based on the development of skills; and
- the supply of health and nutrition services.[36]

This international movement has served as a reference for school health experiences, especially for developing countries. In Brazil, the recognition of the school as a locus for the development of health promotion strategies is detailed in the current National Health Promotion Policy[37] and National Basic Care Policy,[38] in connection with the National Early Childhood Education Policy.[39] The appreciation of the school's role in the territory of health teams, as well as the incentive to the development of intersectoral actions geared towards health promotion in this territory, are examples of strategies defined by these policies. Moreover, work undertaken at schools, such as qualification of oral health care, is also a strategic action of the National Oral Health Policy.[40]

The School Health Program, established in Brazil in 2007 by an intersectoral action between the Ministries of Health and Education, is outlined as a public policy of action in four components: evaluation of the health conditions of students; health promotion and disease prevention; permanent education and training of professionals and of youths; monitoring and evaluation of impact of actions. Although still in the implementation and consolidation phase, this program has the potential to reinforce the development of important intersectoral actions in health promotion in the school environment, in a partnership, now formalized between health and education.

The effectiveness of school health promotion practices with an impact on oral health

Promoting oral health means putting the mouth back into the body, and recognizing the body as part of a person inserted in a particular social context that can increase their vulnerability to diseases or provide support for improving their health. Adapting the expression created by Baelum and Lopez,[41] it is necessary to contextualize "healthy teeth, in healthy individuals, in healthy populations". Sustainable improvements in oral health therefore require effective actions directed at the socio-environmental determinants and at the creation of a social environment, such as the school, which facilitates the maintenance of general and oral health.[14]

Most oral diseases, such as dental caries, periodontal disease oral cancer and dental trauma, are chronic conditions with significant impacts on quality of life. Thus risk factors for other chronic diseases, such diabetes, cardiovascular diseases and cancer, are also risk factors for oral diseases. These risk factors include diet, hygiene, tobacco use and violence. As stated previously, schools are privileged settings for acting on these factors in the context of the lives of children and adolescents, by means of health promotion policies. Evidence has demonstrated that multifaceted approaches developed at schools, especially those that involve the entire school community and act on common risk factors, affecting the "causes of causes" associated with risk behaviours, can have a positive impacts on the general and health of the population.[10-43]

Reviews of reviews on the effectiveness of school health promotion practices geared towards action on common risk factors for chronic diseases present evidence that the health behaviours, such as the use of tobacco and other substances, physical activity, healthy diet, personal hygiene, and others, are interconnected. Therefore, action on one behaviour can have an impact on others. In this way, integrated interventions on multiple factors associated with these behaviours, which act on social influences, on cognitive skills, the training of facilitators, and changes in the school environment, can produce positive results in different behaviours simultaneously[42,43] and can therefore be effective for promoting oral health. On the other hand, there is limited evidence that interventions focused on only one behaviour, such as healthy diet, and on health education actions in an isolated manner, can produce sustained changes in the behaviour of children.[44] Thus, the most effective interventions for promoting healthy behaviours, such as a healthy diet, are those that favour the involvement of the whole school community, teacher training and curricular adaptations, as well as the definition of a sustainable policy for general health at school.[45] Likewise, there appears to be greater effectiveness of tobacco control programs at schools when there is a combination of interventions focused on action on social influences and competences, such as inclusion in the curriculum of actions that offer information; associated with actions that use social influence approaches, such as work with peers; with those that develop generic social competences, such as self-esteem and autonomy; and those that include interventions that involve the family and the community.[46]

Reviews of the impact of school health promotion actions on mental health and aggressive behaviours, which can be associated with greater vulnerability to dental trauma, have demonstrated that the improvement of social relationships and skills can be more effective than interventions designed to teach individualized skills to avoid provocative situations.[47] Effective interventions include the development of participative educational skills, starting early with younger children and continuing with older children, having sustainability over time, working with multimodal approaches and for the entire school, which includes curricular changes, improvements in the school environment, further education for teachers, involvement of parents and community, education of parents, and coordinated actions with institutions outside the school.[48]

The direct impact of school health promotion on oral health in children was explored by Moysés et al.[10] The implementation of health promotion policies at state schools from districts on the outskirts of Curitiba, in southern Brazil, was effective in the control of caries and of dental trauma in children. Schools developing a whole curriculum based on healthy policies, such as the combating of smoking and drugs, the encouragement of healthy eating, and focused on participative education and the development of cooperative projects for the improvement of the school´s physical environment, exhibited a higher percentage of caries-free children and less dental trauma. In addition, schools that demonstrated a commitment to health and safety through the designation of individuals responsible for school health promotion, greater involvement of the parents and development of school safety strategies, recorded a significantly lower number of children who had suffered dental trauma.

Therefore, school health promotion appears to be an important strategy to be developed in collective oral health promotion programs for children, enabling a positive impact on health inequities.

Evidence for practice

Support for the development of practices based on evidence of effectiveness of oral health promotion at schools has ensured the diversification of practices in different contexts. Successful experiences seek to incorporate components of initiatives such as that of HPS and FRESH, putting into practice actions focused on health promotion values and principles. An example is the Fit is School Program,[49] developed in the Philippines and summarized in figure 19.2.

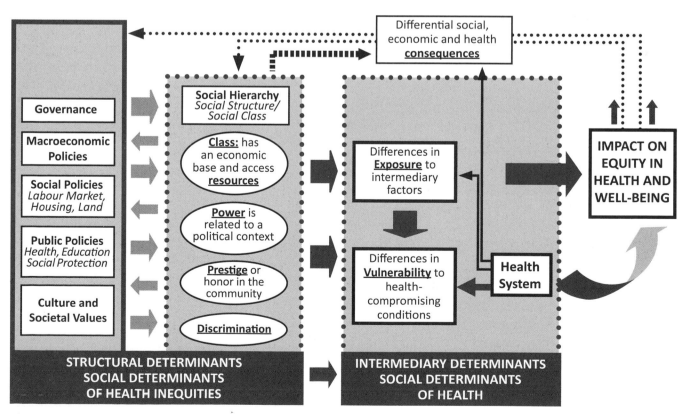

Fig. 19.2 – The role of intermediary determinants of health.

Examples of oral health policies developed at schools show how specific actions can be part of an expanded approach to health promotion in the school environment (Fig. 19.3). The integrated development of several policies can potentiate their effects and effectiveness to achieve significant gains in oral health.

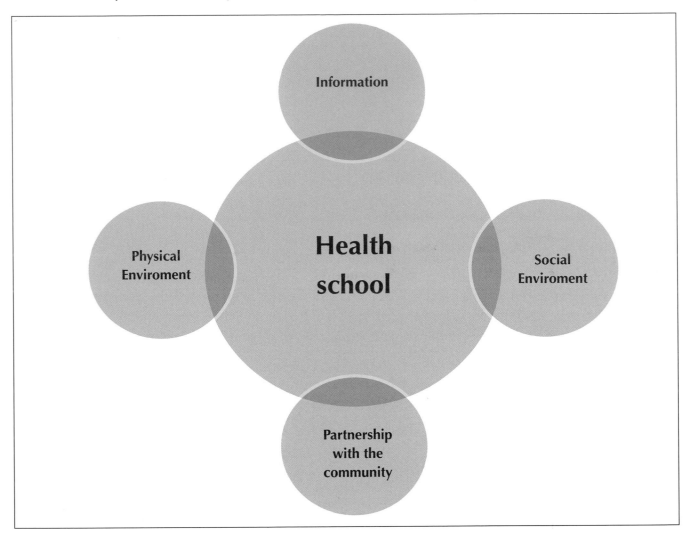

Fig. 19.3 – Basis for a healthy school.[26]

Conclusion

The promotion of oral health at schools favours actions on the socio-environmental determinants of health of children and adolescent and details the political commitment to the reduction of social and health inequities.

Efforts targeting health promotion in this environment should consider the characteristics of its political and pedagogic project, the school´s social context, environmental safety, the health services offered at the school and partnerships with the community, thus creating opportunities for the development of potentials and skills for individual and collective choices that promote health.

Box 19.1 – Fit for School.

In spite of political frameworks that favour integrated school health programs, there are few known examples where these have been put into practice on a large scale. An excellent example is the Essential Health Care Program (EHCP) of the Department of Education of the Philippines (DEPED). EHCP institutionalizes hand washing with soap and brushing with fluoride toothpaste as daily group activities, as well as biannual de-worming to tackle diseases related to hygiene of high impact on children: respiratory infections, diarrhoea, worm infestations and rampant caries, which have a negative effect on the school attendance of children, their academic performance and quality of life. The program currently has around 2 million children as a target and is expanding rapidly. At a United Nations event for South-South Cooperation, EHCP received an award from the World Bank, UNDP and WHO for the construction of a model of application of established concepts, such as FRESH and Health Promoting Schools, put into action.

Based on the Fit for School action model, the program is characterized by three "S's" – simplicity, scalability and sustainability. Clearly defined roles and responsibilities facilitate intersectoral collaboration between the government agencies linked to health and education. Program execution leadership is in the hands of the Department of Education. Incorporating the principles of School-Based Management, it is the role of the school management to ensure the implementation of the program in its respective schools, with teachers supervising daily activities. The responsibility of the school health professionals is limited to the initial training and regular monitoring of the program. The program is funded by the local government (Local Government Units - LGUs) – generally by means of its health budgets. The low cost of the program materials (about USD 0.50 per child per year for toothpaste, toilet soap and toothbrush) guarantees the long-term public commitment that goes far beyond a traditional approach based on corporate donations and sponsorships. The continuous involvement of parents and communities also contributes to the sustainability and local appropriation. Besides contributing towards the initial construction, maintenance and modernization of the necessary facilities, they also participate in the regular monitoring of the program. The guilt-free self-evaluation process motivates and guides them to improve and maintain the quality of execution of actions. Information gathered is coded in an online monitoring system, making the performance of each school transparent in the program implementation.

Since 2009, the NGO Fit for School Inc. (FIT) and Deutsche Gesellschaft für Internationale Zusammenarbeit (GIZ) have contributed to the development of capacities in the Department of Education and in the Local Government Units (LGUs) for the management of EHCP, particularly by means of protocols, manuals and models that facilitate the program implementation. The main activities of FIT are the reinforcement of intersectoral collaboration relative to school health programs between the Department of Education and Provincial Health Offices in each province, which includes intensive advocacy for the funding of the program by local governments. A longitudinal study of results in health, carried out in collaboration with national and international universities, provides the evidence of the program´s impact. After just one year, oral infection, malnutrition rates and worm infections have been significantly reduced among children at schools where the program is implemented.

The success of the program led to requests for technical support from other countries in Southeast Asia. The German Ministry for Economic Cooperation and Development (BMZ), appointed GIZ to support the Ministries of Education of Cambodia, Indonesia and Laos in the adoption of the Fit for Schools approach. A partnership with SEAMEO INNOTECH, the regional centre of the Southeast Asian Ministers of Education Organization (SEAMEO), supports this process and the necessary development of capacities. Moreover, UNICEF, AusAID, GIZ and FIT joined forces to investigate and develop sustainable models for the integration of the school sanitation component in the Fit for School approach.

Box 19.2 – Oral health promotion policies in school.

Healthy school environment
- safe buildings and recreational areas to prevent accidents
- availability of treated and fluoridated water
- ban on the sale of unhealthy food in the vicinity of the school
- psychosocial environment of care and respect
- protocol for treating cases of violence and interpersonal conflicts

School ethos
- commitment to a school integrated to the community
- role of the school in the discussion of local health topics, e.g., fluoridation of water
- support for health promotion activities

Development of policies
- training in development of policies and action plans

- involvement of students, teachers, employees, families and members of the community in planning, development and evaluation of processes
- frequent meetings between the management of the school, Parent-Teachers Association, community councils and health and education managers

Healthy eating
- availability of healthy food in the school canteen
- drinking water fountains at the school
- training for cooks and food providers in healthy eating
- assessment and monitoring of the nutritional condition

Sugar, alcohol and tobacco
- ban on sugar-based foods and beverages on the school premises
- ban on the use of alcohol and tobacco on the school premises

- availability of counselling services and support for quitting smoking

Oral health education
- oral health education as part of the curriculum content
- daily supervised tooth brushing
- training of parents in oral health and encouragement of their involvement in health promotion actions
- training of teachers and employees

Oral health services
- integrated work and activity with local and regional health services
- response to dental emergencies
- role of health professionals in the control of oral diseases

- monitoring of complaints and absenteeism related to oral problems

Oral trauma
- accident prevention
- first aid protocol
- monitoring of trauma incidence

Physical activity in school
- commitment to the availability of safe equipment and settings for sports and leisure activities
- physical activity as a compulsory item in the curriculum
- protocol for safe practice in sports

Adapted from Kwan et al, 2005 (5).

References

1. WHO - World Health Organization, Commission on Social Determinants of Health. Closing the gap in a generation: Health equity through action on the social determinants of health. Geneva: WHO. 2008.
2. WHO. Early child development: a powerful equalizer. Final report of the Early Child Development Knowledge Network of the Commission on Social Determinants of Health. Geneva: World Health Organization. 2007.
3. Watt RG. From victim blaming to upstream action: tackling the social determinants of oral health inequalities. Community Dentistry and Oral Epidemiology. 2007 Feb; 35(1):1-11.
4. Peres MA, Latorre MRO, Sheiham A, Peres KG, Barros FC, Hernandez PG, et al. Social and biological early life influences on severity of dental caries in children aged 6 years. Community Dentistry and Oral Epidemiology. 2005; 33(1):53-63.
5. Kwan SY, Petersen PE, Pine CM, Borutta A. Health-promoting schools: an opportunity for oral health promotion. Bull World Health Organ. 2005; 83(9):677-85.
6. Gray G, Young I, Barnekow V. Developing a health-promoting school. A practical resource for developing effective partnerships in school health, based on the experience of the European Network of Health Promoting Schools. London: European Network of Health Promoting Schools. 2006.
7. WHO. The World Health Organisation's Global School Health Initiative. Geneva: WHO. 1996.
8. Assis SG, Pesce RP, Avanci JQ. Resiliência: enfatizando a proteção dos adolescentes. São Paulo: Artmed. 2006.
9. St Leger AS, Kolbe L, Lee A, et al. School health promotion - achievements, challenges and priorities. In: McQueen D, Jones CM, editors. Global Perspectives on Health Promotion Effectiveness. New York: International Union For Health Promotion and Education. 2007. p.107-24.
10. Moysés ST, Moysés SJ, Watt RG, Sheiham A. Associations between health promoting schools policies on some indicators of oral health. Health Promotion International. 2003; 18(3):209-18.
11. WHO, Commission on Social Determinants of Health. Closing the gap in a generation: health equity through action

on the social determinants of health. Final Report of the Commission on Social Determinants of Health. Geneva: World Health Organization. 2008.

12. WHO - World Health Organization, editor. Fifth Global Conference for Health Promotion, 2000 5-9 June; Mexico: WHO.

13. Hamilton K, Saunders L. The health promoting school: a summary of the ENHPS evaluation project in England. London: Health Education Authority. 1997.

14. Moyses ST. A importância das ações de prevenção e promoção em saúde bucal para a comunidade escolar. Revista Brasileira Saúde da Familia. 2008; 20:70-4.

15. Beattie A. The health promoting school: from idea to action. In: Scriven A, Orme J, editors. Health promotion; professional perspectives. Hampshire: MacMillan The Open University. 1996; p.129-43.

16. Hagquist C, Starrin B. Health education in schools - from information to empowerment models. Health Promotion International. 1997; 12(3):225-32.

17. Lister-Sharp D, Chapman S, Stewart-Brown S, Sowden A. Health promoting schools and health promotion in schools: two systematic reviews. Health Technology Assessment. 1999; 3(22):1-207.

18. Kay EJ, Locker D. Effectiveness of Oral Health Promotion: A Review. London: Health Education Authority. 1997.

19. Kay E, Locker D. A systematic review of the effectiveness of health promotion aimed at improving oral health. Community Dentistry and Oral Epidemiology. 1998; 15(3):132-44.

20. Sprod A, Anderson R, Treasure E. Effective oral health promotion: literature review. Cardiff: Health Promotion Wales. 1996.

21. Wright FAC, Satur J, Morgan MV. Evidence Based Health Promotion; Resources for Planning. Victoria. 2000.

22. Satur JG, Gussy MG, Morgan MV, Calache H, Wright FAC. Review of the evidence for oral health promotion effectiveness. Health Education Journal. 2010; 69(3):257-66.

23. Young I, Willians T. The Healthy School. Edinburgh: SHEG/SCC WHO(Euro) 1989 Nov,1989.

24. Curitiba. Secretaria Municipal da Educação. Programa Comunidade Escola: termo de referência. Curitiba: Prefeitura Municipal de Curitiba. 2005.

25. Canada, Ministry of Education. Healthy Schools. Ottawa2012 [cited 2012 20 de fevereiro]; Available from: http://www.edu.gov.on.ca/eng/healthyschools/foundations.html.

26. WHO - World Health Organization. Promoting health through schools. Technical report series. Geneva: WHO,1997. Report No: 870.

27. St Leger L, Nutbean D. Effective health promotion in schools. In: Boddy D, editor. The evidence of health promotion effectiveness: shaping public health in Europe. Brussels: European Union. 1999; p.110-22.

28. WHO. WHO's Global School Health Initiative: Health Promoting Schools; a healthy setting for living, learning and working. Geneva: WHO. 1998.

29. WHO - World Health Organization. Ottawa Charter for Health Promotion. Health Promotion. 1987; 1(4):iii-v.

30. Nations U-U. Convention on the Rights of the Child. United Nations; 1989 [cited 2011 19 de dezembro]; Available from: http://www2.ohchr.org/english/law/crc.htm.

31. ENHPS. First Conference of the European Network of Health Promoting Schools. The Health Promoting School - an investment in education, health and democracy: conference report, Thessaloniki-Halkidiki, Greece, 1-5 May 1997. Copenhagen: WHO Regional Office for Europe. 1997.

32. Jamison J, Ashby P, Hamilton K, Lewis G, MacDonald A, Saunders L. The health promoting school: final report of the ENHPS evaluation project in England. London: Health Education Authority. 1998.

33. Moon AM, Mullee MA, Thompson RL, Speller V, Roderick P. Health-related research and evaluation in schools. Health Education. 1999; (1):27-34.

34. Mukoma W, Flisher AJ. Evaluations of health promoting schools: a review of nine studies. Health Promotion International. 2004 September 1, 2004; 19(3):357-68.

35. OMS, UNESCO, UNICEF, Mundial B. Focusing Resources on Effective School Health:a FRESH Start to Enhancing the Quality and Equity of Education.: UNICEF; 2000 [cited 2012 20 de janeiro]; Available from: http://www.unicef.org/lifeskills/files/FreshDocument.pdf.

36. Brasil, Ministério da Saúde. Política Nacional de Promoção da Saúde. Brasília: Ministério da Saúde, Série Pactos pela Saúde. 2006.

37. Brasil, Ministério da Saúde. Política Nacional de Atenção Básica. Brasília: Ministério da Saúde, Série Pactos pela Saúde. 2006.

38. Brasil, Educação Md. Política Nacional de Educação Infantil: pelo direito das crianças de zero a seis anos à Educação. Brasilia: MEC SEB. 2006.

39. Brasil, Ministério da Saúde, Coordenação Nacional de Saúde Bucal. Diretrizes da Política Nacional de Saúde Bucal. Brasília: Ministério da Saúde. 2004.

40. Baelum V, Lopez R. Periodontal epidemiology: towards social science or molecular biology? Community Dentistry and Oral Epidemiology. 2004 Aug; 32(4):239-49.

41. Peters LWH, Gerjo K, Dam MGT, Buijs GJ, Paulussen TGWM. Effective elements of school health promotion across behavioral domains: a systematic review of reviews. BMC Public Health. 2009; 9(182):1-14.

42. Jepson RG, Harris FM, Platt S, Tannahill C. The effectiveness of interventions to change six health behaviours: a review of reviews. BMC Public Health. 2010; 10:538-54.

43. Cauwenberghe E, Maes L, Spittaels H, Lenthe FJ, Brug J, Oppert JM, et al. Effectiveness of school-based interventions in Europe to promote healthy nutrition in children and adolescents: systematic review of published and 'grey' literature. British Journal of Nutrition. 2010; 103(6):781-97.

44. Souza EA, Filho VCB, Nogueira JAD, Júnior MRA. Atividade física e alimentação saudável em escolares brasileiros: revisão de programas de intervenção. Cad Saúde Pública. 2011; 27(8):1459-71.

45. Thomas RE, Perera R. School-based programmes for preventing smoking: The Cochrane Library,2012 Contract No.: Art. No. CD001293. DOI: 10.1002/14651858. CD001293.pub4.

46. Mytton JA, DiGuiseppi C, Gough D, Taylor RS, Logan S. School-based secondary prevention programmes for preventing violence. Cochrane Database of Systematic Reviews. 2012(1):Art. No. CD004606.

47. Weare K, Nind M. Mental health promotion and problem prevention in schools: what does the evidence say? Health Promot Int. 2011; 26(Suppl 1):i29-69.

48. Benzian H, Monse B, Jr VB, Schratz A, Sahin M, Helderman WvP. Public health in action: effective school health needs renewed international attention. Glob Health Action. 2012;5(14870). http://www.globalhealthaction.net/index.php/gha/article/view/14870/pdf_1

Chapter **20**

Evaluating Oral Health Promotion: a practical guide

Andrea de Silva
Lisa Gibbs
Elizabeth Waters
Richard Watt

Overview

Evaluation of oral health promotion interventions is critical to answer the important questions of what works, for whom, under what circumstances and at what cost? With strong evaluations, and widely disseminated findings, both consumers and decision makers alike are better equipped to understand which strategies are likely to improve oral health, and what investment is likely to result in what kind of outcomes. In some situations it will also enable greater clarity about those that are not effective.

This chapter has been designed to assist health promotion practitioners to evaluate their efforts by providing a practical guide to developing and undertaking an evaluation.

Background: What are health promotion interventions?

The World Health Organisation defines health promotion as "the process of enabling people to increase control over, and to improve their health"[1] and that peace, shelter, education, food, income, a stable ecosystem, sustainable resources, social justice and equity are fundamental prerequisites for health.[1,2] The health of individuals is influenced by a range of political, economic, social, cultural, environmental, behavioural and biological factors. Health promotion aims to influence these factors in a range of ways to make it easier for individuals to achieve good health.[2] The Ottawa Charter for Health Promotion[1] outlines five priority areas of health promotion action:
- Build healthy public policy
- Create supportive environments
- Strengthen community actions
- Develop personal skills
- Reorient health services

Health promotion: from individuals to populations

Whilst health promotion interventions can be used to improve individual care, health promotion is intended to have its greatest impact when operationalised for effects at the population level. If the above health promotion strategies are implemented in an integrated way, there is a much greater chance of having a sustainable and equitable impact at the population level.

Oral Health Promotion Interventions

In addition to the Ottawa Charter, the conceptual models that guide our understanding of how the population level interventions might work to improve oral health are the socio-ecological model of health and for oral health, more specifically, the recent model from Fisher-Owens et al. (Fisher-Owens 2007). These frameworks recognise the multidimensional and multi level nature of the **influences and causal factors** on health.

Fisher-Owens specifically describes five domains of influence on child oral health (genetic and biological factors, the social environment, the physical environment, health behaviours, and dental and medical care). Given the variety of influences, oral health promotion interventions can be broad, and involve multiple strategies.

Cross-cutting across the five priority areas of the Ottawa Charter, three broad areas of **health promotion action** have been described by Nutbeam:[3]

- **Education:** Strategies which create opportunities for learning and are intended to improve personal health and thereby the capacity of individuals and communities to act to improve and protect their health (eg professional development, workforce training, and role expansion, social marketing)

- **Facilitation:** Action taken in partnership with individuals or social groups to mobilise social and material resources for health (eg central management of waiting lists and workforce, and resource reallocation)
- **Advocacy:** Action taken on behalf of individuals and/or communities to overcome structural barriers to the achievement of health (eg advocating for and supporting the implementation of community water fluoridation, examining local need and advocating for additional clinical services in underserved communities)

Using an outcomes model, the types of outcomes that can be anticipated with successful implementation of the health promotion actions is shown in figure 20.1 (adapted from[3,4]). To determine if these outcomes have been fully, partially or not at all achieved we need evaluation.

Overview of evaluation to generate health promotion evidence

Health promotion evaluation based evidence can answer several key questions. Some of these questions relate to effectiveness:

Does the intervention work or not work? Who does it work for?

while others relate more to the generalisability of the intervention:

How does the intervention work?
Is the intervention appropriate?
Is the intervention feasible?
Is the intervention relevant for another context?

Evaluation determines the significance, worth or condition of […] by careful appraisal and study. Practically, the focus of the evaluation can vary and includes health promotion programs, policies, organisational practices, social marketing etc. In general evaluations are useful for three primary purposes:

Fig. 20.1 – Categories of health promotion outcomes with oral health related examples.

Health & Social outcomes

- **Morbidity**
  - eg reduced caries
- **Quality of life**
  - eg reduced episodes of toothache
- **Equity**
  - eg improved access for vulnerable communitirs

Intermediate Health outcomes

- **Morbidity Lifestyles**
  - eg reduced intake of sweet foods and drinks
- **Effective dental health services**
  - eg workforce, models of care, scope of practice, reduced waiting times
- **Healthy enviroments**
  - eg community water fluoridation programs, changes in foods and drinks available in chidren's settings

Health Promotion outcomes

- **Health literacy**
  - eg incresed oral health, related knowledge and skills
- **Social Influence & action**
  - eg community support for oral health promotion and water fluoridation activities
- **Healthy public policy & organisational practice**
  - eg nutrition policies in chidren's settings, enhanced service co-ordination across the region

1. **To judge merit or worth**
   1.1. Accountability
   1.2. Value for money
   1.3. Health benefits
   1.4. Measure the results of an intervention
   1.5. Reduce inefficiencies or duplication
   1.6. Measure harms or unintended negative consequences
2. **To improve programs or policies and inform decision making**
   2.1. Inform planning and resource allocation
   2.2. Inform practice and policy decisions
   2.3. Advocacy and awareness raising
   2.4. Enable evidence-based decision making
3. **To generate knowledge**
   3.1. Increase knowledge of effective treatments or preventive measures
   3.2. Build the evidence base and inform future research
   3.3. Disseminate findings and share the knowledge gained

One of the often overlooked areas is the issue of potential harms resulting from actions – these may be otherwise known as unintended consequences, but measuring harms is particularly important given the focus of health promotion on health improvement and enhancement. Previous health promotion research has clearly demonstrated that there is a risk that the potential for health promotion programmes to cause harm or increase inequity could be underestimated[5,6] or missed without formal evaluations, which provide an opportunity to capture and measure harms using a variety of methodologies.

Types of evaluations

There are a number of different types of evaluation, and each captures different information and answers different questions. Primarily these are process, impact and outcome evaluation. They each align with a different level of the program or intervention plan (see Table 20.1) which thus provides a reference or guide to what should be evaluated.

Process Evaluation

Process evaluation focuses on the process of the strategies being used for implementation. Ideally it should capture how an intervention (policy or program) was implemented, what activities occurred, under what conditions, by whom and with what level of effort or resources, as well the acceptability of the activities.

The broad areas of process evaluation are: **context** (social and cultural environment and particular political and organisational system in a society,[7] **reach** (the degree to which the intended target group participated in the intervention), 'dose' delivered or intended (level of intervention activity) and **'dose' received** (extent of engagement of participants with the intervention activities), **fidelity** (was the intervention implemented as planned), **level of implementation achieved** (overall rating), and **recruitment** (the procedures used to engage intended participants in intervention activities).[7]

Table 20.1 – Alignment of planning levels with evaluation type.

Planning level	Evaluation type
Goals or Aims	Outcome
Objectives	Impact
Strategies	Process

Ideally process evaluation should provide information which can be used to inform implementation improvements and transferability, identify the barriers and facilitators to implementation, identify departures from program design (and reasons) and document the operations of the intervention. To broaden our understanding of the impacts of oral health promotion interventions, and explore the vital questions of applicability and transferability, detailed process evaluations are required.

A commonly used framework to guide process evaluation reporting is the RE-AIM framework,[8] capturing the following elements:
- **Reach:** Proportion of target group that the intervention reached
- **Efficacy:** Success rate (biological, behavioural and quality of life outcomes)
- **Adoption:** Settings that adopt a policy or program
- **Implementation:** Extent to which the intervention is implemented as intended

- **Maintenance:** Extent to which a program is sustained over time

Process evaluation can be used during the life of the program, from planning through to the end of delivery of the program, or implementation of a policy or organisational change. During planning (formative) and piloting stages, a process evaluation can focus on the development, quality and appropriateness of the strategies, for example, the development and pilot testing of a cultural competence training course for dental practitioners. In the implementation phase, process evaluation can be useful for tracking the reach of the program and the extent to which the intervention has been implemented, for example how many practitioners have completed the cultural competence training.

Process indicators can also assist with redeveloping or redefining the intervention by identifying the enablers and barriers to successful and effective intervention planning and implementation, incorporating client satisfaction and facilitator reports.

Process evaluation data is also critical in understanding, interpreting and explaining much of the data collected through impact and outcome evaluation.

Impact evaluation

Impact evaluation is focused on assessing the changes that occurred as a result of the intervention. In general, impact evaluation is used to examine the short or mid-term impacts of an intervention in the target setting/s or on the target population and others (Davis and MacDowell). Impact evaluation is often used to determine the degree to which program objectives have been achieved, and has been used to assess a variety of effects including:

- behaviours and practices (e.g. infant feeding, drinking, oral hygiene, tobacco use)
- health literacy, knowledge, attitudes and skills (of children, adults, health professionals etc)
- government, organisational or setting policies and practices (e.g. tobacco cessation, fluoridation policy)
- harm associated with the intervention
- cost effectiveness or costs of the intervention
- organisational or environmental change
- service delivery
- workforce capacity
- community capacity

In order for impact evaluation to be possible, it is critical that the program or strategy being evaluated has 'SMART' objectives. A SMART objective is one that is

Specific: identifies a precise outcome or behaviour linked with a number (eg percent, rate, frequency),

Measurable: progress towards and achievement of the objective can be measured

Achievable: the objective can be achieved with a reasonable amount of effort or time

Relevant: the objective is relevant to the intervention goals, community context and stakeholders

Time-bound: there is a date or age etc by which the objective is to be achieved

Two examples of SMART objectives are below:

- To decrease by 20% the proportion of primary school aged children who drink more than 500ml of carbonated sweet drinks each day.
- To increase by 30% the proportion of children who visit a dental professional for preventive measures by age three.

Outcome Evaluation

Outcome evaluation is used to measure the longer-term effects of policies or programs and is often used to determine the degree to which the goal of the intervention has been achieved. The long-term effects may include reductions in the incidence or prevalence of health conditions, changes in mortality, sustained behaviour change, or improvements in quality of life, equity or environmental conditions. In oral health promotion interventions, outcomes which have been measured include:

- dental caries (including early childhood caries, white spot lesions, decayed, missing and filled teeth or surfaces, the decayed, missing and filled teeth (dmft/DMFT) index
- periodontal disease measurement (gingival/periodontal infection, gingival/periodontal index, attachment loss)
- oral health status
- quality of life and oral pain

How do you 'do' an oral health promotion evaluation? (see Box 20.1 for an overview of the five steps, adapted from[9]):

Step 1: Identify the stakeholders early and engage with them to help guide the evaluation and dissemination plans

It is critical to the success of the evaluation to identify and engage with stakeholders. This requires broad and strategic thinking to identify people, groups and organisations with vested interest in the intervention program, its evaluation and the findings (eg community dental clinics, government departments, academics, children's services, funders). Once identified, the evaluators will need to work with the stakeholders to identify the purpose and objectives of the evaluation and to develop the evaluation plan. In many cases there are 'gatekeepers' to the target group, and not engaging with and consulting these individuals and their managers early can limit the evaluators ability to collect the required data.

Box 20.1 – Overview of the steps in evaluation:

Evaluation steps:
1. Identify the stakeholders early and engage with them to help guide the evaluation and dissemination plans
   - Think broadly and strategically to identify people, groups and organisations with vested interest in the intervention program, its evaluation and the findings (eg community dental clinics, government departments, academics, children's services)
   - Work together to identify the purpose and objectives of both the intervention and the evaluation
2. Define the program being evaluated and map its components
   - Define the program context and target group(s)
   - Identify the current stage of the project (eg planning, pilot, implementation, maintenance)
   - Develop a program logic model, or an intervention pathway map to identify the flow of resources, pathways operating and planned impacts and outcomes
3. Plan the evaluation and gather high quality and useful evidence
   - Determine the purpose of the evaluation and stakeholder perspective
   - Determine measures of program success that are shared and agreed upon by the stakeholder group. There may be measures of success identified at community, organisation, service and individual levels.

- Ensure the evaluation aligns with the theoretical underpinnings and purpose of the intervention
- Identify the likely program impacts and outcomes and determine the data needed to measure if these have been achieved
- Identify appropriate methods to collect or gain access to this data
- Consider equity and have a planned approach for reaching the 'hard to reach'

4. Report on the process, impacts and outcomes of the intervention
   - Analyse the data, interpret the results
   - Report on the evaluation findings within the context of the intervention
   - Compare results with comparable published studies, previously reported performance indicators or recommended guidelines/standards
   - Explore sustainability of impacts and outcomes and integration of intervention components into systems, services and practices

5. Communicate and disseminate the findings
   - Synthesise the findings for multiple stakeholder viewpoints and in the most appropriate formats for the various stakeholders (eg technical reports, executive summary, community reports, newsletters for schools, policy briefs)
   - Have a planned approach to communication and dissemination that involves the stakeholders and utilises their networks

Step 2: Define the program or strategy being evaluated

Scrutiny of the early community-based interventions which were large-scale but largely unsuccessful (e.g. Stanford Heart Disease prevention project) enhanced our understanding of the unique nature of such types of health promotion interventions and also demonstrated the importance of conceptualising changes that may occur in complex health interventions.[10] Health promotion interventions are by nature interactive, and quite distinct from medical interventions. Health program interventions can be considered as interactions between the interests of those delivering or receiving the intervention (the actors) and the technical components of the program (eg the education curriculum, the policy being implemented)[10-14] and the interaction between the intervention and the context or setting into which it is delivered (eg disadvantaged community compared to affluent community).

Without an understanding of these interactions there can be disconnect between the complex nature of the behaviours and practices, service systems and environments targeted by the health promotion interventions, and the experimental designs and methods used for evaluation. Program logic models and intervention mapping can take a variety of forms but in general they provide a means of capturing the connections between components of the intervention and articulating the putative pathways by which they will lead to the anticipated impacts and outcomes. They should provide an overview, rather than the detail of the program. These models are often in the form of graphics or schematics and are best developed through a consultative process involving stakeholders. The logic model usually illustrate the linkages between the elements of the program such as the goal, objectives, resources (or inputs, eg staff, facilities, materials, or funds etc), activities (efforts conducted to achieve the program objectives), process measures, impacts, outcomes and ideally included external factors operating. The logic model is usually presented in an ordered and linear format. In that way, the logic model may not accurately represent the interactive and dynamic nature of most health promotion interventions, which are not usually implemented in a linear way. An alternative approach is to capture all of those same elements but also to map the 'actors', the interactions and exchanges and the flow of inputs across the program. An example is shown in figure 20.2. This more dynamic map also shows the specific links between program components and enables a deeper understanding of the flow of activities, the strength of linkages throughout, potential weak spots in the program, and the variety of levels of evaluation required (eg individual, setting, community). There is also no attempt to present a linear process.

Fig. 20.2 – Example of intervention mapping.

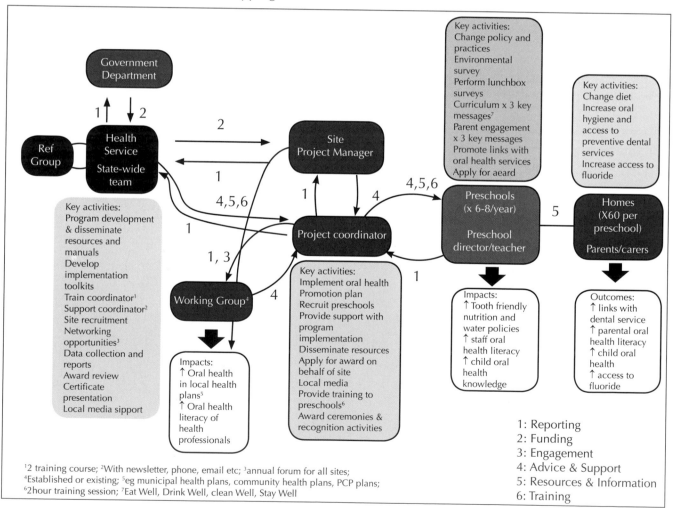

To develop a logic model or intervention map, there is a need for stakeholder engagement, consultation, and an understanding of the intended target groups, intervention components and theoretical underpinnings. The theoretical framework of the intervention may not have been previously articulated, and may require discussion to identify and reach a shared understanding of the underlying paradigms and assumptions driving the approach adopted. There is no set rule in relation to how best to develop a logic model or map, although it is common to start with identification of the outcomes of the program and work backwards. A number of resources are available to support this activity.[9]

Step 3: Plan the evaluation and gather high quality and useful evidence

The planning of the evaluation should be guided by the theoretical framework of the intervention plan and a priori, pre--determined logic models and conceptualisation of the intervention pathways - as discussed above. This guides the evaluator as to the nature of the changes that are expected to occur and the intervention pathways identified as critical to success, thus indicating what should be the focus of the evaluation. For evaluation to be meaningful, there is a need for measurement of changes in the systems involved, going beyond the measurement of individual behaviours, morbidity and mortality on which the 'success' or 'failure' of the intervention may (incorrectly or simplistically) be based.[12] With complex oral health promotion interventions, what appears to be an ineffective intervention, may reflect more on the limited nature of the evaluation and the failure of evaluators of community- or population-level interventions to go beyond reporting (or measuring) individual-level outcomes.

The development of an evaluation plan is critical to bring together all of these factors and ideally, an evaluation plan captures the following elements:

- Identification of the theoretical framework/s and logic models/pathways of the intervention
- Identification of the intervention aims, objectives and strategies
- Evaluation aims and objectives, and evaluation (or research) questions or perspective
- Type of evaluation (process, impact and/or outcome)
- Levels at which data is to be collected (eg individual, setting, organisation, community)
- Methods of data collection
- Instrument/s to be used (if applicable)
- Evaluation output (eg summary of findings, report, conference presentation, research paper, media release)

Methods for data collection

There are both qualitative and quantitative methods of gathering evaluation data.

Qualitative: There are essentially three kinds of qualitative data: Interviews, Observations and Documents.

Examples of methods commonly used to collect this data include focus groups, in--depth interviews, open-ended survey questions, document analysis (eg journals, meeting minutes, implementation diaries), and observation.[15,16]

Quantitative: Quantitative methods are those that assign a number to a concept or phenomenon. This usually involves classification (assigning an item to a category), ranking (assigning items in a rank order according to some feature eg self ratings of oral health), interval scaling (similar to ranking but quantifies the difference between items), and ratio scaling (assign numbers to items using a ratio scale eg one item is 'half' the amount of another).[16]

Examples of methods used to collect such data include questionnaires and surveys, monitoring data, population statistics, document analysis (eg action plans, policy audits). Clinical data or direct measurement can also be collected.

Choice of measurement tool

Independent of the method, the choice of measurement instrument (or tool) should be carefully considered. The choice of method/s depends on the nature of the intervention, the purpose of the evaluation and the resources available. There is also a lot of debate about what evaluation methods are most appropriate for oral health promotion and the instruments used will vary with the purpose of the evaluation, the objectives of the intervention, and the target populations (eg children, adults, marginalized populations).

Measures for oral health promotion: Most of the measures needed for the evaluation of oral health promotion are not straightforward. They include measuring behaviours, attitudes, capacity, quality of life, organisational practices and policies, in addition to clinical outcomes. There is a need for consistent and rigorous methods, and one of the major criticisms emerging from reviews of the oral health promotion literature is the inappropriate nature and poor quality of many evaluation outcome measures used.[17]

Determining the evaluation design and methods

There are a range of important considerations when developing the evaluation methods, which include:

Stage of research and evaluation design - Interventions may go through different stages of research such as feasibility testing and piloting before a larger scale trial to test effectiveness.[18] The evaluation of an intervention undergoing feasibility testing will focus on process measures; whereas evaluating a pilot study will focus on process as well as impact measures. An evaluation of an effectiveness trial that has been through a previous pilot will be able to focus largely on impact and outcome measures.

There are various methods to assess effectiveness. Each has strengths and weaknesses, generating findings with differing degrees of reliability, applicability and transferability. Experimental designs, particularly randomised controlled trials, are considered the gold standard in many areas of health to establish effectiveness. In the evaluation of complex population health and health promotion interventions, the challenges involved with the context, the population groups, the politics and the way of working up sustainable enhancing interventions sometimes render controlled trials impossible, extremely costly, and sometimes inappropriate (see Table 20.1). However, many are demanding an increase in the frequency and rigour of evaluations of health promotion, population health and development programs.[5,19,20] Alternative experimental designs include non-randomised controlled trials, controlled before and after trials, quasi-experimental studies, interrupted time series studies, and pre- and post-studies.

While there may be challenges associated with the application of some study designs to complex health promotion programs, rigorous research is needed to make arguments for the value of oral health promotion.[6] Judgements of rigour (or trustworthiness) may focus on assessing the internal validity (i.e. the risk of bias) and external validity (i.e. the generalisability of the results to a population of interest). The advent of complex interventions, often delivered in 'real-world' scenarios has strengthened the relevance of the available evidence-base. The assessment of either form of validity requires the development of skills and associated assessment tools,[21] which can be a challenge for the oral health promotion workforce.

Feasibility and affordability – Development of the evaluation plan is inevitably influenced by practicality, feasibility, cost, scale, and the level of accuracy and precision required. It may be more useful to evaluate one aspect of the intervention or one element of the evaluation well rather than to try to undertake a comprehensive evaluation without the necessary resources, skills or time.

To inform the decision of which instruments to use, it is important to understand the construct you are trying to measure, as well as how the instrument was developed and validated. The most commonly used instrument may not be most appropriate or best performing, and careful consideration of the factors listed above is recommended. Similarly, evaluators should resist the temptation to develop a new instrument or change an existing, well validated instrumented unless it is essential. Consultation with experts is recommended if at all possible, and the role of monitoring and surveillance data should also be considered. Although not covered here, the approval by bodies which govern the ethical conduct of research and evaluation activities will be required.

Step 4: Report and disseminate the findings

The key consideration in the development of the evaluation report and the dissemination of the evaluation results is identification of the primary stakeholder perspective and key audiences and uses for the findings. The stakeholders will certainly include those who implement the oral health intervention or program, those who fund it, and those who receive it. There are also likely to be a range of other stakeholders with an interest in learning about the results such as clinical colleagues, health service managers, politicians and government agencies, researchers and the media.[16] Consideration of audiences in the early planning stages of the evaluation will help to inform decision making about what data may be useful to collect and analyse in the evaluation.

For example, you may have an interest in using the evaluation findings to increase knowledge and understanding in particular sectors such as government to influence policy, service delivery or funding decisions; or the findings may be used for an academic audience and to contribute to the evidence base. Understanding the intended applications of the findings will also help to inform the development of the evaluation design to ensure that it achieves a sufficiently high level of rigour and scientific quality.

A dissemination plan can help to ensure that the findings are circulated as efficiently and effectively as possible. The same set of findings can be prepared in different formats to suit the information needs and knowledge base of the audience. For example, a detailed evaluation report can also generate a research paper, an executive summary, a conference presentation, and a media release. These different products can then be distributed through the standard academic, professional and community networks as well as via stakeholder networks such as organisational newsletters and email distribution lists.

What does it take to do an evaluation?

Box 20.2 provides an outline of what is needed for an 'ideal' evaluation of a large scale oral health promotion program or intervention. Often not all of these elements are in place, particularly in relation to the available funding, but a realistic view of what it costs for quality evaluation needs to be developed. It is a common error for evaluation planning to begin after the intervention has started or even finished. As most evaluation study designs require baseline data collection, a delayed evaluation makes it very difficult to accurately evaluate the program. Evaluation budgets are also often under-funded due to a common misconception that an evaluation costs approximately 10% of the intervention budget. It is not possible to do a well-conducted, comprehensive evaluation for this amount.

We would suggest that 25-50% of the intervention budget is required to produce meaningful results, and more may be needed for large, complex studies.

Box 20.2 also includes an outline of some of the key skills for an evaluator or evaluation team for evaluating oral health promotion initiatives. Although not all professionals undertaking evaluation will have all of these skills, an evaluation team should have a mix of these skills. Further, early identification of where skills are lacking can be useful to identify the need to recruit additional members to the evaluation team, and also to guide professional development activities to enhance existing skills that exist but are perhaps not fully developed, or to develop skills that are not present. In addition, there is a need for ongoing support of the evaluators by an evaluation advisory group with strong stakeholder engagement.

Box 20.2 – Outline of what is needed for an ideal evaluation of a large scale oral health promotion program or intervention and outline of skills some of the key skills for evaluating oral health promotion initiatives.

The ideal evaluation of large scale, long term health promotion intervention
- 25-50% of total project budget
- Mixed Methods (Qualitative and Quantitative data collected) and data collected across multiple levels
- Process, impact and outcome evaluation conducted and reported
- Process data also includes costs and timeframes, sustainability and equity also captured
- A clearly defined purpose and evaluation perspective
- Guided by concepts of usefulness, integration, feasibility, flexibility, fairness, and accuracy
- Done expertly and independently but not necessarily separately – stakeholder input on preliminary findings can provide invaluable insights without compromising the integrity of the evaluation
- Disseminated strategically and widely
- Aims to improve that being evaluated

Essential evaluation skills for oral health promotion:
- Knowledge of health promotion principles
- An understanding of evaluation principles and data collection methods
- Ability to engage with a variety of stakeholders
- Strong negotiation skills and an ability to develop an understanding of the stakeholder context, perspective and competing priorities
- Project management and organization skills
- Communication and conflict resolution skills
- Knowledge of the determinants of dental diseases and poor oral health

Summary

In summary, evaluation of oral health promotion interventions is critical to answer the important questions of what works for whom, under what circumstances and at what cost? Strong evaluations with findings that are disseminated widely are needed to ensure that effective interventions can be delivered to all who would benefit, and to reduce the implementation of ineffective activities. We have attempted to assist practitioners in their evaluations by providing a practical guide, and we urge the consideration of some level of evaluation alongside the implementation of all new policies, strategies or programs.

REFERENCES

1. World Health Organisation. Ottawa charter for health promotion. Geneva: WHO. 1986.
2. Lincoln P, Nutbeam, D. Philosophy and theory of health promotion. In: Davies M, Macdowall, W., ed. Health promotion theory. New York: Open University Press. 2006.
3. Nutbeam D. Evaluating health promotion - progress, problems and solutions. Health Promot Int. 1998 March 1, 1998; 13(1):27-44.
4. Watt RG, Harnett R, Daly B, Fuller SS, Kay E, Morgan A, et al. Evaluating oral health promotion: need for quality outcome measures doi:10.1111/j.1600-0528.2006.00257.x. Community Dentistry and Oral Epidemiology. 2006; 34(1):11-7.
5. Rosen L, Manor O, Engelhard D, Zucker D. In Defense of the Randomized Controlled Trial for Health Promotion Research. Am J Public Health. 2006 May 30, 2006: AJPH.2004.061713.
6. Macintyre S, Petticrew M. Good intentions and received wisdom are not enough. Journal of Epidemiology and Community Health. 2000; 54(11):802-3.
7. Steckler A, Linnan L, eds. Process evaluation for public health interventions and research. US: Jossey-Bass. 2002.
8. Glasgow RE, Vogt TM, Boles SM. Evaluating the public health impact of health promotion interventions: the RE-AIM framework. Am J Public Health. 1999 Sep; 89(9):1322-7.

9. Centres for Disease Control. Program Evaluation. Office of the Associate Director for Program [cited 2011; Available from: www.cdc.gov/eval/framework/index.htm
10. Atienza AA, King AC. Community-based Health Intervention Trials: An Overview of Methodological Issues. Epidemiologic Reviews. 2002 July 1, 2002; 24(1):72-9.
11. Bisset S, Potvin L. Expanding our conceptualization of program implementation: lessons from the genealogy of a school-based nutrition program. Health Education Research. 2007 October 1, 2007; 22(5):737-46.
12. Potvin L, Gendron S, Bilodeau A, Chabot P. Integrating Social Theory Into Public Health Practice. Am J Public Health. 2005 April 1, 2005; 95(4):591-5.
13. Hawe P, Shiell A, Riley T. Theorising Interventions as Events in Systems. American Journal of Community Psychology. 2009; 43(3):267-76.
14. Shiell A, Hawe P, Gold L. Complex interventions or complex systems? Implications for health economic evaluation. BMJ. 2008 June 7, 2008; 336(7656):1281-3.
15. Patton Micheal Quinn. Qualitative research & evaluation methods. 3rd ed: Sage Publications Inc. 2002.
16. Ovretveit J. Evaluating health interventions: Open University Press. 1998.
17. Petersen PE, Kwan S. Evaluation of community-based oral health promotion and oral disease prevention-WHO recommendations for improved evidence in pu-

blic health practice. Community dental health. 2004 Dec; 21(4 Suppl):319-29.

18. Moore L, Gibbs, L. Considerations in the design of community-based program evaluations: purpose, resources, complexity, stage. In: Waters E SB, Uauy R, Seidell J, ed. Preventing childhood obesity: Evidence, policy and practice: Wiley Blackwell. 2010; 155-66.

19. Hawe P, Shiell A. Use evidence to expose the unequal distribution of problems and the unequal distribution of solutions. The European Journal of Public Health. 2007 October 1, 2007; 17(5):413.

20. Victora CG, Habicht J-P, Bryce J. Evidence-Based Public Health: Moving Beyond Randomized Trials. Am J Public Health. 2004 March 1, 2004; 94(3):400-5.

21. Green LW, Glasgow RE. Evaluating the Relevance, Generalization, and Applicability of Research. Evaluation & the Health Professions. 2006 March 1, 2006; 29(1):126-53.

Chapter 21

Oral Health Research to Promote the Oral Health of Children

Aubrey Sheiham
John Spencer

Introduction

Most dental research funding worldwide is spent on developing new methods of prevention, new treatments and dental materials, and on individual health education efforts to increase individual knowledge and awareness. Such research benefits a relatively small section of the world population - 'the 10/90 gap' where only 10% of research funds are spent on 90% of health problems.[1-3] Whilst significant contributions have been made to improve oral health using fluorides, very little effective theory-based research has been conducted on oral health promotion and virtually none on an integrated common risk factor approach and on tackling social determinants of oral diseases in children.

Dentistry is largely dominated by a treatment philosophy derived from the medical model. When prevention has been implemented, it is mainly an individualized high-risk approach to prevent dental disease solely through a clinical and behavioral approach.[4] Consequently, a shortcoming of dental research is that it is frequently on beha-vioural mediators with an undue focus on individuals, individual psychology and high-risk strategies despite evidence from systematic reviews of the literature on oral disease prevention that such an approach is ineffective in achieving sustained improvements in oral health outcomes, or at tackling oral health inequalities (See Chapter 3).

There is something intrinsically flawed with an approach, such as the dominant one used in dentistry, that calls for regular annual check-ups, treatment and re-education from infancy to old age. Although evidence-based clinical care can reduce suffering, disability and prolong life or increase retention of a natural dentition for life, the aggregate impact of these interventions is limited by lack of access, erratic or unpredictable adherence, and imperfect effectiveness. Not only does such an approach lead to unjustified policies to concentrate on improving access to dental services to improve oral health at considerable cost in developed countries, but this ineffective approach is adopted by developing countries where its high cost makes even surgical treatment to alleviate oral pain unavailable to the vast majority of people. Research on public health approaches to promoting oral health in children are urgently needed. Such approaches must be based upon contemporary public health evidence and underpinned by a sound theoretical framework.[4] Therefore, WHO and the IADR and many countries are responding by developing public oral health policies and expanding their oral health research agendas to include research on oral health promotion.[5] Moreover there are international discussions on the social determinants of health following on the WHO Commission on the Social Determinants of Health[6] report and a growing recognition that despite the considerable amount of money spent on biological and clinical research, relatively little attention has been paid to ensuring that the findings of research are implemented to prevent the major noncommunicable diseases, including oral diseases.[7,8]

Re-orienting research on oral health

The WHO Commission on the Social Determinants of Health6 highlighted the need to address the underlying causes of population disease, because the research evidence highlights the overriding importance of macro-level factors such as political, environmental, social, and community factors in determining population health, the so-called upstream factors.[9,10] Unfortunately, oral health professionals trained in an education system dominated by the medical model fail to understand the importance of these underlying determinants of health, and, as a consequence, have focused their preventive efforts and research at an individual level. Yet, sustained improvements in health and reductions in

inequalities will be secured only through health promotion strategies that tackle the causes of the causes of diseases.

As outlined in this book, the principal shortcoming of oral health approaches to prevention and to reducing inequalities in oral health is the failure of dental researchers and policy makers to collaborate with groups involved in doing research and implementing policies on the determinants of health that are common to most diseases, namely, the Common Risk Factor Approach to preventing noncommunicable disease. Moereover, there are links between oral and general health and an increasing belief of the importance of oral health within the larger framework of general health programs.[11] Petersen[12] pointed out that one of the objectives of the WHO Global Oral Health Programme is to place greater emphasis on developing global policies based on common risk factor approaches and which are coordinated more effectively with other programmes in public health because a core group of modifiable proximal causes of oral disease are common to the major chronic diseases.[13] That is the basis for the Common Risk Factor Approach. The distal causes of oral diseases and the major chronic diseases are socio-environmental factors. Therefore the highest priority is for integrated research on strategies that address both oral disease prevention and the promotion of oral health integrated with chronic disease prevention and general health promotion using the Common Risk Factor Approach within a social determinants framework as the distal and proximal risks to health are linked.

This view is also recommended by the WHO. The WHO considers that more research should be devoted to "Modifiable common risk factors to oral health and chronic disease, particularly the role of diet, nutrition and tobacco."[12] WHO, at the Sixtieth World Health Assembly,[14] also urged that Member States should "… adopt measures to ensure that oral health is incorporated as appropriate into policies for the integrated prevention and treatment of chronic noncommunicable and communicable diseases, and into maternal and child health policies; to take measures to ensure that evidence-based approaches are used to incorporate oral health into national policies as appropriate for integrated prevention and control of noncommunicable diseases; …".[12]

The shortfall of oral health research on social determinants and risk factors common to a number of diseases needs to be remedied. Little research is directed at the determinants of health compromising proximal behaviours, and most importantly, underlying distal social and environmental conditions making healthy choices easier and unhealthy ones more unacceptable. Such research is important as "this link between social conditions and health is not a footnote to the 'real' concerns with health – health care and unhealthy behaviours – it should become the main focus."[15] Unfortunately, when behaviours are investigated by dental researchers the research questions asked are mainly about problems of compliance; how to attract high-risk individuals to dental surgeries because the preventive measures they apply require regular reinforcement and lifelong attention and monitoring by dental professionals.

Dental researchers should be aware of the conclusions of the WHO Assembly that "We know what works, we know what it costs and we know that all countries are at risk. We have an Action Plan to avert millions of premature deaths and help promote a better quality of life for millions more." "Much is known about the prevention of noncommunicable diseases. Experience clearly shows that they are to a great extent preventable through interventions against the major risk factors and their environmental, economic, social and behavioural determinants in the population. Countries can reverse the advance of these diseases if appropriate action is taken."[16] This gap between what is known by epidemiologists and policy makers involved in other noncommunicable diseases and not implemented by dental policy makers is repeatedly emphasized by the WHO. Petersen[12] and Petersen and Kwan8 of the WHO say: "The major challenges of the future will be to translate knowledge and experiences of disease prevention and health promotion into action programmes." "Global health urgently needs to apply the body of evidence based policies, strategies and approaches of health promotion developed over the past twenty years. Two global health promotion charters (Ottawa and Bangkok), conference declarations and WHO Regional Committees and World Health Assembly (WHA) resolutions endorse the importance of health promotion; yet the evidence for their implementation in countries is lacking."[8] We should consider the words of Radford.[17] Radford said "The greatest deficiency of twentieth century medicine is not the lack of resources to develop new high cost technology. It is the failure to distribute the simple, effective methodologies of prevention and cure that are based on an appropriate cultural template, together with the failure to concentrate on health promotion activities as part of the general development plan." That also applies to dentistry.

The causes of the causes captured in social determinants of health are demonstrated in comparisons between countries and over time. Such comparisons highlight that the more distal social context shapes and maintains a population distribution of the proximal risk and protective exposures. In comparing countries in the early part of the 20th Century, Barmes[18,19] described the dramatic increase in caries in children in developed countries many decades ahead of developing countries. These cross-country variations emerged with the changes in the social context in those countries which shape their dietary pattern, particularly the increased availability of refined sugars. The emergence of high caries experience countries within the developed nations is further evidence of the upstream social determinants. Cross-country comparisons can reveal much about the causes of the causes of dentally-sicker populations.[20]

The second half of the 20th Century saw a remarkable change in oral health in nearly all developed countries.[21] Dramatic declines in dental caries to the end of the 20th Century demonstrate that marked improvements in dental caries status can be achieved within a generation. Caries experience in 12 year olds has declined from a DMFT of about 6 to a DMFT of 1 in 25 years. A remarkable improvement in a relatively short period. No other chronic disease has declined so rapidly and throughout large national populations.

The improvement has been credited to the introduction of fluoridated toothpaste in all of these developed countries and to the implementation of either water or salt fluoridation in many, albeit with sometimes restricted population coverage.[22] While fluoridation may not have been so widely available, there is evidence that it had a substantial effect.[23] The population level promotion of tooth brushing as a personal hygiene measure with sensory and social reward has seen oral cleanliness improve and fluoride being provided to the oral cavity regularly. As dentistry and the numbers of dentists also rapidly developed across this same period it has been easy to mistakenly attribute the remarkable improvement in child caries experience to the delivery of dental services by organized dentistry. Two more recent events emphasize the lack of strong connection between dental services and child caries experience. First, while the delivery of dental services has continued to increase in many developed countries in the first decade of the 21st Century child caries experience has begun to increase.[24-26] The increase is inadequately researched, but it is hypothesized that it is due to population wide changes in diet pattern (for instance changes also associated with the obesity epidemic) and to a reduction in exposure to fluoride in water through the decreased consumption of reticulated tap water and/or reduced frequency of tooth brushing. The second event is the increase in child caries experience in developing countries at the same time as there has been rapid growth in the numbers in the dental profession. This is dramatically illustrated in India and China.

A further illustration of the influence of social context in shaping the population distribution of proximal risk and protective factors for child caries is the finding that the social gradient of child caries varies from positive, through neutral, to negative in countries at different stages of development. Caries varies from a disease of affluence in many still less-developed countries to a disease of deprivation in many highly developed countries.[27] The importance of contextual factors in shaping disease experience is frequently acknowledged in health, especially for communicable diseases, but it has received less attention in oral disease.

A rigorous research program on the determinants of the major decline in caries and periodontal disease across countries would provide information that can be applied to sustaining the improvements, extending them into other countries and reducing inequalities in oral health. It will also point to the greater importance of health and oral health promotion; a subject with a low priority in dental research. There are very few reports on the effectiveness of community-wide preventive strategies, apart from those on water fluoridation.

The vast bulk of research on caries and periodontal disease is conducted around associations and their statistical significance. There is a need to add an interpretive step between measures of strength of association and the statements on the implications of the research. This interpretive step involves the calculation of population impact measures.[28] Such measures combine information on the exposure in a population to a risk or protective factor, the strength of association of the factor with the presence of disease and the population distribution of disease. The resulting measures like Population Attributable Risk or Fraction are useful in setting priorities on what factors, and their causes, should be the focus of attention to improve health.[29,30] The principle that such measures illustrate is that a relatively weak 'risk' factor (in terms of strength of association) that is quite prevalent could account for a greater fraction of the total disease in a population than a stronger risk factor that is less frequently present. Conversely, a protective exposure that has a relatively weak association with disease prevention but is highly prevalent may account for a substantial gain in health. This provides emphasis to population-level interventions pursuing the preventive paradox first described by Rose.[31]

The dramatic reductions in the major oral disease, caries, and a sustained decrease in the second most important disease, periodontal disease, and a remarkable increase in the percentages of adults retaining their natural teeth for their lifetime has come about as a result of either exploiting population-wide behaviours such as through fluoridation or changes in behaviours in populations together with an alteration in manufacturing practices and the addition of fluoride to toothpaste. The common dental view, that modern dentistry can take much of the credit by having identified the causes and methods of prevention, is a misinterpretation. Dental services explained 3% of the variation in changes in 12-year-old caries levels in the 1970s and early 1980s whereas broad socioeconomic factors explained 65%.[32] The implication of these findings is that major improvements in the prevention of disease tend to follow social changes - alterations in dietary patterns and breastfeeding, smoking, oral cleanliness, contraception and in the availability of key resources such as fluoridated toothpaste. There is no reason why a similar approach should not prove equally successful in the future. The improvements in oral health demonstrate that the means for effectively controlling caries are known and sometimes widely used by populations. Declines in periodontal disease are most probably due to declines in smoking and availability of anti-calculus toothpastes.[33,34]

Despite the large decline in caries in many developed countries, relatively little has changed in priorities for dental research. Indeed, now more resources than previously are allocated to research on new risk factors and categorization of individuals according to personal disease risk. McMichael[35] puts risk factor epidemiology in perspective when he suggests that "Modern epidemiology is thus oriented to explaining and quantifying the bobbing of corks on the surface waters, while largely disregarding the stronger undercurrents that determine where, on average the cluster of corks ends up along the shoreline of risk." The limitations associated with individual level risk factor intervention approaches are that they divert limited resources away from upstream healthy public policies instead of a social policy approach to healthy lifestyles.[36]

The gap between what is being widely discussed and implemented by other health disciplines and the WHO and the dental fraternity needs to be addressed. The dental care systems worldwide lack a coherent framework for addressing the remarkable decline in dental caries experienced by many in developed countries through non--clinical approaches and their reliance on expensive unnecessary clinical approaches. Research on what changes are needed to clinical guidelines and workforce planning models to treat and carry out prevention on cohorts with low levels of oral disease is an imperative. Another research question is what is the cost-effectiveness of current preventive measures when applied to low disease populations? Indeed, Hausen et al.[37] has stated that it is doubtful whether further reductions in caries can be achieved using current chairside caries preventive measures

on populations with DMFT of one at 12 years of age.

No other health discipline has such detailed scientific knowledge, as dentistry has, on the causes of the diseases they are concerned about. The causes of dental caries and periodontal disease are very well established. They are diet and dirt (plaque). The additional element is the body's defense, influenced by the psychological distress and resilience. Moreover, there are countless clinical trial studies on how to prevent the two major oral diseases. The fundamental gap in knowledge and understanding in dentistry is how to translate the findings on prevention into sustainable effective programs for groups and populations. The reasons for the gap are the widespread conceptual gulf among dental researchers and policy makers regarding fundamental research and implementing findings in populations.

The limitations of most current approaches to improve oral health and reduce inequities in oral health is cogently summed up by Kwan and Petersen.[38] They concluded that "Measures that focus on downstream factors only, such as lifestyle and behavioural influences, may have limited success in reducing oral health inequities. These victim--blaming approaches assume that knowledge and skills automatically lead to behavioural change. Such approaches may be counterproductive; they are often ineffective and costly and fail to address the wider social determinants that cause people to get ill in the first place. People in more privileged social positions tend to benefit from the interventions more than those in disadvantaged groups. Hence, inappropriate interventions can widen inequities. It is necessary to address the root causes, tackling social determinants and the environment. Approaches that take into account the principles of the common risk factor approach, which promotes coordinated work across a range of disciplines, and the Ottawa Charter for Health Promotion, may be promising." This promise will only be fulfilled if the Common Risk Factor Approach is interpreted and acted upon at a population level and not at an individual level where the emphasis is on individual behavior modification.[39] There is a need to understand the population distribution of common risks and for integrated strategies to be pursued that act on the causes and shift the distribution of common risks in the population.

Research on Reducing Inequalities in Health

Health and oral health are socially patterned.[40] Health and oral health is unequally distributed by social circumstance, with poorer health being more frequent among those with less advantaged social circumstances. However, the key feature is a gradient not a threshold relationship between health and social circumstance. The key features of a social gradient in health are captured in the observation that there is no threshold in socioeconomic circumstance above which the risk of disease is negligible and only a minority of those in the most disadvantageous socioeconomic circumstance are likely to have a disease.[41] "The evidence on the links between people's socioeconomic circumstances and their health has generated two kinds of policy responses. The first focuses on those in the poorest circumstances and the poorest health: those with most risk factors. In policy and intervention terms, this leads to approaches that attempt to lift the worst off out of their extreme situation. If effective, such interventions help only a relatively small part of the population. The second approach recognizes that, while those in the poorest circumstances are in the poorest health, this is part of a broader social gradient in health. This means that it is not only the poorest groups and communities who have poorer health than those in the most advantaged circumstances. In addition, there are large numbers of people who, while they could not be described as socially excluded, are relatively disadvantaged in health terms. Preventive and other interventions could produce major improvements in their health and proportionate savings for the healthcare system."[42]

A social determinants approach would give the highest priority to altering the slope of the gradient and to closing the gaps between people at different steps along the social gradient ladder. It is unlikely to be able to eliminate the social gradient in health completely, but it is possible to have a shallower social gradient in health and well-being than is currently the case in most countries. Strategies need to vary in scale and intensity that is proportionate to the level of disadvantage. "To reduce the steepness of the social gradient in health, actions must be universal, but with a scale and intensity that is proportionate to the level of disadvantage. We call this proportionate universalism."[43] That implies that groups of people who are worse off should be brought up to those who are better off.[44] "Greater intensity of action is likely to be needed for those with greater social and economic disadvantage, but focusing solely on the most disadvantaged will not reduce the health gradient, and will only tackle a small part of the problem."[43]

"Most interventions (both at the individual and community levels) remain focused on "downstream" tertiary treatments or one-on-one interventions. These efforts have their origins in the biomedical paradigm and risk factor epidemiology and the behavioral science research methods that serve as their handmaidens."[36] That prevailing paradigm is being challenged. Dental researchers need to move beyond these "downstream" efforts towards research on a more appropriate whole population public health approach to health policy.[31]

The WHO CSDH framework indicated that there are four points of entry for action to reduce health inequities: structural inequities; differential exposure to health threats; differential vulnerabilities and differential consequences of illness.[6] They are outlined in detail in the WHO report on "Equity, social determinants and public health programmes."[45] Although there is research on inequalities in health and numerous studies on interventions to reduce inequalities, few have been successful. Therefore it would be unrealistic to expect that a social determinants approach to reduce inequalities in oral health would be effective unless it is linked to a strategy to reduce inequalities in general health. It will be important to consider a mix of strategies combining both upstream (distal) and downstream (proximal) interventions. Therefore a population, rather than a high risk strategy focusing on disadvantaged groups, should be adopted.[31,46] As the most common noncommunicable diseases such as obesity, chronic heart disease, cancers and dental caries and periodontal disease have major risk factors in common, the main strategy, and the one that requires considerably more dental research, is how to reduce the intake of sugars and increase fruit and vegetables consumption and reduce smoking. That will require a shift in the emphasis of dental research to population-level health promotion research to investigate methods of increasing the likelihood of health enhancing decisions being the easy or default decisions.[47]

Inadequate access to essential evidence-based health services is one of the social determinants of health. While the attenuation of the social gradient in health and oral health attributable to health services may not be as great as clinicians expect, it is posited that 20-30% of the gradient can be reduced by good access to health services. Variation in access to health services is inequality. If a value judgement is made that the variation is unfair or unjust, for instance in relation to needs, then access may be inequitable. The concept of inequality and inequity in access to health services is captured by the Inverse Care Law,[48] which states that, "The availability of good medical care tends to vary inversely with the need for it in the population served." Therefore the role of the health system becomes particularly relevant through the issue of access and good quality care being equitably accessible. The health system can directly address differences in exposure and vulnerability not only by improving equitable access to care, but also in the promotion of intersectoral action to improve health status. The health system is capable of ensuring that health problems do not lead to a further deterioration of people's social status and should facilitate sick people's social reintegration. The health system has three obligations in confronting inequity:

- to ensure that resources are distributed between areas in proportion to their relative needs;

- to respond appropriately to the health care needs of different social groups;
- to take the lead in encouraging a wider and more strategic approach to developing healthy public policies at both the national and local level, to promote equity in health and social justice.[49]

The implications of the reports such as the WHO Commission on Social Determinants of Health and inequality for research on oral health, are profound.[16,49] Therefore, in the light of the WHO CSDH's report, there is an ethical human rights imperative for dental researchers and oral health planners to study and adopt and study and use a social determinants approach to reduce inequalities in oral health.

Inequalities in oral health mirror those in general health.[4] The social gradient is consistently found for most common diseases, as well as oral diseases.[38,50-52] "If social gradients in general and oral health are universal, then the determinants of the gradient need to be addressed."[4] There is abundant evidence demonstrating the underlying influence of psychosocial, economic, environmental and political determinants of health inequalities. There is a need for dental researchers to embed their research and policies with those working on the social determinants of health inequalities.

It is increasingly recognized that the dominant individualistic oral health preventive model alone will not be effective in achieving sustainable oral health improvements across the population, nor in reducing oral health inequalities. That model focuses on individual risk factors to address health inequalities and has major limitations.[4] Yet it is the dominant approach used in oral disease prevention. The limitations of the individual 'lifestyle' approach have been extensively reviewed. The reviews conclude that:

- the lifestyle approach is ineffective and costly;
- 'lifestyle' interventions fail to acknowledge and address the underlying social determinants of health inequalities and are 'victim-blaming' in nature;
- many oral health education interventions lack a sound theoretical basis;
- the 'lifestyle' approach diverts limited resources away from upstream factors.[4]

A paradigm shift is needed to one which addresses the underlying social determinants of oral health through a combination of complementary public health strategies.[4] A range of issues need to be addressed before significant progress is likely in reorienting dental public health research, practice and policy towards a social determinants model. Among them are barriers such as the "lifestyle drift – the tendency for policy to start off recognizing the need for action on upstream social determinants of health inequalities only to drift downstream to focus largely on individual lifestyle factors."[53] This emphasis on lifestyle factors distracts attention away from the determinants of the behaviours – the upstream causes of the causes. Therefore strategies should resist individualized victim-blaming lifestyle drift. Effective action to tackle oral health inequalities can only be developed when the underlying causes of the problem are identified and understood.[12] Public health research into the social determinants of health inequalities has identified causal pathways linking the biological, psychosocial, behavioural, environmental and political factors to health and disease outcomes. Building up suitable capacity among the dental public health workforce so that it is trained in a social determinants and population strategy framework is therefore a key priority.[12,54,55] A need also exists for better co-ordination of research efforts, both within and between countries.

Despite the declines in caries in many developed countries, in some communities there are sections of the population who have relatively high caries rates. The higher level of caries in vulnerable groups suggests that they may be exposed to multiple risks and are likely to have other health problems. Research on prevention should therefore be re-oriented to a broad community perspective which tackles the causes; the determinants of diseases, and makes healthy choices easier and unhealthy choices more difficult for most people. Reducing caries in the high caries group is linked to reducing the rates in the majority of the child population at low risk. Why? Because the distribution of caries is a continuum; one cannot separate the high caries tail of the frequency distribution from the body of the populations' distribution. However, those in the high disease tail of the frequency distribution are found more frequently in low socioeconomic positions or immigrant and refugee groups. These vulnerable groups may be exposed to numerous adverse social and economic conditions.[56-58]

It unreasonable to expect that people will change their behaviours when so many forces in the social, cultural and physical environment work against change. On the other hand, if the social determinants of health are changed for the better then there will be dramatic improvements in health equity between and within countries. To change people's behaviours requires a change in their environment. So, strategies to prevent disease should pay attention not only to the behaviour of individuals, but also to the environmental context within which people live.[59] Therefore, when deciding on priorities for prevention, the health pyramid suggested by Frieden[47] should be used to decide on priorities for action and research. Efforts to address socioeconomic determinants are given the highest priority followed by public health community-wide enabling measures that change the context for health by making healthy choices the easier default decisions. Protective interventions with long-term benefits have higher priority than clinic-based prevention because an environ¬ment-based strategy offers greater scope for improvements in oral health than a strong commitment to individual dental care. In dental practice, however, even the best programs at the pyramid's higher levels achieve limited public health impact, largely because of their dependence on long-term individual's behavior change.[47] Therefore emphasis should be given to research on policies that make healthy choices the easier choices and health compromising choices more difficult and socially unacceptable.[60]

Translational, transformational and transdisciplinary research for reducing inequalities in oral health

Commitment to knowledge translation represents a major opportunity for reduction of health inequalities. Knowledge translation is defined as: "the synthesis, exchange and application of knowledge by relevant stakeholders to accelerate the benefits of global and local innovation in strengthening health systems and improving people's health".[61] Knowledge translation and exchange can influence health inequalities through one or more policy entry points as defined by Diderichsen, Evans, and Whitehead:[62]

- reducing social stratification;
- reducing differential exposure;
- reducing differential susceptibility/ vulnerability;
- reducing differential consequences by enhancing quality, accessibility, affordability, and availability of health care.

"Differential exposure refers to the evidence that disadvantaged populations are exposed to greater health risks. Differential vulnerability implies that exposure to the same health risks may result in greater health damage in disadvantaged populations due to interacting factors. For example, lower education may result in less resilient psychosocial status which could increase vulnerability to health risks such as smoking and commercial sex work."[63] Programmes to reduce vulnerability could focus on improving psychosocial strategies along the life course. Differential consequences of ill health on social and economic circumstances can be mitigated by policies to reduce the out-of-pocket expenses for health care.[63]

A new paradigm recommended by the National Center on Minority Health and Health Disparities is that there should be a shift to integration of translational, transformational and transdisciplinary research.[64] "The term translational research is defined to mean translation of knowledge or science from the molecular or biological level

to practical use, including clinical practice and applied technology. Health disparities researchers have appropriately adopted the phrase "from bench to bedside to curbside" to include the important aspect of outreach and dissemination research. Translational health disparities research is bidirectional and cyclical, not linear; it occurs along a continuum from discovery to development to delivery and back to development and discovery and involves the following domains:

- basic science discovery;
- testing and applications in developmental stages;
- outreach and dissemination of findings; and
- adoption and implementation.

"Transformative or transformational research is a term that has been used by the National Science Foundation and defined as: Research driven by ideas that have the potential to radically change our understanding of an important existing scientific or engineering concept or leading to the creation of a new paradigm or field of science or engineering. Such research is also characterized by its challenge to current understanding or its pathway to new frontiers. … Transdisciplinary health disparities research is the application of an integrative approach to addressing and solving health disparities".[64]

Dental and oral health research and approaches to improve oral health are out of step with current priorities for research on the determinants of health and reducing inequalities in health. Most dental and oral health research and approaches to improve oral health is on individual risk factors and linking oral health with general health. If the logic of linking oral health with general health is to be addressed, then studying the determinants of the causes - causes of causes – of oral and dental diseases would have a higher priority than it does at present.

How to decide on health research priorities

There is a growing need for a sound and informed process to make decisions on health research priorities in general and for research on oral health promotion in particular, both globally and at regional, national, and local community levels, and at single health facilities. The current approach to research priority setting is a closed circle set to increasingly favour basic and clinical research and risks generating ever-increasing inequity. It is driven by criteria such as interests of different advocacy groups, media exposure, interests of donors, individual biases of the members of policy-making panels,

novelty of proposed research and potential for publication in high-impact journals. The application of such criteria to what research should be done results in gross under achievement of improvements in health and may increase inequalities in health. We should keep in mind that health research is the generation of new knowledge, using scientific methods, to identify and deal with health problems.[2]

A major underlying problem in research priority setting is lack of clear criteria and principles that would guide oral health research investments based on a vision of what should be the endpoints of such investments. Therefore one important objective of a research community is to agree that the ultimate endpoint of any oral health research should be reduction of disease burden and improvement of health. Then some of the criteria needed for prioritization of investments should include:

1) Usefulness of the proposed research in terms of its potential to lead to development of new or improved oral health interventions;
2) True effectiveness of those interventions;
3) Their deliverability, affordability, and sustainability in the context of interest; and
4) Their maximum potential to reduce persisting disease burden in an equitable way.

The Child Health and Nutrition Research Initiative (CHNRI) and the Commission on Health Research for Development identified four components, as "essential health research":[2]

1. Assessment of existing and averted disease burden - achieved through epidemiological research. Analysis of the burden of illnesses and their determinants to identify and set priorities among health problems;
2. Further reduction of disease burden - research to guide and accelerate the implementation of research findings to tackle key health problems;
3. Research to improve existing interventions. The development of new tools and methodologies to measure and promote equity; and
4. Research for development of new health interventions. Basic research to advance understanding of disease and disease mechanisms.

"The key challenge in setting investment priorities for health research is to find the right balance of investments into those four different "instruments" of health research. The major advance of the CHNRI's methodology was the recognition that health research should not be limited to generating new knowledge but to implementation of strategies that would reduce the disease burden - deliverability of available interventions.

There has been a neglect of research on how to implement cost-effective interventions. The same can be said for research on oral health promotion. The gap between what is known and implemented on oral health promotion is repeatedly emphasized.[8,12,65] Petersen[12] said that "Global health urgently needs to apply the body of evidence based policies, strategies and approaches of health promotion developed over the past twenty years."

The methodology outlined by the CHNRI is a challenge to the dental research community. They should apply the priority setting approaches and identify dental research priorities that will reduce the dental illness burden. High on the list of priorities for dental research should be:

> 1.   A more detailed analysis of the social determinants of oral health burden; the causes of the causes;
> 2.   Analysis of the current approaches to reduce the disease burden;
> 3.   Research on implementation of effective oral health interventions working collaboratively with others by integrating oral health promotion with those directed at other noncommunicable diseases; and
> 4.   A rigorous scientific exploration of the determinants of the major decline in caries and periodontal disease would provide information that can be applied to reducing inequalities in oral health. It will also point to the greater importance of health and oral health promotion.

Summary

1.   Dental and oral health research and approaches to improve oral health out are out of step with current priorities for research on the determinants of health and reducing inequalities in health. Most dental and oral health research and approaches to improve oral health is on individual risk factors and linking oral health with general health.

2.   The logic of linking oral health with general health is addressed by giving high priority to studying the determinants of the causes - the causes of causes - of oral and dental diseases.

3.   There is a social gradient in health – the lower a person's social position, the worse his or her health. Action should focus on reducing the gradient in health.

4.   Reducing health inequalities is a matter of fairness and social justice.

5.   Variation in determinants between groups suggests that health inequalities may not be unavoidable.

6.   The root causes of health inequalities are to be found in the social, economic and political mechanisms that give rise to a set of hierarchically ordered socioeconomic positions within society, whereby groups are stratified according to income, education, occupation, gender, race/ethnicity and other factors.

7.   Three broad approaches to reducing health inequities can be identified, based on: (1) targeted programmes for disadvantaged populations; (2) closing health gaps between worse-off and better-off groups; (3) addressing the social health gradient across the whole population.

8. A consistent equity-based approach to the social determinants of health must ultimately lead to a gradients focus and a proportionate universalism approach. However, strategies based on tackling health disadvantage, health gaps and gradients are not mutually exclusive. They can complement and build on each other.

9. The main categories of mid- and downstream determinants of health are: material circumstances; psychosocial circumstances; behavioral and/or biological factors; and the health system itself as a social determinant.

10. Interventions and policies to reduce health inequities must not limit themselves to mid- and downstream determinants, but must include policies specifically crafted to tackle underlying structural determinants: the social mechanisms that systematically produce an inequitable distribution of the determinants of health among population groups.

11. Intersectoral policymaking and implementation are crucial. This is because structural determinants can only be tackled through strategies that reach beyond the health sector.

Recommendations for research to promote health and oral health

1. There is an urgent need for oral health research to shift emphasis from what is largely basic biomedical and clinical research to community-based determinants of health research.

2. Research is needed on strategies to close the implementation gap in prevention (primary, secondary and tertiary) and treatment by getting research findings (distilled systematically as best evidence) into both practice and policy, specifically aimed at tackling social determinants, common risk factors and social inequalities.

3. To strengthen oral health research and use evidence-based oral health promotion and disease prevention to consolidate and adapt oral health programmes, and

to encourage the intercountry exchange of reliable knowledge and experience of community oral-health programmes.

4. Research is needed to build an evidence-base at all levels for various population-based oral health interventions to improve child oral health.

5. Establish a database or registry to identify all clinical trials and other types of community-based trials to assist computer-assisted searches. Continue to facilitate and up-date systematic reviews of single and multiple intervention studies that are designed to reduce oral health inequalities. Disseminate those findings in a regular and timely manner to enhance the probability of building a systematic body of evidence.

6. Research on oral health should be incorporated as appropriate into policies for the integrated prevention and treatment of chronic noncommunicable and communicable diseases, and into maternal and child health policies.

7. The Common Risk Factor Approach (CRFA) has strengths that come from the potential synergies of numerous health groups and working with others who may be already innovative and experienced in approaches to change the population distribution to common risk factors. Thus research should look at how we might combine forces and leverage our ability to change environmental, cultural, and individual factors through joint effort.

8. Strengthen the collaborations among investigators in different countries – developed and underdeveloped - to broaden the understanding of various strategies, their applicability in operational settings, and the explanatory power in various societies and political structures. The desirability for combined approaches that create and maintain a role and commitment for all parts of the profession.

9. Intervention research should be designed to address social determinants of oral diseases/conditions. The identification of strategies to improve oral health and reduce oral health inequalities within the context of general health is

an important first step. Research on interventions needs to be accompanied by measurement of their impact on the social gradient. Attention should be addressed to changes in the distribution of health/disease as a result of interventions and recognition of the absolute as well as relative preventive benefits from an intervention in sub-groups of the population. There is however an important second step which must be added, namely what is the evidence base that these strategies are indeed effective, feasible, acceptable, affordable and sustainable in the long term.

10. Targeted research strategies for communities lower down the social gradient should be specifically designed for less developed countries and underserved community settings to support the proportionate universalism approach. The focus should be targeted on the type and mix of interventional strategies and the workforce needed to deliver them.

11. There is an urgent need for more research to test whether one approach/strategy might be better than another or whether combined strategies might be appropriate.

12. Interventional strategies, whether focused on changes in health professions education, oral health promotion, or in health systems strengthening, need to measure health outcomes as dependent variables and process-oriented activity as intermediate, qualifying variables.

13. To assess to what extent evidence-based approaches are used to incorporate oral health into national policies as appropriate for integrated prevention and control of noncommunicable diseases.

14. In strengthening of health systems, strategies to be researched should focus on policy changes to enhance prevention, provider education consistent with this objective, incentives inherent in financing mechanisms to sustain such interventions, and self-care incentives to reduce disease and promote health. Linkages between oral health and systemic health strategies also should reinforce health system effects.

15. Re-orientation of oral health services towards prevention and health promotion. High quality research on oral health systems may be instrumental to adjustment of programmes and services in both developed and developing countries.

References

1. Global Forum for Health Research. The 10/90 Report on Health Research 2000. Geneva: Global Forum for Health Research. 2000.

2. Global Forum for Health Research. The 10/90 Report on Health Research 2001-2002. Geneva: Global Forum for Health Research, 2002. http://www.globalforumhealth.org/about/1090-gap/

3. Sheiham A. Setting priorities in dental research in developing countries; reducing the "10/90" gap in research funding. The Jairam Reddy Dedication Lecture 2008. South African Dent J. 2008; 63:494-499.

4. Watt RG. From victim blaming to upstream action; tackling the social determinants of oral health inequalities. Community Dent Oral Epidemiol. 2007; 35:1-11.

5. Williams DM. Global Oral Health Inequalities: The Research Agenda. Adv Dent Res. 2011; 23:198-200.

6. World Health Organization. Closing the gap in a generation. Health equity through action on social determinants of health. Commission on Social Determinants of Health Final Report. World Health Organization. Geneva. 2008. http://www.who.int/social_determinants/thecommission/finalreport/en/index.html.

7. Bero LA, Grilli R, Grimshaw JM, Harvey E, Oxman AD, et al. Closing the gap between research and practice: an overview of systematic reviews of interventions to promote the implementation of research findings. BMJ. 1998; 317:465-468.

8. Petersen PE, Kwan S. The 7th WHO Global Conference on Health Promotion - towards integration of oral health (Nairobi, Kenya 2009). Community Dental Health. 2010; 27(Supplement 1): 129–36.

9. McKinlay JB. A case for refocussing upstream – the political economy of illness, In: AJ Enelow and JB Henderson (eds) Applying behavioural science to cardiovascular risk. Washington: American Heart Association. 1975.

10. McKinlay, JB. The promotion of health through planned sociopolitical change: challenges for research and policy. Soc Sci Med. 1993; 36:109-17.

11. Lancet. Editorial. Oral health: prevention is key. The Lancet. 2009; 373:1 (one page only) January 3, 2009.

12. Petersen PE. Global policy for improvement of oral health in the 21st century – implications to oral health research of World Health Assembly 2007, World Health Organization. Community Dent Oral Epidemiol. 2009;37:1-8.

13. Sheiham A, Watt RG. The common risk factor approach: a rational basis for promoting oral health. Community Dent Oral Epidemiol. 2000; 28:399-406.

14. World Health Organization. Oral health: action plan for promotion and integrated disease prevention. Sixtieth World Health Assembly WHA60.17 Agenda item 12.9 23 May 2007a. http://www.bfsweb.org/documents/A60_R17--en1.pdf.

15. Marmot M. Fair Society, Healthy Lives The Marmot Review Strategic review of health inequalities in England post-2010 Published by The Marmot Review February 2010. www.ucl.ac.uk/gheg/marmotreview/Documents.

16. World Health Oganization. 2008-2013 Action Plan for the Global Strategy for the Prevention and Control of Noncommunicable Diseases. World Health Assembly document A61/8 (18 April 2008) http://www.who.int/nmh/Action-plan-PC-NCD-2008.pdf.

17. Radford AJ. The inverse care law in Papua New Guinea. In: Changing disease patterns and human behaviour. Ed. NF Stanley and RA Joske, London: Academic Press. 1980; p.340.

18. Barmes DE. International perspectives for the first quarter of the twenty-first century. Swed Dent J. 1989; 13:1-6.

19. Barmes DE. International trends in oral health. J Can Dent Assoc. 1986; 25:379-81.

20. Rose G. Sick individuals and sick populations. Int J Epidemiology. 1985; 14:32-38.

21. Whelton H. Overview of the impact of changing global patterns of dental caries experience on caries clinical trials. J Dent Res. 2004; 83 (Spec Iss C):C29-34.

22. Petersen PE. Improvement of global oral health—the leadership role of the World Health Organization. Community Dent Health. 2010; 27:194-8.

23. Spencer AJ. Contribution of fluoride vehicles to changes in caries severity in Australian adolescents. Community Dent Oral Epidemiol. 1986; 14:238-41.

24. Haugerjordan O, Birkeland JM. Evidence for reversal of the caries decline among Norwegian children. Int J Paediatr Dent. 2002; 12:306-15.

25. Armfield JM, Spencer AJ. Quarter of a century of change: caries experience in Australian children, 1977-2002. Aust Dent J. 2008; 53:151-9.

26. Dye BA, Tan S, Smith V, Lewis BG, Barker LK et al. Trends in oral health status: United States, 1988-1994 and 1999-2002. Vital Health Stat. 2007; 11(248):1-92.

27. Do LG. Distribution of caries in children: variations between and within countries. J Dent Res (forthcoming).

28. Fletcher RH, Fletcher SW, Wagner EH. Clinical epidemiology. 2nd Ed. Baltimore: Williams and Wilkins. 1988.

29. Rockhill B. Theorizing about the causes of disease at the individual level while estimating effects at the population level: implications for prevention. Epidemiol and Society. 2005; 16:124-9.

30. Rockhill B, Kawachi I, Colditz GA. Individual Risk Prediction and Population-wide Disease Prevention. Epidemiological Reviews. 2000; 22:176-80.

31. Rose G. Roses' Strategy of Preventive Medicine. Oxford: Oxford University Press. 2008.

32. Nadanovsky P, Sheiham A. The relative contribution of dental services to the changes in caries levels of 12 year-old children in 18 industrialized countries in the 1970s and early 1980s. Community Dent Oral Epidemiol. 1995; 23:231-9.

33. Netuveli, GS. Public Health aspects of dental calculus. An analysis of trends and future scenarios. PhD Thesis. London: University of London. 2002.

34. Sheiham A, Netuveli GS. Periodontal diseases in Europe. Periodontology 2000. 2002; 29:104-21.

35. McMichael AJ. The health of persons, populations, and planes: Epidemiology comes full circle. Epidemiology. 1995; 6:633-5.

36. McKinlay JB. Paradigmatic obstacles to improving the health of populations: implications for health policy. Salud Publica Mex. 1998; 40:369-79.

37. Hausen H, Kärkkäinen S, Seppä L. Application of the high risk strategy in controlling dental caries. Community Dent Oral Epidemiol. 2000; 28:26-34.

38. Kwan S, Petersen PE. Oral health: equity and social determinants. In: Equity, social determinants and public health programmes. Edited E Bias and AS Kurup. Geneva: World Health Organization. 2010; p.159-76.

39. http://whqlibdoc.who.int/publications/2010/9789241563970_eng.pdf.

40. Starfield B, Hyde J, Gervas J, Heath I. The concept of prevention: a good idea gone astray? J Epid Community Health. 2008; 62:580-3.

41. Sanders AE. Social determinants of oral health: conditions linked to socioeconomic inequalities in oral health in the Australian population. ARCPOH Population Oral Health Series No. 7. Adelaide: University of Adelaide. 2007.

42. Marmot MG. Understanding social inequalities in health. Perspect Biol Med. 2003;46(3 Suppl):S9-S23. http://www.ucl.ac.uk/gheg/marmotreview/FairSocietyHealthyLives.

43. Graham H, Kelly MP. Health inequalities: concepts, frameworks and policy. Briefing paper. London: NHS and Health Development Agency, 2004. http://www.nice.org.uk/niceMedia/documents/health_inequalities_concepts.pdf.

44. Marmot M. Fair Society, Healthy Lives The Marmot Review Strategic review of health inequalities in England post-2010. Published by The Marmot Review February 2010 ISBN 978–0–9564870–0–1 http://www.ucl.ac.uk/gheg/marmotreview/FairSocietyHealthyLives. www.ucl.ac.uk/gheg/marmotreview/Documents.

45. Whitehead M, Dahlgren G. Levelling up (Part 1): a discussion paper on concepts and principles for tackling social inequities in health. Studies on social and economic determinants of population health, No 2.World Health Organization Regional Office for Europe, Copenhagen, Denmark. 2006.

46. World Health Organization. Equity, social determinants and public health programmes. Edited by Erik Blas and Anand Sivasankara Kurup. World Health Organization. Geneva. 2010. http://whqlibdoc.who.int/publications/2010/9789241563970_eng.pdf.

47. Batchelor P, Sheiham A. The limitations of a 'high-risk' approach for the prevention of dental caries. Community Dent Oral Epidemiol. 2002; 30:302-12.

48. Frieden TR. Framework for public health action: The Health Impact Pyramid. Am J Public Health. 2010; 100:590-595.

49. Tudor Hart J. The inverse care law. The Lancet. 1971; 297,Issue 7696:405- 412.

50. World Health Organization. Commission on Social Determinants of Health. A Conceptual Framework for Action on the Social Determinants of Health. Discussion paper for the Commission on Social Determinants of Health. DRAFT April 2007b. CSDH Framework for action. Last version.

51. Adler NE, Ostrove JM. Socioeconomic status and health: what we know and what we don't. Ann NY Acad Sci. 1999; 896:3-15.

52. Sanders AE, Slade GD, Turrell G, Spencer AJ, Marcenes W. The shape of the socioeconomic-oral health gradient: implications for theoretical explanations. Community Dent Oral Epidemiol. 2006; 34:310–9.

53. Sabbah W, Tsakos, G, Chandola, Sheiham A, Watt RG. Social gradients in oral and general health. J Dent Res. 2007; 86:992-6.

54. Popay J, Whitehead M, Hunter DJ.. Injustice is killing people on a large scale – but what is to be done about it? J Public Health. 2010; 32:148-9.

55. Petersen PE. The World Oral Health Report 2003: Continuous improvement of oral health in the 21st Century – the approach of the WHO Global Oral Health Programme. Community Dent and Oral Epidemiol. 2003; 31(Suppl 1):3–24.

56. Petersen, PE. Priorities for research for oral health in the 21st Century - the approach of the WHO Global Oral Health Programme. Community Dent Health. 2005; 22:71-4.

57. Pattussi MP, Marcenes W, Croucher R, Sheiham A. Social deprivation, income inequality, social cohesion and dental caries in Brazilian school children. Soc Sci Med. 2001; 53:915-25.

58. Thomson WM, Poulton R, Milne BJ, Caspi A, Broughton JR, Ayers KM. Socio-economic inequalities in oral health in childhood and adulthood in a birth cohort. Community Dent Oral Epidemiol. 2004; 32:345-53.

59. Frohlich KL, Potvin L. Transcending the known in public health practice. The Inequality Paradox: The Population Approach and Vulnerable Populations. Amer J Public Health 2008;98:216-21.

60. World Health Oganization. Socio-environmentally determined health inequities among children and adolescents. Summary of outcomes, background papers and country case studies. WHO/HBSC FORUM 2009. World Health Organization Regional Office for Europe. 2009.

61. http://www.euro.who.int/__data/assets/pdf_file/0009/135891/e94866.pdf.

62. Milio N. Making healthy public policy; developing the science of art: an ecological framework for policy studies. Health Promotion. 1988; 2:236-74.

63. World Health Organization. Preventing chronic diseases: A vital investment. Geneva: World Health Organization, 2005. http://www.who.int/chp/chronic_disease_report/contents/en/index.html.

64. Diderichsen F, Evans T, Whitehead M. The social basis of disparities in health. In Challenging inequities in health: from ethics to action. ed. Whitehead M, Evans T, Diderichsen F, Bhuiya A, Wirth M. New York: Oxford University Press. 2001; p.13-23.

65. Tugwell P, Robinson V, Morris E. Mapping global health inequalities: challenges and opportunities. Mapping Global Inequalities, Center for Global, International and Regional Studies, UC Santa Cruz, 2007. http://escholarship.org/uc/item/2f11d67c.

66. Dankwa-Mullan I, Rhee KB, Williams K, Sanchez I, Sy FS, et al. The science of eliminating health disparities: summary and analysis of the NIH Summit recommendations. Am J Public Health. 2010; 100(Supplement 1):S12–S18.

67. Sheiham A, Alexander D, Cohen L, Marinho V, Moyses S, et al. Global Oral Health Inequalities: Task Group - Implementation and delivery of oral health strategies. Adv Dent Res. 2011 23: 259-7. http://adr.sagepub.com/content/23/2/259.